FIRST AID FOR THE® NBDE PART I

DEREK M. STEINBACHER, MD, DMD
University of Pennsylvania School of Dental Medicine
Class of 2001

Resident in Oral and Maxillofacial Surgery
Massachusetts General Hospital
Boston, Massachusetts

STEVEN R. SIERAKOWSKI, DMD, MDSc
University of Pennsylvania School of Dental Medicine
Class of 2001

Diplomate, American Board of Periodontology
Private Practice
Philadelphia, Pennsylvania

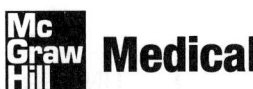
Medical

New York / Chicago / San Francisco / Lisbon / London / Madrid / Mexico City
Milan / New Delhi / San Juan / Seoul / Singapore / Sydney / Toronto

The McGraw·Hill Companies

First Aid for the® NBDE Part I

Copyright © 2007 by The McGraw-Hill Companies, Inc. All rights reserved. Printed in the United States of America. Except as permitted under the United States Copyright Act of 1976, no part of this publication may be reproduced or distributed in any form or by any means, or stored in a data base or retrieval system, without the prior written permission of the publisher.

First Aid for the® is a registered trademark of The McGraw-Hill Companies, Inc.

1 2 3 4 5 6 7 8 9 0   QPD/QPD   0 9 8 7 6

ISBN 13: 978-0-07-145637-1
ISBN 10: 0-07-145637-6
ISSN: 1931-2407

NOTICE

Medicine is an ever-changing science. As new research and clinical experience broaden our knowledge, changes in treatment and drug therapy are required. The authors and the publisher of this work have checked with sources believed to be reliable in their efforts to provide information that is complete and generally in accord with the standards accepted at the time of publication. However, in view of the possibility of human error or changes in medical sciences, neither the authors nor the publisher nor any other party who has been involved in the preparation or publication of this work warrants that the information contained herein is in every respect accurate or complete, and they disclaim all responsibility for any errors or omissions or for the results obtained from use of the information contained in this work. Readers are encouraged to confirm the information contained herein with other sources. For example and in particular, readers are advised to check the product information sheet included in the package of each drug they plan to administer to be certain that the information contained in this work is accurate and that changes have not been made in the recommended dose or in the contraindications for administration. This recommendation is of particular importance in connection with new or infrequently used drugs.

This book was set in Palatino by International Typesetting and Composition.
The editors were Catherine Johnson and Christie Naglieri.
The production supervisor was Phil Galea.
Project management was provided by International Typesetting and Composition.
Quebecor World Dubuque was printer and binder.

This book is printed on acid-free paper.

DEDICATION

To our families and loved ones who supported us through this endeavor,

and

To those mentors who sparked our enthusiasm for learning.

Derek M. Steinbacher, MD, DMD
Steven R. Sierakowski, DMD, MDSc

CONTENTS

Acknowledgments — vii
How to Contribute — ix
How to Use This Book — xi
Introduction — xiii

SECTION I — ANATOMIC SCIENCES — 1

Gross Anatomy — 3
General Histology — 157
Oral Histology — 195
Developmental Biology — 211

SECTION II — BIOCHEMISTRY–PHYSIOLOGY — 243

Physical-Chemical Principles — 245
Biological Compounds — 247
Metabolism — 265
Molecular Biology — 283
Membranes — 293
Neurophysiology — 297
Muscle Physiology — 329
Circulatory and Cardiac Physiology — 337
Respiratory Physiology — 361
Renal, Fluid, Acid-Base Physiology — 375
Gastrointestinal Physiology — 389
Nutrition — 399
Endocrine Physiology — 405

SECTION III — MICROBIOLOGY–PATHOLOGY — 431

Microbiology — 433
Oral Microbiology and Pathology — 477

Reactions to Tissue Injury	485
Immunology and Immunopathology	497
Systemic Pathology	513
Neoplasia	585

SECTION IV — DENTAL ANATOMY AND OCCLUSION — 615

Tooth Morphology	617
Eruption	645
Occlusion and Function	649
Tooth Anomalies	659
Index	663

ACKNOWLEDGMENTS

We are grateful to the Albert Einstein Medical Center (Philadelphia, Pennsylvania), division of orthodontics, for use of their models and casts. We also extend our sincere gratitude to our photographic models (including Sandra Sierakowski and Jennifer Fox). Thanks to Julie Paquette for her support, encouragement, and humor.

Thanks to our publisher, McGraw-Hill, for recognizing the need for this book and for the assistance of their staff. Thanks to Catherine Johnson, our editor, for her continued support and guidance. Thanks to Christie Naglieri for her fine editorial work, and to the graphics team for illustration reproductions.

Derek M. Steinbacher, MD, DMD
Steven R. Sierakowski, DMD, MDSc

HOW TO CONTRIBUTE

We welcome your comments, suggestions, ideas, corrections, or other submissions to help with this and future editions of *First Aid for the® NBDE Part I*. What information can you contribute?

- Test-taking tips and study strategies for the exam
- Suggestions for mnemonics, diagrams, figures, and tables
- Critiques related to the content or arrangement of facts contained herein
- Other sources of study material you find useful

Contributions used will result in a personal acknowledgement in the next edition of this book.

If you wish to contribute, e-mail your entries or suggestions to the following address. Please include your name, address, email address, and school affiliation.

nbde_firstaid@yahoo.com

NOTE TO CONTRIBUTORS

All contributions become property of the authors and are subject to editorial manipulation. In the event that similar or duplicate entries are received, only the first entry received will be used. Please include a reference to a standard textbook to verify the factual data.

HOW TO USE THIS BOOK

We feel that this book is an organized and resourceful guide to help you prepare for the NBDE Part I.

It is recommended that you use this book as early as possible, preferably in conjunction with your basic science and dental anatomy curriculum. The information contained within this book highlights the major facts and concepts commonly used in the NBDE Part I. Determine your own study strategy using not only this book, but also the materials you find most appropriate: concise review texts, the internet, or your own class notes.

First Aid for the® NBDE Part I is not meant to be a comprehensive review text; nor is it meant to be used as a substitute for a lack of studying during the first two years of dental school. As you study each topic, refer to the corresponding section in this book for a concise review or self-test. You may even want to make your own notes in the margins or highlight particular facts.

Some of the information found in the NDBE Part I is repeated in different sections. Many of the Key Facts in this book will guide you in cross-referencing a particular topic to another section. Use this to test yourself and integrate these facts into your body of knowledge.

During the last week before the exam, review the topics about which you feel the most unsure. The tables and figures in this book will help you keep the heavily-tested information fresh in your memory.

As soon as possible after you take the exam, we recommend that you review the book to help us create an even-better second edition. Tell us what information should be revised, included, or removed. You may even send in your own annotated book.

INTRODUCTION

The National Board Dental Examination (NBDE) Part I is the first of two national standardized examinations administered by the Joint Commission on National Dental Examinations. Its purpose is to provide state dental licensing boards an objective method of evaluating the qualifications of prospective applicants. The NBDE Part I is intended to assess competency in the pre-clinical dental and basic biomedical sciences.

WHY DO WELL ON THE EXAM?

Achieving a passing score is a necessary requisite for both graduation from a dental school accredited by the Commission on Dental Accreditation, and for obtaining dental licensure in the United States. Although each state reserves the authority to use the scores from the NBDE as a requisite to fulfill its written examination requirement, all 50 states, the District of Columbia, Puerto Rico, and the Virgin Islands use the NBDE for their licensing protocol. Additionally, each jurisdiction may have its own minimum NBDE Part I score requirement in order to obtain a dental license. It is essential that the future dentist be aware of the licensure requirements for each state in which he or she wishes to practice. A score of 85 or above is adequate in every state.

The NBDE Part I scores are also a major criterion used to gauge the quality of students applying to postdoctoral training programs. Since this examination is usually taken after the second year of dental school, it is often the only objective method of comparing soon-to-be graduates for such programs. Performing well on the NBDE Part I gives the student more bargaining potential when applying for these programs, as well as positions in academic, military, or private practice settings. In short, it behooves you to earn a good score on the NBDE Part I. Much diligence and a targeted study strategy, using materials like this book, will help you accomplish this goal.

STRUCTURE OF THE EXAMINATION

The NBDE Part I is given in print format at prescribed testing locations in the United States and Canada on the same date, always on a Monday. It is administered twice per year, usually in July and December. A computerized format is now also offered only in the United States at Prometric Test Centers throughout the country. This version is administered on most business days throughout the year. The locations of the certified testing centers can be found at www.2test.com.

The exam consists of four test sections of approximately 100 questions each, for a total of 400 questions. The questions are strictly in the form of multiple-choice test items, each with 4 to 5 possible answer choices, and are covered from four broad categories:

- Anatomic Sciences (100 questions)
- Microbiology and Pathology (100 questions)
- Biochemistry and Physiology (100 questions)
- Dental Anatomy and Occlusion (100 questions)

The total testing time is seven hours. For the written examination, candidates are to report to the testing center for orientation and instructions by 8:30 A.M. Both the Anatomic Sciences and Biochemistry/Physiology sections are completed together in one session from 9:00 to 12:30. The Microbiology/Pathology and Dental Anatomy/Occlusion sections are then taken in the afternoon from 1:30 to 5:00. One hour is provided as a lunch break between the examination sessions. A similar time schedule allowing flexibility between the two morning and two afternoon sections is available if the computerized version is taken.

SCORING OF THE EXAMINATION

The NBDE Part I is scored on a scale of 49–99. Scores are scaled based on both the historical distribution of scores, and the performance of other students taking the examination for the first time. The total number of questions you answered correctly (your raw score) determines your scaled score. There is no penalty for answering a question incorrectly. Furthermore, up to 15% of the questions may be discarded as they may be used for other evaluation purposes. A scaled score of 75 for each section is considered the minimum passing score for the NBDE Part I. Roughly 50–55 questions in each section need to be answered correctly to achieve a passing score.

Your score report will be mailed in approximately 6–8 weeks if you take the written examination or 3–4 weeks if you take the computerized version. You will receive a total of five scores: an individual score for each of the four subject areas, and one combined average score. The scaled scores can be then be converted into percentiles using the printed table included with your score report. The dean of your dental school will also receive a copy of your scores. Requesting additional copies of score reports is possible on written request, and is necessary for both post-doctoral program and state licensure applications.

REGISTERING FOR THE EXAM

An active or former dental student is eligible for the NBDE Part I after your dental school certifies, either by signature or electronic approval, that the student has successfully completed all subjects included in Part I. For US and Canadian students, the signature of the dean or school designee is the only requirement. For graduates of international dental schools, Educational Credential Evaluators, Inc. (ECE) must verify their official dental school transcripts.

You can request an application in writing, by telephone, or online. For more information, or to request a Candidate's Guide, contact the address below:

The Joint Commission on National Dental Examinations
American Dental Association
211 East Chicago Avenue, 6th Floor
Chicago, Il 60611
(312) 440-2678
www.ada.org

PREPARATION FOR THE EXAMINATION

The best preparation for the NBDE Part I is of course performing as well as possible in your pre-clinical dental school courses. The examination will address each of the subjects you have encountered during years one and two of dental school, although sometimes more or less depending on the specifics of your curriculum.

Make a concerted effort to master the material when it is initially presented at your school. Be organized. Keep your notes for each course and have them arranged by topic or theme. Be aware of the subjects covered on NBDE Part I and create your study sheets accordingly. Use this book as an outline or an umbrella under which you can incorporate the pertinent details of each individual dental school course. For instance, when taking dental school microbiology in first year, cross-reference the subject matter with the outlines and material presented here in First Aid. In this way you will create organized study materials that will be easy to reference when you go back to study for the NBDE Part I.

If you are now just a few months away from taking the NBDE Part I and have not prepared in the manner just mentioned over the past 2 years, do not fret. The major obstacle is the disparate location of information. There is a lot of material to cover, but what is most important is that all facts are compiled in one place. Choose your study materials and then cross-reference and combine information pertaining to each topic in one location. Try and decide on a study method that has worked for you. This could be note cards, subject outlines, or categorical maps. The process of organizing the information in one place will force you to learn it. A combination approach that we find helpful is looking at the broad categories of topics with study sheets or maps and focusing on the particular details with note cards or lists. For example, when studying microbiology it is useful to first divide bacteria generally into classes based say on Gram stain (outline this on one sheet), then prepare flashcards with more specifics, e.g., organism names on one-side and pertinent descriptive details on the other.

If you are only days or weeks away from the exam you need to do some self-reflection. Now that the exam is computerized you can postpone the date of the exam with relative ease. If, for some reason, you cannot push back the exam you must focus on quickly hammering out the high yield facts. Recognition and recall are essential for last minute cramming. Go through lists of buzzwords. Try to organize these in different categories if possible. Visualize their interrelationships. If you are in a private place, it may help to talk aloud. The mantra is: "repetition to create recognition and recall."

STUDY TACTICS

It is ideal to plan well ahead and orchestrate your exam date at a convenient time. You should allow for ample time to address all subject areas and review thoroughly. As mentioned, the best situation is to concurrently use the First Aid book as a study aid while taking each pre-clinical course. You will want to commit to memory all of the topic headings and buzzwords. This is made more tangible by linking concepts to associations and looking at the interrelationships of different ideas.

Set up a schedule at least 1–2 months ahead of time. The laxity of the schedule depends on your circumstances. If you are very busy during the spring semester of your second year, you may want to arrange for a longer study phase with less information covered each day. Alternatively, your school may set aside dedicated NBDE study time. You can plan to complete most of your rigorous studying during this period and concentrate on your dental school classes up until then. If you know you are weak in a particular subject area, it would be prudent to spend some extra time reviewing that topic earlier in the semester.

Do not jeopardize a healthy lifestyle at the expense of studying. It is important to eat well, exercise regularly, and get ample sleep each night. All of these things will allow you to be maximally efficient during your studying. Feeling good and maintaining yourself personally will help your mind absorb all of the meticulous information required. When studying, take regular breaks. Some advocate a breather every 45 minutes or so. You should take a 15-minute break at least every hour and a half to 2 hours. Get up and stretch. Have a snack. Take a power nap. Do something to distract yourself from pre-clinical dental and basic science courses.

An important tenet to follow is to start your studying with areas that you find most difficult or that will require the most time to master. Set your schedule with time allotted for each subject and goals you want to achieve with each session. For example, you may want to allow 2 weeks to study pathology and each night you will cover a subset thereof—e.g., cellular injury. At the end of each session it is a good idea to test yourself; either with released test questions or with questions you derive on your own during the course of studying. Equally important is taking time to review. Before each new study session, take 15–20 minutes to review the material you have learned last time. Your study timeline should allow for 1–2 weeks prior to the exam for a comprehensive review. You can use your cross-referenced summary study sheets or lists and take old examinations. Taking loads of old exams the last week is very helpful. For one, you get into the groove of taking 8-hours worth of questions in a single day. Secondly, you will gain familiarity with the writing style of NBDE questions. Lastly, you will be able to witness your deficiencies and take time to work them out.

Lore has it that the day prior to the exam should be reserved for leisurely activity and getting a good night's rest. True: you should engage in some stress-relieving activity and be sure to go to bed early. However, it is completely reasonable to review material for a few hours that day. This may mean reading over your review sheets for each subject, listing aloud high-yield buzzwords, or going through the practice questions that you got wrong. Do not try to learn brand new material or complete a rigorous study session during these final hours!

In the end, try to relax. It is only an exam and if anything happens to go wrong it is not the end of the world. The vast majority of students pass on their first try. If you have a bad day—and we all have had one—the exam will be there for you to take again. It may set you back some money, but spend some time preparing and you will make it through dental school perfectly fine and go into the field you have always imagined.

DAY OF THE EXAM

Be sure to set your alarm with plenty of time allowed. You need to perform your morning routine in an unhurried fashion. Do some light stretching and eat a healthy breakfast. Plan on arriving at the test site with 10–15 minutes to spare. Bring ample snacks with you. We would advise that you take a break between at least every other section. Use this time to go to the restroom, eat a banana, or breathe some fresh air. Save time to take at least a 25-minute lunch break.

During the exam, relax. Read each question carefully from start to finish. Do not jump to the answer choices until you have read the entire question. As you process the question in your mind you should be thinking about the possible answers. Try and deduce what the answer should be and see if it matches with the available choices. If you look at the answer choices prior to fully processing the question you are apt to be swayed by the "trap answers." Go with your first instinct. If you are not sure about the correct answer do not worry. Mark the question so you can return to it later. Do not get bogged down and spend 10-minutes on a single question. Move on to the next question and continue until you have gone through all the items for a single pass. Then you can return to the questions you have marked. Pay attention to the clock. You want to divide your marked questions by the available time. Go through with your best choice or best guess and be done. By all means, answer every question—there is no penalty for wrong answers.

You have studied hard and prepared well. This book will help guide your studying. Good luck.

SECTION 1
Anatomic Sciences

- Gross Anatomy
- General Histology
- Oral Histology
- Developmental Biology

CHAPTER 1

Gross Anatomy

Head: Cranial Anatomy and Osteology	6
CRANIUM	6
CRANIAL FOSSAE	8
FACE AND VISCEROCRANIUM	12
SCALP	21
MENINGES	22
PTERYGOID PLEXUS OF VEINS	25
VENTRICULAR SYSTEM	25
BLOOD-BRAIN BARRIER	27
INTRACRANIAL CIRCULATION	27
Oral Cavity and Pharynx	29
ORAL CAVITY	29
PHARYNX	39
Nasolacrimal Apparatus	41
NASOLACRIMAL APPARATUS	41
Mastication and TMJ	47
MASTICATION	47
TEMPOROMANDIBULAR JOINT (TMJ)	50
Neck Anatomy	54
CERVICAL VERTEBRAE	54
LAYERS AND FASCIA OF THE NECK	55
TRIANGLES OF THE NECK	59
SCM, TRAPEZIUS MUSCLES	62
HYOID BONE	62
SUPRA- AND INFRAHYOID MUSCLES	63
CERVICAL PLEXUS (OF NERVES)	65
CERVICAL PLEXUS	65
PHRENIC NERVE	66
BLOOD SUPPLY TO FACE	66
EXTERNAL CAROTID ARTERY	66
VENOUS DRAINAGE FROM THE FACE	69
LYMPH NODES IN THE FACE	71

Thyroid	72
Parathyroid Glands	74
Larynx	74
Respiratory System	76

Brachial Plexus and Upper Extremities — 77
Axilla	77
Brachial Plexus	79
Limb Muscles and Functions by Joint	81

External Thorax and Abdomen — 83
Sternum	83
Clavicle	83
Ribs	83
Intercostal Space	83
Muscles of Respiration	84
Abdominal Regions	85
Rectus Sheath	86
Breast	86
Dermatomes	87
Reflexes	87
Femoral Triangle	88

Thoracic and Abdominal Viscera — 88
Body Cavities	88
Lung	89
Heart and Great Vessels	90
Atria	91
Ventricles	92
Veins of the Heart	93
Mediastinum	93
Thymus	94
Aorta	95
Azygous System	96
Splanchnic Nerves	97
Superior Vena Cava	98
Inferior Vena Cava	98
Portal Vein	98
Portal Triad	99
Lymphatic System	100
Peritoneum	101
Mesentery	101
Peritoneal Ligaments	101
Gastrointestinal Tract	102
Stomach	104
Liver	106
Spleen	107
Gallbladder	107
Small Intestine	108

Large Intestine	108
Retroperitoneal Structures	109
Posterior Abdominal Muscles	110
Pancreas	110
Adrenal Gland	110
Urinary System	111
Kidney	111
Pelvic Cavity	112
Inguinal Canal	113

Neuroanatomy 113

Nervous System	113
Brain	113
Cranial Nerves	118
CN II—Optic Nerve	124
CNs III, IV, VI—Oculomotor, Trochlear, Abducens	125
CN V—Trigeminal Nerve	129
Facial Reflexes (Involving CN V)	136
CN VII-Facial Nerve	137
CN VIII—Vestibulocochlear	141
CN IX—Glossopharyngeal	143
CN X—Vagus	145
CN XI—Accessory	147
CN XII—Hypoglossus	147
Spinal Cord	149
Peripheral Nervous System	151

HEAD: CRANIAL ANATOMY AND OSTEOLOGY

Cranium

- The neurocranium encloses the brain and the viscerocranium comprises the face.

There are four unpaired bones of the cranium: ethmoid, sphenoid, frontal, occipital.

Bones of the viscerocranium (except the mandibular condyle) form by intramembranous growth.

Neurocranium	Viscerocranium
Frontal bone	Maxillae (2, then fuse)
Parietal bones (2)	Nasal bones (2)
Temporal bones (2)	Zygomatic bones (2)
Occipital bone	Palatine bones (2)
Sphenoid bone	Lacrimal bones (2)
Ethmoid bone	Inferior conchae (2) Vomer Mandible Hyoid

Anterior Skull

See Figure 1–1 for the anterior aspect of the skull.

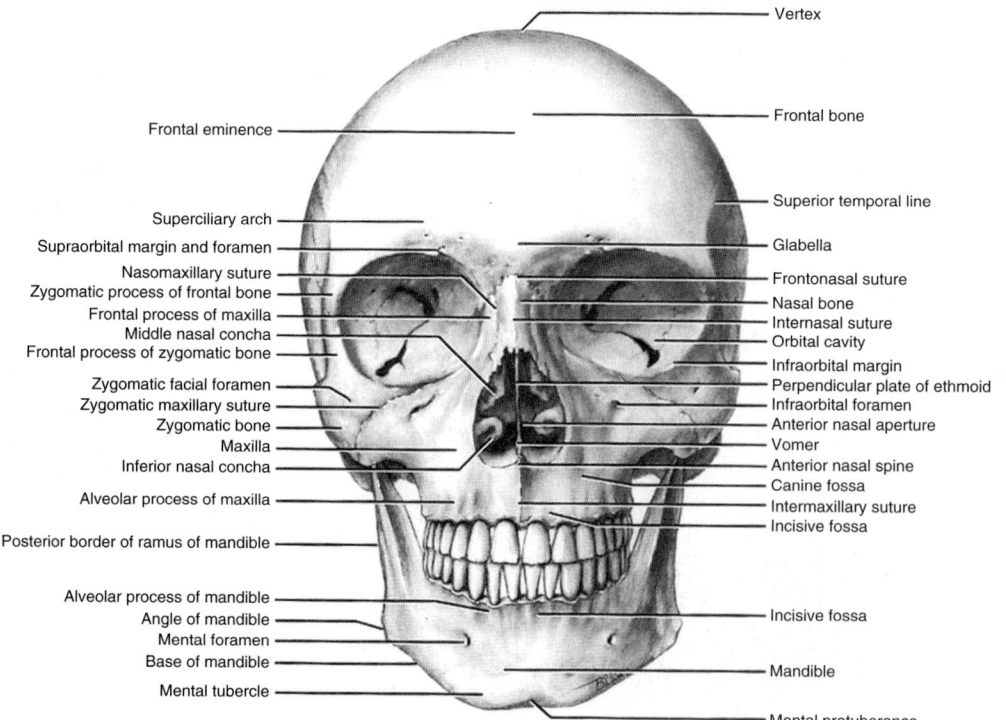

FIGURE 1–1. Anterior aspect of the skull.

Reproduced, with permission, from Montgomery RL. *Head and Neck Anatomy: With Clinical Correlations.* New York: McGraw-Hill, 1981.

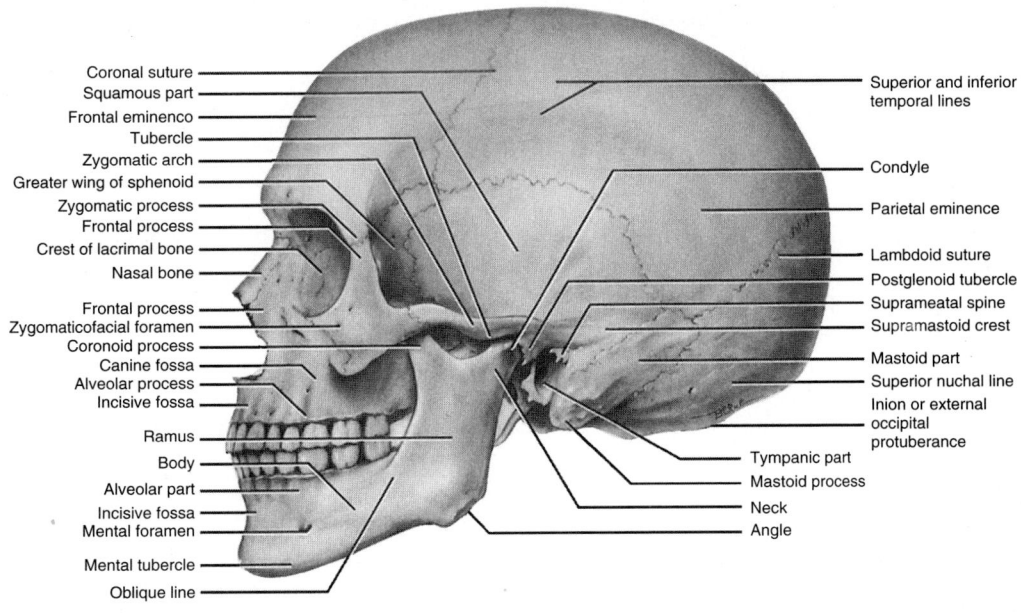

FIGURE 1-2. Lateral aspect of the skull.

Reproduced, with permission, from Montgomery RL. *Head and Neck Anatomy: With Clinical Correlations*. New York: McGraw-Hill, 1981.

LATERAL SKULL

See Figure 1–2 for the lateral aspect of the skull.

POSTERIOR SKULL

See Figure 1–3 for the posterior aspect of the skull.

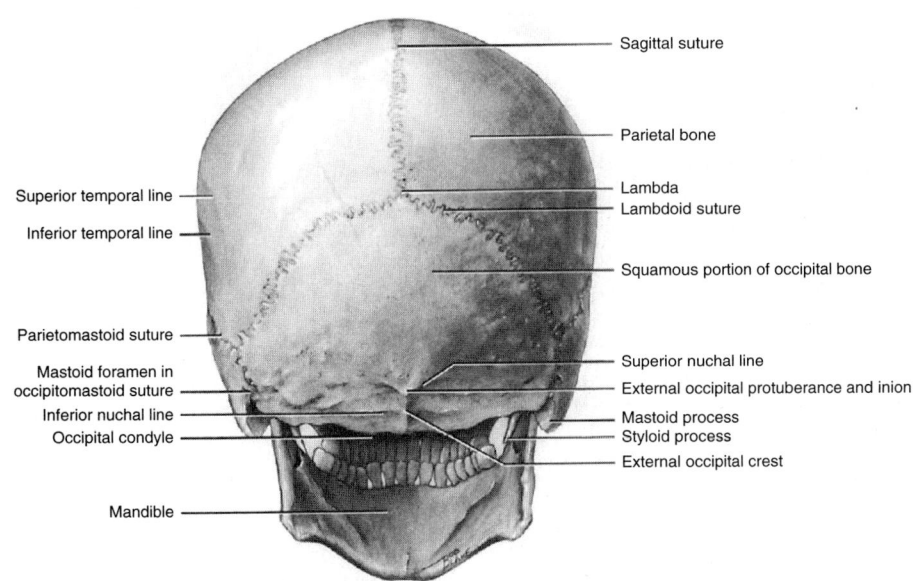

Petrous temporal bone forms the floor of the middle cranial fossa and separates middle and posterior cranial fossae.

Middle meningeal artery is located in middle cranial fossa (exits foramen spinosum).

FIGURE 1-3. Posterior aspect of the skull.

Reproduced, with permission, from Montgomery RL. *Head and Neck Anatomy: With Clinical Correlations*. New York: McGraw-Hill, 1981.

Cranial Fossae

See also the section "Internal Skull."

	Anterior Cranial Fossa	Middle Cranial Fossa	Posterior Cranial Fossa
Formed by	Frontal and ethmoid bone and parietal bones	Sphenoid, temporal,	Occipital and temporal bones
Contents	Frontal lobes Cribriform plate Foramen cecum Crista galli	Temporal lobes Pituitary Optic foramen Superior orbital fissure Carotid canal Trigeminal ganglion Foramen rotundum Foramen ovale Foramen spinosum	Occipital lobes Brainstem Cerebellum Internal acoustic meatus Jugular foramen Foramen magnum Hypoglossal canal

See also the sections "Internal Skull" and "Cranial Base."

Important Cranial Foramina

Foramina	Bone(s)	Contents Passed
Foramen cecum	Frontal and ethmoid	Emissary vein
Greater palatine foramen	Palatine	Greater palatine nerve, artery, vein
Lesser palatine foramen	Palatine	Lesser palatine nerve, artery, vein
Incisive canal	Maxilla	Nasopalatine nerve
Supraorbital foramen	Frontal	Supraorbital nerve, artery, vein
Infraorbital foramen	Sphenoid and maxilla	Infraorbital nerve (V-2), artery, and vein
Optic canal	Sphenoid	Optic nerve (II) and ophthalmic artery

Foramina	Bone(s)	Contents Passed
Superior orbital fissure	Sphenoid (between greater and lesser wings)	Oculomotor (III), Trochlear (IV), Abducens (VI), Trigeminal (V-1–lacrimal, frontal, and nasociliary nerves) and superior ophthalmic vein
Inferior orbital fissure (leads to infraorbital foramen)	Spehenoid, maxilla	V-2, infraorbital vessels, ascending branches of sphenopalatine ganglion
Foramen rotundum	Sphenoid	V-2
Foramen ovale	Sphenoid	V-3, lesser petrosal nerve
Foramen spinosum	Sphenoid	Middle meningeal artery and vein
Petrotympanic fissure	Temporal	Chorda tympani, anterior tympanic artery
Foramen lacerum	Temporal and sphenoid	Greater and deep petrosal nerves (internal carotid artery runs over top)
Internal acoustic meatus	Temporal (petrous)	VII and VIII
Stylomastoid foramen	Temporal	Facial nerve (VII)
Jugular foramen	Temporal and occipital	IJV, glossopharyngeal (IX), vagus (X), and spinal accessory (XI) nerves
Foramen magnum	Occipital	Medulla oblongata/spinal cord, vertebral arteries, spinal accessory nerve
Mandibular foramen	Mandible	Inferior alveolar nerve, artery, vein
Mental foramen	Mandible	Mental nerve, artery, and vein

INTERNAL SKULL

See Figure 1–4 for the internal skull base.

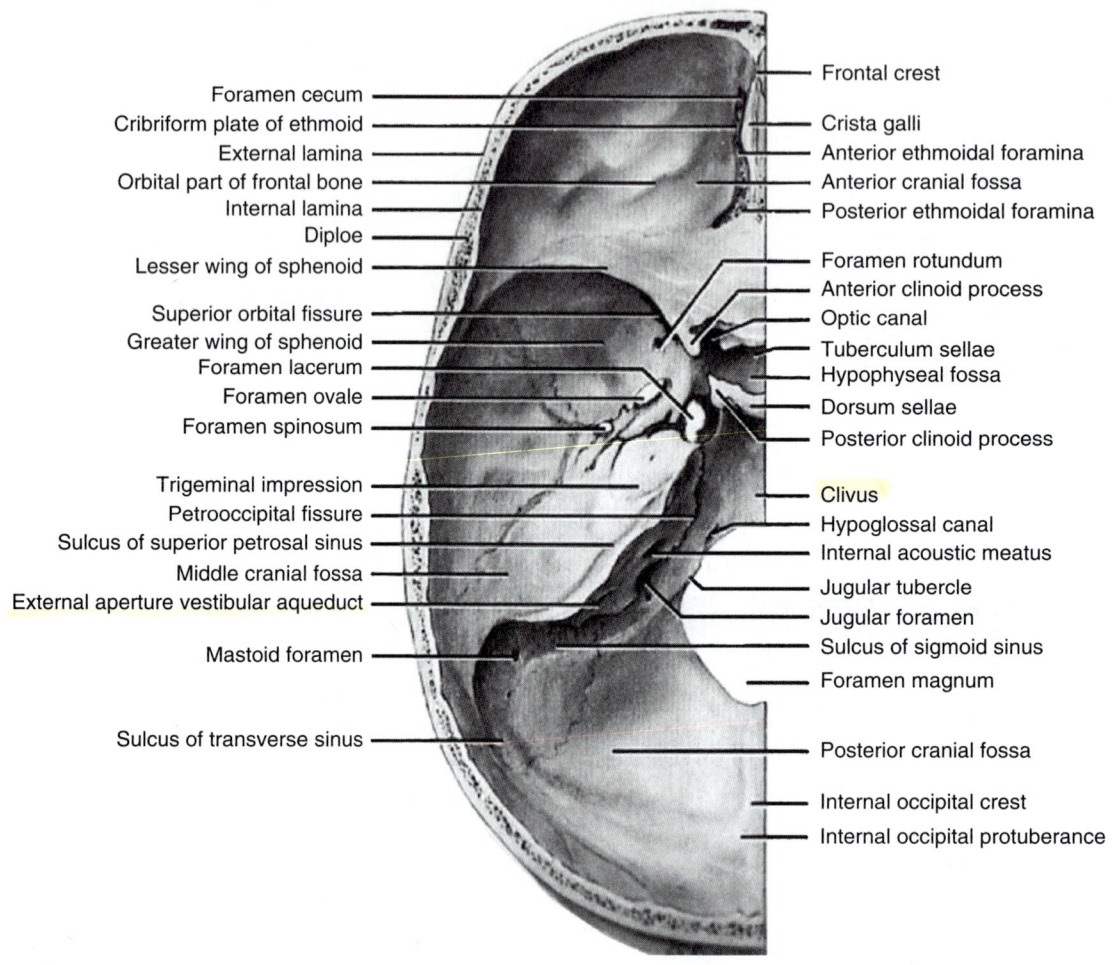

FIGURE 1-4. Internal skull.

Reproduced, with permission, from Montgomery RL. *Head and Neck Anatomy: With Clinical Correlations.* New York: McGraw-Hill, 1981.

CRANIAL BASE

See Figure 1–5 for the cranial base.

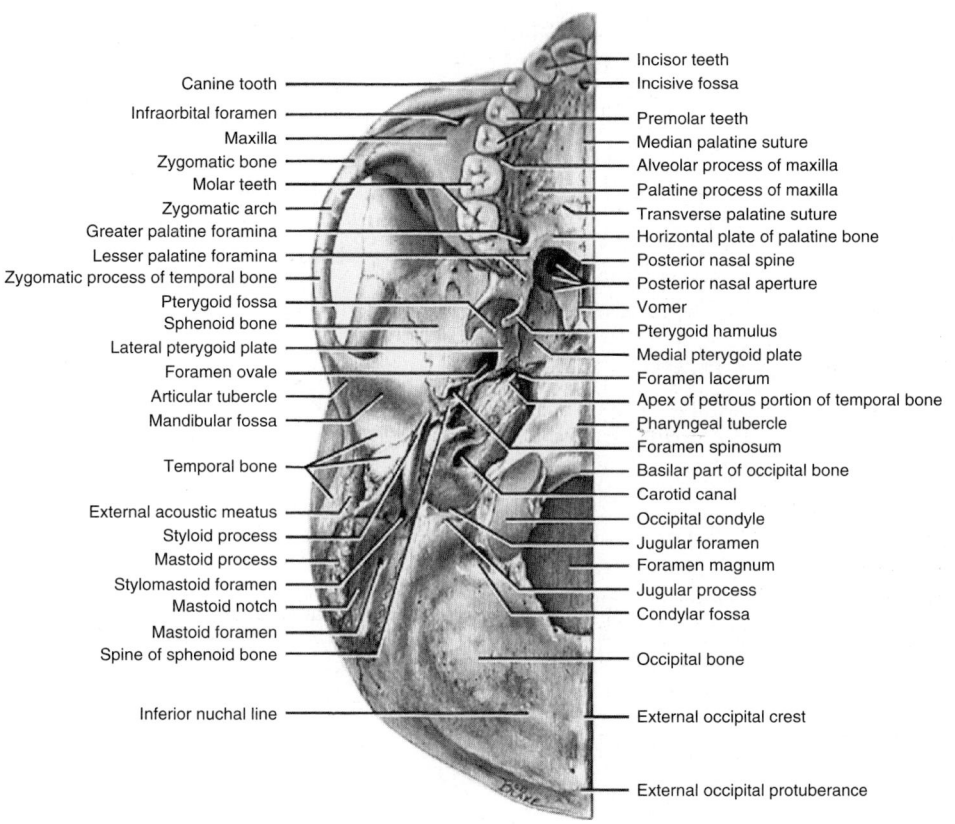

FIGURE 1-5. **The internal cranial base.**

Reproduced, with permission, from Montgomery RL. *Head and Neck Anatomy: With Clinical Correlations*. New York: McGraw-Hill, 1981.

ETHMOID AND SPHENOID BONES

- Single (unpaired) midline, bilaterally symmetric bones.
- Contribute both to the neurocranium and viscerocranium.

The inferior nasal conchae is its own bone.

The greater wing of sphenoid contains three foramina: rotundum, ovale, spinosum (middle cranial fossa).

	Component	Function
Ethmoid	Cribriform plate	Olfactory foramina.
	Crista galli	Attaches to falx cerebri.
	Lateral plates	Contain ethmoid sinuses, lamina papyracea, superior and middle nasal conchae.
	Perpendicular plate	Superior part of nasal septum.
Sphenoid	Hollow body	Sella turcica and sphenoidal sinuses.
	Greater wings	Lateral orbital wall and roof of infratemporal fossa.
	Lesser wings	Roof of orbit and superior orbital fissure (contains optic foramen).
	Medial and lateral pterygoid plates	Lateral pterygoid plate is attachment for both medial and lateral pterygoid muscles; medial pterygoid plate ends as a hamulus (tensor veli palatine muscle hooks around this).

Face and Viscerocranium

BONES OF THE ORBIT

See Figure 1–6 for the orbit, which comprises seven bones:

- Frontal
- Maxilla
- Zygoma
- Ethmoid
- Sphenoid
- Lacrimal
- Palatine

See the chart on important cranial foramina.

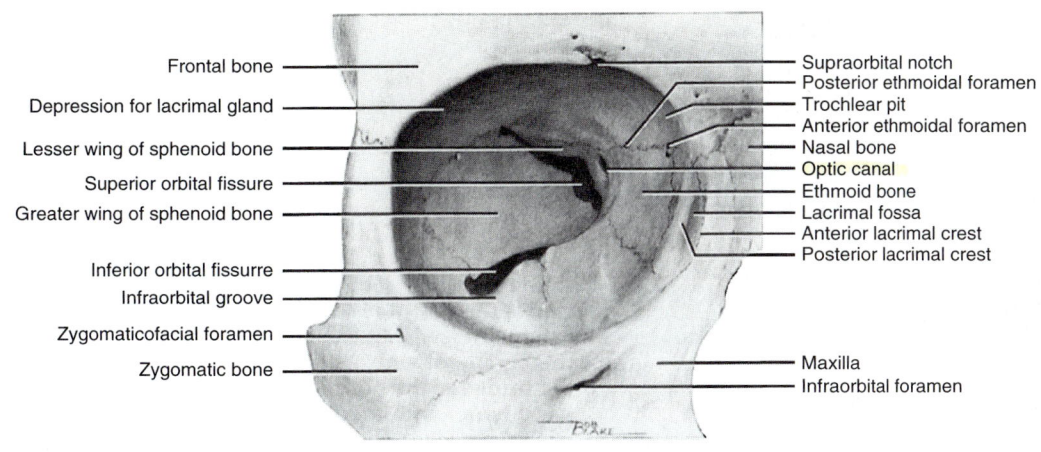

FIGURE 1-6. The orbit.

Reproduced, with permission, from Montgomery RL. *Head and Neck Anatomy: With Clinical Correlations*. New York: McGraw-Hill, 1981.

ORBITAL CONTENTS

See Figure 1-7 for orbital contents.

ZYGOMA

The zygomatic bone is also referred to as the malar and the cheekbone.

- Located in the upper and lateral part of the face.
- Prominence of the cheek.
- Part of the lateral wall and floor of the orbit.
- Parts of the temporal and infratemporal fossae.
- Articulates with the maxilla (anteriorly) and the temporal bone (posteriorly).

ZYGOMATIC ARCH

- Formed by temporal process of zygomatic bone and zygomatic process of temporal bone.
- Temporalis muscle passes deep to zygomatic arch.
- Masseter muscle originates from the zygoma and zygomatic arch.

The ophthalmic artery (a branch of the internal carotid artery, ICA) is the major blood supply to the orbit and eye. It enters the orbit with the optic nerve via the optic canal.

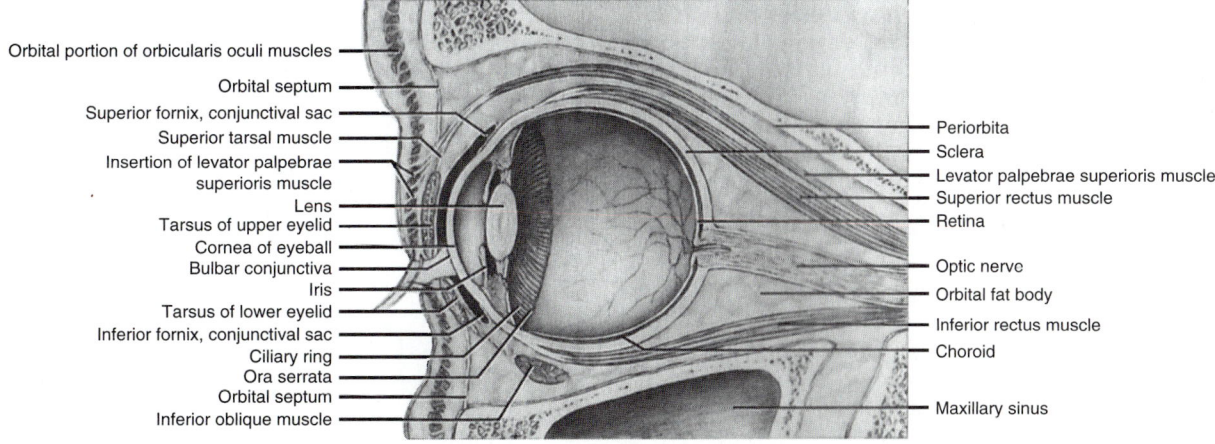

FIGURE 1-7. The orbit, sagittal view.

Reproduced, with permission, from Montgomery RL. *Head and Neck Anatomy: With Clinical correlations*. New York: McGraw-Hill, 1981.

Maxilla

- Upper jaw.
- Consists of a body and four processes: zygomatic, frontal, alveolar, and palatine.
- Forms boundaries of three cavities.
  - Roof of the mouth (palate).
  - Floor and lateral wall of the nose.
  - Floor of the orbit.
- Forms of two fossae (See Table 1–1).
  - Infratemporal (See Figure 1–8).
  - Pterygopalatine.
- Forms two fissures.
  - Infraorbital.
  - Pterygomaxillary.

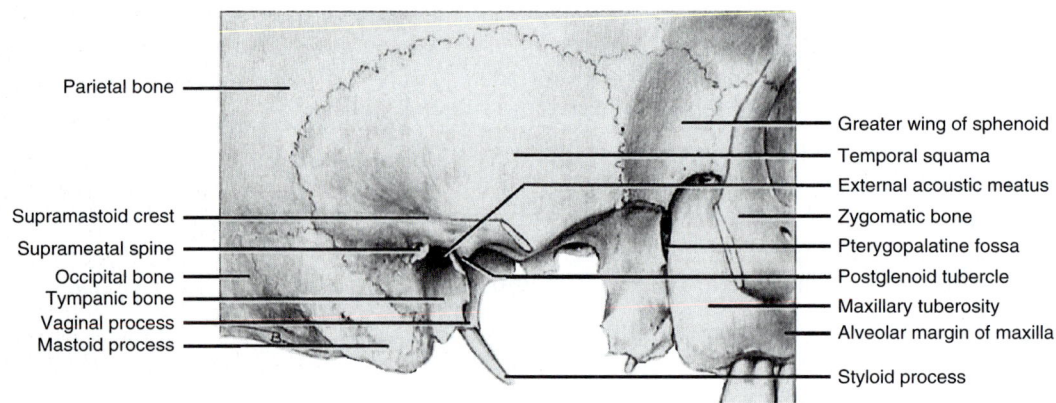

FIGURE 1–8. Infratemporal fossa.

Reproduced, with permission, from Montgomery RL. *Head and Neck Anatomy: With Clinical Correlations.* New York: McGraw-Hill, 1981.

TABLE 1-1. Infratemporal and Pterygopalatine Fossae

Fossae	Boundaries						Contents
	Anterior	Posterior	Medial	Lateral	Roof	Floor	
Infratemporal fossa	Posterior maxilla	Temporal bone (tympanic portion, mastoid, and styloid process)	Lateral pterygoid plate (sphenoid)	Mandibular ramus	Greater wing of sphenoid (with foramen ovale →CN V-3)	Medial pterygoid muscle (superior surface where inserts into mandible)	Temporalis and pterygoid muscles; Maxillary artery (and branches, e.g., middle meningeal); Pterygoid plexus of veins; Mandibular nerve (V-3); Chorda tympani (VII); Otic ganglion (IX)
Pterygopalatine fossa	Maxilla	Pterygoid plates	Nasal fossa	Infratemporal fossa	Greater wing of sphenoid; opens into inferior orbital fissure	Pyramidal process of palatine bone; inferior end contains palatine canals	Pterygopalatine (3rd) part of maxillary artery and its branches; Maxillary nerve (V-2); Nerve of pterygoid canal; Pterygopalatine ganglion and branches[a]

[a]For pterygopalatine ganglion, see the parasympathetic ganglia chart.

Pterygopalatine Fossa Major Communications

Direction	Passageway	Contents Passing	Space
Lateral	Pterygomaxillary fissure	Posterior superior alveolar NAV, maxillary artery	Infratemporal fossa
Anterosuperior	Inferior orbital fissure	CN V-2	Orbit
Posterosuperior	Foramen rotundum and pterygoid canal	CN V-2; nerve of pterygoid canal (formed by deep and greater petrosal nerves)	Middle cranial fossa
Medial	Sphenopalatine foramen	Sphenopalatine artery and vein, nasopalatine nerve	Nasal cavity
Inferior	Palatine canals	Greater and lesser palatine NAVs	Oral cavity

See Figure 1–9 for lateral scheme of the pterygopalatine fossa.

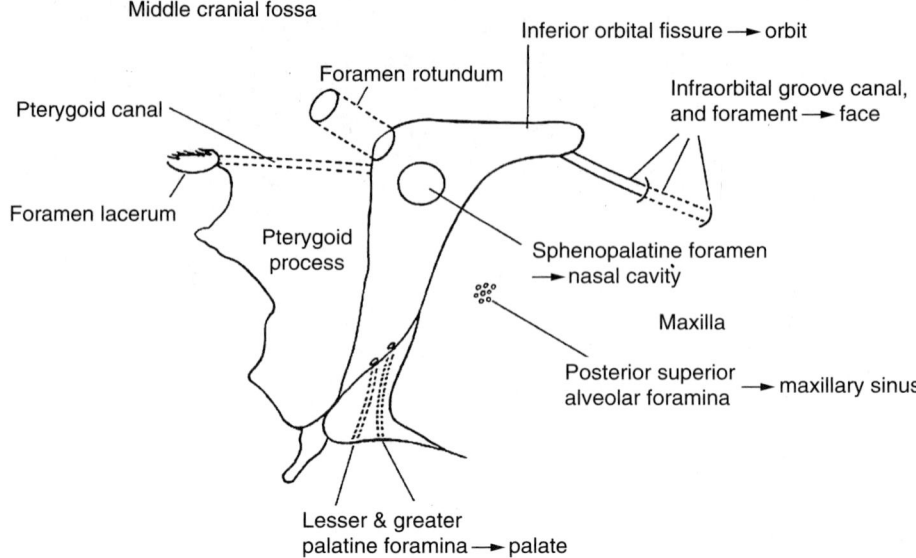

FIGURE 1–9. Lateral scheme of the pterygopalatine fossa to show the entrances and exits.

Reproduced, with permission, from Liebgott B. *The Anatomical Basis of Dentistry*. Toronto: BC Decker, 1986.

HARD PALATE

The palate forms the roof of the oral cavity and the floor of the nasal cavity.

- Maxilla are palatal processes (anterior two thirds).
- Palatine bones are horizontal palates (posterior one third).
- Pterygoid plates of the sphenoid articulate with the maxillary tuberosity (posterior palate).

Palatal Foramen

- Incisive foramen (Scarpa, midline; Stenson, lateral)—descending palatine vessels and the nasopalatine nerves (of V-3)—anterior palatal block.
- Greater and lesser palatine foramen—descending palatine vessels and anterior palatine nerve (of V-3)—site of palatal anesthetic block.

Nasal Cavity

Boundary	Contributing Structures
Floor	Hard palate (maxilla and palatine bones)
Roof	Cribriform plate of ethmoid, anterior body of sphenoid, nasal spine of frontal bone, nasal bones, lateral nasal cartilages
Lateral wall	Nasal, ethmoid, sphenoid, maxilla, palatine, and inferior conchal bones
Medial wall	Nasal septum
External nose	Two nasal bones, nasal cartilages

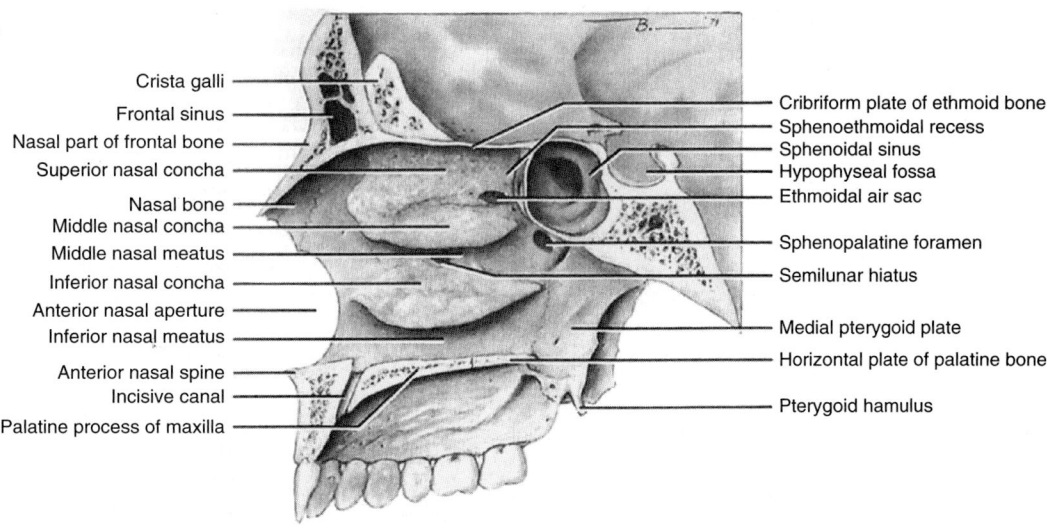

FIGURE 1-10. Lateral nasal cavity and hard palate.

Reproduced, with permission, from Montgomery RL. *Head and Neck Anatomy: With Clinical Correlations.* New York: McGraw-Hill, 1981.

Nasal Cavity

See Figure 1–10.

- Sensory innervation is from branches of V-2.
  - Nasopalatine
  - Infraorbital
  - Greater palatine
- Some sensory branches are from V-1 (ophthalmic division).
  - Anterior ethmoidal nerve
- Parasympathetic to secretory glands supplied by branches of the pterygopalatine ganglion.
- Olfactory epithelium (roof of the nasal cavity) is innervated by the olfactory nerve (I).
- Blood supply—sphenopalatine branch of maxillary artery, anterior ethmoidal branch of ophthalmic artery, and septal branch of superior labial branch of facial artery.
- Superior nasal conchae and upper third of septum contain yellowish olfactory mucosa.

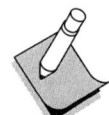

CN I (olfactory nerve) projects to the primary olfactory cortex (pyriform cortex).

Conchae	Meatuses
Superior and middle (ethmoid bone) Inferior (its own bone)	Areas below each conchae are the superior, middle, and inferior meatuses, respectively
Increase air turbulence for warming, filtering, olfaction	Drainage points for sinuses and nasolacrimal apparatus

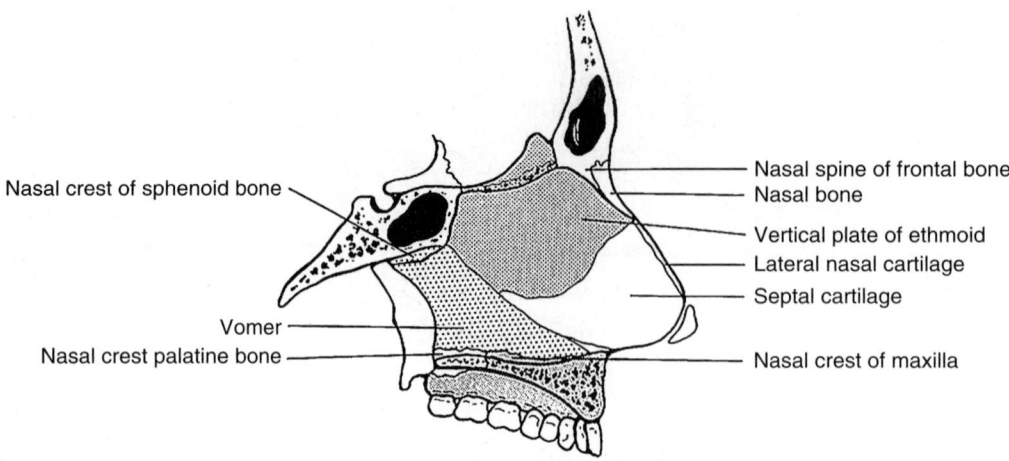

FIGURE 1-11. The cartilaginous and bony components of the nasal septum.

Reproduced, with permission, from Montgomery RL. *Head and Neck Anatomy: With Clinical Correlations.* New York: McGraw-Hill, 1981.

NASAL SEPTUM

The nasal septum comprises five bones and one cartilage.

See Figure 1-11.

- Vertical plate of ethmoid
- Vomer
- Nasal crest of maxilla and palatine bones
- Nasal crest of sphenoid bones
- Septal cartilage

KIESSELBACH'S PLEXUS

- This plexus is the anastomosis of five arteries:
    - Sphenopalatine
    - Greater palatine (of maxillary artery)
    - Superior labial (of facial artery)
    - Anterior ethmoid arteries (of ICA) (in the anteroinferior part of the nasal septum)
    - Lateral nasal branches of facial artery

Most cases of epistaxis arise from this area.

The maxillary sinus is lined by the Sniderian membrane.

PARANASAL SINUSES

See Figure 1-12.

- Frontal
- Maxillary
- Ethmoid
- Sphenoid

System	Location of Drainage
Nasolacrimal apparatus	Inferior meatus (below inferior concha)
Frontal sinuses	**Middle meatus:** Hiatus semilunaris (below middle concha)
Maxillary sinuses	**Middle meatus:** Ostium (below middle concha) (within hiatus semilunaris)
Ethmoid sinuses: anterior, middle, posterior	**Middle meatus** (within hiatus semilunaris and ethmoidal bullae, respectively) Superior meatus
Sphenoid sinuses	Sphenoethmoidal recess of nasal cavity

A surgical approach to pituitary gland is via the sphenoid sinus.

The middle meatus contains openings for the frontal sinus, anterior and middle ethmoidal sinuses, and maxillary sinuses.

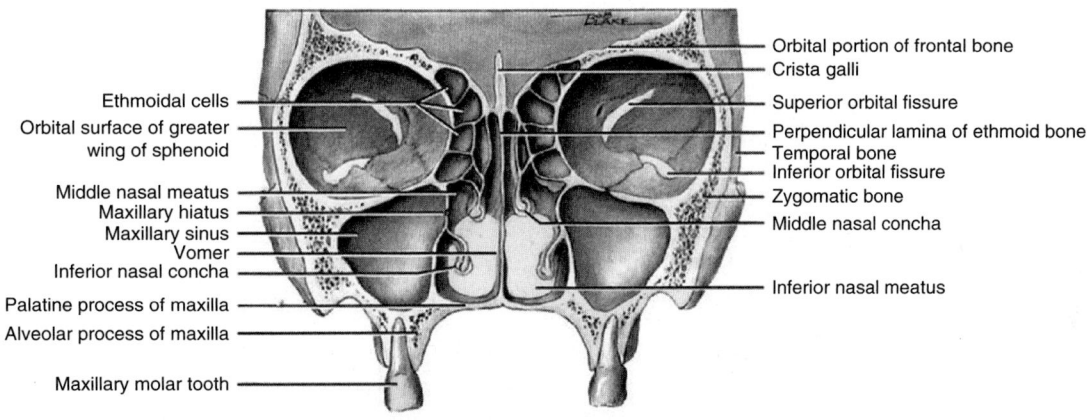

FIGURE 1-12. Paranasal sinuses.

Reproduced, with permission, from Montgomery RL. *Head and Neck Anatomy: With Clinical Correlations.* New York: McGraw-Hill, 1981.

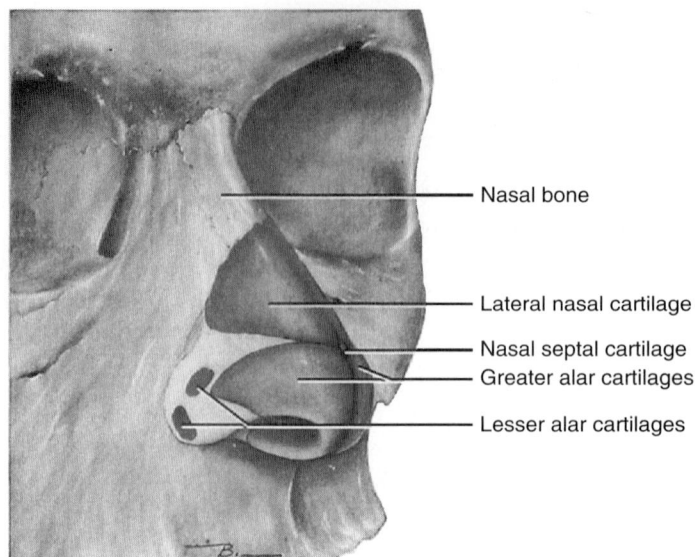

FIGURE 1–13. The nose.

Reproduced, with permission, from Montgomery RL. *Head and Neck Anatomy: With Clinical Correlations.* New York: McGraw-Hill, 1981.

Cartilage of the external nose is hyaline.

EXTERNAL NOSE

See Figure 1–13.

- Nasal bones
- Septal cartilages
- Lateral cartilages
- Alar cartilages

MANDIBLE

- Largest and strongest bone of the face.
- Lower jaw; houses lower teeth.
- Consists of:
  - Body (curved, horizontal).
  - Rami (two perpendicular portions).
    - Body and rami unite at angle (nearly 90 degrees).
  - Coronoid process (attachment of temporalis muscle).
  - Condyle.

See Section 4 of this chapter for information on temporomandibular joints and the muscles of mastication.

The mandibular canal traverses the mandibular body and opens anteriorly at the mental foramen.

FORAMINA

Mandibular Foramen

- Is located on the medial side of the ramus (just below lingula), midway between anterior and posterior borders of the ramus.
- It passes
  - Inferior alveolar nerve (IAN.) (of V-3).
  - Inferior alveolar artery and vein.

Mental Foramen

- Is located below the second premolar on each side.
- It passes
  - Mental nerve, an inferior alveolar nerve that exits as a mental nerve. It supplies skin and mucous membrane of the mental region.
  - Incisive branch, which supplies the pulp chambers of the anterior teeth and adjacent mucous membrane.

Scalp

See Figure 1–14. A mnemonic device to remember the components of the scalp is:

- **S**kin
- **C**onnective tissue
- **A**poneurosis (galea aponeurotica, epicranial aponeurosis)
- **L**oose connective tissue
- **P**eriosteum

The lingula is a tongue-shaped projection above the mandibular foramen where the sphenomandibular ligament attaches.

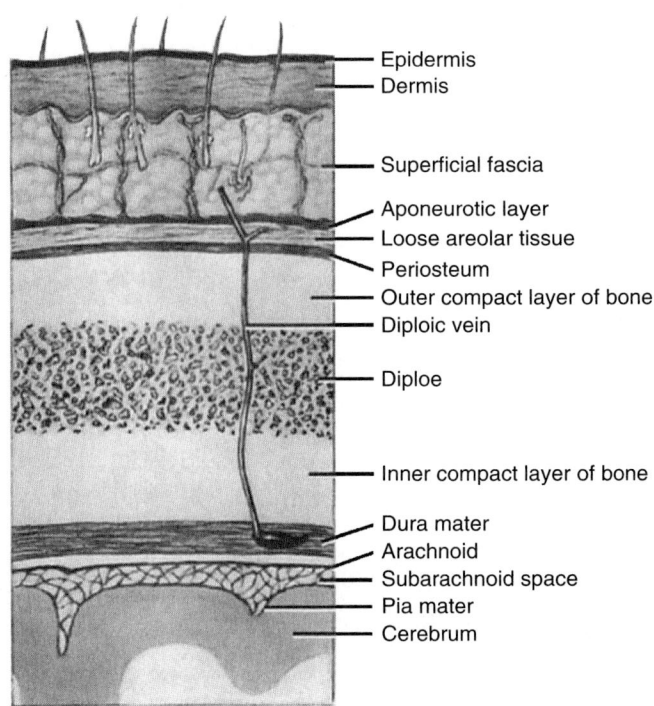

FIGURE 1–14. The scalp.

Reproduced, with permission, from Montgomery RL. *Head and Neck Anatomy: With Clinical Correlations.* New York: McGraw-Hill, 1981.

Meninges

- Three layers surround the brain and spinal cord.

Meningitis is inflammation of the meninges. For more information, see the "Systemic Pathology" section in Chapter 22.

Meninge	Space	Description
	Epidural space	Potential space between periosteum of inner surface of skull and dura; middle meningeal artery is in this location.
Dura mater		Tough membranous, outermost layer, continuous with the periosteum within the skull; forms the venous sinuses in the cranial cavity. Endosteal layer is continuous with cranial periosteum. Meningeal layer folds between brain.
	Subdural space	Between dura and arachnoid; bridging veins and cranial venous sinuses are located here.
Arachnoid		(Spiderlike) weblike lattices interposed between dura and pia; does not follow the sulci; bridges them.
	Subarachnoid space	Between arachnoid and pia; is filled with Willis CSF; cerebral circulation is here (circle of Willis). This is the space entered with a lumbar puncture ("spinal tap").
Pia mater		Layer adherent to the brain and ; spinal cord follows the sulci.

Blood surrounds the meninges in the following ways:

- **Epidural hematoma** involves the middle meningeal artery.
- **Subdural hematoma** involves a bridging vein.
- **Subarachnoid hemorrhage** often involves a ruptured aneurysm (e.g., anterior communicating artery).

DURAL FOLDS

See Figure 1–15 for the folds of the dura mater.

Fold	Description
Vertical Falx cerebri	Vertical, midline. Separates the cerebral hemispheres. Forms the superior and inferior sagittal sinuses.
Falx cerebelli	Separates cerebellar hemispheres. Contains occipital sinus.
Horizontal Tentorium cerebelli	Separates cerebral hemispheres (occipital lobes) from cerebellum below. Contains straight, transverse, and superior petrosal sinuses. **Uncus** (medial parahippocampal gyrus); amygdala lies beneath; herniates below tentorium.
Diaphragma sella	Roof of the sella turcica. Small hole allows passage of the pituitary stalk.

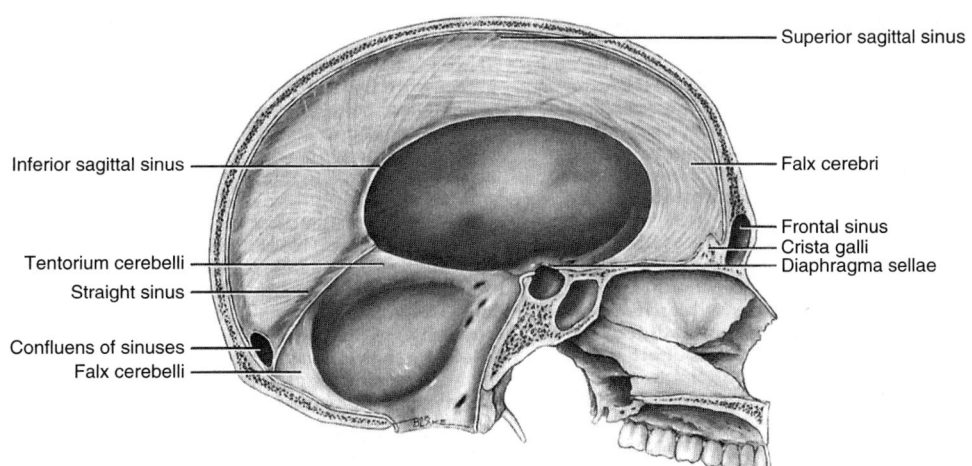

FIGURE 1–15. The folds of the dura mater.

Lumbar puncture (from outside to in):
- Skin
- Subcutaneous tissue
- Supraspinous ligament
- Interspinous ligament
- Ligamentum flavum (if not midline)
- Epidural space (fat, venous plexus)
- (Subdural space— potential space)
- Subarachnoid space with cerebrospinal fluid (CSF)

Reproduced, with permission, from Montgomery RL. *Head and Neck Anatomy: With Clinical Correlations.* New York: McGraw-Hill, 1981.

Venous Sinuses

See Figure 1–16. The **dural sinuses** are:

- Superior sagittal sinus
- Inferior sagittal sinus
- Straight sinus
- Cavernous sinus (2)
- Superior petrosal sinus (2)
- Inferior petrosal sinus (2)
- Occipital sinus
- Transverse sinus (2)
- Confluence of sinuses (torcular of herophile)
- Sigmoid

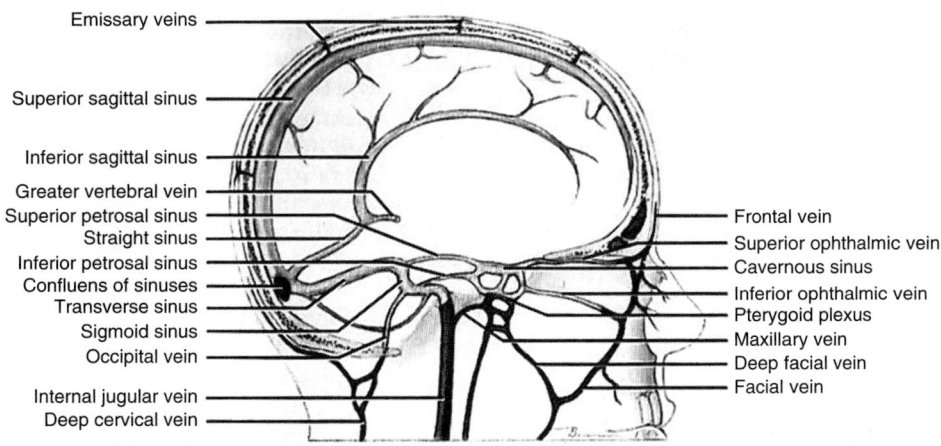

FIGURE 1–16. The venous sinuses.

Reproduced, with permission, from Montgomery RL. *Head and Neck Anatomy: With Clinical Correlations.* New York: McGraw-Hill, 1981.

Drainage of the head/brain is via the internal jugular vein (IJV).
*IJV forms from the inferior petrosal and simoid sinuses.

Tributaries of Dural Sinuses

Emissary veins	Drain scalp into dural sinuses.
Diploic veins	Drain the diploe of the skull into dural sinuses.
Meningeal veins	Drain meninges into dural sinuses.

CAVERNOUS SINUS

Location	Connections	Contents	Description
Middle cranial fossa (on either side of sella turcica)	**Anterior:** superior and inferior ophthalmic veins, pterygoid plexus of veins (via facial vein)	Lateral wall: CNs III, IV, V-1, V-2	Route of infection to brain (e.g., zygomycosis)
	Posterior: superior and inferior petrosal, intercavernous sinus	Running through cavernous sinus: CN VI, ICA	Cavernous sinus thrombosis (see the "Path" section in Chapter 22)

Ophthalmic veins (superior and inferior) can communicate with the cavernous sinus. Because there are no valves, retrograde flow occurs.

- Inferior ophthalmic vein; two branches. (See Figures 1–16, 1–17, and 1–18.)
  - One branches into the cavernous sinus (or joins with superior ophthalmic vein).
  - One branches into pterygoid plexus of veins.

The superior petrosal sinus connects the cavernous and sigmoid sinuses.

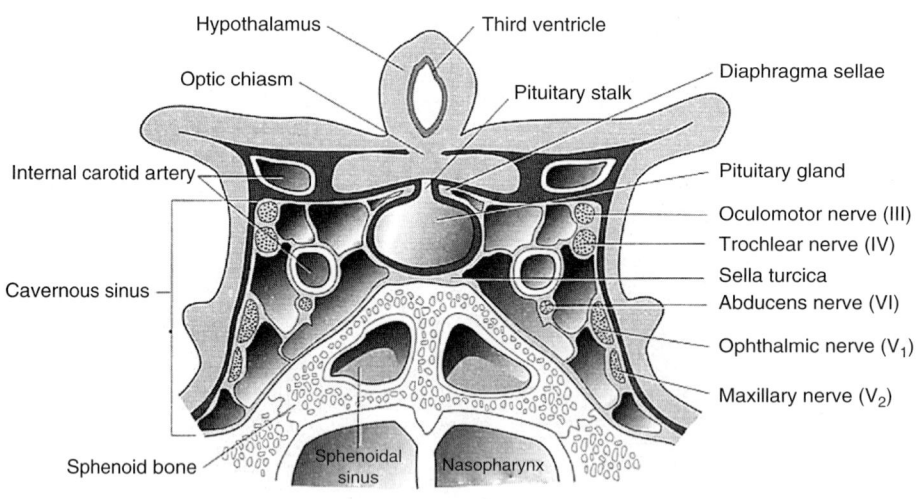

FIGURE 1–17.

Reproduced, with permission, from Bushhan V, et al. *First Aid for the USMLE Step 1.* New York: McGraw-Hill, 2003. Adapted from Stobo J, et al. *The Principles and Practice of Medicine,* 23rd ed. Stamford, CT: Appleton & Lange, 1996:277.

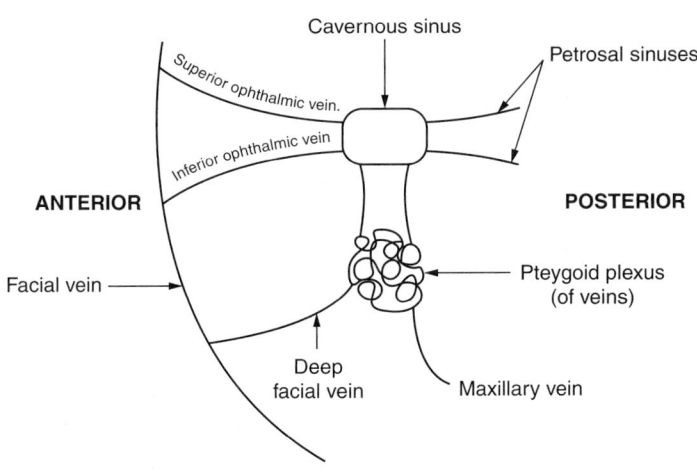

FIGURE 1-18. Cavernous sinus and its communications.

The abducens nerve is most likely affected from laterally expanding pituitary tumor because it is medially located within the cavernous sinus.

Pterygoid Plexus of Veins

Location	Receives	Drains
Located in the infratemporal fossa. Surrounds the maxillary artery. Associated with the pterygoid muscles.	Venous branches corresponding with those of the maxillary artery	Maxillary vein posteriorly. Deep facial vein into the facial vein anteriorly.

Deep facial vein connects anterior facial vein and pterygoid plexus.

Ventricular System

See Figure 1-19.

- This system is lined with ependymal cells; ventricular system consists of these parts: lateral ventricle, interventricular foramen, third ventricle, cerebral aqueduct, fourth ventricle (releases CSF into subarachnoid space).

The choroid plexus and ventricular system regulates intracranial pressure.

Ventricle	Nearby Anatomical Structure
Lateral ventricle	Caudate nucleus
Lateral ventricle (inferior horn)	Hippocampus
Third ventricle	Hypothalamus
Floor of fourth ventricle	Pons

Ependymal cells can also produce cerebrospinal fluid.

Hydrocephalus results from excess buildup of CSF.

- Noncommunicating—obstruction in the ventricular system (e.g., blocked cerebral aqueduct).
- Communicating—obstruction in subarachnoid space.

CSF Circulation

- The CSF flows from lateral ventricles (produced in choroids plexus) through the ventricular system to the subarachnoid space, where it enters the venous circulation.

- *Pathway*

  Lateral ventricles
  ↓
  Foramen of Monro
  ↓
  Third ventricle
  ↓
  Cerebral aqueduct
  ↓
  Fourth ventricle
  ↓
  Foramina of Magendie and Lushka (exits ventricular system into subarachnoid space)
  ↓
  Bathes the cisterns in the subarachnoid space
  ↓
  Arachnoid granulations protrude into the superior sagittal sinus and empty CSF into the venous circulation.

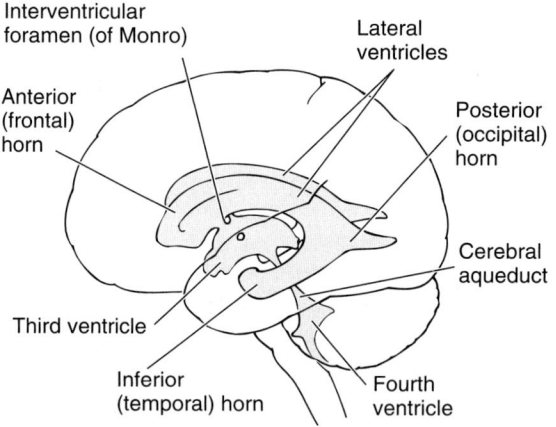

FIGURE 1-19. The ventricular system.

Reproduced, with permission, from Waxman SG. *Clinical Neuroanatomy*, 25th ed. McGraw-Hill, 2003.

Blood-Brain Barrier

- The blood-brain barrier (BBB) consists of three (3) parts.

Blood-CSF Barrier	Vascular-Endothelial Barrier	Arachnoid Barrier
CSF produced in choroid plexus in ventricles. Choroid plexus epithelial cells are joined by tight junctions, allowing selective passage.	Tight junctions between endothelial cells	Arachnoid cells form a barrier, preventing substances from dural vessel from diffusing in toward brain.

Intracranial Circulation

- Blood is supplied to the brain via many arteries.

CIRCLE OF WILLIS

See Figures 1–20 and 1–21.

- Contents:
    - Posterior cerebral artery
    - Posterior communicating artery
    - Internal carotid artery
    - Anterior cerebral artery
    - Anterior communicating artery
- Four arteries contribute: vertebral arteries (2) and carotid arteries (2).

BBB is absent in hypothalamus, pineal gland, area postrema (of fourth ventricle), and areas near third ventricle.

Circle of Willis

Feeder Arteries	Branches	Supplies
Internal carotid artery (2) Enters through carotid canal, passes over foramen lacerum.	Anterior cerebral artery.	Medial aspect of cerebral hemispheres.
	Middle cerebral artery; connects to ACA by anterior communicating artery.	Lateral convexity of brain.
Vertebral arteries (2).	Posteroinferior cerebellar.	Medulla, cerebellum.
Basilar artery (1) Formed from the converging vertebral arteries (2).	Anteroinferior cerebellar.	Pons, cerebellum.
	Superior cerebellar.	Pons, cerebellum.
	Posterior cerebral artery connects to MCA by posterior communicating artery.	Occipital cortex (visual area).

Vertebral arteries are branches of the subclavian artery.

The ICA has no branches in the neck.

The ophthalmic artery is a branch of the ICA (follows optic nerve through optic foramen into orbit); it gives off the anterior ethmoidal branch that supplies the nasal cavity.

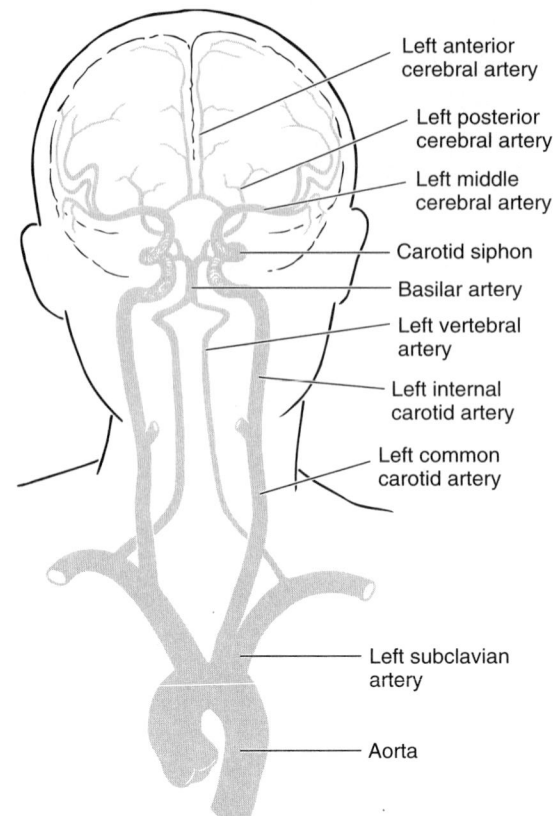

FIGURE 1-20. Major cerebral arteries.

Reproduced, with permission, from Waxman SG. *Clinical Neuroanatomy*, 25th ed. McGraw-Hill, 2003.

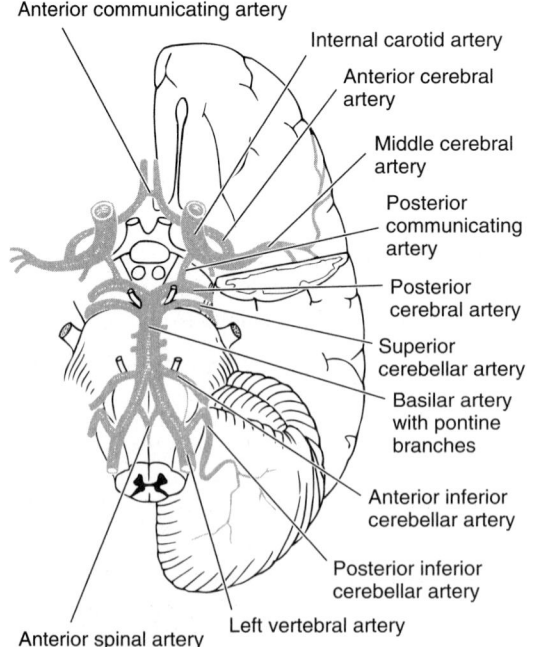

FIGURE 1-21. Circle of Willis and principal arteries of the brainstem.

Reproduced, with permission, from Waxman SG. *Clinical Neuroanatomy*, 25th ed. McGraw-Hill, 2003.

MIDDLE CEREBRAL ARTERY

- Largest branch of the ICA.
- Middle cerebral artery **is not** part of the circle of Willis. If blocked, it causes the most ischemic injury.
- Leticulostriate arteries, branches of the MCA, are often involved in stroke, are thin-walled, and can rupture.

▶ ORAL CAVITY AND PHARYNX

Oral Cavity

See Figure 1–22, which shows the mouth and oral cavity.

Components	Description
Oral vestibule	Slitlike space between lips and cheeks and the facial surfaces of teeth and gingivae.
Oral cavity proper	Space posterior and medial to dental arches (deep to lingual surfaces of teeth). Posterior termination is palatoglossal arch. Roof is the palate. Tongue occupies this space at rest with mouth closed.

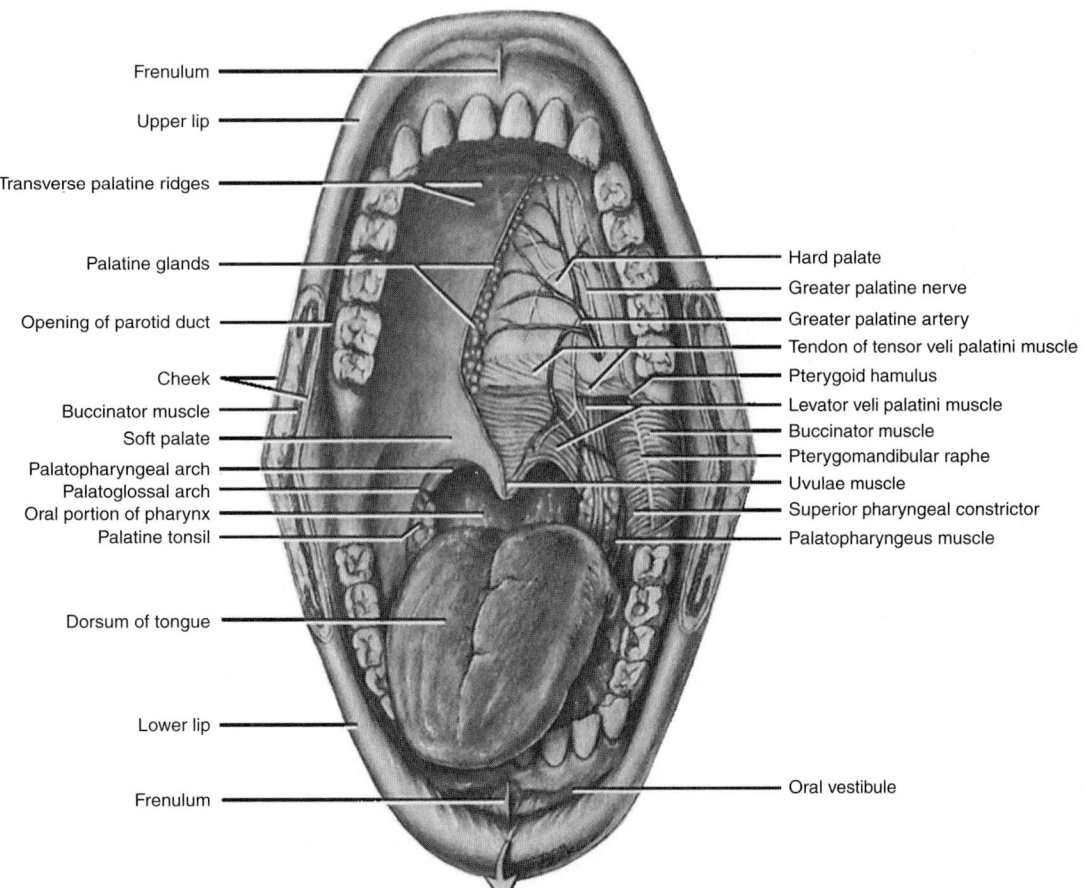

FIGURE 1–22. **The mouth of the oral cavity.**

Reproduced, with permission, from Montgomery RL. *Head and Neck Anatomy: With Clinical Correlations.* New York: McGraw-Hill, 1981.

Tongue

Function	Innervation
Motor	CN XII
Sensation	CN V-3, IX, X
Taste	CN VII, IX, X

General Sensation of the Tongue

See Figure 1–23 for the innervation of the tongue, which is mediated by these cranial nerves (CNs):

- V-3
- IX
- X

Taste Sensation of the Tongue

The sense of taste is mediated by the following CNs:

- VII
- IX
- X

See embryology. The tongue is derived from the first four pharyngeal arches and is innervated by associated nerves of those arches: arch 1 (V), arch 2 (VII), arch 3 (IX), and arch 4 (X).

Location	Nerve	Pathway			
Anterior 2/3	CN VII Chorda tympani nerve travels via lingual nerve (of V-3) to the geniculate ganglion	Solitary tract	Nucleus of solitary tract (gustatory nucleus)	VPM	Gustatory cortex next to the somatosensory representation of the tongue (frontal-parietal operculum, insula)
Posterior 1/3	CN IX	Same as above	Same as above	Same as above	Same as above
Epiglottis	CN X	Same as above	Same as above	Same as above	Same as above

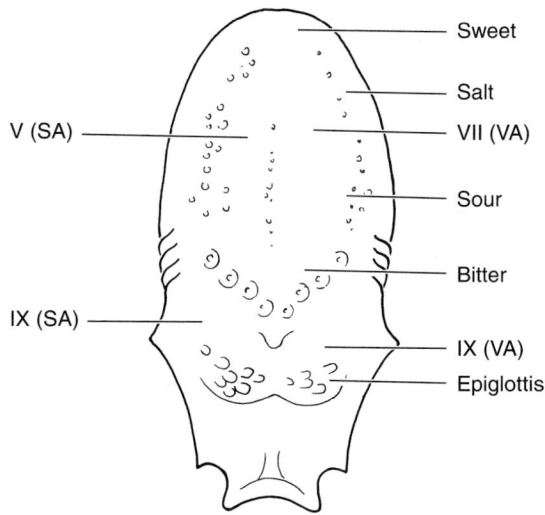

FIGURE 1–23. Sensory innervation of the tongue.

Reproduced, with permission, from Waxman SG. *Clinical Neuroanatomy*, 25th ed. McGraw-Hill, 2003.

CHORDA TYMPANI NERVE

- This nerve is part of the structure of the facial nerve (CN VII).

Course

- Nucleus of solitary tract (accepts taste fibers).
- Superior salivatory nucleus (parasympathetic to submandibular, sublingual glands).
- Chorda tympani nerve arises from the geniculate ganglion.
- Emerges from petrotympanic fissure.
- Crosses the medial surface of the tympanic membrane.
- Joins the lingual nerve (of V3) in the infratemporal fossa.

Components

- **Taste** (pathway): See Figure 1–24.
    - Anterior two thirds of tastebuds.
    - Chorda tympani (travels with lingual nerve).
    - Cell bodies are located in the geniculate ganglion (within facial canal or petrous temporal).
- **Preganglionic parasympathetic**
    - Synapse in submandibular ganglion.

INFERIOR SURFACE OF THE TONGUE

- Lingual frenulum: vertical fold in the midline.
- Plica fimbriata: fold of mucous membrane, lateral to the frenulum.
- Wharton's and Rivian ducts: openings of the submandibular and sublingual glands.
- (Blood supply of the tongue: see external carotid artery.)

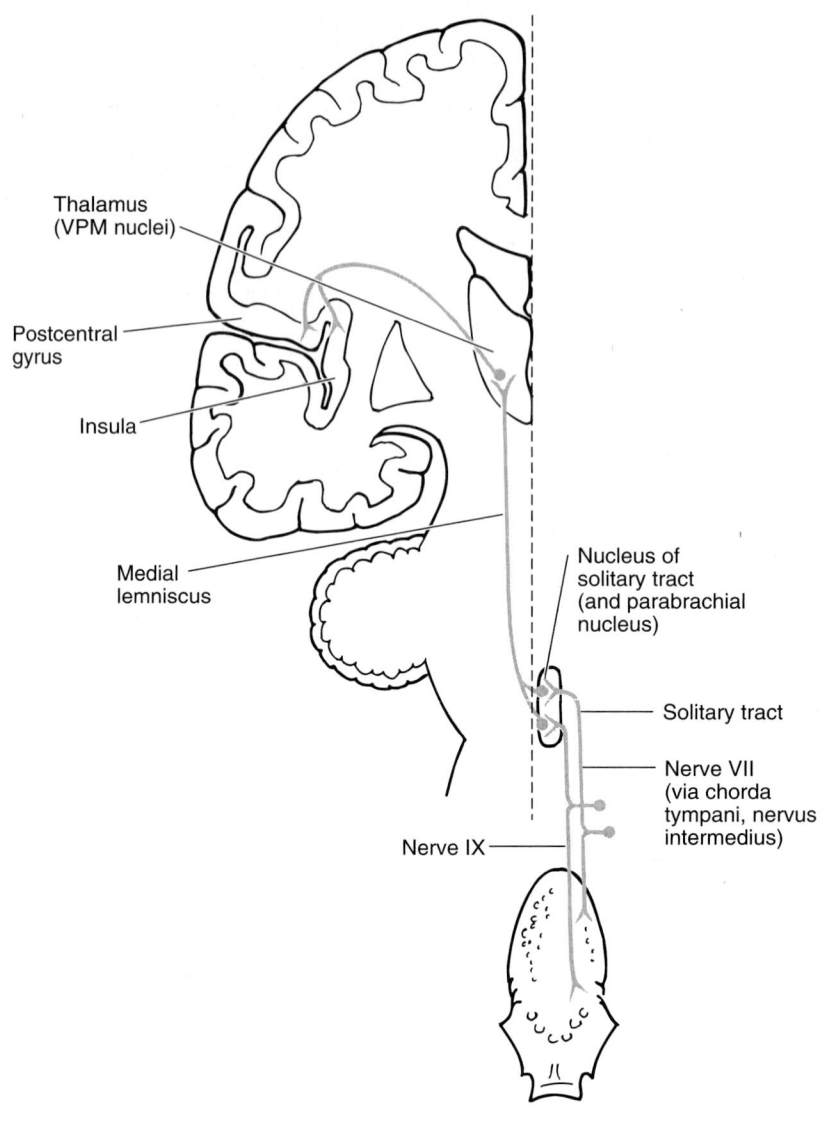

FIGURE 1-24. Diagram of taste pathways.

Reproduced, with permission, from Waxman SG. *Clinical Neuroanatomy*, 25th ed. McGraw-Hill, 2003.

All tastebuds except filiform are vascular.

TASTEBUDS

Tastebud Type[a]	Description
Filiform papillae	Rough texture of tongue; found in rows; avascular; most numerous papillae of tongue; do not contain tastebuds.
Fungiform papillae	Mushroom-shaped; scattered among filiform papillae; *usually* contain tastebuds.
Circumvallate papillae	Seven to nine large circular structures *with tastebuds*; serous-only salivary glands within (von Ebner glands).
Foliate papillae	On lateral surface of tongue in ridges; rudimentary and nonfunctional.

[a]Listed from smallest to largest.

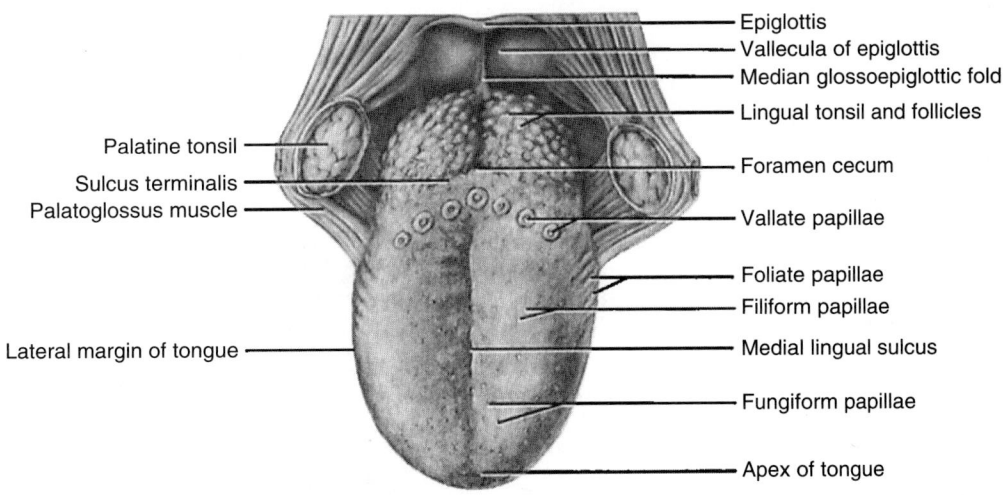

FIGURE 1-25. **The tongue, dorsal view.**

Reproduced, with permission, from Montgomery RL. *Head and Neck Anatomy: With Clinical Correlations.* New York: McGraw-Hill, 1981.

OTHER SURFACE COMPONENTS OF THE TONGUE

See Figure 1–25 for the dorsal view of the tongue.

- Foramen cecum
    - Upper part of thyroglossal duct
- Sulcus terminalis
- Lingual tonsils (See the section "Waldeyer's Ring.")
- Glands
    - Mucous (back, front, and sides)
    - Serous (posteriorly)
    - Anterior lingual glands (of Nuhn)

LYMPHATIC DRAINAGE OF THE TONGUE

See Figure 1–26 for an illustration of the lymph nodes of the tongue. Also see lymphatic drainage of head and neck.

MUSCLES CONTROLLING THE TONGUE

See Figure 1–27.

Bony Attachments

- Genial tubercles
- Styloid process
- Hyoid bone

All tongue muscles, except palatoglossus, are innervated by CN XII.

The muscles attaching to genial tubercles are the genioglossus and the geniohyoid.

The tongue's blood supply is via lingual artery; veins drain into IJV.

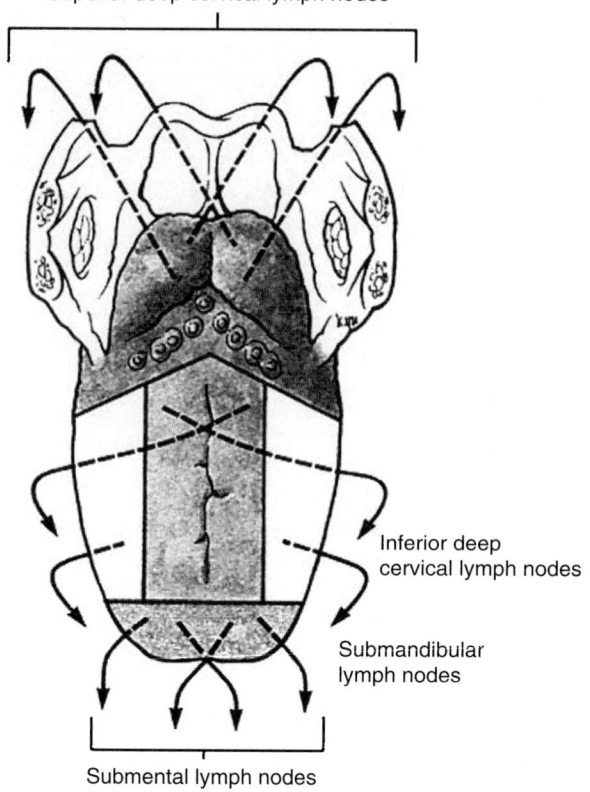

FIGURE 1-26. Lymph drainage of the tongue.

Reproduced, with permission, from Moore K, Agur A. *Essential Clinical Anatomy*, 2nd ed. Lippincott Williams & Wilkins, 2002.

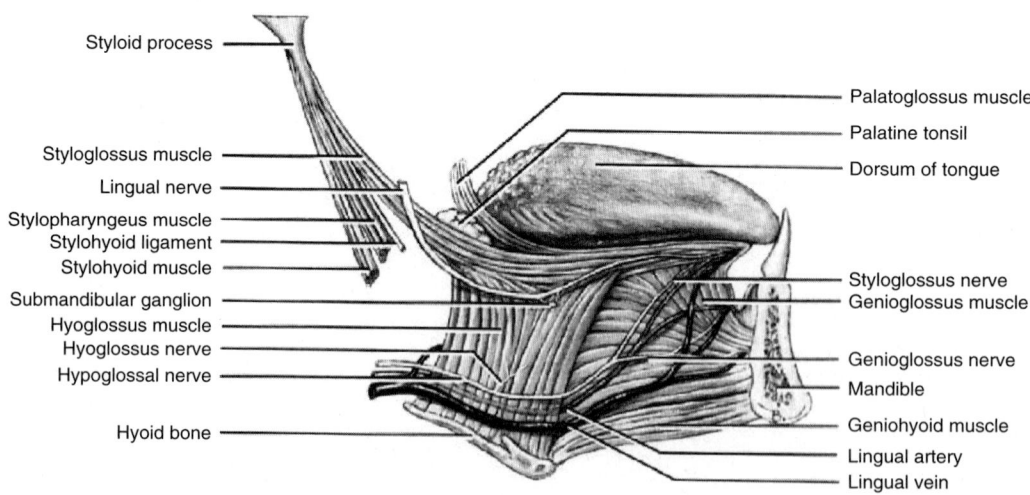

FIGURE 1-27. Muscles controlling the tongue.

Reproduced, with permission, from Montgomery RL. *Head and Neck Anatomy: With Clinical Correlations.* New York: McGraw-Hill, 1981.

EXTRINSIC MUSCLES

Muscle	Origin	Insertion	Action	Innervation
Genioglossus	Genial tubercles	**Inferior:** Hyoid **Superior:** Tongue	Protrude tongue	XII
Hyoglossus	Hyoid (body, greater cornu)	Side of tongue, medial to styloglossus	Depress tongue, pull down sides (retracts)	XII
Styloglossus	Styloid process	Side of tongue	Pull tongue up and back	XII
Palatoglossus	Anterior soft palate	Side and dorsum of tongue	Pull tongue up and back (toward palate)	X (pharyngeal plexus)

INTRINSIC MUSCLES

- These muscles lie within the tongue itself.

Longitudinals (superior and inferior)	Underneath mucosa; shorten the tongue (both); make dorsum concave (superior); make dorsum convex (inferior).
Transversus	Arise from median fibrous septum and pass laterally; narrows and elongates the tongue.
Verticalis	Flattens and broadens the tongue.

SPEAKING SOUNDS

- "La-la" CN XII moves tongue against roof of mouth.
- "Mi-mi" CN VII moves lips.
- "Kuh-kuh" CN X raises the palate.

RELATIONSHIP OF LINGUAL ARTERY, VEIN, AND SUBMANDIBULAR DUCT

The relationships to the hyoglossus muscle are:

- Medial to the hyoglossus.
    - Lingual artery
- Lateral to the hyoglossus.
    - Lingual vein
    - Lingual nerve
    - Submandibular duct
    - Hypoglossal nerve

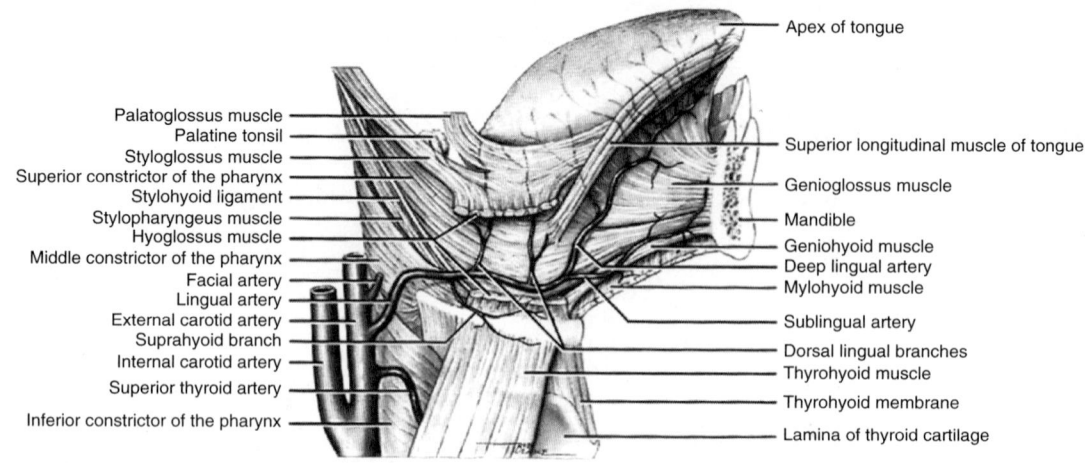

FIGURE 1-28. Branches of the lingual artery.

Reproduced, with permission, from Montgomery RL. *Head and Neck Anatomy: With Clinical Correlations.* New York: McGraw-Hill, 1981.

The palatal salivary glands are mostly mucous, are located beneath the mucous membrane of hard and soft palates, and contribute to oral fluid.

See Figure 1–28 for branches of the lingual tongue.

PALATE

- Roof of oral cavity, floor of nasal cavity.

Innervation

- Motor
  - Pharyngeal plexus (except tensor veli palatine, CN V-3).
- Sensory
  - CN V-2
    - Greater palatine nerve is located posteriorly; it travels anteriorly.
    - Nasopalatine nerves are located anteriorly; they join the greater palatine posteriorly.

Blood Supply

- Third part of the maxillary artery (branch of ECA).
  - Greater palatine artery travels with nerve and vein from the greater and lesser palatine foramina.
  - Sphenopalatine vessels travel with nasopalatine nerves from the incisive foramen.

Hard Palate	Soft Palate (Muscles)
Maxillary bone (palatine processes) Palatine bones (horizontal plates)	Palatopharyngeus Palatoglossus Levator veli palatini Tensor veli palatini Uvular

Covered by keratinized mucosa (with rugae anteriorly)
 Palatal salivary glands (beneath mucosa)
	Covered by nonkeratinized mucosa
	 Submucosa
	   Anterior zone of palatal submucosa contains fat
	   Posterior zone contains mucous glands
	 Palatal aponeurosis: Fibrous connective tissue of soft palate (muscles beneath)

The soft palate attaches to the tongue by the glossopalatine (palatoglossal) arches and to the pharynx by the palatopharyngeal arches.

Uvula

- Suspended from soft palate.
- Bifid uvula results from incomplete fusion of palatine shelves.
- Unilateral damaged pharyngeal plexus causes uvula to deviate to contralateral side. Contraction on intact side pulls it to functional side.

Fauces

- The fauces are between anterior and posterior pillars, and they house the palatine tonsils.

Remember: Most muscles of the soft palate attach to the palatal aponeurosis.

Pillar	Muscle	Muscle Function
Anterior pillar	Palatoglossus (palatoglossal fold)	Draws tongue and soft palate closer together (with swallowing). Narrows isthmus of fauces.
Posterior pillar	Palatopharyngeus (palatopharyngeal fold)	Elevates pharynx. Helps close the nasophatrynx. Aids in swallowing.

Tonsils

Tonsil	Location	Description
Pharyngeal tonsils (adenoids)	Nasopharynx (posterior wall and roof)	**No lymph, sinuses, nor crypts** Surrounded in part by connective tissue and in part by epithelium
Palatine tonsils	In isthmus of fauces (between palaotglossal and palatopharyngeal folds) on either side of the posterior oropharynx	Reach maximum size during childhood then diminish Contain **crypts and lymphoid follicles** (No sinuses) Covered partly by connective tissue, partly by epithelium
Lingual tonsils	Dorsum of tongue (posteriorly)	**Lymphoid follicles**, each with a **single crypt**

(See Peyers patches in GI section).

The tensor and levator veli palatini muscles prevent food from entering the nasopharynx. (See Figure 1-29 for parasagittal view of the soft palate and pharynx).

WALDEYER'S RING

Ring of lymphoid tissue

- Lingual tonsil (inferiorly)
- Palatine tonsils (faucial tonsils) (laterally)
- Nasopharyngeal tonsils (adenoids) (superiorly)

Tensor Versus Levator Veli Palatini

Muscle	Origin	Insertion	Action	Innervation
Tensor veli palatini	Greater wing of sphenoid (scaphoid fossa), lateral cartilage of auditory tube	Wraps around hamulus to insert onto midline palatal aponeurosis (with contralateral fibers)	Tenses palate, opens auditory tube with mouth opening	CN V-3
Levator veli palatini	Inferior petrous temporal bone, medial auditory tube	Palatine aponeurosis	Elevates/raises palate (during swallowing)	CN X

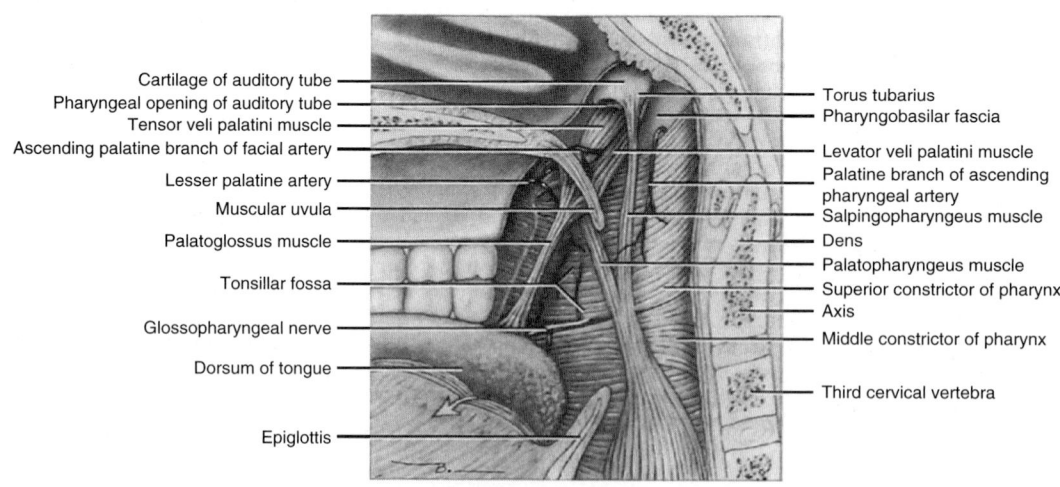

FIGURE 1-29. Parasagittal view of soft palate and pharynx.

Reproduced, with permission, from Montgomery RL. *Head and Neck Anatomy: With Clinical Correlations.* New York: McGraw-Hill, 1981.

Pharynx

See Figures 1–30 and 1–31 for views of the throat and Table 1–2 for locations and descriptions.

- Pharynx is behind nasal and oral cavities.
- Pharynx shares conduit to larynx and esophagus.

Pharyngeal Muscles

Muscle	Origin	Insertion	Action	Innervation
Constrictors				
Superior	Pterygomandibular raphe and pharyngeal tubercle; mylohyoid line of mandible.	Midline pharyngeal raphe (posteriorly); pharyngeal tubercle.	Contract in waves (to propel food).	**Sensory:** CN X **Motor:** CN XI (via X)
Middle	Hyoid bone (greater and lesser horns).	Midline pharyngeal raphe (posteriorly).	Contract in waves (to propel food).	**Sensory:** CN X **Motor:** CN XI (via X)
Inferior	Thyroid and cricoid cartilages.	Midline pharyngeal raphe.	Contract in waves (to propel food).	**Sensory:** CN X **Motor:** CN XI (via X)
Cricopharyngeus	Lower fibers of inferior constrictor.	Midline raphe.	Constant contraction (serves as UES).	**Sensory:** CN X **Motor:** CN XI (via X)
Longitudinal muscles				
Palatopharyngeus	Palatal aponeurosis.	Posterolateral pharynx.	Raise pharynx and larynx during swallowing	CN XI (via X) (pharyngeal plexus)
Salpingopharyngeus	(part of palatopharyngeus); cartilage of auditory tube.	Muscles of pharynx.	Elevate nasopharynx, open auditory tube.	CN XI (via X) (pharyngeal plexus)
Stylopharyngeus	Styloid process.	Pass between superior and middle constrictors; blend with palatopharyngeus.	Raise pharynx and larynx during swallowing.	CN IX

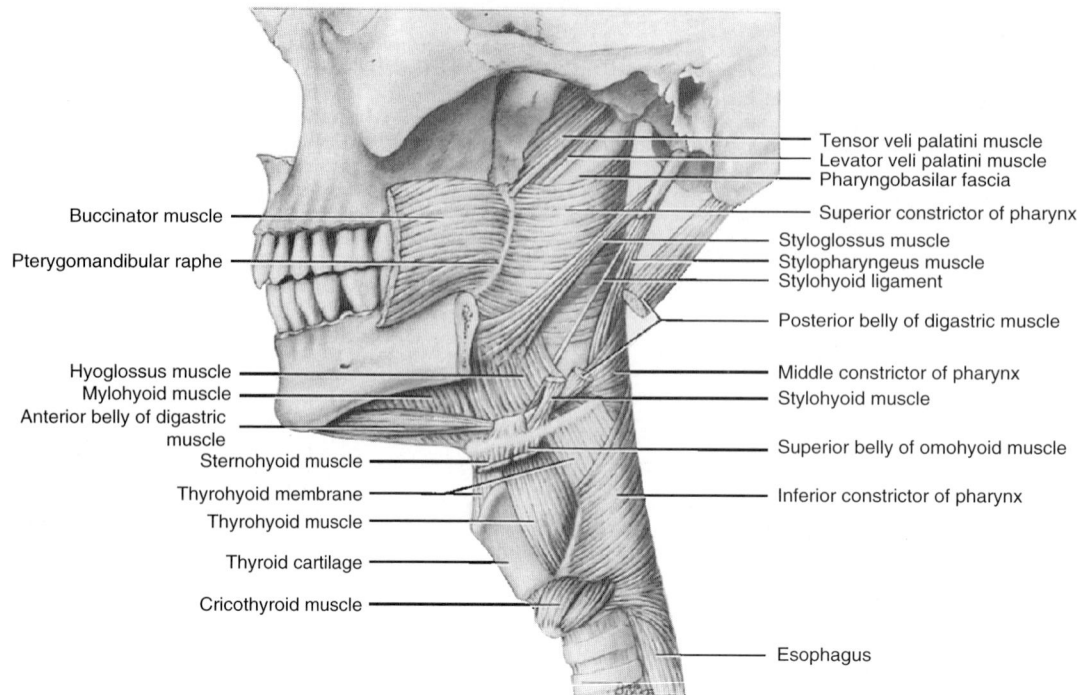

FIGURE 1-30. External view of the pharynx.

Reproduced, with permission, from Montgomery RL. *Head and Neck Anatomy: With Clinical Correlations.* New York: McGraw-Hill, 1981.

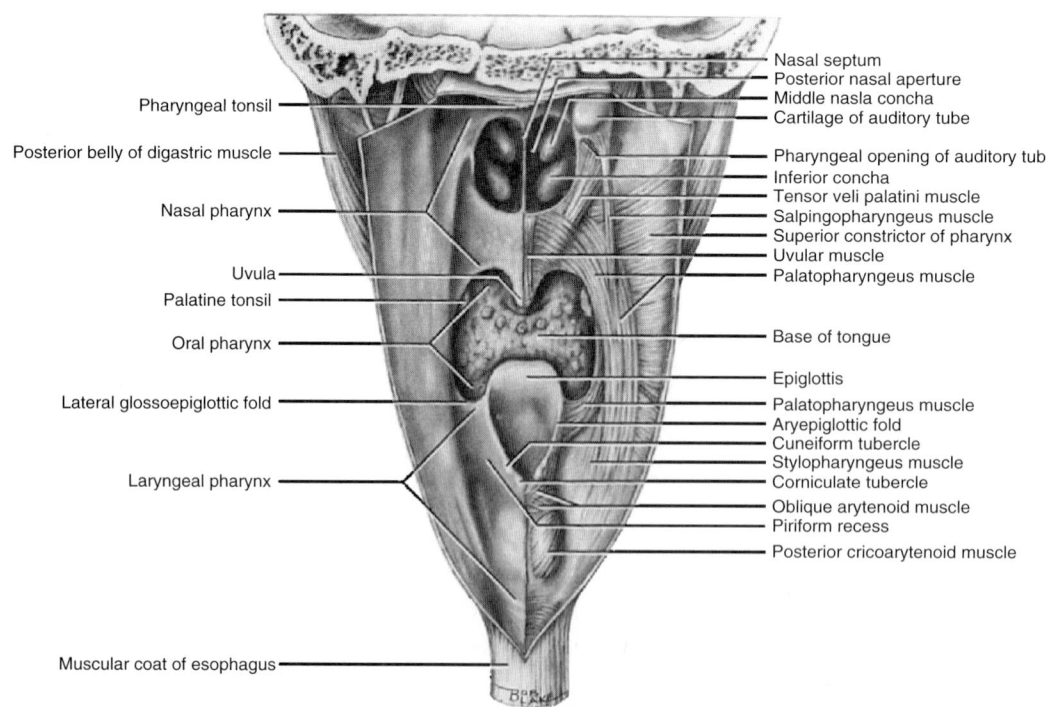

FIGURE 1-31. Posterior view of the soft palate and pharynx.

TABLE 1–2.

	LOCATION	DESCRIPTION
Nasopharynx	Above the soft palate; continuous with nasal passages; soft palate and uvula form anterior wall.	Auditory tube connects nasopharynx with middle ear.
Oropharynx	Extends from anterior pillars to larynx.	Communicates with oral cavity via fauces; food and air from mouth; air and sinus drainage from nasopharynx; contains palatine and lingual tonsils.
Laryngopharynx	Area inferior to oropharynx containing entrance to both larynx and esophagus.	Allows food into esophagus; air into larynx.

Pharyngeal plexus = CNs IX, X, XI. Provides innervation to constrictors, palatoglossus, palatopharyngeus, and cricopharyngeus.

Stylopharyngeus muscle is the only muscle supplied by CN IX. This muscle is a landmark for finding the nerve.

SWALLOWING

Close Palate

This prevents velopharyngeal incompetence.

- Raise velum:
    - Palatoglossal (CN X)
    - Levator veli palatini (CN X)
- Tense velum:
    - Tensor veli palatini (CN V)
- Depress velum, raise/constrict pharynx:
    - Palatopharyngus (CN XI)
- Shorten velum:
    - Muscularis uvula (CN XI)

Food can get caught in the vallecula or pyriform recesses.

Propel Food Down Pharynx

- Plunger action of tongue is most important.
- Pharyngeal constrictors perform wavelike action (CN IX, X, XI).
- Hyoid and pharynx pull up (epiglottis closes over airway).
- Cricopharyngeus (functional upper esophageal sphincter) relaxes.

▶ **NASOLACRIMAL APPARATUS**

Nasolacrimal Apparatus

See Figure 1–32.

Sensory information goes to the swallowing center (nucleus ambiguous in medulla oblongata). Nucleus ambiguous sends motor information (SVE), via CNs IX, X, XI, XII, to facilitate swallowing.

- **Lacrimal gland**
    - Located in the lacrimal sulcus in the superolateral aspect of the orbit.
    - Produces tears that wash across the globe superolateral to inferomedially.
- **Lacrimal puncta** collects tears and drains into the
- **Lacrimal canals** (superior and inferior), which join the
- **Lacrimal sac**, which drains down the
- **Nasolacrimal duct** to empty underneath the inferior nasal concha in the
- **Inferior meatus.**

Postganglionic nerves from the pterygopalatine ganglion exit via the inferior orbital fissure and join the lacrimal nerve (of V-1) to supply the lacrimal gland.

The lingual artery and facial artery are both braches of the external carotid artery (ECA).

Lymphatic drainage: Parotid gland, through parotid nodes, then superior deep cervical lymph nodes. Submandibular and sublingual glands, through submandibular and deep cervical nodes.

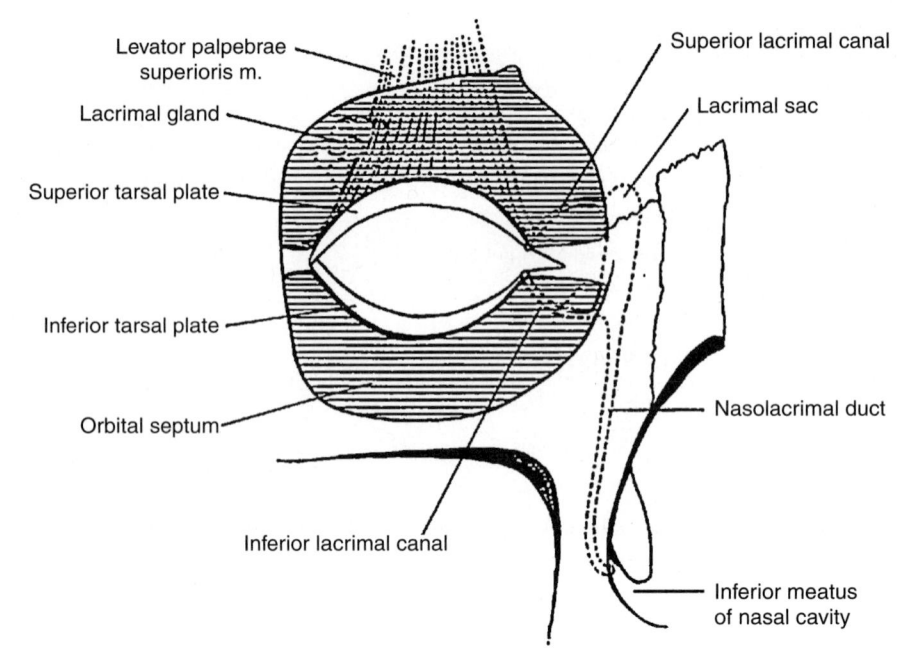

FIGURE 1-32. The lacrimal apparatus.

Reproduced, with permission, from Liebgott B. *The Anatomical Basis of Dentistry*. Toronto: BC Decker, 1986.

LACRIMAL GLAND

- Paired serous glands.
- Involved in tear production.
- Parasympathetic innervation.
    - **Superior salivatory nucleus** (brainstem)
    - **Greater petrosal nerve** (of CN-VII) (preganglionic synapses at pterygopalatine ganglion)
    - **Lacrimal nerve** (of V-1) (postganglionic parasympathetics from pterygopalatine ganglion)

Salivary Glands

Gland	Location	Secretion	Duct	Innervation	Blood Supply
Parotid gland (See Figure 1–33.)	Parotid region, between posterior border of mandibular ramus and anterior border of SCM. (Below and anterior to ear.)	Serous	Stensons (parotid duct) goes anterior along lateral masseter, rolls over anterior border of masseter and pierces cheek, buccinator muscle; empties next to maxillary second molar.	**Preganglionic:** Lesser petrosal nerve (of CN IX). **Synapse:** Otic ganglion. **Postganglionic:** Leaves otic ganglion, travels with auriculotemporal nerve (of V-3) to parotid.	Glandular branches of superficial temporal artery and transverse facial artery.

Salivary Glands (Continued)

Gland	Location	Secretion	Duct	Innervation	Blood Supply
Submandibular gland (See Figure 1–34.)	**Superficial portion** Between lateral aspect of mylohyoid muscle and submandibular fossa of mandible (submandibular triangle). **Deep portion:** In floor of mouth between base of tongue and sublingual gland (between mylohyoid and hyoglossus)	Serous and mucous	Submandibular duct continues forward from deep portion of gland, crosses lingual nerve (near the sublingual gland), and empties into oral cavity at the sublingual caruncle (papilla) (next to sublingual frenulum; behind lower central incisors).	**Preganglionic:** Chorda tympani (of VII) **Synapse:** Submandibular ganglion **Postganglionic:** Leaves ganglion and passes to gland.	Glandular branches of facial and lingual arteries.
Sublingual gland (See Figure 1–35.)	Floor of mouth medial to sublingual fossa of mandible (above mylohyoid muscle).	Mucous	Sublingual (Rivian) ducts open directly into oral cavity through openings in sublingual fold; anterior ducts open medially into submandibular duct (the single Bartholin's duct empties into submandibular duct at sublingual papilla).	**Preganglionic:** Chorda tympani (of VII) **Synapse:** Submandibular ganglion **Postganglionic:** Leaves ganglion and passes to gland.	Glandular branches of lingual artery (sublingual artery).

(Adapted, with permission, from Liebgott B. The Anatomical Basis of Dentistry. Toronto: BC Decker, 1986:346.)

Minor Salivary Glands

Gland	Location	Secretion
Labial and buccal minor salivary glands	Labial and buccal mucosa	Mucous only
Von Ebner glands	At base of circumvallate papillae (rinse food away from papilla)	Serous only saliva
Glands of Blandin-Nuhn (anterior lingual glands)	Anterior lingual	Mixed serous-mucous

The submandibular gland emits the highest volume of salivary fluid per day. The parotid gland is second in volume to submandibular gland.

Going from largest to smallest, the major salivary glands go from serous to mixed to mostly mucous (parotid, submandibular, and sublingual respectively).

Minor salivary glands: See the "Pathology" section in Chapter 19 for neoplasms, mucocele, ranula, and so on.

Parotid and von Ebner glands are the only glands to secrete serous-only saliva.

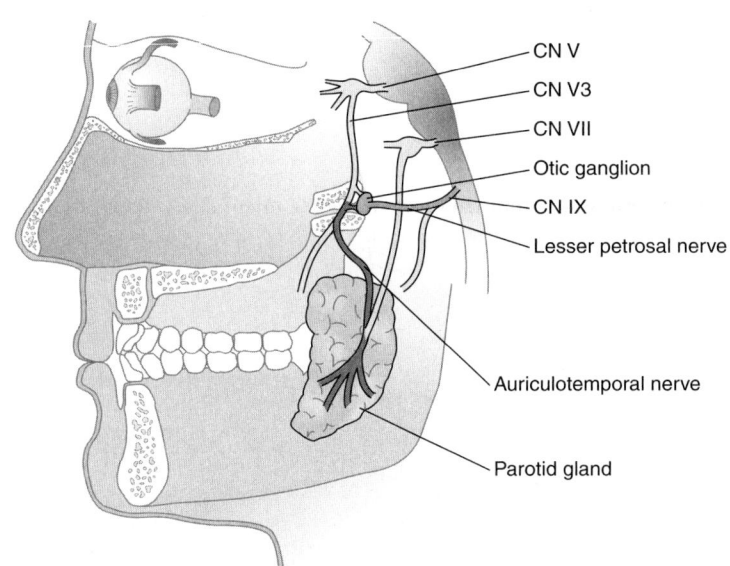

FIGURE 1–33. Schematic of the innervation of the parotid gland by the glossopharyngeal nerve.

Solid black: Preganglionic parasympathetic nerves leave the brainstem with the glosopharyngeal nerve (CN IX) and run with the lesser petrosal nerve to the otic gangion.

Hatched segment: Postganglionic parasympathetic nerves travel with the auriculotemporal branch of CN V3 and then the facial nerve to reach the parotid gland. (Reproduced, with permission, from Lalwani AK. (ed). *Current Diagnosis & Treatment in Otolaryngology–Head & Neck Surgery.* New York: Lange Medical Books/McGraw-Hill, 2004.)

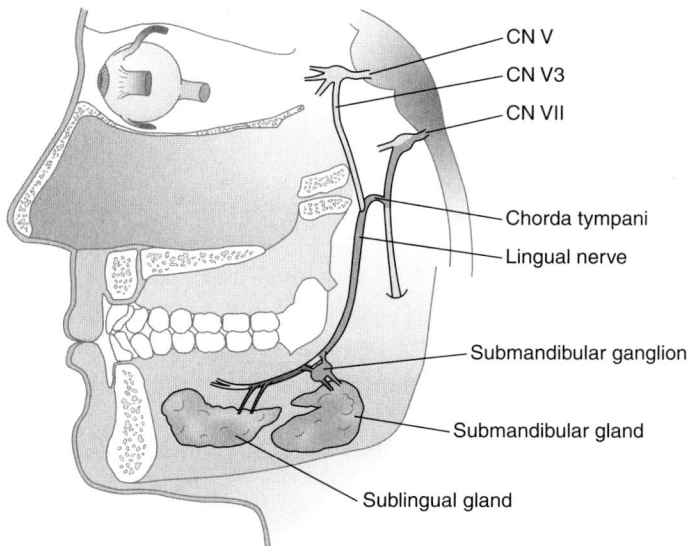

FIGURE 1-34. Schematic of the innervation of the submandibular and sublingual glands by the facial nerve.

Solid black: Preganglionic parasympathetic nerves leave the brainstem with the facial nerve (CN VII) and run with the chorda tympani and the lingual branch of CN V3 to the submandibular ganglion.

Hatched segment: Postganglionic parasympathetic nerves travel either directly to the submandibular gland or back to the lingual branch of CN V3 to the sublingual gland. (Reproduced, with permission, from Lalwani, AK. [ed]. *Current Diagnosis & Treatment in Otolaryngology–Head & Neck Surgery*. New York: Lange Medical Books/McGraw-Hill, 2004.)

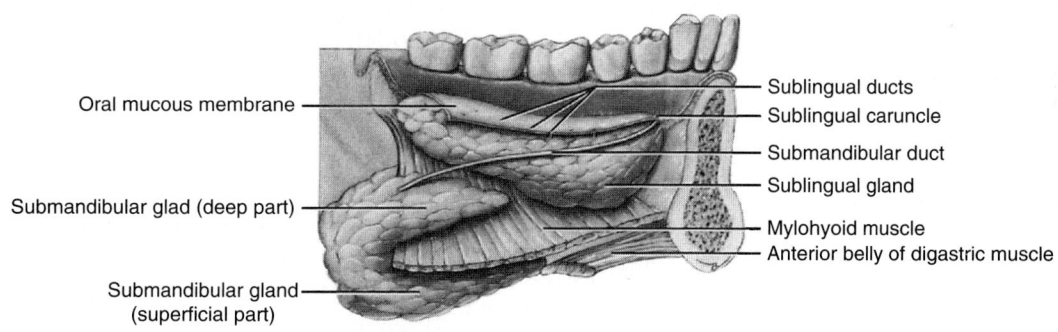

FIGURE 1-35. The sublingual gland.

Reproduced, with permission, from Montgomery RL. *Head and Neck Anatomy: With Clinical Correlations.* New York: McGraw-Hill, 1981.

FASCIAL SPACES

See Figure 1–36.

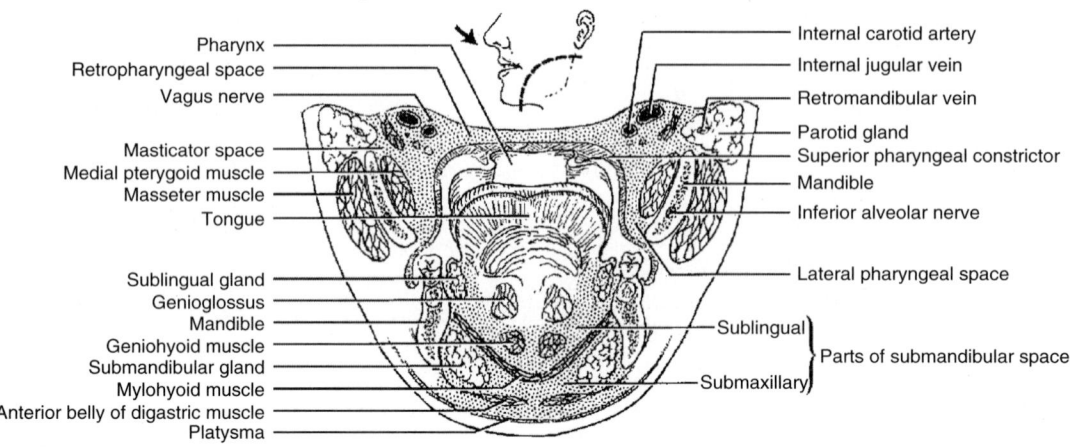

FIGURE 1–36. Canine, buccal, masticator, temporal, and pterygomandibular spaces, space of body of the mandible, and parotid, submaxillary, submental, submandibular, and sublingual spaces of the face and jaws.

Reproduced, with permission, from Montgomery RL. *Head and Neck Anatomy: With Clinical Correlations.* New York: McGraw-Hill, 1981.

Space	Boundaries	Contents
Parotid	**Superfical:** Skin. **Deep:** Styloid process. **Superior and inferior:** Parotid capsule. **Posterior:** Sternocleidomastoid. **Anterior:** Posterior mandibular ramus, stylomandibular ligament.	Parotid gland Facial nerve External carotid artery (and terminal branches) Retromandibular vein
Submandibular	**Lateral:** Superficial fascia, body of mandible. **Medial:** Mylohyoid muscle. **Superior:** Mylohyoid line. **Inferior:** Hyoid bone.	Submandibular gland Lymph nodes Hypoglossal nerve Nerve to mylohyoid Facial artery
Sublingual	**Lateral:** Mandibular body. **Medial:** Base of tongue. **Superior:** Floor of mouth mucosa. **Inferior:** Mylohyoid.	Sublingual gland Deep submandibular gland and duct Lingual nerve (and submandibular ganglion) Lingual artery Hypoglossal nerve

Space	Boundaries	Contents
Tonsillar	**Anterior:** Palatoglossus. **Posterior:** Palatopharyngeus. **Lateral:** Pharyngobasilar fascia. **Medial:** Oropharyngeal mucosa.	Palatine tonsil Glossopharyngeal nerve Tonsillar and ascending palatine branches of the facial artery
Masticator	**Lateral:** Lateral side of cervical fascia, masseter fascia, and temporalis fascia (all blend) to superior temporal line. **Medial:** Deep fascia—deep to mandibular ramus and medial pterygoid. **Posterior:** Stylomandibular ligament. **Anterior:** Anterior mandibular ramus, temporalis tendon (part of the fascia blends with buccopharyngeal fascia of buccinator). **Superior:** Limited by roof of infratemporal fossa and superior aspect of temporalis muscle.	Mandibular ramus and TMJ Muscles of mastication Mandibular nerve Maxillary artery Pterygoid plexus of veins Chorda tympani nerve
Parapharyngeal ■ Retropharyngeal space	**Anterior:** Neck viscera. **Posterior:** Vertebral column. **Lateral:** Sternocleidomastoid muscle. Posterior aspect of parapharyngeal space. Extends from the skull base to the superior mediastinum component.	Carotid sheath Deep cervical chain of lymph nodes

▶ **MASTICATION AND TMJ**

Mastication

- Mastication is the process of biting and chewing food to make it soft enough to swallow.
- Muscles of mastication, which are all controlled by CN V-3:
    - Masseter
    - Temporalis
    - Medial and lateral pterygoids
- Accessory muscles of mastication include the supra- and infrahyoids.
- Tongue and buccinator are essential for controlling the food bolus and propelling it posteriorly for swallowing (CNs XII, VII, respectively).

Left lateral pterygoid muscle moves mandible to the right; the right condyle is pivot point. Injury to left lateral pterygoid causes the mandible to deviate toward the left, the injured side. Subcondylar fracture: Mandible deviates to affected side for same reason. Only the contrateral lateral pterygoid is functional, pulling the mandible to fractured side.

MUSCLES OF MASTICATION

See Figures 1–37, 1–38, and 1–39.

Muscle	Origin	Insertion	Action
Masseter	**Superficial:** Zygomatic process of maxilla, anterior 2/3 zygomatic arch. **Deep:** Zygomatic arch (inner posterior 1/3).	**Superficial:** Angle of mandible. **Deep:** Lateral ramus.	Elevation Retrusion Ipsilateral excursion
Temporalis	Curvilinear lower temporal line. Temporal fossa. Temporal fascia.	Medial coranoid, anterior ramus (passing deep to zygomatic arch).	Elevation (anterior and superior fibers) Retrusion (posterior fibers) Ipsilateral excursion
Medial pterygoid	Medial side of lateral pterygoid plate.	Medial side of mandibular angle.	Elevation Protrusion Contralateral excursion
Lateral pterygoid	**Superior:** Roof of infratemporal fossa. **Inferior:** Lateral side of lateral pterygoid plate.	**Superior:** Articular capsule and disc. **Inferior:** Anterior condylar neck.	Protrusion Depression Contralateral excursion

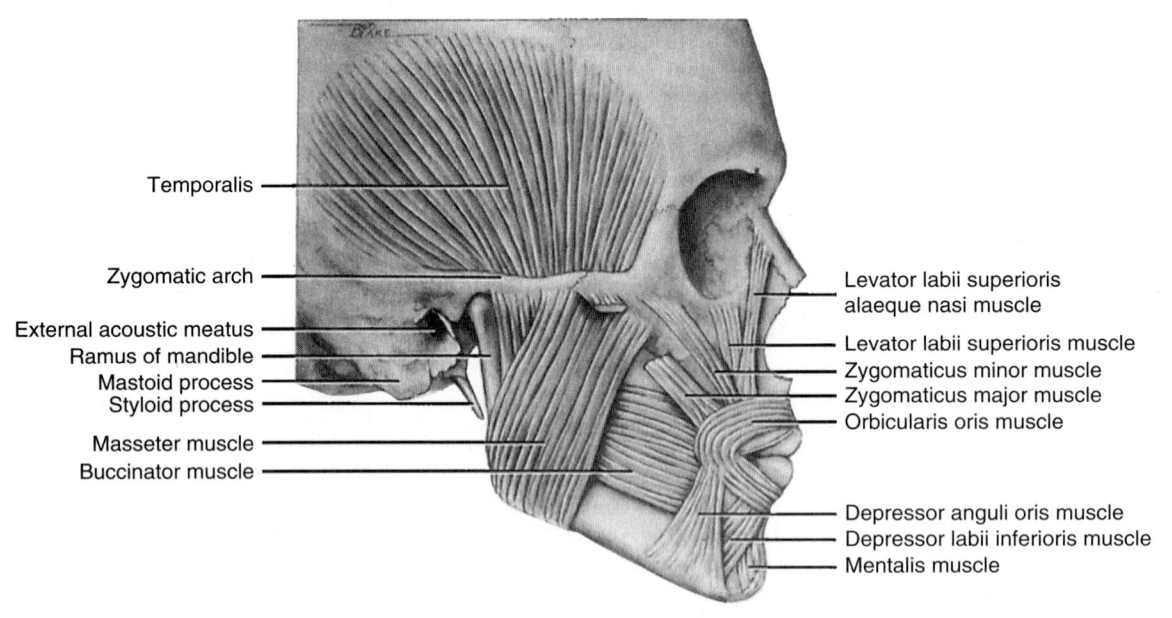

FIGURE 1–37. The masseter muscle.

Reproduced, with permission, from Montgomery RL. *Head and Neck Anatomy: With Clinical Correlations.* New York: McGraw-Hill, 1981.

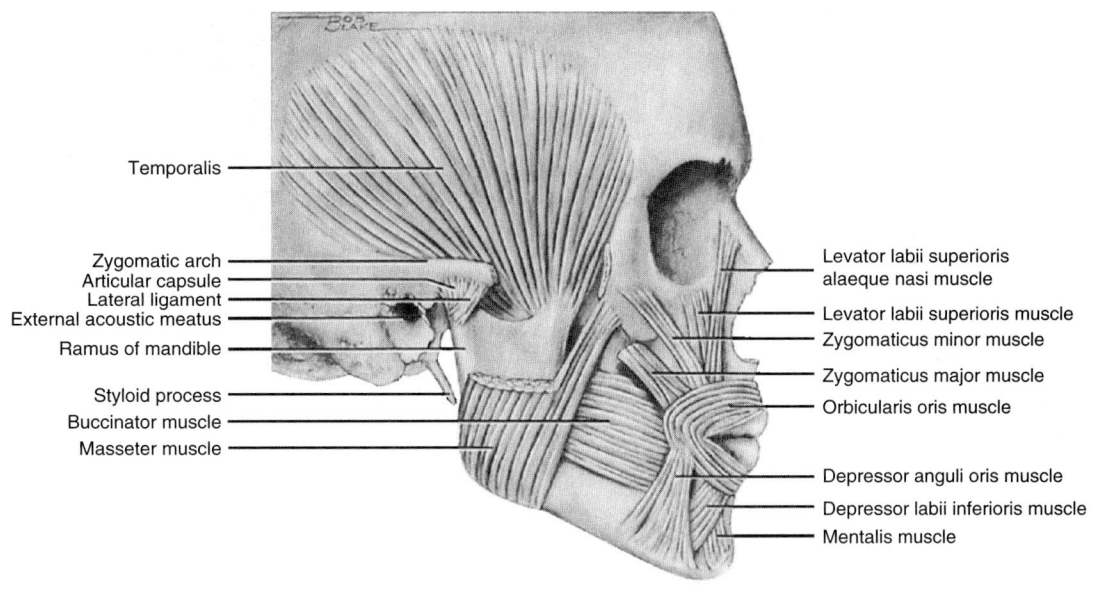

FIGURE 1-38. The temporalis.

Reproduced, with permission, from Montgomery RL. *Head and Neck Anatomy: With Clinical Correlations.* New York: McGraw-Hill, 1981.

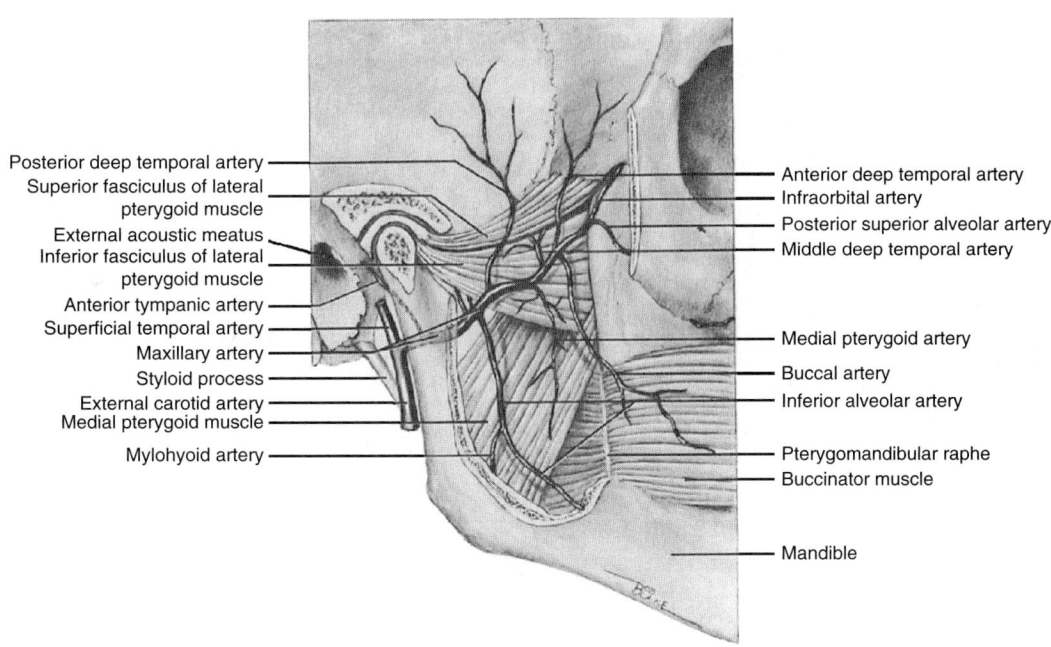

FIGURE 1-39. Lateral and medial pterygoid muscles.

Reproduced, with permission, from Montgomery RL. *Head and Neck Anatomy: With Clinical Correlations.* New York: McGraw-Hill, 1981.

Mandibular Functions for Mastication

Function	Muscles Involved
Opening	Lateral pterygoids, suprahyoids, infrahyoids
Closing	Temporales, masseter, medial pterygoids
Protrusion	Pterygoids (medial and lateral)
Retrusion	Temporales, masseters (deep)
Excursion	Ipsilater masseter, temporalis; contralateral pterygoids (medial and lateral)

Masseter and medial pterygoid muscles form a sling at the angle of mandible; both elevate/close the mandible and stabilize laterally.

Temporomandibular Joint (TMJ)

- Bilateral synovial joint (diarthrodial).
- Articulation between mandibular condyles and skull base on both sides. (Other articulation is between maxillary and mandibular teeth.)

Components

- Moving from superior to inferior:
  - Glenoid/mandibular fossa (of temporal bone)
  - Articular cartilage
  - Disc/meniscus
  - Condylar cartlilage cap
  - Condyle of mandible
- Articular capsule surrounds joint, with synovium internally.
  - Ligaments stabilize.

Palpate posterior aspect of mandibular condyle through external auditory meatus and lateral aspect in front of the external auditory meatus (anterior to tragus).

BONY COMPONENTS

- **Condyle** of the mandible
  - Elliptically shaped with long axis oriented mediolaterally.
  - Posterior condyle is rounded and convex.
  - Anteroinferior aspect is concave.
- **Glenoid/mandibular fossa** (of temporal bone)
  - Concave.
- **Articular eminence**
  - Anterior part of glenoid fossa (squamous temporal bone).
  - Articular eminence (tubercle) is convex.
- Articular sufaces
  - Glenoid fossa and condyle are lined with dense fibrocartilage.
  - **Not** hyaline cartilage like most synovial joints.

Articular Disc (Meniscus)

- Fibrocartilaginous biconcave disc.
- Lies between articular surfaces of condyle and mandibular fossa.
- Divides disc space into superior and inferior compartments.

Lateral pterygoid attaches to neck of condyle, capsule and articular disc of TMJ. Damage to disc where lateral pterygoid inserts can render lateral pterygoid non-functional on that side. (mandible will deviate to the damaged side)

- Attaches peripherally to the capsule and anteriorly to the lateral pterygoid muscle.
- Attaches to medial and lateral poles of the condyle via collateral ligaments.
- Regions
  - Thin intermediate zone.
  - Thick anterior and posterior bands.
  - Posterior band is contiguous with the posterior attachment tissues (bilaminar zone).
  - Bilaminar zone is vascular, innervated tissue (role in allowing condyle to move forward).

ARTICULAR CAPSULE

- Fibrous capsule that surrounds the TMJ.
- Attaches superiorly to the glenoid fossa (tubercle of articular eminence).
- Attaches inferiorly to the condylar neck.
- **Synovium**
  - Lines the internal surface of the joint capsule.
  - Secretes synovial fluid for joint lubrication.
  - Does **not** cover the articular surfaces or articular disc.

TMJ IMAGING

Bony Structures of TMJ

- Panorex x-ray
- CT scan
- Plain films

Soft Tissue of TMJ

- MRI (magnetic resonance imaging)
  - Especially the position of the articular disc

MRI uses a magnetic field to alter energy levels of water in tissues. The advantage of MRI is the lack of x-ray radiation exposure, with no harmful effects being shown.

NERVES OF THE TMJ

TMJ receives only **sensory** innervation (motor is to the muscles).

- **Auriculotemporal nerve** (of V-3) conducts primary innervation to the TMJ.
  - Transmits pain in capsule and periphery of disc.
  - Also provides parasympathetics to the parotid gland.
- **Nerve to masseter** (of V-3)
  - A few sensory fibers to anterior part of TMJ.
- **Posterior deep temporal nerve** (of V3)
  - Also supplies anterior part of TMJ.

LIGAMENTS OF THE TMJ

- TMJ ligaments stabilize the mandible.

To reduce luxated TMJ, apply pressure inferiorly and posteriorly. Stand behind patient; thumbs on patient's occlusal surfaces, fingers below chin; press thumbs inferiorly while fingers close the mandible; condylar head then slides back into articular fossa.

Ligament	Description
Temporomandibular ligament (lateral ligament)	Thickened fibrous band connecting lateral thickening of the joint capsule. Helps prevent excessive lateral or medial movement of the condyle out of the fossa. Prevents posterior and inferior condylar displacement. Only ligament that gives direct support to the TMJ capsule.
Accessory ligaments	
▪ Sphenomandibular ligament	Remnant of Meckel's cartilage. Thickened fibrous band connecting spine of sphenoid with lingual of mandible.
▪ Stylomandibular ligament	Connects styloid process to mandibular angle.

TMJ DISLOCATION

- TMJ can be dislocated anteriorly only (known as "lockjaw").
    - Luxation: requires assistance for reduction.
    - Subluxation: auto-reduces.

TMJ DISC PLACEMENT

- Usually occurs anteromedially.
- Collateral ligaments loosen or tear, allowing the lateral pterygoid to pull the disc anteromedially.

TMJ Noises

Noise	Description
Click	With anterior disc displacment: First click **Open:** The disc clicks over the anteriorly moving condyle (condyle clicks past the thick posterior band of articular disc). Second click **Closed:** Condyle moves posteriorly past the disc. Can also hear this click with lateral excursion to the contralateral side (as the disc is anteromedially located and the condyle is moving medially).
Crepitus	Associated with osteoarthritis of the condyle (degenerative disease).
Dull thud	With self-reducing subluxation of the condyle.

TMJ MOVEMENTS

- Six mandibular movements:
  - Protrusion
  - Retrusion
  - Opening
  - Closing
  - Medial and lateral excursions
- Normal mandibular range of motion (ROM) is 50 mm opening, 10 mm protrusively and laterally.
- See Posselt's envelope of motion.

Hinge-Type Rotation

- With small movements (lower compartment).

Translation

- With larger movements (upper compartment).
- Slides forward out of the mandibular fossa.

See Figure 1–40 for mandibular condyle and meniscus.
See Figure 1–41 for mandibular capsule, temporomandibular ligament, and sphenomandibular ligament.

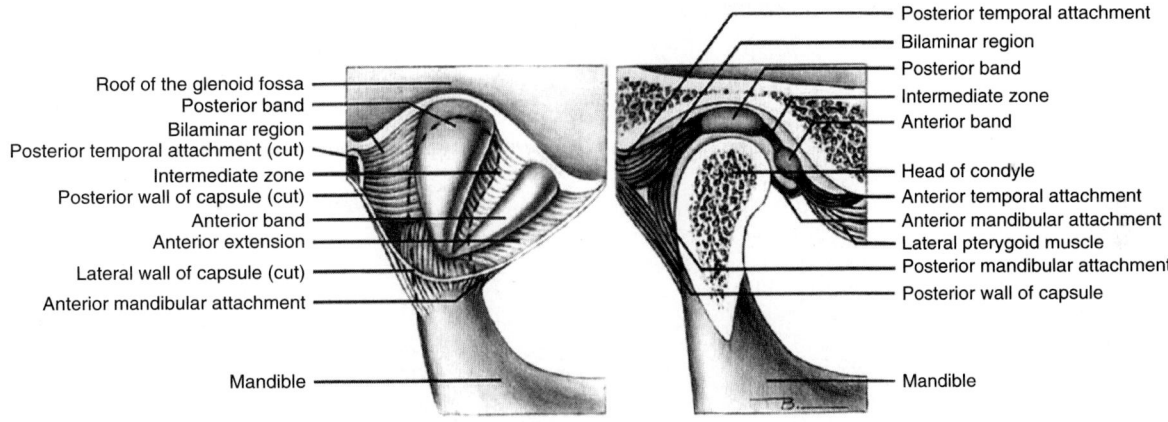

FIGURE 1-40. The mandibular condyle and meniscus.

Reproduced, with permission, from Montgomery RL. *Head and Neck Anatomy: With Clinical Correlations.* New York: McGraw-Hill, 1981.

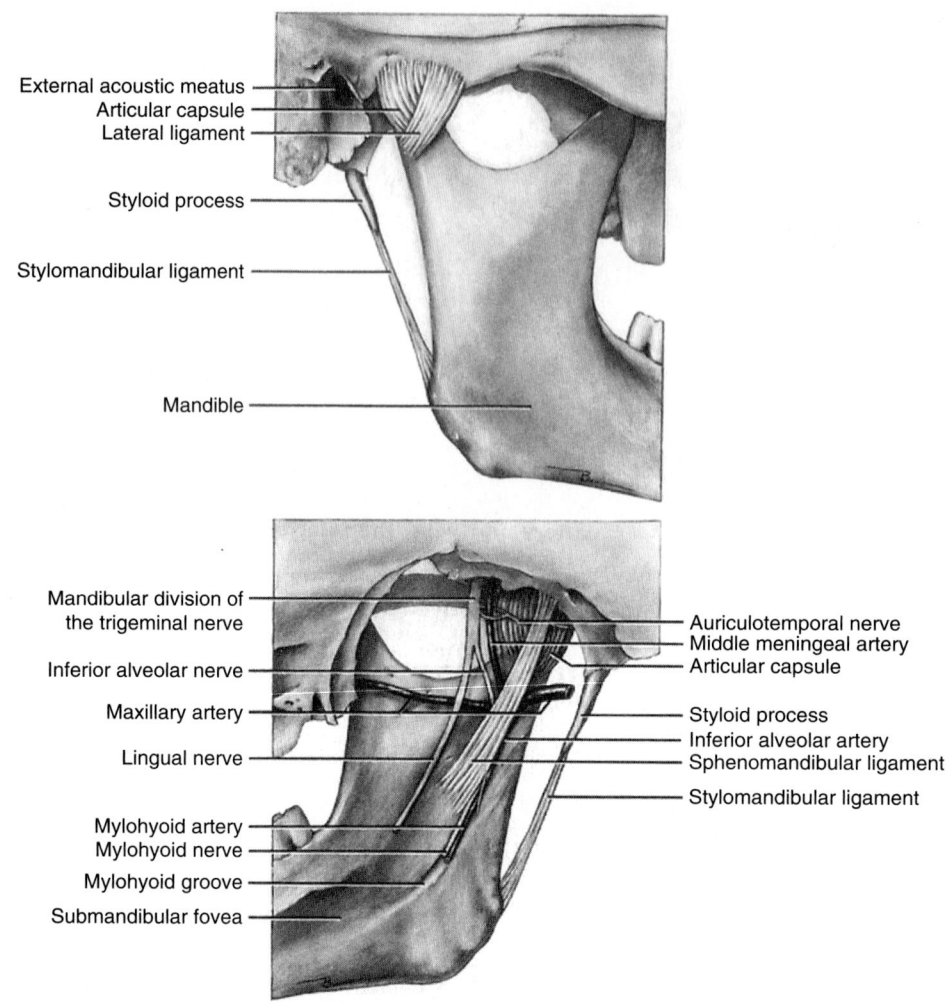

FIGURE 1-41. Mandibular capsule, temporomandibular ligament, and sphenomandibular ligament.

Reproduced, with permission, from Montgomery RL. *Head and Neck Anatomy: With Clinical Correlations.* New York: McGraw-Hill, 1981.

▶ NECK ANATOMY

Cervical Vertebrae

- C1-C7
    - C1 atlas (no vertebral body)
    - C2 axis (dens or odontoid process)
- Transverse foramen allow passage of the vertebral artery (from subclavian; forms basilar).

ATLANTO-OCCIPITAL JOINT

- Articulation between C1 (atlas) superior facets and the occipital condyles of the skull.
    - Allows to say YES.

Atlanto-Axial Joint

- Articulation between C1 vertebrae (atlas) inferior facets and the C2 vertebrae (axis) superior facets.
  - Allows to say NO.

Layers and Fascia of the Neck

Layer	Contents
Skin	
Subcutaneous tissue (superficial cervical fascia).	Cutaneous nerves, blood and lymphatic vessels, fat, platysma (anterolaterally).
Deep cervical fascia (muscular fascia) - Investing - Pretracheal - Prevertebral	Support thyroid gland, muscles, vessels, and deep lymph nodes.

Platysma Muscle

See Figure 1–42.

- Innervated by CN VII; blends with orbicularis oris.
- Superficial to the deep cervical fascia.

Investing Layer of Deep Cervical Fascia

Description	Attachments Superiorly	Attachments Inferiorly
The most superficial deep fascial layer. Splits into superficial and deep layers to invest the SCM and trapezius. Splits to enclose submandibular gland. Splits to form fibrous capsule of parotid gland.	Superior nuchal line (occipital bone) Mastoid process (temporal bone) Zygomatic arches Inferior border of mandible Hyoid bone Spinous processes of cervical vertebrae	Manubrium (sternum) Clavicles Acromions and spines of scapula

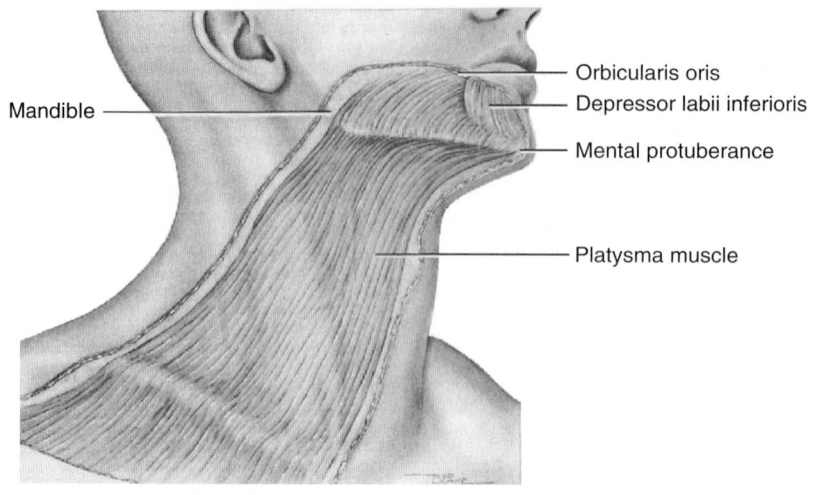

FIGURE 1-42. The platysma muscle.

Reproduced, with permission, from Montgomery RL. *Head and Neck Anatomy: With Clinical Correlations.* New York: McGraw-Hill, 1981.

PRETRACHEAL LAYER (OF DEEP CERVICAL FASCIA)

See Figure 1-43.

- Extends from hyoid bone to thorax (blends with fibrous pericardium).
- Has a thin muscular layer enveloping infrahyoid muscles.
- Visceral layer encloses thyroid gland, trachea, esophagus.
  - Visceral layer is continuous with buccopharyngeal fascia.
- Blends laterally with carotid sheaths.

The prevertebral layer of deep cervical fascia is why the thyroid moves w/ laryngeal movements.

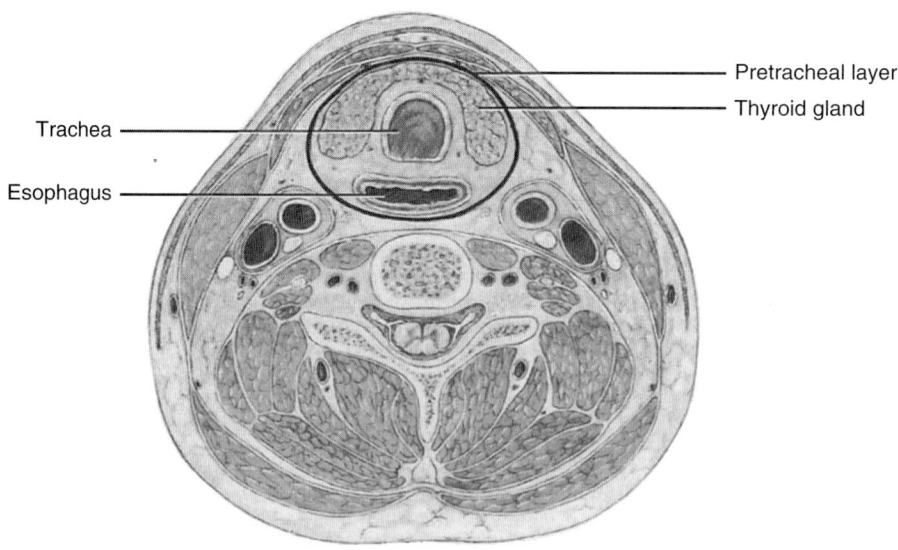

FIGURE 1-43. The pretracheal layer.

Reproduced, with permission, from Montgomery RL. *Head and Neck Anatomy: With Clinical Correlations.* New York: McGraw-Hill, 1981.

CAROTID SHEATH

See Figure 1–44.

- Extends from base of cranium to root of neck.
- Blends with investing and pretracheal fascia anteriorly.
- Blends with prevertebral fascia posteriorly.

Contents

- Common carotid artery
- Internal jugular vein
- CN X
- Also associated with:
    - Lymph nodes
    - Carotid sinus nerve
    - Sympathetic nerves

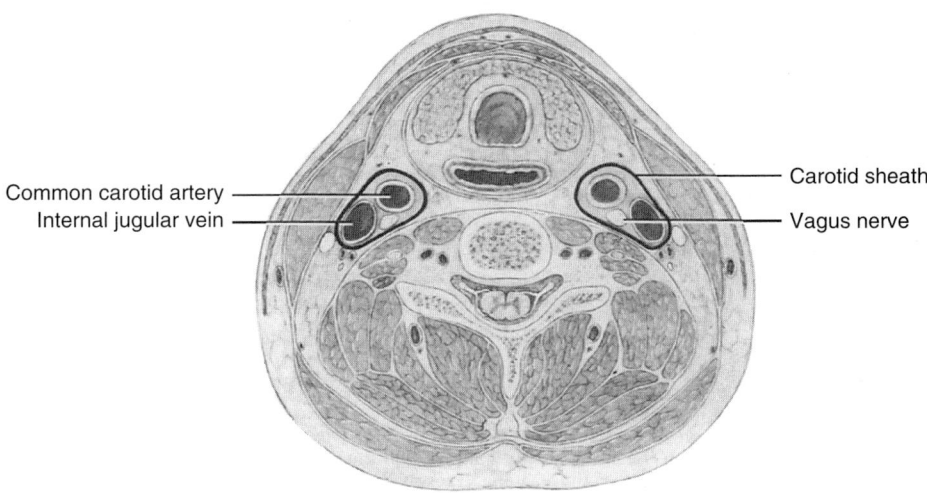

FIGURE 1–44. The carotid sheath.

Reproduced, with permission, from Montgomery RL. *Head and Neck Anatomy: With Clinical Correlations.* New York: McGraw-Hill, 1981.

PREVERTEBRAL LAYER (OF DEEP CERVICAL FASCIA)

- Runs from investing layers in both sides of the lateral neck; splits to enclose the thyroid.
- **Superiorly:** Attaches to laryngeal cartilages.
- **Inferiorly:** Fuses with perichondrium.
- **Posteriorly:** Fuses with anterior longitudinal ligament.

RETROPHARYNGEAL SPACE

See Figure 1–45.

- Between pharynx (buccopharyngeal fascia) and prevertebral fascia.
- Communicates with mediastimum (concern for infection spread, Ludwig's angina).

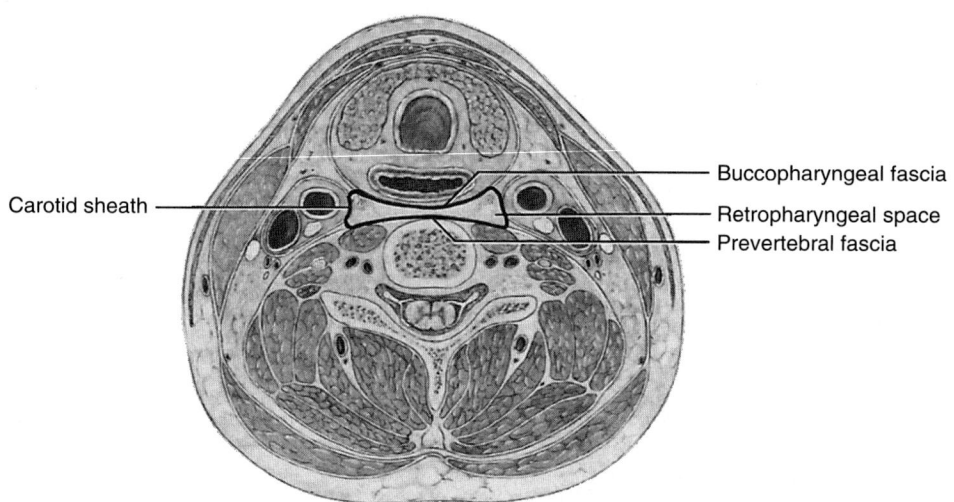

FIGURE 1–45. The retropharyngeal space.

Reproduced, with permission, from Montgomery RL. *Head and Neck Anatomy: With Clinical Correlations.* New York: McGraw-Hill, 1981.

Triangles of the Neck

See Figure 1–46 (A), (B) and (C) for regions of the neck.

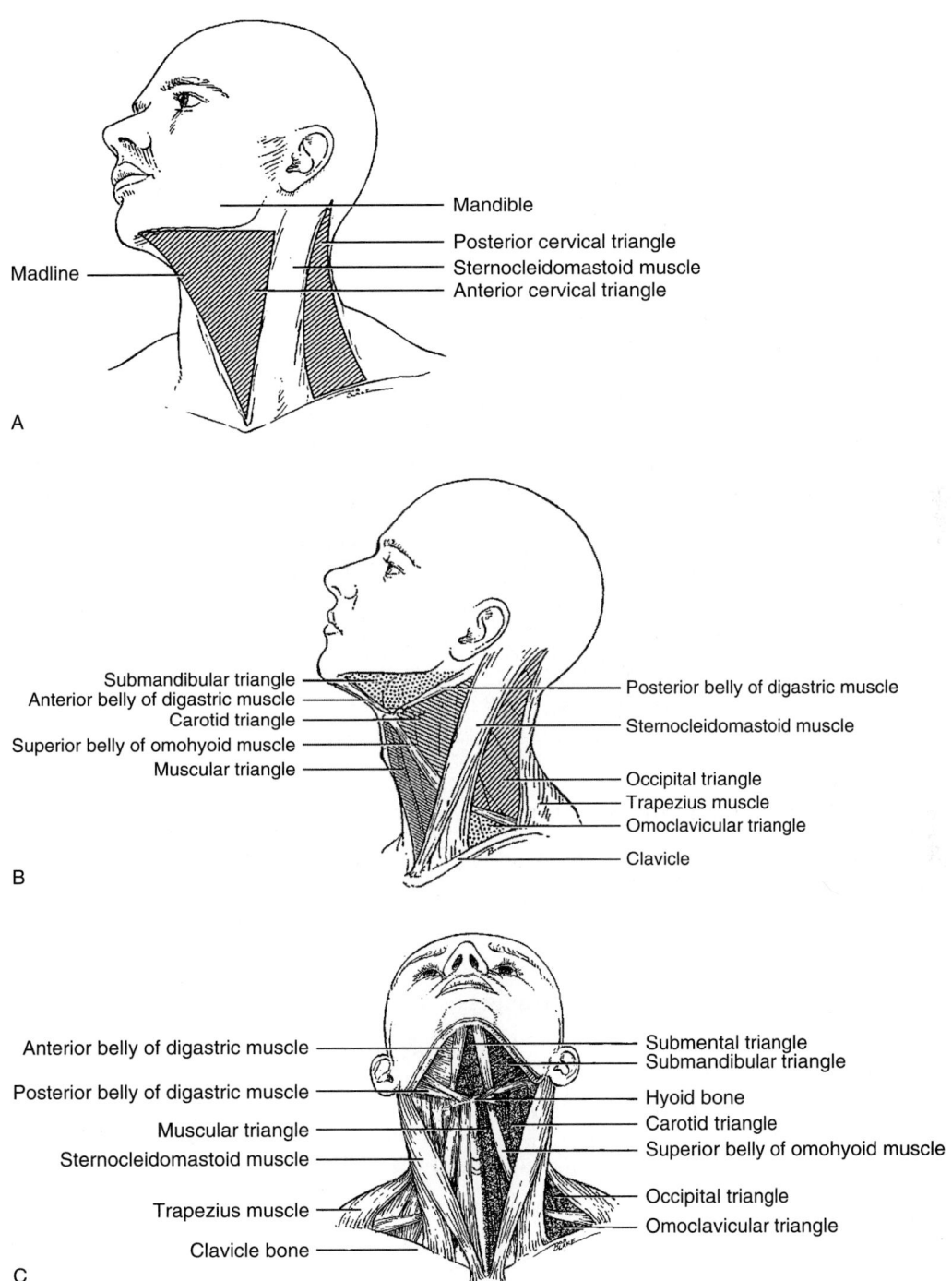

FIGURE 1–46 A, B, & C. **Topographic anatomy: regions of the neck.**

Reproduced, with permission, from Montgomery RL. *Head and Neck Anatomy: With Clinical Correlations.* New York: McGraw-Hill, 1981.

Posterior Triangle

Boundaries					Contents
Anterior	**Posterior**	**Inferior**	**Floor**	**Roof**	
SCM (post border)	Trapezius (anterior border)	Clavicle (middle 1/3)	Splenius capitus Levator scapulae Scalene muscles	Skin Superficial fascia, platysma, Deep investing fascia of neck	Exterior jugular vein Cervical plexus, lesser occipital nerve, great auricular nerve; CN XI, phrenic nerve Subclavian vein, artery, brachial plexus

Anterior Triangle

Boundaries					Contents
Anterior	**Posterior**	**Inferior**	**Floor**	**Roof**	
Neck midline	SCM (anterior border)	Inferior border of mandible	Pharynx, larynx, thyroid	Skin Superficial fascia Platysma Deep investing fascia	Infrahyoid, suprahyoid muscles common, internal, external carotid arteries Internal, external jugular vein Retromandibular vein CNs X, XI, XII, cervical plexus

Submandibular triangle contains two glands (or nodes), two nerves, two arteries, and two veins.

Subsets of the Anterior Triangle

Submandibular Triangle

See Figures 1–47 and 1–48.

Submandibular Triangle

Boundaries				Contents
Inferior	**Superior**	**Floor**	**Roof**	
Bellies of digastric	Inferior border of mandible	Mylohyoid Hyoglossus	Skin, Superficial fascia, Platysma, Deep fascia	Submandibular gland Submandibular lymph nodes Hypoglossal nerve Mylohyoid nerve Lingual and facial arteries and veins

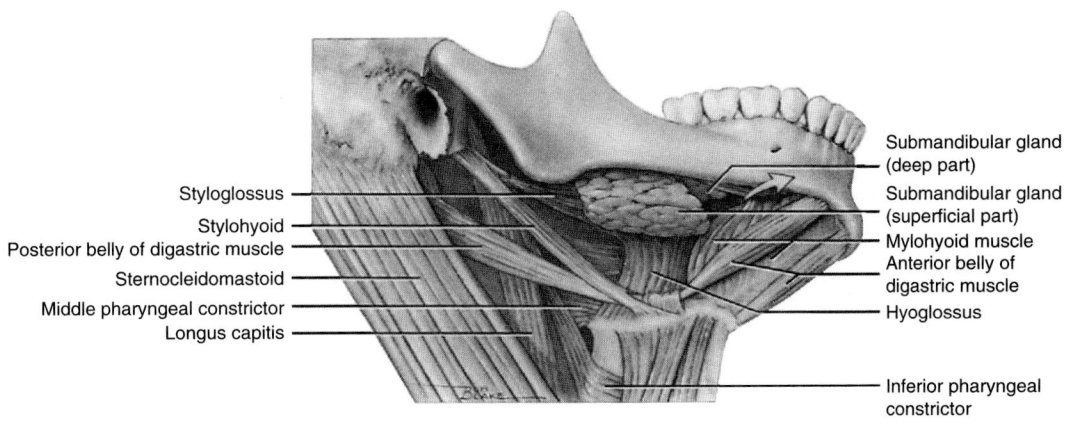

FIGURE 1-47. The submandibular gland.

Reproduced, with permission, from Montgomery RL. *Head and Neck Anatomy: With Clinical Correlations.* New York: McGraw-Hill, 1981.

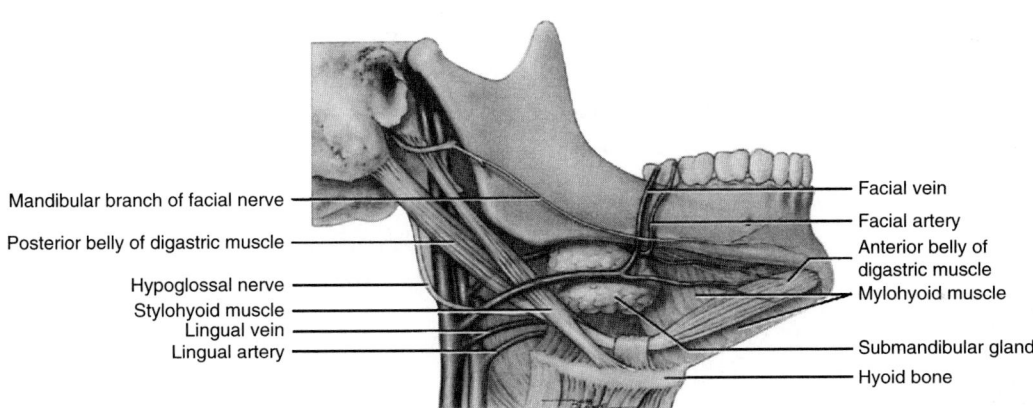

FIGURE 1-48. The submandibular triangle.

Reproduced, with permission, from Montgomery RL. *Head and Neck Anatomy: With Clinical Correlations.* New York: McGraw-Hill, 1981.

The suboccipital triangle (of the posterior triangle) is where the vertebral artery is found.

Subsets of Anterior Triangle (Continued)

	Muscular Triangle
Boundaries	Superior belly of omohyoid, SCM, midline of neck
Contents	Infrahyoid strap muscles
	Carotid Triangle
Boundaries	Superior belly of omohyoid, posterior belly of digastric, SCM
Contents	Common carotid artery, internal jugular vein, CNs X, XI, XII, cervical plexus
	Submental Triangle
Boundaries	Right and left anterior bellies of the digastric, body of hyoid
Contents	Mylohyoid muscle (midline raphe)

SCM, Trapezius Muscles

With damage to CN XI (spinal accessory), in the posterior triangle, you cannot raise an arm above horizontal and cannot shrug shoulder (because of the trapezius).

	Origin	Insertion	Action	Innervation
SCM	Manubrium, medial 1/3 clavicle	Mastoid process, superior nuchal line (lateral)	**Bilateral:** Flexes neck. **Unilateral:** Pulls head to shoulder, turns head to opposite side.	CN XI
Trapezius	Thoracic and cervical spines Ligamentum nuchae Superior nuchal line	Scapula (spine and acromion) Lateral 1/3 clavicle	**Bilateral:** Extends head. **Unilateral:** Chin up to opposite side; elevate acromion (rotates, elevates scapula and clavicle).	CN XI

With injury to SCM, you get torticollis.

Hyoid Bone

- U-shaped floating bone (from second and third branchial arches).
- Composed of body, greater horns, and lesser horns.

Hyoid Attachments

Ligaments	Muscles (Innervation)
Stylohyoid ligament Hypoepiglottic ligament	Mylohyoid (V3) Anterior digastric (V3) Posterior digastric (VII) Stylohyoid (VII) Hypoglossus (XII) Geniohyoid (XII) Omohyoid (ansa cervicalis) Sternohyoid (ansa cervicalis) Thyrohyoid (C1 via the hypoglossal)

Connections to styloid process (of temporal bone):

- Stylomandibular ligament
- Stylopharyngeus muscle
- Stylohyoid muscle
- Styloglossus muscle

Supra- and Infrahyoid Muscles

See Figure 1–49.

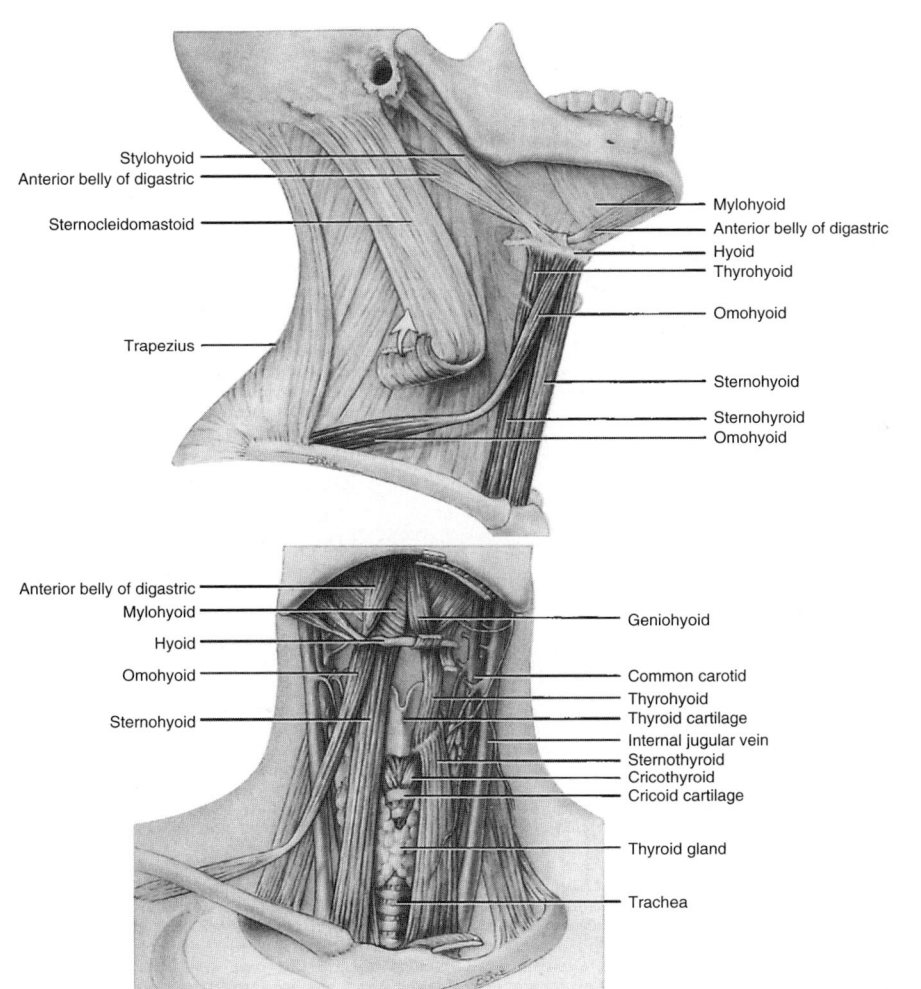

FIGURE 1–49. Infrahyoid muscles.

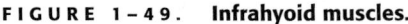

Reproduced, with permission, from Montgomery RL. *Head and Neck Anatomy: With Clinical Correlations.* New York: McGraw-Hill, 1981.

The mylohyoid is the muscle that makes it difficult to place anterior periapical films in the mouth when it is not relaxed.

Muscle	Origin	Insertion	Action	Innervation
Suprahyoids Digastric (anterior)	Intermediate tendon.	Anterior mandible (digastric fossa).	Raises hyoid.	CN V-3 (nerve to mylohyoid)
Digastric (posterior)	Temporal bone (digastric notch).	Intermediate tendon.	Raises hyoid.	CN VII
Mylohyoid	Medial mandible (mylohyoid line).	Median raphe; body of hyoid.	Raises hyoid, base of tongue, floor of mouth.	CN V-3 (nerve to mylohyoid)
Geniohyoid	Genial tubercles (mandible).	Body of hyoid.	Raises hyoid (pulls hyoid forward to open pharynx).	C1 fibers carried by CN XII
Stylohyoid	Styloid process.	Hyoid (greater horn).	Raises hyoid.	CN VII
Infrahyoids Omohyoid	**Superior belly:** Intermediate tendon. **Inferior belly:** Superior scapula.	**Superior belly:** Hyoid (body, lower surface). **Superior belly:** Intermediate tendon.	Depresses hyoid and larynx.	Ansa cervicalis
Sternohyoid	Manubrium of sternum.	Hyoid (lower surface).	Depresses hyoid and larynx.	Ansa cervicalis
Sternothyroid	Manubrium of sternum.	Thyroid cartilage (oblique line).	Depresses larynx.	Ansa cervicalis
Thyrohyoid	Thyroid cartilage (oblique line).	Hyoid (body and greater horn).	Depresses hyoid and larynx.	C1 carried with CN XII

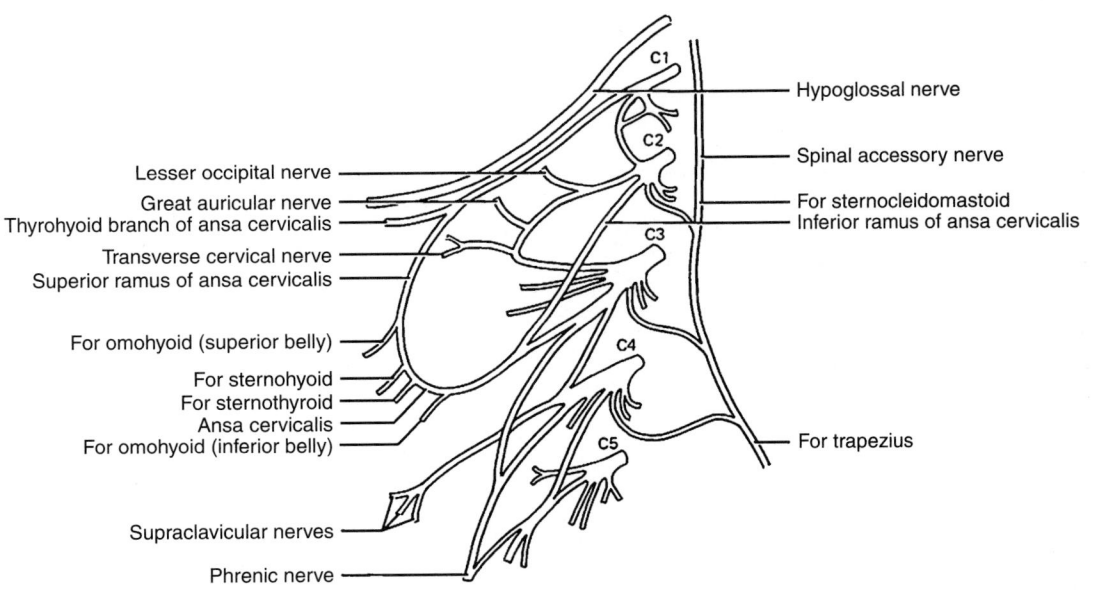

FIGURE 1-50. The cervical plexus.

Reproduced, with permission, from Montgomery RL. *Head and Neck Anatomy: With Clinical Correlations.* New York: McGraw-Hill, 1981.

Cervical Plexus (of nerves)

See Figure 1–50.

Cervical Plexus

- C I-C IV
- Positioned deeply in the neck (lateral to first four cervical vertebra).
- **Cutaneous innervation** to:
  - Skin of neck.
  - Shoulder.
  - Anterior upper chest wall
- **Motor** to:
  - Infrahyoid muscles.
  - Geniohyoid.
- **Phrenic nerve** is contributed to, in part, by ansa cervicalis.
- **Supraclavicular nerves** innervate skin over the shoulder.
- **Transverse cervical nerve** carries sensory innervation to anterior and lateral neck.

ANSA CERVICALIS (MOTOR)

- Motor division of cervical plexus.
- Comes from C I (runs with CN XII), C II, C III.
- Innervates:
  - Infrahyoids (except thyrohyoid, which is innervated by C I).
  - Genioglossus muscle (moves hyoid anteriorly to hold open the pharynx).

See innervation of external ear. Remember, four nerves are involved.

Branches of C2, C3 Loop (Sensory)

Nerve	Supplies
Lesser occipital nerve (C II)	Skin of neck and scalp (posterosuperior to auricle)
Great auricular nerve (C II, C III)	Skin over parotid gland, posterior aspect of auricle, area from angle of mandible to mastoid
Transverse cervical nerve (C II, C III)	Skin of anterior triangle

Phrenic Nerve

- C III, IV, V—"keeps the diaphragm alive."
- Contains motor, sensory, and sympathetic nerve fibers.
- Sole motor innervation to the diaphragm.

Blood Supply to Face

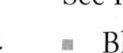

The terminal branches of the ECA are the maxillary and superficial temporal arteries.

See Figure 1–51 for arteries of the head and neck.

- Blood is supplied to the face via the external carotid branches.

External Carotid Artery

Course

In addition to the lingual artery, the tongue receives some blood supply from the tonsillar branch of the facial artery and the ascending pharyngeal artery.

- Branches from the common carotid artery at the level of the upper border of thyroid cartilage.
- Gives off branches and continues to the substance of the parotid gland where it ends as:
- Maxillary artery.
- Superficial temporal branch (superiorly).

Supply

- Supplies most of head and neck (**except** the brain).
  - Face
  - Thyroid
  - Salivary glands
  - Tongue
  - Jaws
  - Teeth
- Carotid sinus (baroreception).
  - At the common carotid bifurcation.
- Carotid body (chemoreception).
  - Posterior to the bifurcation of the CCA.

The mnemonic to remember the branches of the facial artery is TAGS ISLA.

See also the Physiology section in Chapter 12.

BRANCHES OF THE EXTERNAL CAROTID

- The mnemonic to remember the branches of the external carotid artery is **SALFOPSM**.

Branch	Supplies
Superior thyroid	Thyroid gland, gives off SCM branch and the superior laryngeal artery.
Ascending pharyngeal	Pharyngeal wall.
Lingual	Tongue.
Facial	Face and submandibular gland.
Occipital	Pharynx and suboccipital triangle.
Posterior auricular	Posterior scalp.
Superficial temporal	Infratemporal fossa, nasal cavity.
Maxillary	Temple and scalp.

The terminal branch of facial artery is the angular artery.

The facial artery supplies the muscles of facial expression.

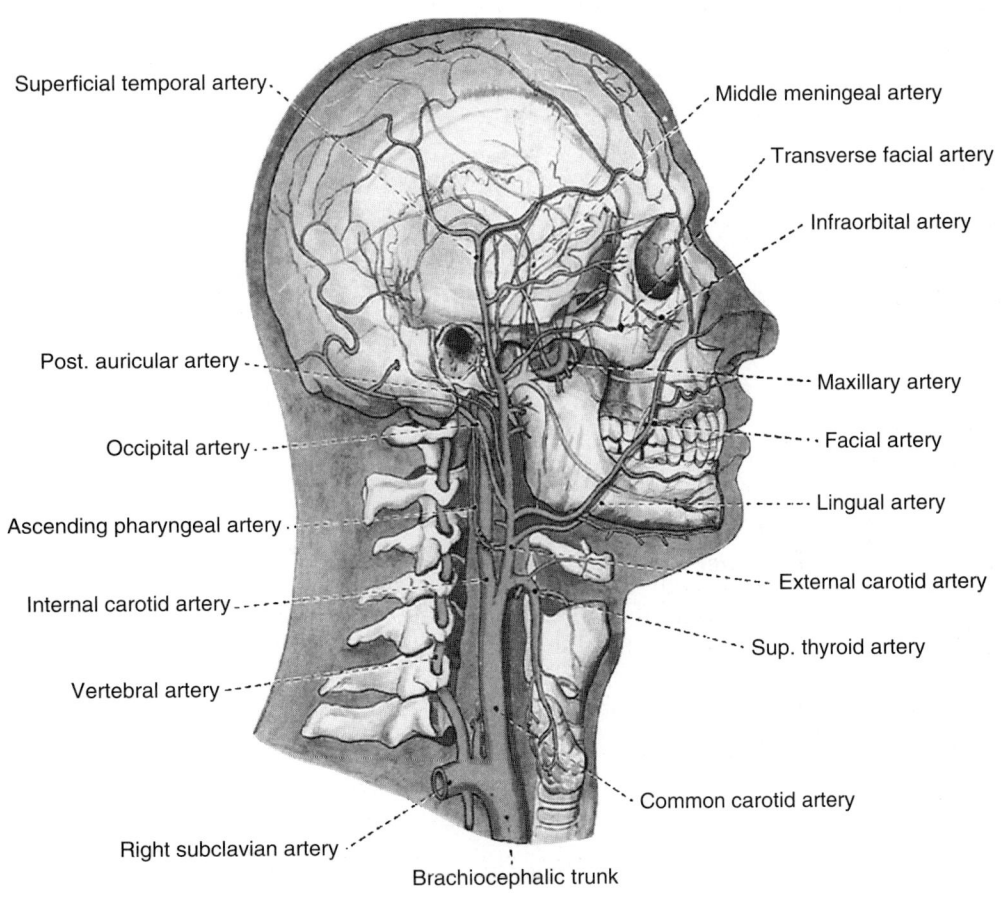

FIGURE 1-51. Arteries of the head and neck.

Reproduced, with permission, from Langman J, Woerdeman MW. *Atlas of Medical Anatomy.* Philadelphia: WB Saunders Company, 1978.

The anterior hard palate is supplied by the nasopalatine artery, a branch of the sphenopalatine, after it exits the incisive foramen.

Epistaxis (nosebleed) occurs because of the anastomoses in the nasal septum (Kiesselbach's plexus, comprising five arteries).

The greater palatine artery (out greater palatine foramen) supplies the hard palate (posterior to the maxillary canines).

The lesser palatine artery (out lesser palatine foramen) supplies the soft palate and tonsils.

The middle meningeal is a branch of the maxillary artery.

LINGUAL ARTERY

- Originates from the ECA at the greater horn of hyoid bone (in the carotid triangle).
- Supplies:
  - Tongue.
  - Sublingual gland.
  - Floor of mouth.
- Branches:
  - Dorsal lingual.
  - Suprahyoid.
  - Sublingual arteries (to sublingual gland).
- Ends as the deep lingual artery
  - Between the genioglossus and inferior longitudinal muscles.
- Passes deep to hyoglossus muscle then supplies tongue.

See also the section "Relationship of Lingual Artery, Vein, Nerve, Hypoglossal Nerve, and Submandibular Duct."

FACIAL ARTERY

- The facial artery is considered in two portions.

Portion	Branches	Supplies
Cervical	Tonsillar Ascending pharyngeal Glandular Submental	Tonsils Pharyngeal wall Submandibular gland Beneath chin
Facial	Inferior labial Superior labial Lateral nasal Angular	Lower lip Upper lip, anterior nose Lateral wall of nose Medial eye; anastomose with ophthalmic artery (of ICA)

MAXILLARY ARTERY

- Divided into three parts by the lateral pterygoid muscle.
- Branches from the ECA at the posterior border of the mandibular ramus.
- Supplies:
  - Muscles of mastication.
  - Maxillary and mandibular teeth.
  - Palate.
  - Most of the nasal cavity.

Maxillary Artery

Portion	Branches	Supplies
Mandibular	Deep auricular Anterior tympanic Middle meningeal Accessory meningeal Inferior alveolar	External auditory meatus. Eardrum. Middle cranial fossa. Cranial cavity. Chin, lower teeth.
Pterygoid	Anterior and posterior deep temporal Pterygoid (medial and lateral branches) Masseteric Buccal	Temporalis muscle. Pterygoid muscles. Masseter muscle. Buccinator muscle.
Pterygopalatine	Posteriosuperior alveolar (PSA) Infraorbital Descending palatine Artery of pterygoid canal Pharyngeal Sphenopalatine	Maxillary molars and premolars. Maxillary canines and incisors. Greater and lesser palatine arteries to posterior palate. Pharynx Terminal branch of maxillary artery; gives rise to nasopalatine artery (out incisive foramen to anterior palate and anastomoses with palatine vessels).

Venous Drainage from the Face

See Figure 1–52.

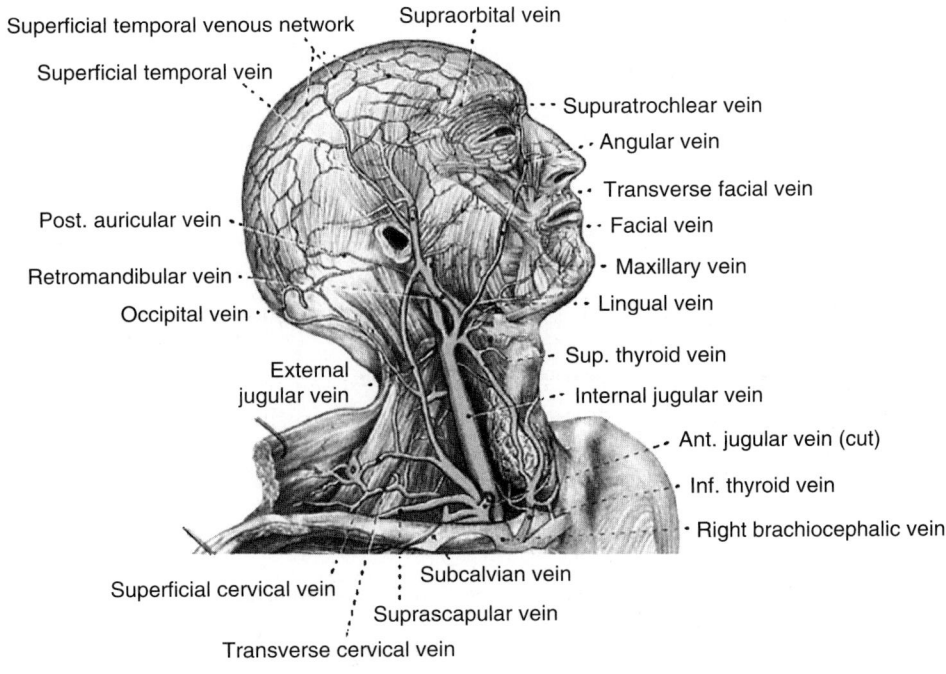

FIGURE 1-52. Veins of the head and neck.

Reproduced, with permission, from Langman J, Woerdeman MW. *Atlas of Medical Anatomy.* Philadelphia: WB Saunders Company, 1978.

Facial Venous Drainage

See Figure 1-53.

Remember: *The scalp can drain superficially (via superficial temporal and posterior auricular veins) or deeply (via emissary veins).*

Superficial Temporal Vein

- Drains scalp and side of head.
- Merges with maxillary vein and plunges into parotid gland.

Maxillary Vein

- Forms from the pterygoid plexus of veins, which is the connection of deep system with superficial venous drainage.

Retromandibular Vein

- Formed by the superficial temporal and maxillary veins.
- Divides at the angle of the mandible into anterior and posterior branches.

External Jugular Vein

- Formed by the posterior auricular and retromandibular veins.
- Crosses the SCM.
- Drains the
  - Skin.
  - Parotid gland.
  - Muscles of the face and neck.
- Empties into the subclavian vein.

Facial Vein (Anterior Facial Vein)

- Forms from the angular vein (which itself forms from the supraorbital and supratrochlear veins).
- Receives infraorbital and deep facial veins.
- Enters into the IJV (directly or by way of the common facial vein).

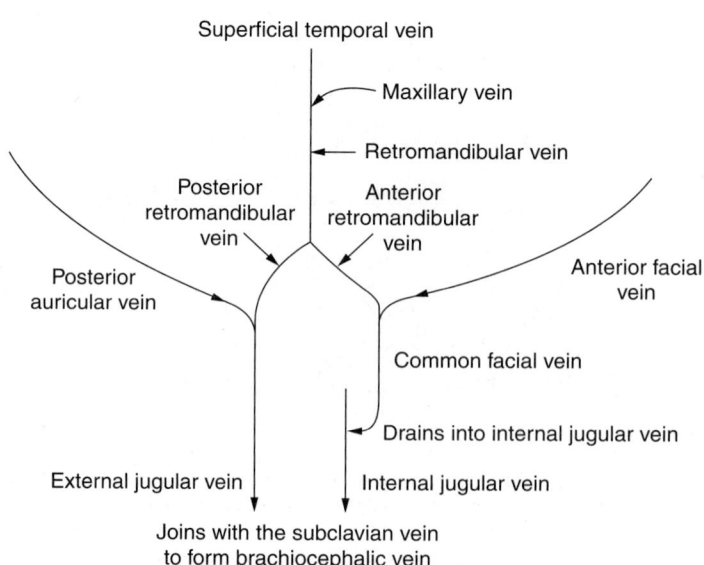

FIGURE 1-53. Facial venous drainage.

Common Facial Vein

- Formed by the anterior facial and retromandibular veins.

Internal Jugular Vein

- Arises from the sigmoid and inferior petrosal sinuses.
- Drains the dural venous sinuses.
- Exits the skull via the jugular foramen (along with CNs XI, X, IX).
- Descends the neck in the carotid sheath.
- Merges with the subclavian vein to form:
  - Large brachiocephalic vein (behind the sternoclavicular joint).
  - Left and right brachiocephalic veins form the superior vena cava.

Danger Triangle of the Face

- Area where superficial facial veins communicate with deep system (dural sinuses).
  - **Base:** Upper lip/anterior maxilla.
  - **Apex:** Infraorbital region.

Lymph Nodes in the Face

See Figures 1–54 and 1–55.
See the section "Tongue" for illustration of tongue lymph drainage.

Important:
Veins of the head and neck contain no valves.

Because there are no valves, retrograde flow can allow infection to spread via the deep facial vein, pterygoid plexus, and ophthalmic veins to the cavernous sinus.

The deep cervical nodes form the jugular lymph trunk (along IJV).

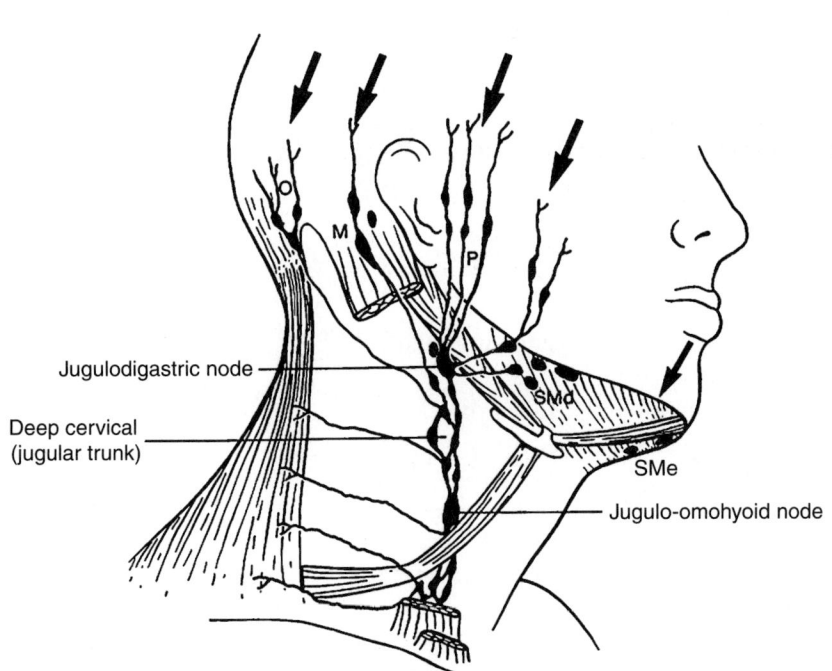

FIGURE 1-54. Lymphatic drainage of the face. M, mastoid nodes: O, occipital nodes; P, parotid nodes; SMd, submandibular nodes; SMe, submental nodes.

Reproduced, with permission, from Liebgott B. *The Anatomical Basis of Dentistry*. Toronto: BC Decker, 1986.

The jugular lymph trunk empties into either

- *The thoracic duct (on left) or the right lymphatic duct (which then empties into the brachiocephalic vein).*
- *Example:*
- *Infection of lower lip*
  - *Enters blood stream at right brachiocephalic vein.*
- *Infection of abdomen*
  - *Enters at left brachiocephalic vein.*

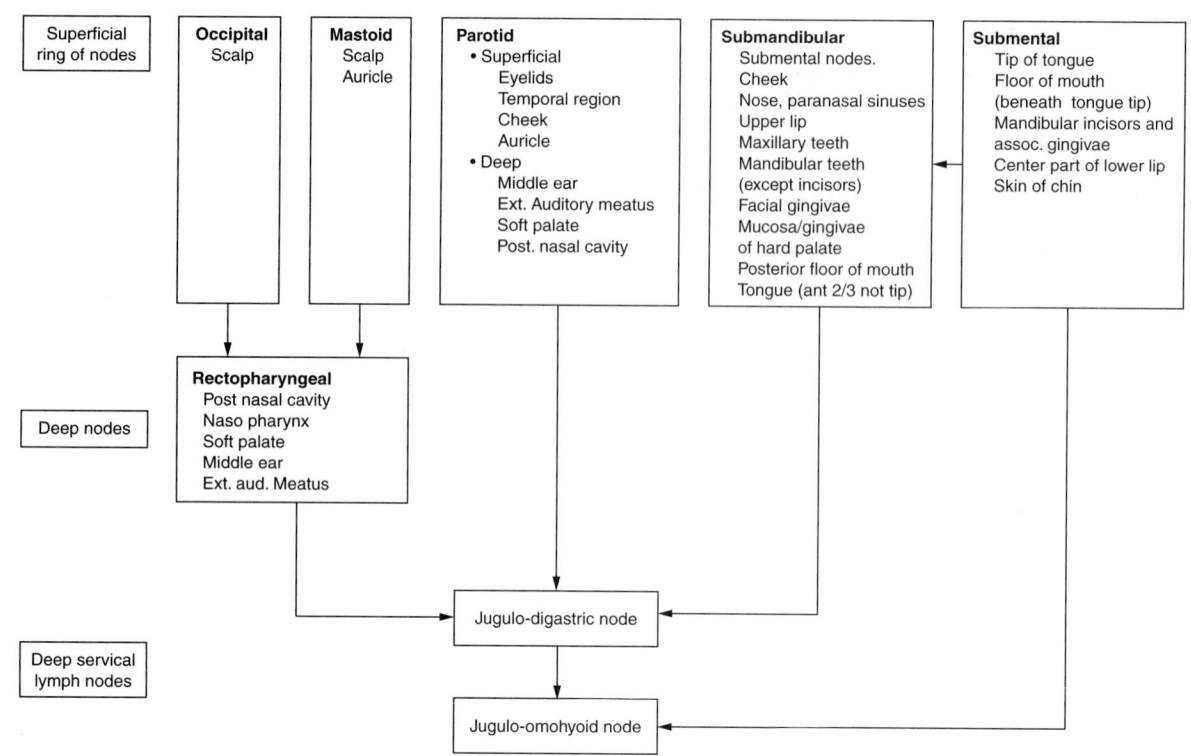

FIGURE 1-55. Lymph nodes in the face.

Thyroid

See Figure 1–56.

- H-shaped gland at laryngotracheal junction at anterior neck.
- Two lobes (right and left) joined by isthmus.
- Largest endocrine gland.
- Produces/secretes
    - Thyroid hormone.
    - Calcitonin.
- **Blood supply:** See the following chart.
- **Nerve supply**
    - Glandular branches of cervical ganglia of sympathetic trunk.

Follicular Cells

- Produce thyroglobulin (tyrosine-containing).
    - Stored in colloid.
    - Precursor to T3 (triiodothyronine) and thyroxine (involved in basal metabolic rate).

Parafollicular (C) Cells

- Produce calcitonin.
    - Lower blood calcium and phosphate.

Thyroglossal Duct

- Connects thyroid gland to tongue development.
- Foramen cecum at base of tongue is proximal remnant.

Important: There is **no** middle thyroid artery.

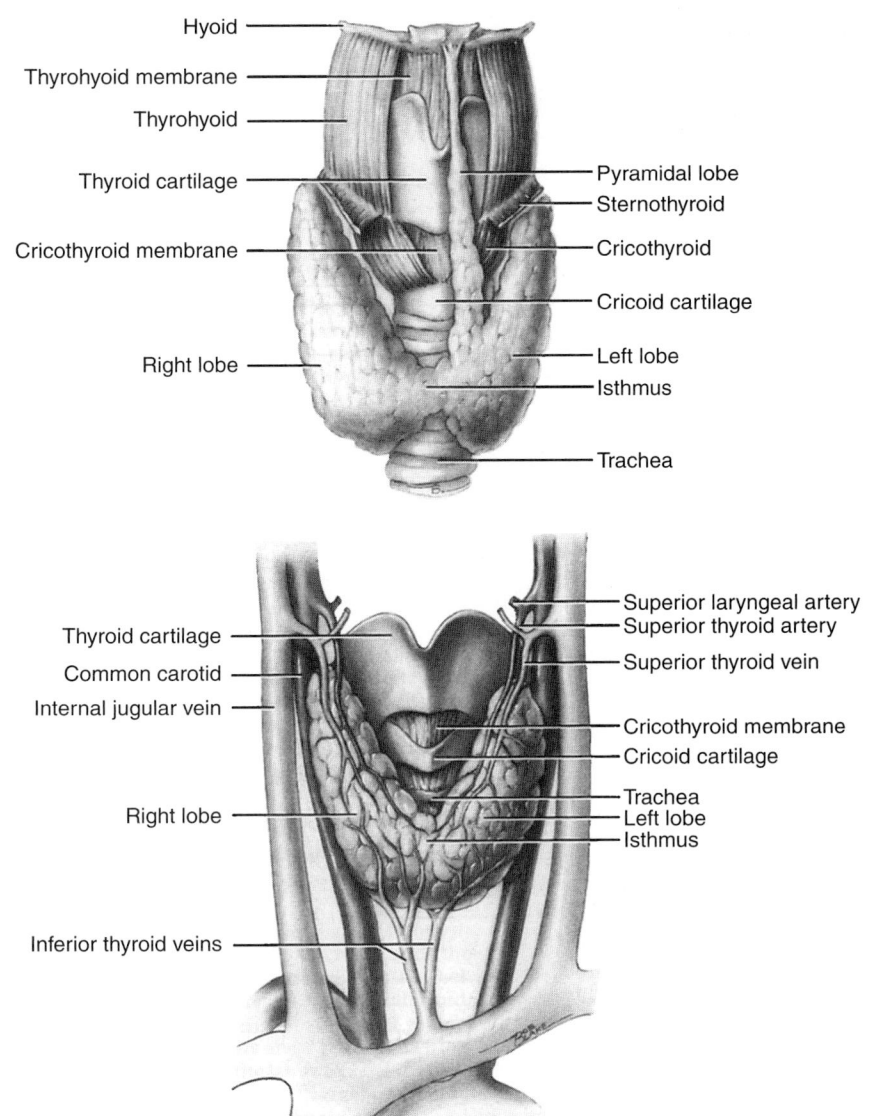

FIGURE 1-56. Thyroid gland.

Reproduced, with permission, from Montgomery RL. *Head and Neck Anatomy: With Clinical Correlations.* New York: McGraw-Hill, 1981.

Thyroid Blood Supply and rainage

Artery	Branch of	Vein	Drains to
Superior thyroid artery	ECA	Superior thyroid vein	IJV
—	—	Middle thyroid vein	IJV
Inferior thyroid artery	Thyrocervical trunk	Inferior thyroiv	Brachiocephalic vein

Parathyroid Glands

- Small pea-shaped organs.
- Two superior parathyroids.
- Two inferior parathyroids.
- Develop from the fourth pharyngeal pouches.
- Encased in the posterior surface of the thyroid.
- **Blood supply**
  - Superior thyroid artery (from ECA) (to superior part of gland).
  - Inferior thyroid artery (from thyrocervical trunk) (to inferior part of gland).
- **Innervation**
  - Postganglionic sympathetic fibers of superior cervical ganglion.
- Produces parathyroid hormone (PTH).
  - Regulates calcium and phosphate metabolism.
  - Deficiency of PTH → decrease Ca^{2+} can cause tetany.

Larynx

- The larynx is responsible for voice production.

Laryngeal Skeleton

The vocal cords attach anteriorly at the lamina of thyroid cartilage and posteriorly at the vocal process of arytenoid cartilages.

- Nine cartilages (three single, three paired)

Cartilage	Description
Thyroid	Largest; forms the laryngeal prominence ("Adam's apple"); superior thyroid notch; superior surface is attached to hyoid by thyrohyoid membrane.
Cricoid	Only laryngeal cartilage to form a complete ring around the airway.
Epiglottic	Fibrocartilage; gives flexibility to epiglottis.
Arytenoid (2)	Vocal cord attaches posteriorly.
Corniculate (2)	
Cuneiform (2)	

The cricothyroid membrane is incised at the midline for an emergent cricothyroidotomy/tracheotomy. The cricothyroid space is entered (inferior to rima glottides where aspirated objects are often lodged or laryngospasm is occurring).

Vocal Folds

- True vocal cords.
- Composed of vocal ligament and vocalis muscle.
- Involved in sound production.
- Sphincter of respiratory tract.

Glottis

- Composed of vocal fold and rima glottis.
- Rima glottis is the opening between vocal folds.

VESTIBULAR FOLDS

- False vocal folds.
- **No** role in vocalization.
- Protective.

EPIGLOTTIS

- Thin leaf-shaped cartilage, covered with mucous membrane, at the root of the tongue.
- Flap closing over the larynx when swallowing.
- Median glossoepiglottic fold (1).
- Lateral glossoepiglottic folds (2).
- Valecullae (2) (lie between the glossoepiglottic folds).
- Taste buds (CN X) are located on superior surface of epiglottis.

LARYNGEAL MUSCLES

Extrinsic Muscles

Muscle Group	Function
Suprahyoids and stylopharyngeus muscle	Raise larynx.
Infrahyoids	Depress larynx.

*All intrinsic laryngeal muscles are supplied by the recurrent laryngeal nerve **except** the cricothyroid muscle, which is innervated by the external laryngeal nerve (a branch of the superior laryngeal nerve).*

Intrinsic Muscles

Muscle	Origin	Insertion	Action	Innervation
Cricothyroid	Anterolateral cricoid cartilage	Thyroid cartilage (inferior margin and inferior horn)	Stretches and tenses vocal fold.	External laryngeal nerve
Posterior cricoarytenoid	Cricoid cartilage (posterior laminae)	Muscular process of arytenoid cartilage	Abducts vocal fold.	Recurrent laryngeal nerve
Lateral cricoarytenoid	Cricoid cartilage (arch)	Muscular process of arytenoid cartilage	Adducts vocal fold.	Same as above
Thyroarytenoid	Thyroid cartilage (posterior surface)	Muscular process of arytenoid cartilage	Relaxes vocal fold.	Same as above
Transverse and oblique arytenoids	Arytenoid cartilage	Opposite arytenoids cartilage	Closes rima glottides.	Same as above
Vocalis	Depression between laminae of thyroid cartilage	Vocal ligament and vocal process of arytenoid scartilage	Relaxes posterior vocal ligament Tenses anterior vocal ligament Antagonist of cricothyroid muscle.	Same as above

Injured nerves (e.g., after thyroid or neck surgery) cause hoarseness.

Laryngeal Nerves

See also Vagus.

Recurrent Laryngeal Nerve

See Figure 1–57.

- Is a branch of the vagus nerve (CN X).
- Comes off the vagus in the mediastinum and ascends to the larynx in the tracheoesophageal groove.
- Has close association with thyroid gland and inferior thyroid artery.
- **Left recurrent laryngeal nerve** wraps around aortic arch (ligamentum arteriosum).
- **Right recurrent laryngeal nerve** wraps around right subclavian.
- **Motor innervation:** Involves all intrinsic muscles of larynx (via the inferior laryngeal branch) except cricothyroid.
- **Sensory innervation:** Involves laryngeal mucosa below vocal folds and upper trachea.

Superior Laryngeal Nerve

- Branch of the vagus nerve arising just after exit from jugular foramen.
- Passes through thyrohyoid membrane.
- **External branch:** Innervates cricothyroid muscle (adducts cords).
- **Internal branch:** Provides sensory information to laryngeal mucosa above the vocal folds.

Respiratory System

- Nasal cavity
- Pharynx
- Larynx
- Trachea
- Bronchi
- Bronchioles
- Alveoli

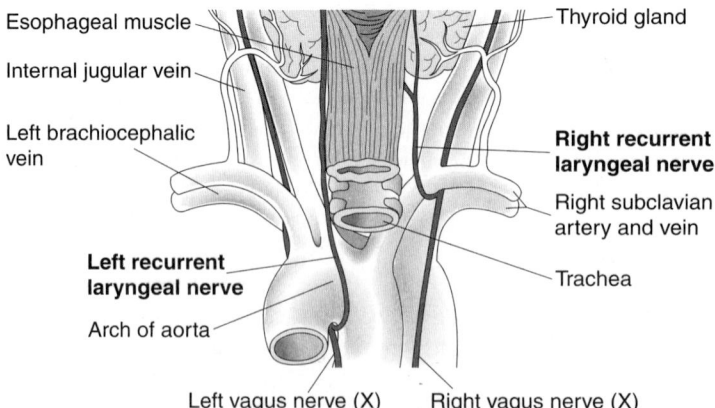

FIGURE 1–57. Course of the recurrent laryngeal nerve (posterior view).

Reproduced, with permission, from Bushhan V, et al. *First Aid for the USMLE Step 1.* New York: McGraw-Hill, 2003.

TRACHEA

- Air tube of tracheal rings.
- Lined with respiratory epithelium.
- Formed from hyaline cartilage.
- ~10 cm long.
- ~2.5 cm diameter.
- Extends from:
  - C5-C6 level (base of larynx—starts as ligamentous attachment to cricoid) to Sternal angle (of Louis) T4/5 level (second rib level).
- Branches into left and right mainstem bronchi (at Carina).

Branching Pattern

Trachea
↓
Primary bronchi: two mainstem bronchi (one per lung)
↓
Secondary bronchi: five lobar bronchi (three in right lung; two in left lung)
↓
Tertiary bronchi
↓
Terminal bronchioles
↓
Respiratory bronchioles
↓
Alveoli

▶ BRACHIAL PLEXUS AND UPPER EXTREMITIES

Axilla

Boundaries	
Medial	Upper 4–5 ribs Intercostal muscles Serratus anterior muscle
Lateral	Humerus Coracobrachialis and biceps muscles Within intertubercular groove
Posterior	Subscapularis Teres major Latissimus dorsi
Anterior	Pectoralis major and minor Subclavius muscles
Base	Axillary fascia Skin

The subclavian arteries supply the upper extremities.

Contents
- Axillary vessels
- Brachial plexus
- Biceps brachii (both heads)
- Coracobrachialis

AXILLARY ARTERY

- Continuation of subclavian artery.
  - Named axillary artery as it passes lateral border of first rib.
- Travels close with the medial cord of the brachial plexus.
  - Aneurysm can compress the medial cord.
- Passes posterior to pectoralis minor muscle.
- Becomes brachial artery.
  - As it passes inferior border of teres major and enters the arm.

BRACHIAL ARTERY

Profunda brachii artery arises from brachial artery in proximal arm.

- Continuation of axillary artery in the arm.
- Immediately medial to tendon of biceps brachii at elbow.

AXILLARY VEIN

Brachial and basilic veins merge to form the axillary vein.

- Formed from the brachial veins and the basilic vein at the inferior border of teres major.
- Changes name to subclavian vein at the lateral border of the first rib.

CEPHALIC VEIN

- Drains into the axillary vein.
- Found in deltopectoral groove.
  - Located between deltoid and pectoralis major.
- Drains superficial arm.
  - Drains blood from the radial side of arm.

Thoracic outlet syndrome *results from compression of the lower trunk of the brachial plexus and the subclavian artery between the anterior and middle scalene.*

BRACHIAL VEIN

- Drains blood from the deep arm.

BASILIC VEIN

- Drains blood from the superficial arm.

SCALENE MUSCLES

- There are three scalene muscles per side:
  - Anterior
  - Middle
  - Posterior
- Phrenic nerve and subclavian vein pass on the surface of the anterior scalene.
- Brachial plexus and subclavian artery pass between the anterior and middle scalene.

See Figure 1–58 for the dorsal scapular artery.

Brachial Plexus

- The brachial plexus innervates the shoulder girdle and upper limb (ventral rami C5-T1).

OTHER BRANCHES OF THE BRACHIAL PLEXUS

See Figure 1–59.

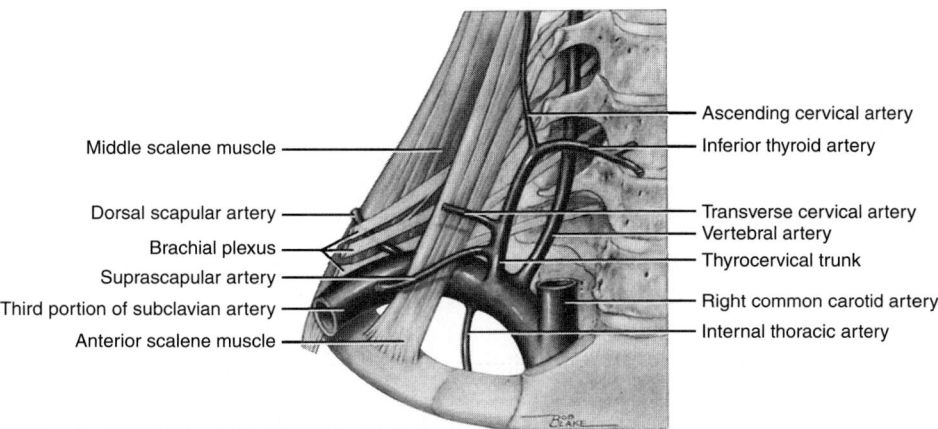

FIGURE 1-58. The dorsal scapular artery.

Reproduced, with permission, from Montgomery RL. *Head and Neck Anatomy: With Clinical Correlations.* New York: McGraw-Hill, 1981.

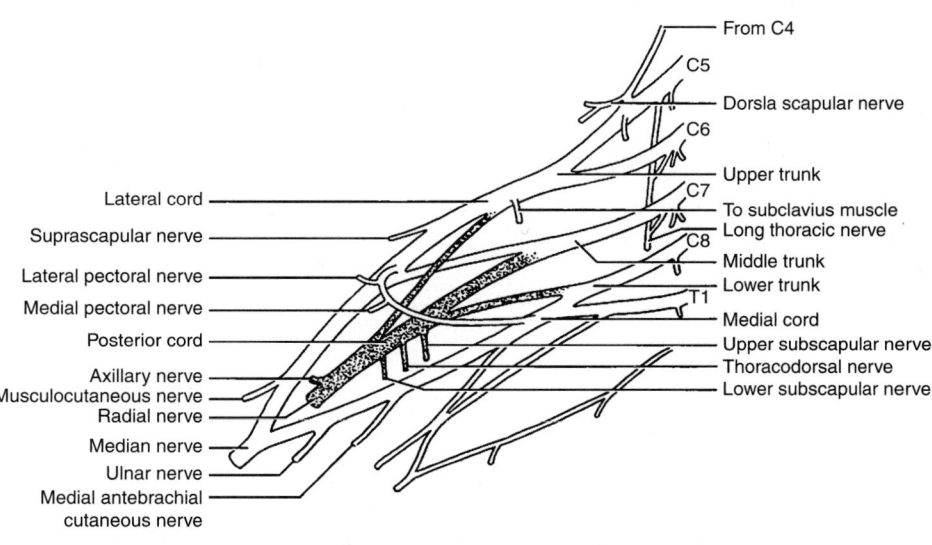

FIGURE 1-59. The brachial plexus.

Reproduced, with permission, from Montgomery RL. *Head and Neck Anatomy: With Clinical Correlations.* New York: McGraw-Hill, 1981.

Major Terminal Nerves of the Brachial Plexus

Nerve	Course	Motor	Sensory
Median (C5-T1) (from lateral and medial cords)	Lateral and medial cords. Passes between two heads of pronator teres. Enters carpal tunnel in wrist between. Palmaris longus Flexor carpi radialis	Forearm flexors: Flexor carpi radialis Palmaris longus Pronators Digital flexors Thenar muscles Lateral two lumbricals (thumb side).	Anterior arm Lateral palm (radial 2/3; thumb side) Lateral $3\frac{1}{2}$ digits (thumb, 2, 3, including nailbeds)
Ulnar (C8-T1)	Medial cord. Behind medial epicondyle (elbow). Between flexor carpi ulnaris and flexor digitorum profundus (wrist). Superficial to flexor retinaculum in wrist.	Flexors of wrist and fingers (including flexor carpi ulnaris). Ulnar two lumbricals. Interosseous muscles.	Medial arm/forearm Medial palm Medial $1\frac{1}{2}$ digit (pinky)
Radial C6-C8)	Posterior cord. Musculospiral groove (posterior humerus). Passes between brachioradialis and brachialis muscles.	Extensors of arm/forearm: <ul><li>Triceps.</li><li>Brachioradialis.</li><li>Extensor carpi radialis.</li><li>Extensor carpi ulnaris.</li><li>Extensors of wrist/fingers.</li><li>Adductor pollicus.</li><li>Supinator (BEST).</li></ul>	Posterior arm Forearm Hand (not fingers)
Axillary	Comes off in axilla.	Deltoid. Teres minor.	Skin of lower $\frac{1}{2}$ of deltoid
Musculocutaneous (C5-C7)		Arm flexors.	Anterolateral arm Forearm

Summary of Brachial Plexus Actions by Roots

Root(s)	Action(s)
C5	Shoulder Flexion Abduction Lateral rotation Elbow Flexion
C5, C6	Elbow ■ Extension
C6, C7	Wrist ■ Flexion
C7, C8	Shoulder ■ Extension Elbow ■ Pronation Fingers ■ Extension

Nerve	Supplies
Long thoracic (C5–7)	Serratus anterior
Suprascapular (C4–6)	Supraspinatus Infraspinatus Glenohumeral joint

The thenar (thumb) region of the hand and nailbeds of thumb, index, and middle fingers (and half of ring finger) are supplied by palmar digital nerves of the median nerve.

The hypothenar (pinky) region of the palm is supplied by the ulnar nerve.

The posterior cord gives rise to the radial and axillary nerves.

The radial nerve is the "great extensor nerve." It is motor to all muscles of the posterior arm. It is the most often injured nerve in a mid-humeral shaft fracture because it runs in the radial (spiral) groove of the humerus. Radial nerve deficit includes wrist drop, inability to make a tight fist, and sensory deficit to the radial hand and lower part of thumb and digits 2 and 3 (and half of 4).

Limb Muscles and Functions by Joint

MOVEMENT OF THE ARM AT THE SHOULDER

■ This movement involves the glenohumeral joint.

Muscle(s)	Movement
Pectoralis major Deltoid Biceps Coracobrachialis	Flexion
Triceps Teres major Pectoralis major Deltoid Latissimus dorsi	Extension
Deltoid Supraspinatus	Abduction

The posterior cord gives rise to the radial and axillary nerves.

Axillary nerves are often injured by falling on an outstretched arm when the glenohumeral joint is dislocated because the nerve runs immediately inferior to the glenohumeral joint.

One can damage the lower part of the brachial plexus if the arm is abruptly extended above the head (e.g., when grabbing a fixed object to slow a fall, as with a skier grabbing a tree).

The long thoracic (nerve of Bell) supplies the serratus anterior (C5, 6, 7 or "wings of heaven").

The interosseous membrane holds radius and ulna together.

Muscle(s)	Movement
Pectoralis major Latissimus dorsi Teres major Triceps Coracobrachialis	Adduction
Teres major Pectoralis major Latissimus dorsi Subscapularis Deltoid	Medial rotation
Infraspinatus Teres minor Deltoid	Lateral rotation

MOVEMENT OF THE ARM AT THE ELBOW

- This movement involves the humeroulnar joint.

Muscle(s)	Movement
Biceps Brachialis Coracobrachialis	Flexion
Triceps Anconeus	Extension

MOVEMENT OF THE HAND AT THE ELBOW

- This movement involves the radioulnar joint.

Muscle(s)	Movement
Pronator quadratus, pronator teres	Pronation
Supinator, biceps	Supination

ROTATOR CUFF

- **Supraspinatus:** Abduction of arm at shoulder
- **Infraspinatus:** External roation of arm at shoulder
- **Teres minor:** External rotation of arm at shoulder
- **Subscapularis:** Internal rotation of arm at shoulder

The mnemonic for the muscles of the rotator cuff is SITS.

► EXTERNAL THORAX AND ABDOMEN

Sternum

- Anterior rib articulation (upper seven ribs articulate directly with sternum).
- Three parts (from superior to inferior):
  - Manubrium.
  - Body.
  - Xiphoid process.
- Jugular notch (suprasternal notch).
  - Superior border of manubrium.
- Angle of Louis (sternal angle).
  - Articulation of manubrium and body at second rib.

Clavicle

- S-shaped bone.
- Articulates with:
  - Acromion of scapula (laterally).
  - Manubrium of sternum (medially).
- Posterior dislocation at sternoclavicular joint can damage:
  - Trachea.
  - Subclavian vessels.
  - Nerves to arm (brachial plexus).
- Subclavius muscle helps prevent fractured clavicle from doing this damage.
- Clavicle forms by membranous bone formation.

If one stabs the fourth intercostal space near sternal border, the right ventricle is injured.

If one fractures the tenth and eleventh ribs, the spleen is injured.

Ribs

- Twelve total:
  - Ribs 1–6 are true.
  - Ribs 7–10 are false.
  - Ribs 11 and 12 float.

Intercostal Space

- The intercostal NVB runs on the inferior surface of the rib.
- Going from the closest undersurface of the rib inferiorly:
  - **Vein**
    - Intercoastal vein drains into the hemiazygos and azygos veins.
  - **Artery**
    - Anterior intercostal artery arises from internal thoracic artery.
    - Posterior intercostals arteries arise from thoracic aorta.
  - **Nerve**
    - Nerve is most exposed; least protected by costal groove.
    - Nerve at angle of rib is at inferior surface in costal groove, so you can anesthetize here.
- Intercostals muscles are involved in respiration.

Muscles of Respiration

- Diaphragm.
- Intercostals.
- Accessory muscles.

DIAPHRAGM

The phrenic nerve travels through the thorax between pericardium and pleura.

- Main muscle for breathing.
- Flat, domelike muscle.
- Muscular tent divides thoracic and abdominal cavities.
- Upper surface contacts heart, lungs.
- Lower surface contacts liver, stomach, spleen.
- Contraction (inspiration)
    - Flattens; moves inferiorly into abdomen.
    - Creates negative intrathoracic pressure/vacuum.
- Relaxes (exhalation/expiration).
    - Forms dome; moves up.
    - Positive intraabdominal pressure pushes it up.
    - Contract abdominal muscles for forceful exhalation.
- Openings and passageways:
    - **Aortic opening**
        - Aorta (passes through two crura).
        - Thoracic duct (passes through with aorta).
        - Azygos and hemiazygos veins.
    - **Caval opening**
        - Inferior vena cava.
    - **Esophageal opening**
        - Esophagus.
    - Other things that pass:
        - Posterior and anterior vagal trunks.
        - Splanchnic nerves.
        - Sympathetic trunk.
        - Superior epigastric artery.
- Innervation
    - Phrenic nerve (C3, C4, C5).
- Blood supply to diagphragm and lower anterior intercostals spaces.
- Musculophrenic artery.

INTERCOSTAL MUSCLES

- All are innervated by the intercostals nerves.

Muscle	Orientation
External intercostal	Run from rib to rib in "hands-in-pocket" direction (homologous to external obliques).
Internal intercostal	Run from dib to rib 90 degrees from external intercostals; continue toward vertebral column *as* posterior intercostals membrane.
(NVB *lies here*)	
Innermost intercostal	Same direction as internal intercostals but the intercostals NVB lies in between.

ACCESSORY MUSCLES OF RESPIRATION

- Sternocleidomastoid.
- Scalenes.
- Subcostals.
- Transversus thoracis.
- These latter two are innervated by intercostals nerves.

Muscles of the Thorax

Muscle	Origin	Insertion	Action	Innervation
Pectoralis major	Medial half of clavicle; sternum and costal cartilages 1–6	Greater tubercular crest (crest leading downward from greater tubercle)	Medially rotates, flexes, and adducts humerus.	Lateral and medial pectoral nerves
Pectoralis minor	Anterior ends of ribs 3–5	Coracoid process	Protracts and depresses glenoid of scapula.	Lateral and medial pectoral nerves
Subclavius	Anterior end of rib 1	Underside of clavicle	Protracts and depresses clavicle.	Nerve to subclavius

MUSCLES OF THE PECTORAL GIRDLE

- Serratus anterior
- Pectoralis minor
- Subclavius
- Trapezius
- Levator scapulae
- Rhomboideus major
- Rhomboideus minor

Abdominal Regions

- **Umbilical:** Central around the umbilicus.
- **Lumbar:** Right and left of umbilical region.
- **Epigastric:** Midline region above umbilicus (subxiphoid, area of stomach).
- **Hypochondriac:** Left and right of epigastric regions (beneath rib cage).
- **Hypogastric (pubic):** Midline below umbilicus.
- **Iliac (inguinal):** Right and left of hypogastric region.

Abdominal Muscles

Muscle	Origin	Insertion	Action	Innervation
External oblique	Superficial aspect of lower 8 ribs	Iliac crest, linea alba	Increases abdominal pressure.	Lower intercostal nerves
Internal oblique	Lumbodorsal fascia, iliac crest, inguinal ligament	Costal cartilages of last 3 ribs, linea alba	Same as above.	Lower intercostals, iliohypogastric, ilioinguinal nerves

Abdominal Muscles (Continued)

Muscle	Origin	Insertion	Action	Innervation
Transversus abdominis	Internal surface of lower 6 costal cartilages, lumbodorsal fascia, iliac crest, inguinal ligament	Linea alba	Same as above.	Lower intercostals, iliohypogastric, and ilioinguinal nerves
Rectus abdominis	Pubic symphysis	External surface xiphoid process, external surface costal cartilages 5–7	Increases abdominal pressure, flex vertebral column.	Lower intercostal nerves

POINTS

- **External oblique fibers** (like external intercostals)
    - Run in a "hands-in-pocket" fashion.
    - Obliquely; lateral to medial going superior to inferior.
- **Internal oblique fibers** (like internal intercostals fibers)
    - Run opposite (perpendicular) to external oblique fibers.
    - Obliquely from lateral to medial going inferior to superior.
- **Cremaster muscle**
    - Derived from internal oblique muscle.

Rectus Sheath

- Aponeurotic sheath covering the rectus muscle.
- **Anterior rectus sheath**
    - Formed from the tendinous continuations of the external oblique and internal oblique.
- **Posterior rectus sheath**
    - Formed from the aponeurosis from the internal oblique and tranverse abdominis.
- **Linea alba**
    - Midline fusion of the anterior and posterior rectus sheath.
    - At the midline of two bellies of the rectus.

Fascia

- Covers muscles.
- Attaches to nearby bones by blending with covering periosteum.

Breast

- Mammary glands.
- Modified sweat glands.
- Lie in superficial fascia.
- Myoepithelial cells (star-shaped)
    - Encircle some of the secretory cells.
    - Force secretion toward the ducts.
- Suspensory ligamaments (Cooper's ligaments)
    - Strong fibrous processes.
    - Run from dermis to deep layer of superficial fascia through breast.

- Support the breasts.
- Can cause dimpling of overlying skin and nipple retraction in breast cancer.
■ Innervation:
- Fourth intercostal nerve (T4) (to the nipple).
■ Blood supply:
- Lateral thoracic (branch of axillary).
- Internal thoracic arteries.
■ Lymph drainage.
■ To lymph nodes (LNs) in axilla.

Dermatomes

See Figure 1–60. A dermatome is an area of skin supplied by a single nerve.

- CN V: Head and face.
- CN V, VII, IX, X: Ear.
- C1: **Does not** supply a dermatome.
- C2 (greater occipital nerve): Posterior scalp (posterior half of skull cap).
- C3: Neck.
- C4: Low collar.
- T4: Nipple
- T7: Xiphoid.
- T10: Umbilicus.
- L1: Inguinal ligament.
- L4: Knee caps.
- S2, S3, S4: Erection, sensation of penile and anal zones.

> *Cranial nerve dermatomes **do not** overlap.*
> - Spinal nerve dermatomes overlap by as much as 50%.
> - May require loss of three spinal nerves to produce anesthesia in middle dermatome.
> - For example, lesion to dorsal root of T7, T8, and T 9 to produce numbness of T8 dermatomal distribution.

Reflexes

- C5, C6: Biceps
- C7: Triceps
- L4: Patella
- S1: Achilles

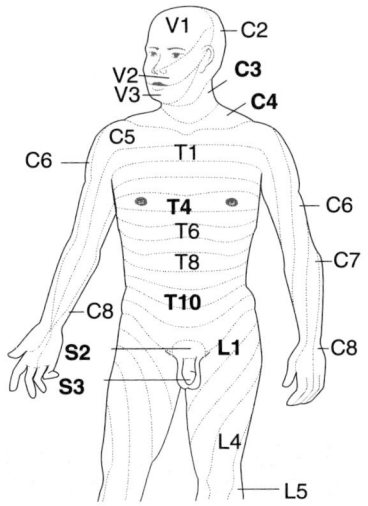

FIGURE 1-60. Areas of skin supplied by a single nerve.

Reproduced, with permission, from Bushhan V, et al. *First Aid for the USMLE Step 1.* New York: McGraw-Hill, 2003.

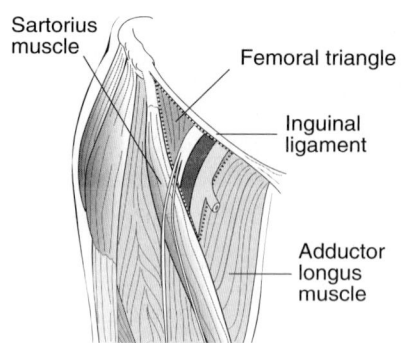

FIGURE 1-61. Femoral triangle.

Reproduced, with permission, from Bushhan V, et al. *First Aid for the USMLE Step 1.* New York: McGraw-Hill, 2003.

Femoral Triangle

See Figure 1–61. The femoral triangle has the following boundaries:

- **Lateral:** Sartorius.
- **Medial:** Adductor longus.
- **Superior:** Inguinal ligament.
- **Floor:** Iliopsoas and pectineus.
- **Femoral:** NVB.
- **From lateral to medial:** Nerve, artery, vein.

▶ THORACIC AND ABDOMINAL VISCERA

Body Cavities

Posterior	Anterior
Cranial: Contains brain. **Spinal:** Contains spinal cord. These two cavities communicate via foramen magnum. Lined by meninges. Bathed in CSF.	**Thoracic** **Pericardial cavity:** Surrounds heart. **Pleural** (right and left). ■ Surrounds each lung. ■ Mediastinum lies between two pleural cavities. **Abdominopelvic Abdominal** ■ Stomach. ■ Spleen. ■ Liver. ■ Gallbladder. ■ Pancreas. ■ Small and large intestines. **Pelvic cavity** ■ Rectum. ■ Urinary bladder.

Lung

- Housed in left and right pleural cavities.
- **Visceral pleura:** Covers the lungs.
- **Parietal pleura:** Covers the thoracic cavity.
- Pleural cavity.
  - Between the two layers of pleura.
  - Filled with serous fluid.

Right Lung	Left Lung
Three lobes - Superior - Middle - Inferior Three lobar bronchi (secondary bronchi) Ten bronchial segments (tertiary bronchi) One bronchial artery Larger capacity than left lung	Two lobes - Superior - Inferior Lingula - Tongue-shaped part of superior lobe corresponding to middle lobe of right lung Two lobar bronchi (secondary bronchi) Eight bronchial segments (tertiary bronchi) Cardiac notch - Medial side of the superior lobe of left lung Two bronchial arteries

LUNG HILUM (ROOT)

- Pulmonary artery
- Pulmonary vein
- Bronchus

OTHER STRUCTURES PASSING INTO THE HILUM

Bronchial Arteries

- Supply the lung tissues with oxygen.
- Also pass into the hilum.
- Follow the bronchial tree.

> *Describes where the pulmonary artery sits in relation to the bronchus:*
>
> **RALS**
>
> **R**ight
> **A**nterior
> **L**eft
> **S**uperior

Aspiration occurs more often in the right lung (apical aspect of right lower lobe) because the right mainstem bronchus is straighter, shorter, and larger than the left. The left mainstem takes a more acute angle.

See the "Physiology" section in Chapter 13 for Hering-Breuer and cough reflexes.

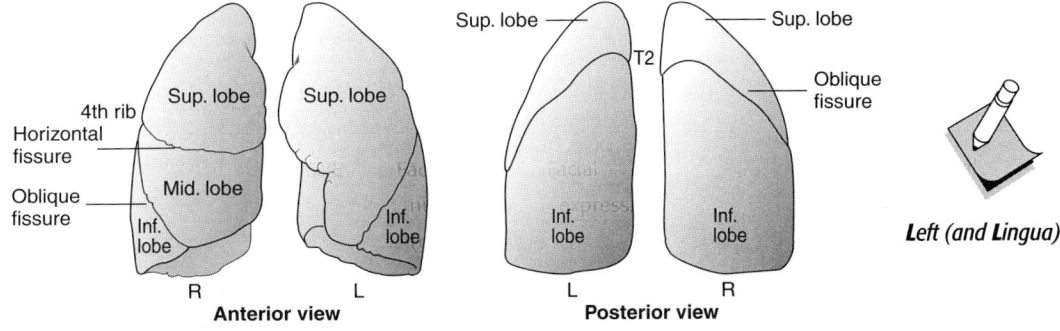

Left (and **L**ingua).

FIGURE 1-62. Anterior and posterior view of the lungs.

Reproduced, with permission, from Bushhan V, et al. *First Aid for the USMLE Step 1*. New York: McGraw-Hill, 2003.

Branches of the Vagus Nerve

- Also pass into the root of the lung.

Heart and Great Vessels

See Figure 1–63.

	From Body (Deoxy)	**From Lungs (Oxy)**
Chamber	Right atrium	Left atrium
Valve	Tricuspid valve	Mitral valve
Chamber	Right ventricle	Left ventricle
Valve	Pulmonic valve	Aortic valve
	To Lungs	To body

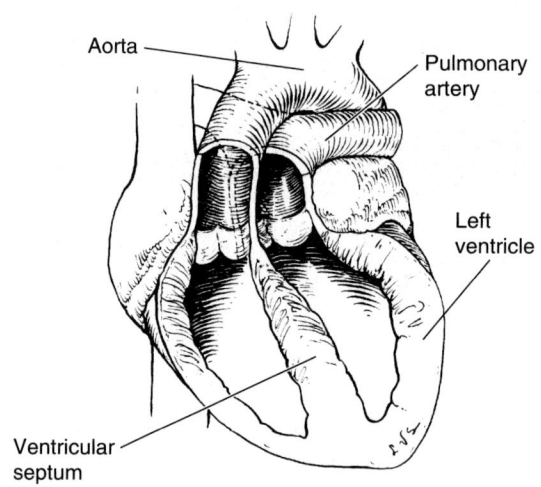

FIGURE 1–63. Heart and great vessels.

Reproduced, with permission, from Way LW, Doherty GM (eds). *Current Surgical Diagnosis and Treatment*, 11th ed. New York: McGraw-Hill, 2002.

VALVES

SEMILUNAR

- Each has three semilunar cusps.
- No chordae tendineae or papillary muscles are associated with semiluar valves.
- **Pulmonic valve**
  - Right ventricle (RV) to pulmonary arteries.
  - Hear at left sternal border, second intercostal space.
- **Aortic valve**
  - Left ventricle (LV) to aorta.
  - Hear over right sternal border, second intercostal space.

ATRIOVENTRICULAR

- **Tricuspid valve**
  - Right atrium (RA) to right ventricle (RV).
  - Hear over left sternal border, fifth intercostal space.
- **Mitral valve**
  - Left atrium (LA) to left ventricle (LV).
  - Hear over fifth intercostal space, midclavicular line.

Atria

RIGHT ATRIUM

- Incoming deoxygenated blood from vena cavae.
- **Fossa ovalis**
  - Depression remnant of the foramen ovale.
  - Lies on atrial septum (interatrial); dividing the left and right atria.
  - Anulis ovalis is the upper margin of the fossa.
- **Crista terminalis**
- Vertical ridge between vena cavae orifices.
  - Sinoatrial (SA) node is located here.
  - Junction of sinus venosus and the heart in the developing embryo.
- **Sulcus terminalis**
  - Vertical groove on external heart represents crista terminalis (internally).
- **Pectinate muscles**
- Radiate from crista terminalis to atrial appendage.
- **Right auricle**
  - Appendage of right atrium.
- **Conduction system**
  - SA node.
  - AV node.
  - Coronary sinus

LEFT ATRIUM

- Incoming blood from pulmonary veins.

Ventricles

RIGHT VENTRICLE

- Responsible for the pulmonic circulation.
  - Pumps deoxygenated blood through the pulmonic valve to pulmonary artery and lungs for oxygenation.
- Trabeculae carnae.
  - Ridges of cardiac muscle in the ventricles.
- Chordae tendinae.
  - Thin tendinous cords passing from valve cusps to papillary muscles.
- Papillary muscles.
  - Anchor chordae tendinae to heart wall.

LEFT VENTRICLE

- Apex of the heart.
  - Auscultate fifth intercostals space at midclavicular line.
- Responsible for the systemic circulation.
  - Receives oxygenated blood from the lungs and pumps it out to the rest of the body.
  - Out the aortic valve to aorta.
- Thicker than RV because of systemic circulation.
- Same internal features as RV.

PERICARDIUM

- Tough, double-walled covering of the heart
- **Parietal pericardium:** Outer fibrous
- **Visceral pericardium:** Inner serous

CORONARY ARTERIES

See Figure 1–64.

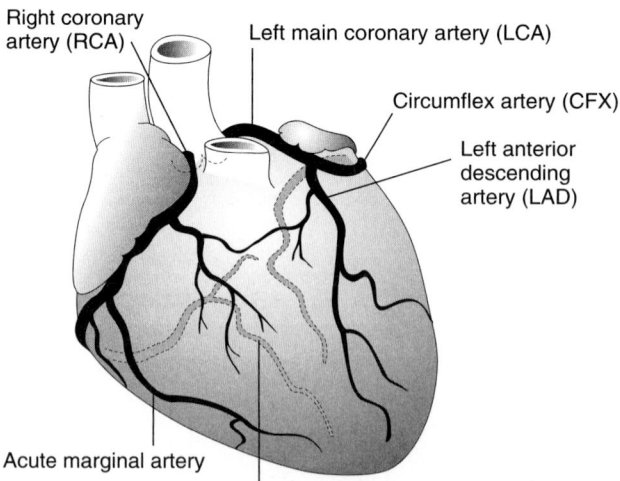

FIGURE 1-64.   Coronary arteries.

Reproduced, with permission, from Bushhan V, et al. *First Aid of the USMLE Step 1.* 2003:91; Adapted from *Ganong Review of Medical Physiology*, 19th ed. Stamford CT: Appleton & Lange, 1999:592).

*The chordae tendinae and papillary muscles do **not** help the AV valves close. They prevent the valve from everting back into the atria.*

See the "Pathology" section in Chapter 19. Heart strain and hypertrophy secondary to increased resistance to flow:

- Left heart
  - Coarctation of the aorta
  - Systemic hypertension
- Right heart
  - Pulmonary hypertension

The pericardial cavity lies between the two layers of pericardium.

- First branches of the aorta.
  - Coronary ostia located within aortic valve leaflets.
  - Drain to coronary sinus which drains back to RA.
- Coronary arteries fill during diastole.
- Blockage; thrombus on disrupted plaque can lead to:
  - Ischemia (angina).
  - Infarction (heart attack).

Vessel	Area Supplied
Left circumflex	LV lateral wall
Left anterior descending artery (LAD)	Anterior wall LV Interventricular septum
Right coronary artery (RCA)	Right ventricle AV node Posterior, inferior walls of LV

Veins of the Heart

- Cardiac veins lie superficial to the arteries.
- **Coronary sinus**
  - Continuation of **great cardiac vein.**
  - Opens into the right atrium between the IVC and the tricuspid orifice.
  - All veins drain into the coronary sinus **except** the **anterior cardiac veins** (drain directly into the right atrium).

Mediastinum

- The mediastinum is the area between and medial to lungs in the thorax.

The superior vena cava (SVC), the inferior vena cava (IVC), and coronary sinus all empty deoxygenated blood into the RA.

Mediastinum	Location	Contents
Anterior	Anterior to pericardium	Thymus Connective tissue Lymph nodes Branches of internal thoracic artery
Middle	Within pericardium	Pericardium Heart Roots of great vessels Phrenic nerve
Posterior	Posterior to pericardium	Thoracic duct Descending aorta Azygous vein Hemiazygous vein Esophagus Vagus nerves Splanchnic nerves Lymph nodes

The thymus is located in both the anterior and superior mediastinum.

The inferior mediastinum is split into anterior, middle, and posterior.

Mediastinum	Location	Contents
Superior	Above manubiosternal junction (T4)	Thoracic duct Ascending aorta Aortic arch Branches of aortic arch Descending aorta SVC Brachiocephalic veins Thymus Trachea Esophagus Cardiac nerve Left recurrent laryngeal nerve

Zinc is the most important element for immunity (involved in almost all aspects of immunity).

The thymus has no afferent lymphatics or lymphatic nodules.

*All lymphoid organs are derived exclusively from mesenchyme **except** for the thymus.*
***Remember:** The thymus has a double embryologic origin:*

- *Mesenchyme*
  - *Lymphocytes (hematopoietic stem cells)*
- *Endoderm*
  - *Hassall's corpuscles (epithelium)*
    - *Derived from the third pharyngeal pouch.*

Thymoma is associated with MG.

Thymus

FUNCTION

- A primary lymphoid organ.
  - Along with spleen, tonsils, lymph nodes, Peyer's patches.
- Master organ of immunogenesis in young.
  - Proliferation and maturation of T cells (cell mediated immunity).
- Releases factors important in development of immune system:
  - Thymopoietin.
  - Thymosin.
  - Thymic humoral factor.
  - Thymic factor.
- Zinc, B12, Vitamin C are important for thymic hormones.

ANATOMY

- Located inferior to thyroid, ventral/anterior to heart.
- Deep to sternum in **superior mediastinum.**
- Two lobes (soft, pinkish).
- Inner medulla
  - Lymphocytes.
  - Hassall's corpuscles (epithelial vestiges with unknown function).
- Blood supply
  - Internal thoracic artery.
  - Inferior thyroid arteries.
- Nerve supply
  - Vagus nerve.
  - Phrenic nerve.

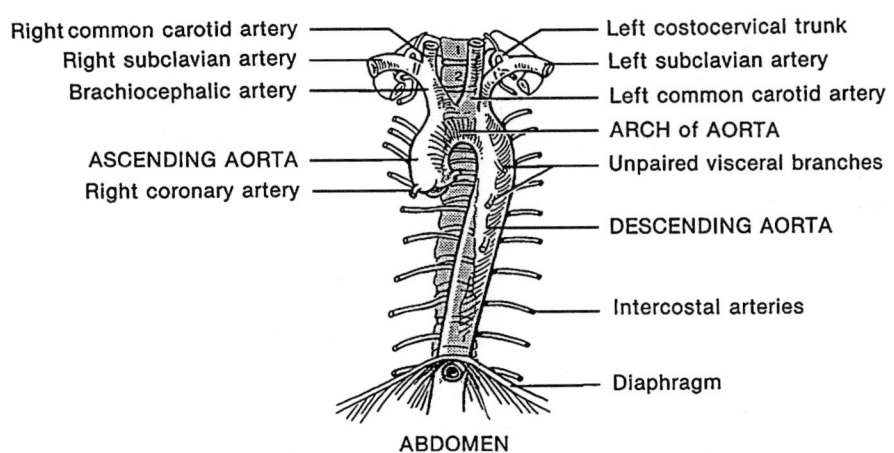

FIGURE 1-65. The thoracic aorta and its branches.

Remember: There is one brachiocephalic artery, two brachiocephalic veins.

Reproduced, with permission, from Liebgott B. *The Anatomical Basis of Dentistry.* Toronto: BC Decker, 1986.

Aorta

See Figure 1–65.

- Descending thoracic aorta extends from T4 to T12.
- Descending abdominal aorta extends from T12 to L4.
- Aorta terminates around L4 when it divides into left and right common iliac arteries (supplying lower limbs and pelvic viscera).

Parts	Major Branches	Supplies
Ascending	Right and left coronary arteries	Heart
Aortic arch	Brachiocephalic artery Left common carotid Left subclavian	Head, neck, upper limbs
Descending thoracic aorta	Posterior intercostals	Posterior thorax, diaphragm
Descending abdominal aorta	**Midline** celiac trunk SMA IMA **Paired** Renal Gonadal	Abdominal viscera

Common Carotid

- Supplies head and neck.
- Bifurcates into external and internal carotid arteries at superior border of the thyroid cartilage.

See the "Neck" section for branches.

SUBCLAVIAN ARTERY

- Supplies the upper extremity.
- Continues as the axillary artery past the inferior margin of the first rib.

BRANCHES OF SUBCLAVIAN ARTERY

- Vertebral (forms basilar—circle of Willis)
- Thyrocervical
- Internal thoracic
- Costocervical

INTERNAL THORACIC ARTERY

- Runs underneath the sternum.
- Gives off anterior intercostals (meets posterior intercostals off the aorta).
- Extends inferiorly as superior epigastric artery.

SUPERIOR EPIGASTRIC ARTERY

- Continuation of the internal thoracic artery.
- Enters rectus sheath and supplies rectus muscle.
- Anastomoses with inferior epigastric artery (branch of the external iliac artery) near the umbilicus.

ABDOMINAL AORTA

Midline ranches

If the celiac trunk is blocked, blood can still reach the foregut by way of anastomoses between the superior pancreaticoduodenal artery (a branch of the gastroduodenal) and the inferior pancreaticoduodenal (a branch of the SMA).

The third part of duodenum passes anterior to the IMA.

Branch	Branches	Structures Supplied
Celiac	Common hepatic, splenic, left gastric	Foregut
SMA	Inferior pancreaticoduodenal, intestinal (ileal, jejunal), right and middle colic arteries	Midgut
IMA	Superior rectal, sigmoid, left colic arteries	Hindgut

Azygous System

See Figure 1–66.

- The azygous system drains the thoracic wall.

Remember:
The right superior intercostal vein drains into the azygos vein.
The left superior intercostal vein drains into left brachiocephalic vein.

Anatomy	Formed by	Drains to
Ascends through aortic orifice of diaphragm. Lies within posterior mediastinum. Leaves a notch in the right lung as it passes over the hilum.	Right ascending lumbar vein. Right subcostal vein.	Empties into the superior vena cava (SVC).

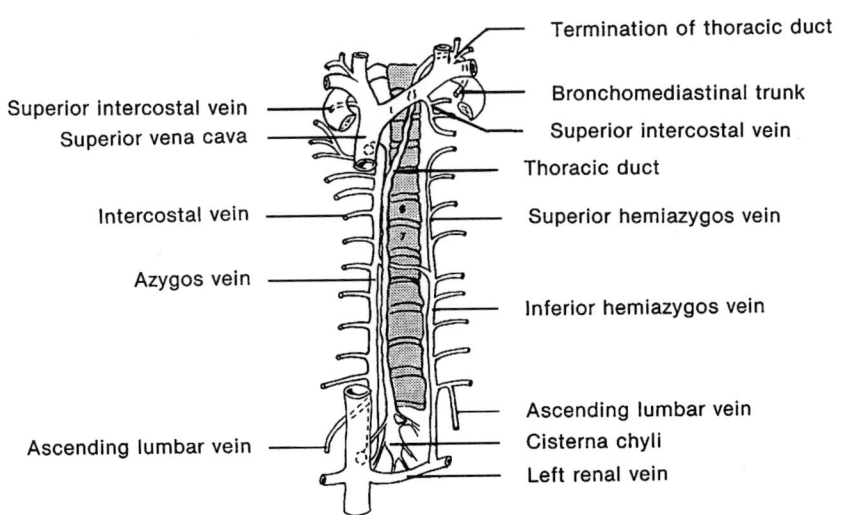

FIGURE 1-66. The azygous system of veins and the thoracic duct.

Reproduced, with permission, with Liebgott B. *The Anatomical Basis of Dentistry*. Toronto: BC Decker, 1986.

Hemiazygos Vein (Inferior Hemiazygos Vein)	Accesory Hemiazygos Vein (Superior Hemiazygos Vein)
Formed by: ■ Left ascending lumbar vein ■ Left subcostal vein ■ Empties into the azygos vein	Formed by: ■ 4th to 8th intercostal veins ■ Empties into the azygos vein

Splanchnic Nerves

- Sympathetic nerves to the abdominal viscera.
    - Counteract vagal/parasympathetic inputs.
- Arise from thoracic ganglia
    - T5–12.
    - All pass through the diaphragm.
- Preganglionic sympathetic fibers pass through ganglia of the sympathetic trunk **without** synapsing.
    - This is the exception to the short preganglionic, long postganglionic.
    - They synapse with small ganglia in the tissues/effector organs which give off short postganglionics.
- Distribute to smooth muscle and glands of viscera.

Nerve	Components	Innervates
Greater splanchnic nerve	T5–T9	Synapse at cervical plexus (foregut)
Lesser splanchnic nerve	T10, 11	Synapse with superior mesenteric plexus; aorticorenal ganglion (midgut)
Least splanchnic nerve	T12	Inferior mesenteric plexus/renal plexus (hindgut)

Superior Vena Cava

- Drains the
  - Head.
  - Neck.
  - Upper extremities.
  - Upper chest.
- No valve.
- Formed by
- Left and right brachiocephalic veins (merging in the superior mediastinum).
- Brachiocephalic veins are formed from
  - Internal jugular vein.
  - Subclavian vein.
- Azygos vein empties into SVC.
- SVC empties into RA.

> **SVC Syndrome**
> - Example: Compression of SVC with lung cancer
> - Dyspnea
> - Facial swelling and flushing
> - Jugular venous distention
> - Mental status changes

Inferior Vena Cava

Remember: The left gonadal vein drains into left renal vein. The right gonadal vein empties directly into the IVC.

- Larger than SVC.
- Rudimentary, nonfunctioning valve.
- Drains
  - Thorax.
  - Abdomen.
  - Lower extremities.
- Receives blood from the hepatic veins.
- Empties into RA.

The left renal vein is longer than the right and the right renal artery is longer than the left. This is due to the positions of the vena cava and aorta, respectively.

Paired Branches of the IVC

Branch	Structures Supplied
Suprarenal	Adrenal glands
Renal	Kidneys
Gonadal	Testes/ovaries
Lumbar	Lumbar epaxial muscles

A pelvic kidney may be supplied by the common iliac artery.

Portal Vein

See Figure 1–67.

- Transmits venous blood from the abdominal viscera (with absorbed substances) to the liver and, via the portal system, to the heart.

  Portal vein → hepatic sinusoids → central vein → hepatic veins → IVC.

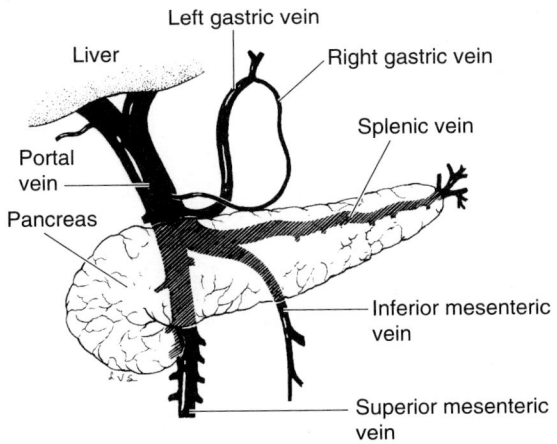

Figure 1-67. Anatomic relationship of portal vein and branches.

Reproduced, with permission, from Way LW, Doherty, GM (Eds). *Current Surgical Diagnosis and Treatment*, 11th ed. New York: McGraw-Hill, 2002.

The portal vein arises from:

- Splenic vein
    - Drains:
        - Spleen.
        - Stomach (L and R gastroepiploic veins, R and L gastric veins).
        - Pancreas (pancreatic vein).
        - Gallbladder (cystic vein).
- Superior mesenteric vein
    - Drains
        - Small intestine.
        - Cecum.
        - Ascending and transverse colon.
- Inferior mesenteric vein
    - Enters into the splenic vein, the SMV, or crotch of the two.
    - Drains:
        - Transverse colon distal to L colic flexure (splenic flexure).
        - Descending colon.
        - Rectum.

Portal blood can also get to the IVC by the azygos and hemiazygos veins.

Portocaval shunt can be created by anastomosing the splenic vein and renal vein (a portal component and a systemic venous component).

Portal Triad

- Consists of:
    - Portal vein.
    - Hepatic artery.
    - Bile duct.
- Lies on free edge of lesser omentum (anterior to epiploic foramen of Winslow).
- Portal vein is posterior while hepatic artery and bile duct are anterior.
- Portal vein carries twice as much blood as the hepatic artery.

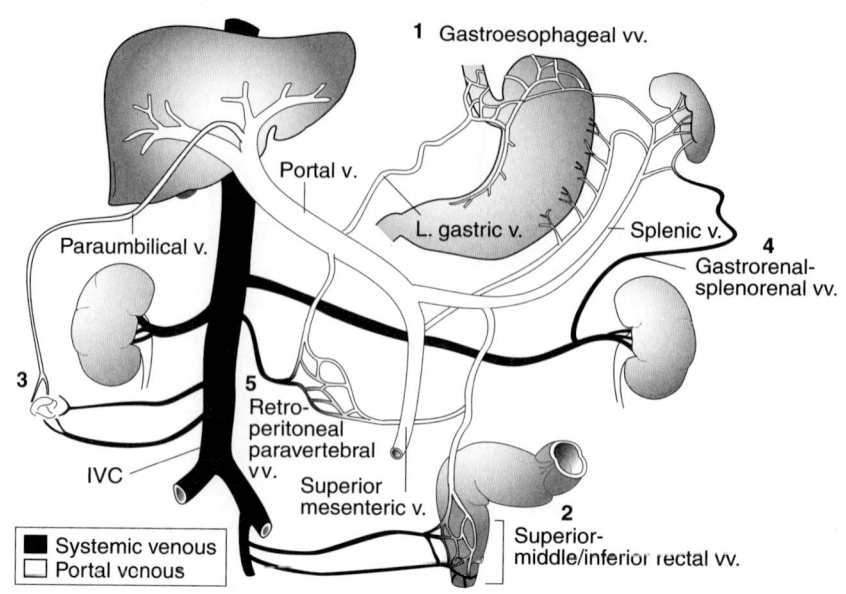

FIGURE 1-68. Portal systemic anastomoses.

Reproduced, with permission, from Bushhan V, et al. *First Aid for the USMLE Step 1*. New York: McGraw-Hill, 2003.

VENOUS ANASTOMOSES

See Figure 1–68.

Lymphatic System

CISTERNA CHYLI

Occlusion of lymph supply (e.g., cancer) leads to intractable edema.

- Located in the para-aortic region below the diaphragm.
- Drains lymph from
    - Abdomen.
    - Pelvis.
    - Inguinal region.
    - Lower extremities.
- Continuous superiorly with the thoracic duct.

THORACIC DUCT

Aside from the right arm, chest, and right head, the rest of the body–including the right leg–is drained by the thoracic duct.

- Continuation of the dilated cisterna chyli.
- Located in posterior and superior mediastinum.
- Drains lymph from
    - Lower limbs.
    - Abdomen.
    - Chest wall.
- Empties into venous system at
    - Junction of the subclavian and internal jugular vein (on the left side only).

Right Lymphatic Duct

- Drains
  - Right arm.
  - Right side of chest.
  - Right side of head.
- Empties into the
- Junction of the right internal jugular vein and right subclavian veins (formation of the right brachiocephalic vein).

Important: The diaphragm divides the thoracic cavity and abdominal cavity.

Peritoneum

- Membrane lining the interior of the abdominopelvic cavity.
- Consists of:
  - Single layer of simple squamous mesothelium.
  - Thin layer of irregular connective tissue.
- **Visceral peritoneum**
  - Covers organs.
- **Parietal peritoneum**
  - Covers body walls.
- **Peritoneal fluid**
  - Fills the peritoneal space/cavity (space between these two serous layers).

Pleura is the analog to peritoneum in the pleural cavity.

Mesentery

- Double-layer fold of peritoneum pushed into peritoneal cavity.
- Suspends most organs of abdominoperitoneal cavity (holds them in place).
- Allows path for blood vessels and nerves.

Embryonic Mesentery	Adult Mesentery
Dorsal mesogastrium	Greater omentum Omental bursa
Dorsal mesoduodenum	Disappears (duodenum lies retroperitoneal)
Pleuropericardial membrane	Pericardium Contribution to diaphragm
Ventral mesentery	Falciform ligament Ligamentum teres Lesser omentum (hepatogastric, hepatoduodenal ligaments)

The **pericardioperitoneal canal** embryologically connects the thoracic and peritoneal cavities.

The **greater omentum** begins at its attachment to the greater curvature of the stomach, drapes over (apronlike) the small and large intestines and loops back to insert on the transverse colon.

Peritoneal Ligaments

- Either a mesentery or omentum.
- Named double fold of the peritoneum and connects
  - Two organs or
  - Organ to the abdominal wall.
- Are associated with the stomach, jejunum, ileum, appendix, transverse colon, sigmoid colon, spleen, liver, and gallbladder.

Ligament	Description
Splenorenal ligament	Connects spleen to posterior abdominal wall. Contains splenic artery, vein, and tail of pancreas. Passes from spleen to parietal peritoneum on the anterior surface of the kidney. Separates the greater peritoneal sac from the left portion of the lesser peritoneal sac.
Gastrosplenic ligament	Part of dorsal mesogastrium between greater curve f stomach and spleen. Separates greater peritoneal sac from left portion of lesser peritoneal sac. Incise to gain access to left side of lesser peritoneal sac.
Gastrocolic ligament	Part of greater omentum, between greater curvature of stomach and transverse colon. Contains gastroepiploic arteries.
Gastroduodenal ligament	Between lesser curve of stomach and duodenum.
Gastrohepatic ligament	**Part of lesser omentum** between liver and lesser curvature. Separates greater peritoneal sac and right part of lesser peritoneal sac. Contains no significant blood vessels (so may be incised for access).
Hepatoduodenal ligament	**Part of lesser omentum** Connects liver to first part of duodenum. Contains CBD, proper hepatic artery (with brachial cystic artery), and portal vein. Separates greater peritoneal sac from right part of lesser peritoneal sac. Forms anterior portion of epiploic foramen.
Falciform ligament	Connects liver to anterior abdominal wall. Contains ligamentum teres (remnant of umbilical vein).

Epiploic Foramen of Winslow

- Inlet to lesser sac.
- Posterior to the free edge of the lesser omentum (hepatoduodenal ligament).
- Portal triad is located over top (anteriorly).

Gastrointestinal Tract

See Figure 1–69 for the cross section of the gastrointestinal tract.

GI Segment	Derivatives	Arterial Supply	Innervation
Foregut	Esophagus Stomach Duodenum (1st part) Liver Gallbladder Pancreas	Celiac trunk	Vagal parasympathetics Thoracic nerve Splanchnic sympathetic nerve
Midgut	Duodenum (2nd–4th parts) Jejunum Ileum Appedix Ascending colon Transverse colon (to Splenic flexure)	Superior mesenteric artery	Vagal parasympathetics Thoracic splanchnic sympathetic nerve
Hindgut	Transverse colon (distal to splenic flexure) Descending colon Sigmoid colon Rectum	Inferior mesenteric artery	Pelvic splanchnic nerve (S2–S4) parasympathetic Lumbar splanchnic sympathetic nerve

See histology for the myenteric nervous system.

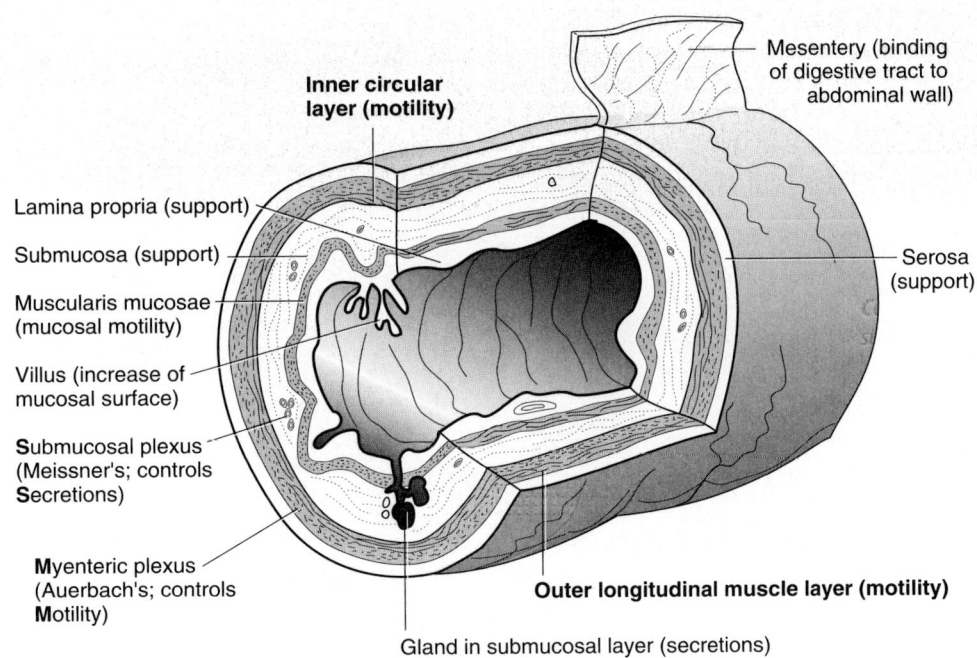

FIGURE 1–69. Cross-section of the gastrointestinal tract.

Reproduced, with permission, from Bushhan V, et al. *First Aid for the USMLE Step 1*. New York: McGraw-Hill, 2003. Adapted from McPhee S, et al. *Pathophysiology of Disease: An Introduction to Clinical Medicine*, 3rd ed. New York, McGraw-Hill, 2000:296

ESOPHAGUS

Description	Blood Supply	Innervation
10-inch muscular tube Peristalsis. Food propelled from pharynx to stomach (pierces diaphragm at cardiac orifice). Posterior to trachea. Travels through the mediastinum (superior and posterior). Upper 1/3 skeletal muscle. Middle 1/3 skeletal and smooth muscle. Lower 1/3 smooth muscle.	Inferior thyroid artery Descending thoracic aorta (direct branches) Left gastric artery	**Parasympathetic:** Vagus (esophageal branches) **Sympathetic:** Esophageal plexus **Motor:** Recurrent laryngeal nerve (of vagus)

Stomach

See Figure 1–70 for the anatomy of the stomach.

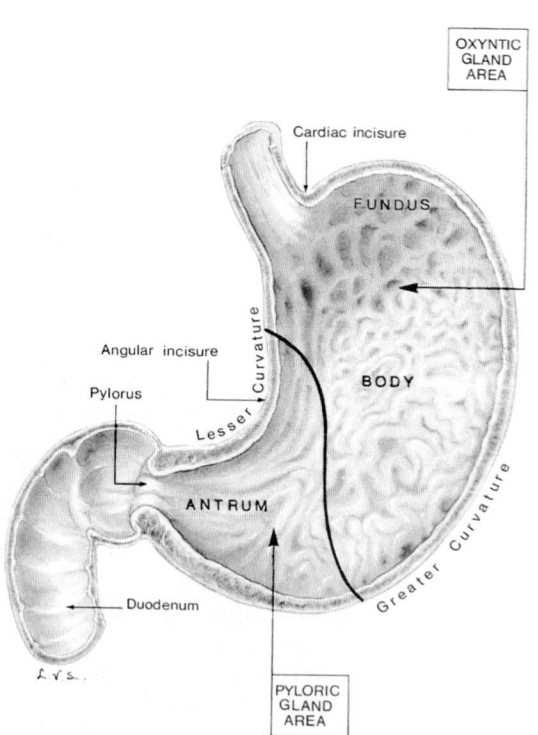

FIGURE 1-70. Names of the parts of the stomach.

The line drawn from the lesser to the greater curvature depicts the approximate boundary between the oxyntic gland area and the pyloric gland area. No prominent landmark exists to distinguish between antrum and body (corpus). The fundus is the portion craniad to the esophagogastric junction. (Reproduced, with permission, from Way LW, Doherty, GM [eds]. *Current Surgical Diagnosis and Treatment*, 11th ed. New York: McGraw-Hill, 2002.)

Sphincters of the Stomach

	Description
Cardiac/lower esophageal sphincter	Composed of: - Internal esophageal sphincter (intrinsic esophageal muscle). - External sphincter (crura of diaphragm).
Pyloric sphincter	Outlet of stomach into duodenum.

Pyloric stenosis in children causes violent, nonbilious projectile vomiting.

Blood Supply to Stomach

See Figure 1–71 for the structures that supply blood to the stomach.

Artery	Description
Splenic artery	Direct branch of celiac trunk. Supplies: - Spleen. - Stomach. Branches: - Short gastrics to fundus. - Left gastroepiploic to left greater curvature.
Left gastric artery	Direct branch of celiac trunk. Supplies: - Left lesser curvature of stomach. - Inferior esophagus.
Right gastric artery	Branch of gastroduodenal (a branch of the hepatic artery proper off the celiac trunk). Supplies: - Right lesser curvature of the stomach.
Right gastroepiploic	Branch of gastroduodenal. Supplies: - Right 1/2 greater curvature of stomach. - Gastric ulcer likely bleeds from this.

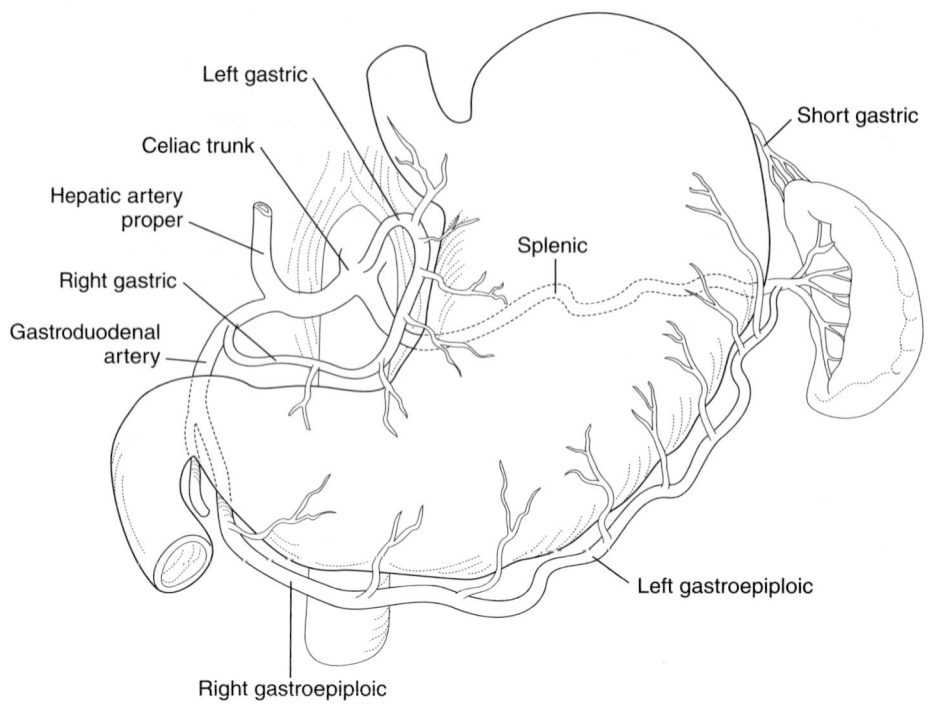

Figure 1-71. Blood supply to the stomach.

Reproduced, with permission, from Bushhan V, et al. *First Aid for the USMLE Step 1*. New York: McGraw-Hill, 2003.

Liver

Function	Anatomy	Blood Flow
Metabolic Produces bile. Involved in cholesterol metabolism. Urea cycle. Produces proteins. Clotting factors. Enzymes. **Detoxification** Liver enzymes. Receives substances from portal blood. **Phagocytosis** **Kupffer cells** (phagocytic); line sinusoids. Filter bacteria and other particles.	Lies under right diaphragm. Two lobes (large right, small left). **Falciform ligament** Attaches to anterior body wall. **Coronary ligaments** Attach liver to diaphragm. **Hepatic sinusoids** With fenestrated endothelial cells. Permit flow of serum across. **Portal triad** Structural unit.	**Arterial supply** Hepatic artery. From common hepatic artery (branch of the celiac trunk). Oxygenated blood to keep liver viable. **Portal venous blood** Drains intestines. Filtering. Detoxification of newly absorbed substances. All blood (hepatic artery and portal blood) is emptied into the same **sinusoids**. Sinusoids empty into **common central vein.** Central vein empties into hepatic veins. **Hepatic veins** empty into **IVC.**

Spleen

- Develops from mesenchymal cells (of the mesentery attached to primitive stomach).
  - **Does not** develop from the primitive gut (i.e., forgut, midgut, hindgut).
- Lies in the left hypochondrium (of the abdominal cavity).
  - Between the stomach and diaphragm.
- Ovoid organ.
- Size of a fist.
- Functions:
  - Blood reservoir.
  - Phagocytosis (foreign particles and red blood cell [RBC] senescence).
  - Production of mononuclear leukocytes.
- Blood supply: Splenic artery (from celiac trunk).
- Venous drainage: Splenic vein (part of portal system).
- Innervation: From celiac plexus.
- Histology.
  - White pulp.
    - Lyphocytes located around splenic artery branches.
  - Red pulp.
  - Blood-filled sinusoids.
  - Phagocytic cells (macrophages, monocytes).
  - Lymphocytes cells.
  - Plasma cells.

Gallbladder

- Pouch on inferior surface of liver.
- Stores and concentrates bile.
- Bile is produced by the liver.
- **Common bile duct** formed by:
  - Cystic duct (from gallbladder).
  - Hepatic duct (from liver).
- Common bile duct empties into duodenum.
- Sphincter of Oddi (ampulla of Vater) (on duodenal papilla).
  - Relaxes:
    - Cholecystokinin; fat into intestine.
    - Gallbladder contracts
    - Bile released into duodenum for fat emulsion.
  - Contracts:
    - No cholecystokinin; intestine is empty.
    - Forcing bile up the cystic duct to the gallbladder for storage.
- Blood supply: Cystic artery (branch of right hepatic).
- Innervation: Vagal fibers (celiac plexus).
- Lymph drains into cystic lymph node, then hepatic nodes, then celiac nodes.

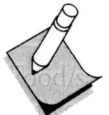

*The gallbladder **does not** contain a submucosa (the stomach and small and large bowel do).*

Bile is composed of bile salts, pigments, cholesterol, and lecithin. Bile serves to emulsify fats, and fat-soluble vitamins (A, D, E, K).

For innervation see foregut, midgut, hindgut table.

Enzymes present in intestinal villi:

- Carbohydrate
  - Maltase
  - Sucrase
  - Lactase
- Protein
- Aminopeptidase
- Dipeptidase
- Activating pancreatic enzymes
  - Enterokinase
    - Converts trypsinogen to trypsin.
  - Trypsin activates other pancreatic enzymes.

Small Intestine

Segment	Blood Supply	Description
Duodenum	Superior pancreaticoduodenal artery (indirect Celiac branch) Inferior pancreaticoduodenal artery (of SMA)	C-shaped. Surrounds pancreas. Shortest and widest part of small intestine. Part of it is retroperitoneal. Connects stomach to jejunum. Common bile duct and pancreatic duct empty into duodenum at duodenal papilla. Contains Brunners glands (submucosal glands) secreting mucous.
Jejunum	SMA—intestinal branches	Valves of Kerckring (plicae circulares). Most villi (for greatest absorption). Thickest muscular wall (of any small intestine segment; for peristalsis).
Ileum	SMA—intestinal branches and ileocolic branch	Peyer's patches. Vitamin B_{12} absorption. More goblet cells and mesenteric fat than jejunum. No plicae circulares in lower Ileum.

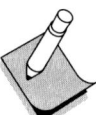

Descending and sigmoid colon, rectum, and anus are part of the hindgut, so they are supplied by the pelvic splanchnic nerves rather than the vagus.

Large Intestine

- Extends from ileocecal valve to anus.
- Site of fluid and electrolyte reabsorption.
- Lack villi (unlike small intestine).
- **Does not** secrete enzymes or have enzymes along brush border (unlike small intestine).
- Has goblet cells, absorptive cells, microvilli (see Chapter 2).

Segment	Blood Supply	Description
Cecum	SMA; cecal branches, appendicular artery (to appendix)	"Blind sac". Ileocecal valve enters. Verminform appendix. Lymphoid tissue.
Colon ■ Ascending ■ Transverse ■ Descending ■ Sigmoid	SMA—Ileocolic, right colic SMA—Middle colic IMA—Left colic IMA—Sigmoid	1/4 length of small intestine. Larger diameter than small intestine. **Teniae coli** (3 smooth muscle bands). **Haustra** (pouches created by teniae). **Epiploic appendages** (fat globules on serosal surface). Ascending and descending colon are retroperitoneal.
Rectum	SMA—Superior rectal artery Internal iliac— ■ Middle rectal arteries (of hypogastric)	From sigmoid to anus. Straight. Located with in pelvic cavity. **No** teniae. **No** Haustra. **No** epiploic appendages.
Anal canal	Internal iliac— ■ Inferior rectal (of internal pudendal)	Last 3–4 cm of rectum. Internal sphincter (involuntary). External sphincter (volunatary).

PEYER'S PATCHES

- Subepithelial, nonencapsulated lymphoid tissue (like tonsils).
- Located in ileum (small intestine).
- Limit numbers of harmful bacteria.

Retroperitoneal Structures

See Figure 1–72.

- **Not** suspended from mesenteries.
- Plastered against posterior body wall, behind the peritoneum.

Each part of the colon alternates between retroperitoneal and intraperitoneal.

- *Ascending colon (retroperitoneal)*
- *Transverse colon (intraperitoneal)*
- *Descending colon (retroperitoneal)*
- *Sigmoid (intraperitoneal)*
- *Rectum (retroperitoneal)*

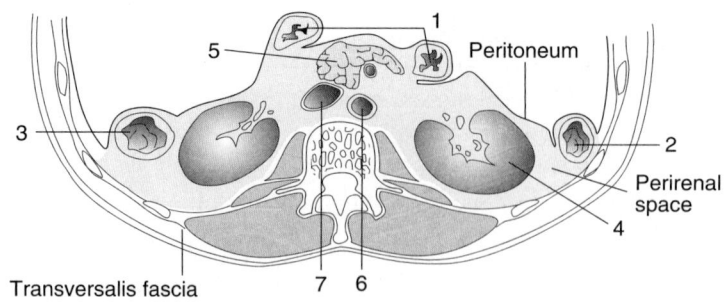

FIGURE 1-72. Retroperitoneal structures.

Reproduced, with permission, from Bushhan V, et al. *First Aid for the USMLE Step 1*. New York: McGraw-Hill, 2003.

Posterior Abdominal Muscles

Muscle	Innervation
Psoas major and minor	Lumbar plexus
Quadratus lumborum	Lumbar plexus
Iliacus	Femoral nerve

Pancreas

Bile and pancreatic enzymes are released at ampulla of Vater into the second part of duodenum.

- Lobulated gland.
- Extends from curve of duodenum to spleen.
- Retroperitoneal (except for small portion of tail).
- **Head** (from ventral bud)
  - Lies in the C (concavity) of the duodenum.
  - Located to right of midline (anterior to origin of SMA).
  - Extends from L1–3.
- **Body:** Extends across; splenic vein lies underneath.
- **Tail:** Abuts spleen hilum (in lienorenal ligament).

PANCREATIC DUCTS

- **Duct of Wirsung** (main pancreatic duct)
  - Begins at tail and joins common bile duct to form ampulla of Vater (hepatopancreatic ampulla), where it empties into duodenum.
- **Santorini's duct** (accessory pancreatic duct)
  - Opens separately into duodenum (when present).

Adrenal Gland

- Triangular glands.
- Located in adipose tissue on superior aspect of kidneys.

ADRENAL CORTEX

- Develops from mesoderm (**unlike** medulla).

ADRENAL MEDULLA

- Modified nervous tissue (like postganglionic sympathetic cells).
- Develops from neuroectoderm.
  - Neural crest cells differentiate into medullary cells (chromaffin cells).
- Releases
  - Epinephrine.
  - Norepinephrine.
- Same effect as direct sympathetic stimulation but lasts longer.
- **Can** live without adrenal medulla because postganglionic cells provide same function and will compensate for the loss.

Urinary System

- Consists of:
  - Kidneys (2).
  - Ureters (2).
  - Urinary bladder.
  - Urethra.
- Lined with transitional epithelium.
- Parasympathetic fibers from pelvic splanchnic nerve.
- Kidneys, ureters, and bladder are all retroperitoneal.

Kidney

See Figure 1–73.

- Retroperitoneal.
- Upper portion protected by ribs 11 and 12.
- Left kidney attached to the spleen by the lienorenal ligament.

URETER

- Long slender muscular tubes (peristalse).
- Transports urine from kidney to urinary bladder.
- Travels in retroperitoneal location.

As ureter enters pelvic cavity it crosses over the top of the common iliac artery (at its point of bifurcation) and dives deep into the pelvis.

URETHRA

- Passes urine from bladder to outside.
- Female: 4 cm; opens into vestibule (between clitoris and vagina).
- Male: 20 cm; travels through penis; also conveys semen.

Females are more prone to urinary infections because of the shorter urethra.

URINARY BLADDER

- Distensible sac in pelvic cavity; posterior to pubic symphysis.
- Holds urine.

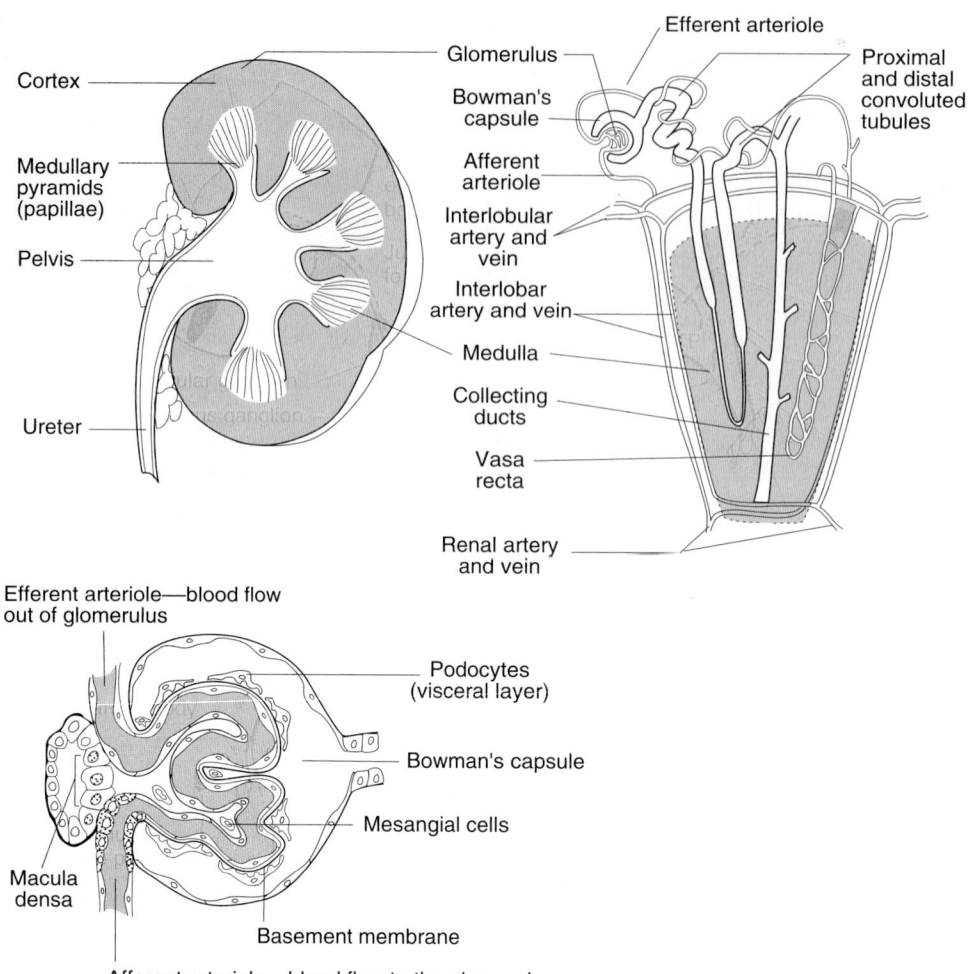

FIGURE 1-73. Structure of the kidney.

Reproduced, with permission, from Bushhan V, et al. *First Aid for the USMLE Step 1*. New York: McGraw-Hill, 2003. (Adapted from McPhee S, et al. *Pathophysiology of Disease: An Introduction to Clinical Medicine*, 3rd ed. New York, McGraw-Hill, 2000:296.)

Pelvic Cavity

- From anterior to posterior:
  - Bladder
  - Uterus
  - Rectum
- **Females:** Paired ovaries and single uterus
  - Vesicouterine pouch
    - Between bladder and uterus
  - Rectouterine pouch
  - Between rectum and uterus
- **Males:** Paired ductus deferens and seminal vesicles, and single prostate
  - Rectovesicle pouch
    - Between rectum and bladder

Inguinal Canal

- **Males:** Spermatic cord.
  - Suspends the testes within the scrotum.
- **Females:** Round ligament of the uterus.
  - Fibromuscular band attached to the uterus extending from fallopian tube, through inguinal canal to labia majora.

The inguinal canal is larger in males than females.

SPERMATIC CORD

Layers	Contents
External spermatic fascia	Ductus deferens
Cremaster muscle	Testicular artery
Internal spermatic fascia	Pampiniform plexus
Loose areolar tissue	Vessels and nerves of ductus deferens
Remnants of the processus vaginalis	

- **Ductus deferens:** Conveys epididymis from testis to ejaculatory duct.
- **Ejaculatory duct** (ductus deferens + seminal vesicle ducts): Empties into prostatic urethra.
- **Pampiniform veins:** Form the testicular vein.
  - Left testicular vein drains into left renal vein.
  - Right testicular vein drains into the IVC.

DEFECATION

- Mediated by pelvic and pudendal nerves.
- Internal sphincter relaxes
  - Pelvic nerve (senses distention then reflexively relaxes internal sphincter).
- External anal sphincter contracts
  - Pudendal nerve.
- Conscious urge to defecate is sensed.

▶ NEUROANATOMY

Nervous System

- Peripheral nervous system = Somatic.
- Autonomic system = Visceral.
- Myenteric nervous system = GI, intrinsic.

Central nervous system = Brain + spinal cord.

Brain

See the "Embryology" section in Chapter 4 for derivation.

CEREBRUM

See Figure 1–74 for functions of the cerebral cortex.

- Is 80% of brain mass.
- Has five paired lobes within two cerebral hemispheres.
- Commands higher function.
- See also the section "Humunculus" in Chapter 4.

Component	Description
Cerebral cortex	Gray matter externally (6 layers)
Cerebral medulla	Internal white matter (myelinated)
Corpus callosum	White matter tracts; connect the two hemispheres

Area	Function
Frontal lobe (precentral gyrus: 4)	Primary motor area
Frontal lobe	Frontal association areas; executive function
Parietal lobe (postcentral gyrus: 3, 1, 2)	Primary sensory area
Parietal lobe	Taste (tongue distribution on homunculus)
Parietal lobe	Integration and interpretation areas
Temporal lobe	Olfaction Hearing/auditory cortex
Occipital	Visual cortext (17)

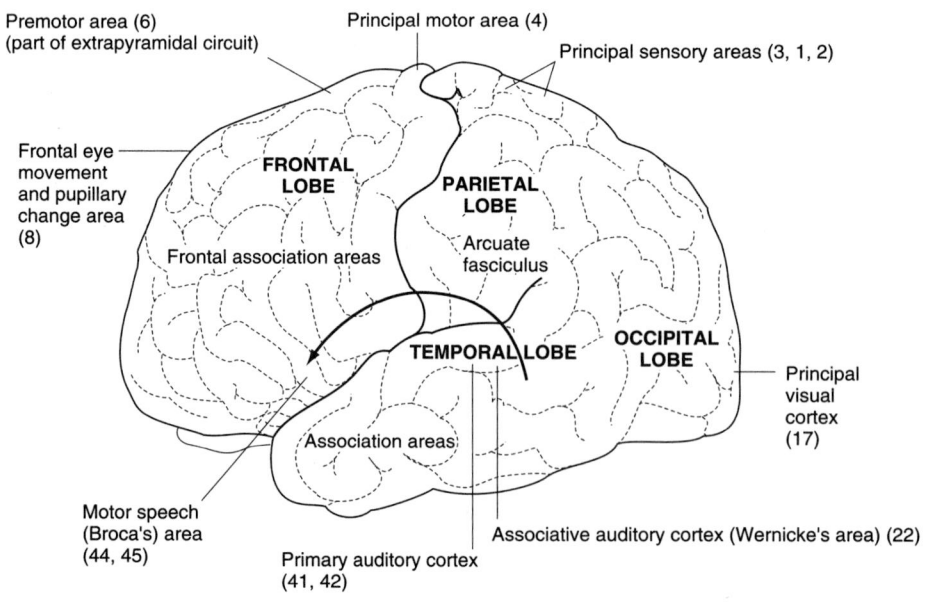

Figure 1–74. Cerebral cortex functions.

Reproduced, with permission, from Bushhan V, et al. *First Aid for the USMLE Step 1*. New York: McGraw-Hill, 2003.

Basal nuclei modulate motor activity first initiated from area 4 precentral gyrus of frontal lobe.

Diencephalon

The diencephalon consists of:

- Thalamus.
- Hypothalamus.
- Epithalamus.
  - Pineal gland is located within epithalamus.
    - Releases melatonin (as does hypothalamus); plays a role in:
      - Circadian rhythms/sleep—wake cycle.
      - Body temperature regulation.
      - Appetite.
- Pituitary gland (See Chapters 2 and 17).

Remember: Diencephalon contributes to Rathke's pouch (forming part of posterior pituitary).

	General	Nuclei	Functions
Thalamus	Sensory relay station	Lateral geniculate	Visual
		Medial geniculate	Auditory
		Ventral posterior lateral (VPL)	Proprioception, pressure, touch, vibration
		Ventral posterior medial (VPM)	**Facial sensation (including pain)**
		Ventral anterior/ventral lateral	Motor
Hypothalamus	Body homeostasis	Ventromedial nucleus	Satiety center (hyperphagia with bilateral destruction; decreases urge to eat with stimulation)
		Lateral nucleus	Hunger center (starvation with destruction; increase eating with stimulation)
		Septal nucleus	Aggressive behavior
		Suprachiasmatic nucleus	Circadian rhythms; input from retina
		Supraoptic nucleus	Water balance; ADH, oxytocin production

Cerebellum

Function	Components
Coordinates muscle movement. Maintains equilibrium and posture. Receives proprioceptive inputs and position sense (e.g., dorsal columns).	**Purkinje cells:** Project to deep cerebellar nuclei (which then project out of cerebellum). **Climbing fibers:** Afferents to cerebellum. **Golgi cell bodies** **Granule cells** **Mossy fibers:** All afferents to cerebellum (except climbing fibers).

Brainstem

See Figure 1–75 for a ventral view of the brainstem.

- Connects cerebrum and spinal cord (fiber tracts to and from spinal cord pass).
- Embryologically is the midbrain + hindbrain.
- Cranial nerves (3–12) originate from brainstem.
- Basic life functions:
  - Respiration.
  - Swallowing.
  - Heart rate.
  - Arousal.

Segment	Comments
Midbrain	Auditory and visual reflex
Pons	Relay station Respiratory center
Medulla oblongata	Relay station Respiratory, cardiac, vasomotor centers Reflexes: coughing, gagging, swallowing, vomiting

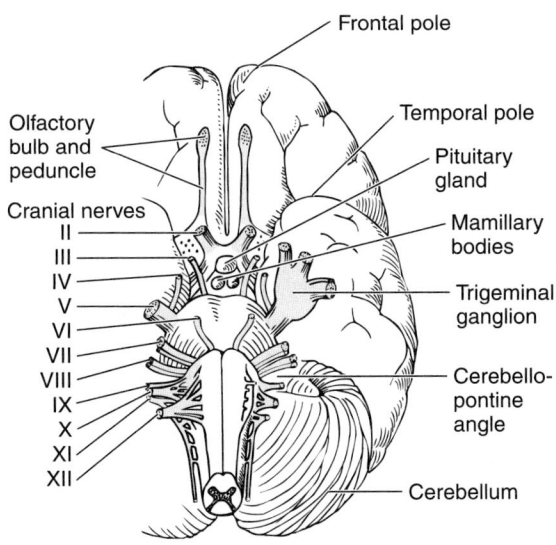

FIGURE 1-75. Ventral view of the brainstem with cranial verves.

Reproduced, with permission, from Waxman SG. *Clinical Neuroanatomy.* 25th ed. McGraw-Hill, 2003.

Important Brainstem Nuclei

		Nuclei (CN)	**Function**
Efferent (motor/ parasympathetic)	Receive higher levels information (e.g., cortical) then project efferent neurons to end organs (via ganglia in the case of parasympathetics).	**Superior salivatory nucleus (VII)**	Salivation (submandibular, sublingual glands), Glandular secretion
		Inferior salivatory nuclei (IX)	Salivation (parotid)
		Nucleus ambiguous (IX, X)	Swallowing
Afferent (sensory)	Receives sensory information and relays this to the thalamus and cortex.	**Nucleus of the solitary tract (VII, IX, X)**	Taste

All cranial nerves (except I and II) originate from the brainstem.
Tracts: Olfactory, Optic; no nuclei for CNs I and II.

All cranial nerve motor nuclei have unilateral corticonuclear connections except:
- *CN VII: Upper third M's facial expression bilateral innervation.*
- *CN XII: Genioglossus M. has bilateral motor innervation.*

All cranial nerve sensory nuclei have unilateral representation except hearing. Hearing is bilateral; you can't go deaf in one ear from a stroke to the unilateral temporal area.

The mnemonic for the cranial nerves is On Old Olympus Topmost Top A Fat Aged German Viewed Some Hops.

Cranial Nerves

- Olfactory (I)
- Optic (II)
- Oculomotor (III)
- Troclear (IV)
- Trigeminal (V)
- Abducens (VI)
- Facial (VII)
- Vestibulocochlear/Auditory (VIII)
- Glossopharyngeal (IX)
- Vagus (X)
- Spinal Accessory (XI)
- Hypoglossal (XII)

CANIAL NERVE COMPONENTS

See Table 1–3 for a complete chart of the cranial nerves.

- **Sensory:** I, II, VIII
- **Motor:** III, IV, VI, XI, XII
- **Sensory and Motor:** V, VII, IX, X

Preganglionic parasympathetics are provided by CN III (ciliary ganglion), VII (pterygomandibular and submandibular ganglia), IX (otic ganglion), and X (small terminal ganglia).

Characteristic		Cranial Nerves
General Afferent	Sensory	V, VII, IX, X
	Proprioceptive	V, VII
Special afferent (*special sense*)		I, II, VII, VIII, IX, XI
Voluntary efferent (*motor to skeletal muscle*)		III, IV, V, VI, VII, IX, X, XI, XII
Involuntary efferent (*parasympathetic to smooth muscle or glands*)		III, VII, IX, X

Parasympathetic Ganglia (and Cranial Nerves)

Ganglion	Location	Parasympathetic Root	Sympathetic Root	Distribution
Ciliary	Lateral to optic nerve	CN III	Internal carotid plexus	Ciliary muscle Spincter pupillae Dilator Pupillae Tarsal muscles
Pterygopalatine	Pterygopalatine fossa (on branch of V2)	Greater petrosal (CN VII) N. of pterygoid canal	Internal carotid plexus	Lacrimal gland Glands in palate and nose
Otic	Just distal to Foramen ovale (on trunk of V3)	Lesser petrosal (CN IX) (and tympanic branch of CN IX)	Plexus associated with middle meningeal artery	Parotid gland
Submandibular	On Hyoglossus muscle (on Lingual n. of V3)	Chorda tympani (CN VII) by way of lingual nerve	Plexus on facial artery	Submandibular Sublingual small salivary glands

Sympathetic Ganglia of the Head and Neck

Ganglia	Location	Comments
Superior cervical ganglia	Lies between ICA and IJV.	Largest and responsible for most sympathetic fibers to head and neck (cell bodies of postganglionics are here); these postganglionics give rise to the plexuses in the parasympathetic ganglia chart.
Middle cervical ganglia	At level of cricoid cartilage.	Related to loop of inferior thyroid artery.
Inferior cervical ganglia	C7 vertebral level.	Fused to first thoracic sympathetic ganglion to forma stellate ganglion.

Preganglionics come from the T1-2 (ciliospinal center of Budge) where they have descended from the brainstem.

TABLE 1-3. Cranial Nerve Chart

Cranial Nerve	(Division)	To/From Skull	Type	Origin of Cell Bodies	Function	Innervated Structures Afferent	Efferent
I-Olfactory		Cribriform plate	SVA	Bipolar cells	Smell	Nasal mucosa	
II-Optic		Optic foramen	SSA	Retinal ganglion cells	Vision, Pupillary light reflexes (with CN III)	Retina	
III-Oculomotor		SOF	GSE	Oculomotor nucleus (rostral midbrain)	Ocular movements		Levator palpebrae, all extraocular muscles, except lateral rectus, superior oblique, pupillary constrictor (ciliary ganglion), ciliary muscle (ciliary ganglion)
			GVE	Edinger-Westphal nucleus (rostral midbrain) (ciliary ganglion)	Miosis, convergence, accomodation		
IV-Troclear		SOF	GSE	Trochlear nucleus (caudal midbrain)	Turns eye down and laterally		Superior oblique
VI-Abducens		SOF	GSE	Abducent nucleus (caudal pons)	Turns eye laterally		Lateral rectus
V-Trigeminal	V1 (Ophthalmic)	SOF	GSA	Trigeminal ganglion and mesencephalic nuc of CN V	Facial Sensation	Upper eyelid, globe, lacrimal gland, paranasal sinus mucous membrane, forehead skin	

TABLE 1-3. Cranial Nerve Chart (Continued)

Cranial Nerve	(Division)	To/From Skull	Type	Origin of Cell Bodies	Function	Innervated Structures Afferent	Efferent
	V2 (Maxillary)	Foramen rotundum	GSA		Sensation	Lower eyelid, mid-face skin, nose, upper lip, nasopharynx, maxillary sinus, soft palate, tonsils, hard palate, upper teeth	
	V3 (Mandibular)	Foramen ovale	GSA		Sensation	Tongue (general not taste sensation!), temporoariclar skin, lower face, lower teeth	
			SVE	Motor nucleus CN V (mid pons)	Chewing, opening, swallowing		Muscles of mastication, tensor veli platini, tensor tympani
VII-Facial		Internal acoustic meatus, stylomastoid foramen	GSA	Geniculate ganglion (facial canal of temporal bone)	Sensation	External ear, soft palate, auditory tube	
			SVA	Geniculate ganglion (facial canal)	Taste	Anterior 2/3 tongue	
			SVE	Facial nucleus (caudal pons)	Facial expression		Ms. Facial expression, stylohyoid, post digastric, stapedius

TABLE 1-3. Cranial Nerve Chart (Continued)

Cranial Nerve	(Division)	To/From Skull	Type	Origin of Cell Bodies	Function	Innervated Structures Afferent	Efferent
			GVE	Superior salivatory nucleus (caudal pons)	Secretomotor		Lacrimal gland, glands of nasopharynx and sinuses (pterygopalatine gangl)
							Submandibular and sublingual glands (submandibular ganglion)
VIII-Vestibulo-cochlear (auditory)		Internal acoustic meatus	SSA	Vestibular ganglion (int. auditory meatus)	Hearing	Organ of corti (cochlea)	
				Spiral ganglion (modiolus)	Balance	Semicircular canals (vestibular)	
IX-Glossopharyngeal		Jugular foramen	GSA	Superior ganglion (jugular foramen)	Sensation	Auricle	
			GVA	Inferior petrosal ganglion (jugular foramen)	Sensation	posterior 1/3 tongue, pharynx, middle ear	
			GVA	Inferior petrosal ganglion (jugular foramen)	Chemo-, baroreception	carotid body, carotid sinus	
			SVA	Inferior petrosal ganglion (jugular foramen)	Taste	Post 1/3 tongue	

TABLE 1-3. Cranial Nerve Chart (Continued)

Cranial Nerve	(Division)	To/From Skull	Type	Origin of Cell Bodies	Function	Innervated Structures Afferent	Efferent
			SVE	Nucleus ambiguus (rostral medulla)	Motor		Stylopharyngeus
			GVE	Inferior salivatory nucleus (rostral medulla)	Secretomotor		Parotid gland (via otic ganglion and aurioculotemporal branch of V3), parasym path of pharynx, larynx
X-Vagus		Jugular foramen	GSA	Superior ganglion (jugular foramen)	Sensation	Posterior meninges, external ear	
			GVA	Nodose ganglion (jugular foramen)	Sensation	Viscera of pharynx, larynx, thoracic and abdominal viscera (to left colic flexure)	
			SVA	Nodose ganglion (jugular foramen)	Taste	Laryngeal additus and epiglottis	
			SVE	Nucleus ambiguus (medulla)	Motor		Pharyngeal constrictors, palatopharyngeus, levator palatini, palatoglossus, laryngeal ms

TABLE 1-3. Cranial Nerve Chart (Continued)

Cranial Nerve	(Division)	To/From Skull	Type	Origin of Cell Bodies	Function	Innervated Structures Afferent	Innervated Structures Efferent
			GVE	Dorsal nucleus of CN 10 (medulla)	Secretomotor		Viscera of neck, thoracic and abdominal cavities (to left colic flexure)
XI-Spinal accessory	Cranial	Jugular foramen	SVE	Nucleus ambiguus (medulla)	Motor		Cranial-ms larynx, pharynx, esophagus
		Foramen magnum					Spinal—SCM, trapezius
	Spinal			Ventral horn C1-6			
XI-Hypoglossal		Hypoglossal canal	GVE	Hypoglossal nucleus (medulla)	Motor		All intrinsic and extrinsic muscle of tongue (not palatoglossus)

CN II—Optic Nerve

See Figure 1–76 and Table 1–3.
See also the "Physiology" section in Chapter 10 for lesions involving the optic nerve.

Course

- Ganglion cells of retina (converge at optic disc to form optic nerve).
- Leaves orbit via optic foramen/canal (sphenoid).
- Optic chiasm (two optic nerves unite at floor of diencephalons; anterior to pituitary stalk).
- Optic tracts.
- Lateral geniculate nuclei (thalamus).
- Geniculocalcarine fibers (optic radiations).
- Calcarine sulcus in the primary visual cortex (area 17) of the occipital lobe.

Important

- Nasal side fibers (most medial) decussate and go with contralateral optic tract.
- Temporal hemiretina fibers stay ipsilateral.
- Left visual field = right optic tract.
- Right visual field = left optic tract (right visual field is interpreted on left brain).

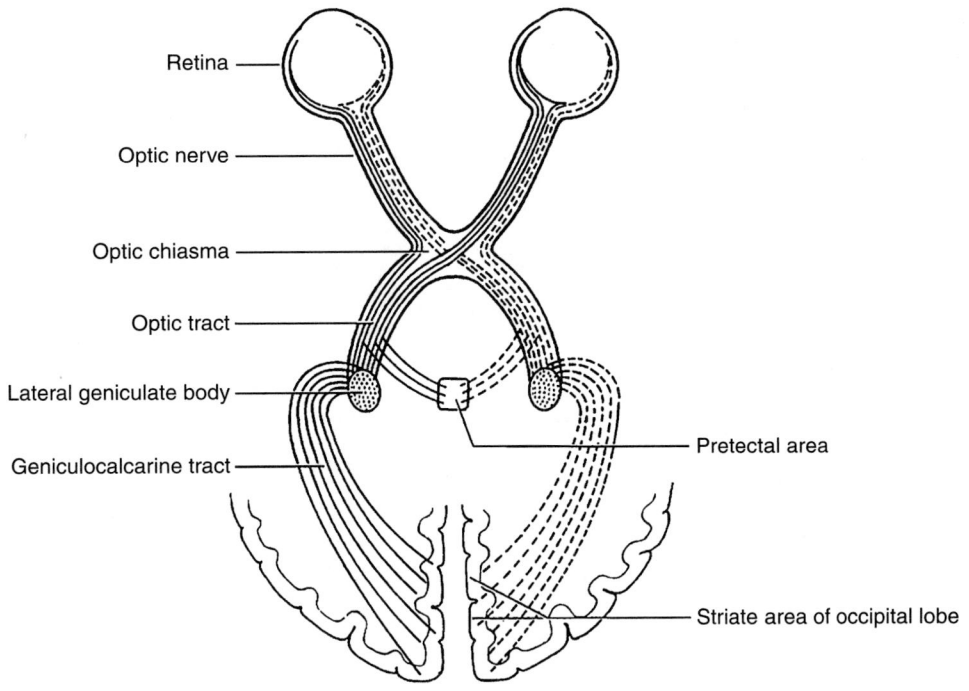

FIGURE 1–76. The optic nerve.

Reproduced, with permission, from Montgomery RL. *Head and Neck Anatomy: With Clinical Correlations.* New York: McGraw-Hill, 1981.

CNs III, IV, VI—Oculomotor, Trochlear, Abducens

See Figure 1–77.

- **Oculomotor nerve:** Controls most of the extraocular muscles, the levator palpebrae superioris, and carries parasympathetic and sympathetic control to the pupil.
- **Trochlear nerve:** Is the smallest cranial nerve and the only cranial nerve that exits from the posterior surface of the brainstem.

Extraocular Movements

Muscle	Nerve	Movement
Medial Rectus	CN III	Adduction (in)
Superior Rectus	CN III	Elevation (after abduction) (up)
Inferior rectus	CN III	Depression (after abduction) (down)
Inferior oblique	CN III	Elevation and adduction (up and in)
Superior oblique	CN IV	Depression and adduction (down and out)
Lateral rectus	CN VI	Abduction (out)

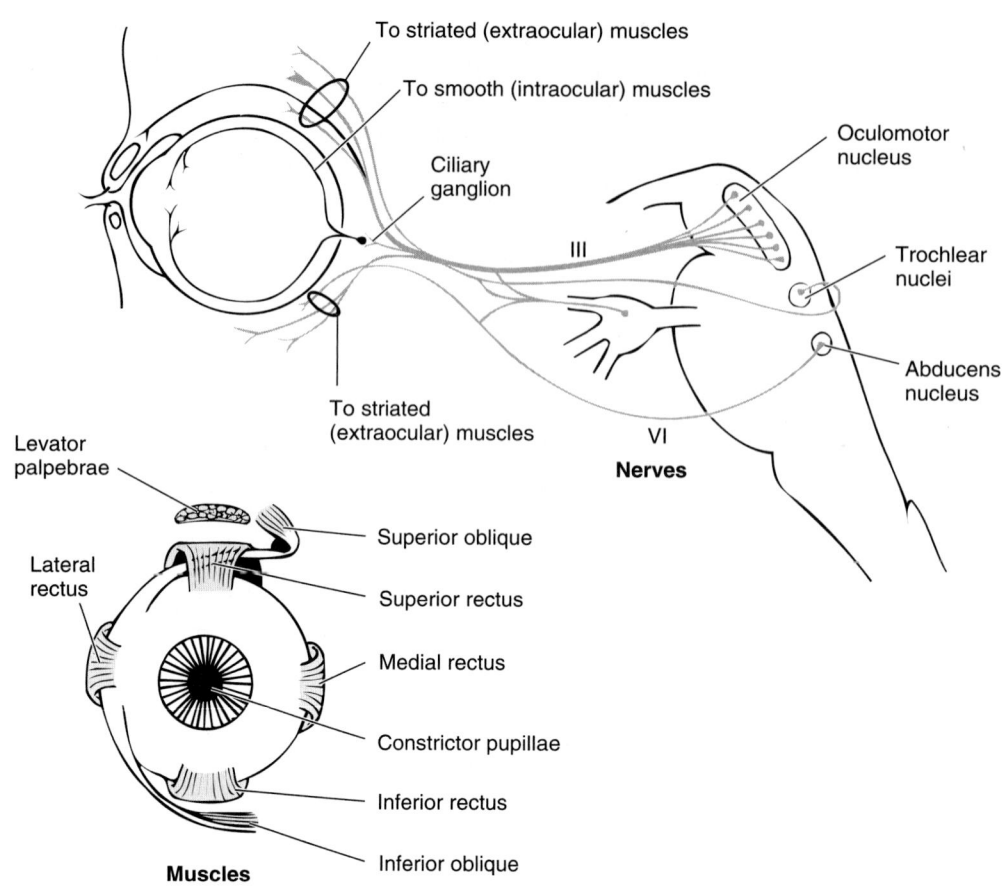

FIGURE 1-77. The occulomotor, trochlear, and abducens nverves; ocular muscles.

Reproduced, with permission, from Waxman SG. *Clinical Neuroanatomy*, 25th ed. McGraw-Hill, 2003.

EYE ELEVATORS

See Figure 1–78 for a diagram of the eye muscle action.

- **Superior rectus:** Adducts and elevates (only muscle that elevates from abducted position).
- **Inferior oblique:** Abducts and elevates (only muscle to elevate from adducted position).

Pupillary Light Reflex

- Direct and consensual papillary responses.
- Does **not** involve cortex.
- Shine light into one eye that eye (direct) pupil constricts as does the pupil of the contralateral eye (consensual).

Response	Afferent	Efferent
Direct response	Optic nerve of eye tested (ipsilateral)	CN III to the eye tested (ipsilateral)
Consensual response	Optic nerve of eye tested (ipsilateral)	CN III of opposite eye (contralateral)

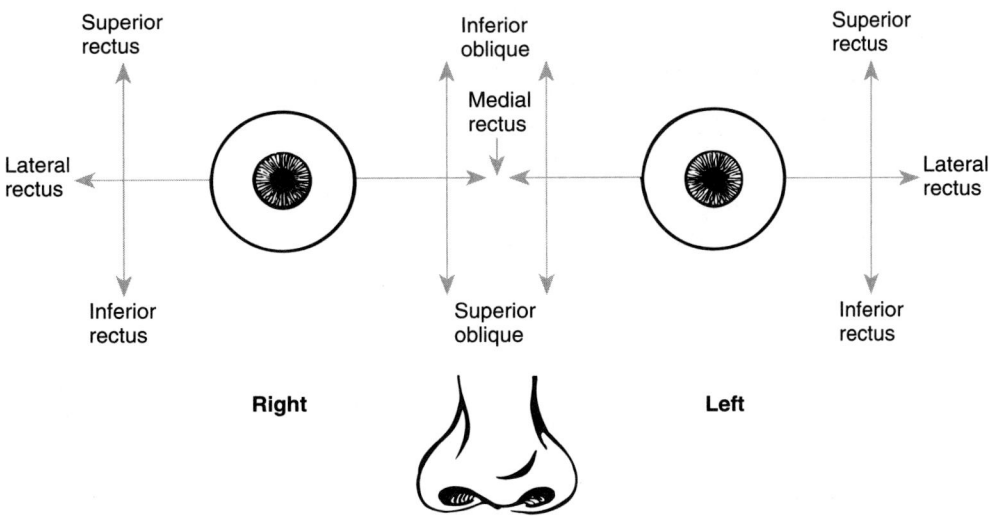

FIGURE 1–78. Diagram of eye muscle action.

Reproduced, with permission, from Waxman SG. *Clinical Neuroanatomy*, 25th ed. McGraw-Hill, 2003.

Pathway/Reflex Arc

See Figure 1–79.

- Optic nerve
- Edinger-Westphal nucleus (midbrain) bilaterally
- Ciliary ganglia
- Short ciliary nerve (post-ganglionic)
- Constrictor pupillae muscle

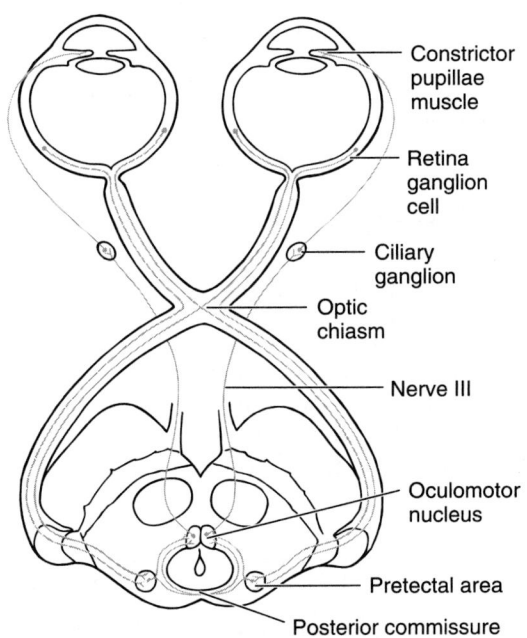

FIGURE 1–79. The path of the papillary light reflex.

Reproduced, with permission, from Waxman SG. *Clinical Neuroanatomy*. 25th ed. McGraw-Hill, 2003.

ACCOMODATION AND CONVERGENCE

- Gazing from distant to near, pupils constrict (accommodate), eyes move midline (converge), lenses become more convex.

Pathway

- Optic nerve
- Geniculate body
- Visual association cortex
- Frontal eye fields
- Edinger-Westphal nuclei and main oculomotor nuclei (both in midbrain)
- Constrictor pupillae muscle and medial recti, respectively

LESION

- Blurred vision with a lesion to any of CN III, IV, VI.
- Ptosis (drooping eyelid) and dilated pupil with CN III injury (levator palpebrae superioris and sphincter pupillae muscle).
- Lesion CN VI eye persistently directed toward nose (because of lateral rectus).

Lesion	Description
Ophthalmoplegia	**Internal:** EOMs spared, selective loss of autonomically innervated sphincter and ciliary muscles (because parasympathetic fibers are more peripheral, can be compressed). **External:** Paralysis of all EOMs (except superior oblique, rectus); sphincter and ciliary muscles spared (as with DM neuropathy).
Internuclear ophthalmoplegia	Lesion within the medial longitudinal fasciculus—lose connection III, IV, VI. If lesion on right—look laterally to the right, both eyes move look laterally to left, only left eye moves (right eye medial rectus does not pull it medially); however with accommodation, both medial recti work.
Relative afferent (Marcus-Gunn) pupil	Lesion in optic nerve (afferent limb of papillary light relflex, e.g., MS optic neuritis). Swinging flashlight test—both pupils constrict when shine light in good eye; quickly swing to contralateral eye and both pupils dilate.
Horner's syndrome	Lesion of oculosympathetic pathway (sympathetics don't come from CNs but run with them; come from superior cervical ganglion, ciliospinal center of Budge); miosis, ptosis, hemianhidrosis, apparent enophthalmos.
Argyll Robertson pupil (pupillary light-near dissociation)	Think prostitute's pupil—accommodates but does not react; also associated with syphilis. No miosis (papillary constriction) with either direct or consensual light; does constrict with near stimulus (accommodation-convergence). Occurs in syphilis and diabetes.

CN V—Trigeminal Nerve

- Largest cranial nerve.
- Trigeminal or gasserian ganglion—in the middle cranial fossa.
- Three divisions leave through foramina in the sphenoid bone.
- **Sensory (GSA):** Facial sensation (light touch; pain and temperature; proprioception)
  - Divisions V1, V2, V3.
- **Efferent (SVE):** Motor to muscles of mastication, tensor veli palatini, tensor tympani.
  - Division V3.
- **No** parasympathetic fibers are contained with the trigeminal nerve at its origin; other nerves distribute parasympathetic preganglionics by way of trigeminal branches.
  - Oculomotor (III).
  - Facial nerve (VII).
  - Glossopharyngeal nerve (IX).

V1 and V2 are purely sensory; V3 is both sensory and motor.

Remember: *The buccinator nerve of V-3 provides sensation to the cheek; whereas the buccal branch of CN VII is motor to the buccinator muscle.*

TRIGEMINAL NERVE DIVISIONS

See Figure 1–80 for the trigeminal nerve and its branches.

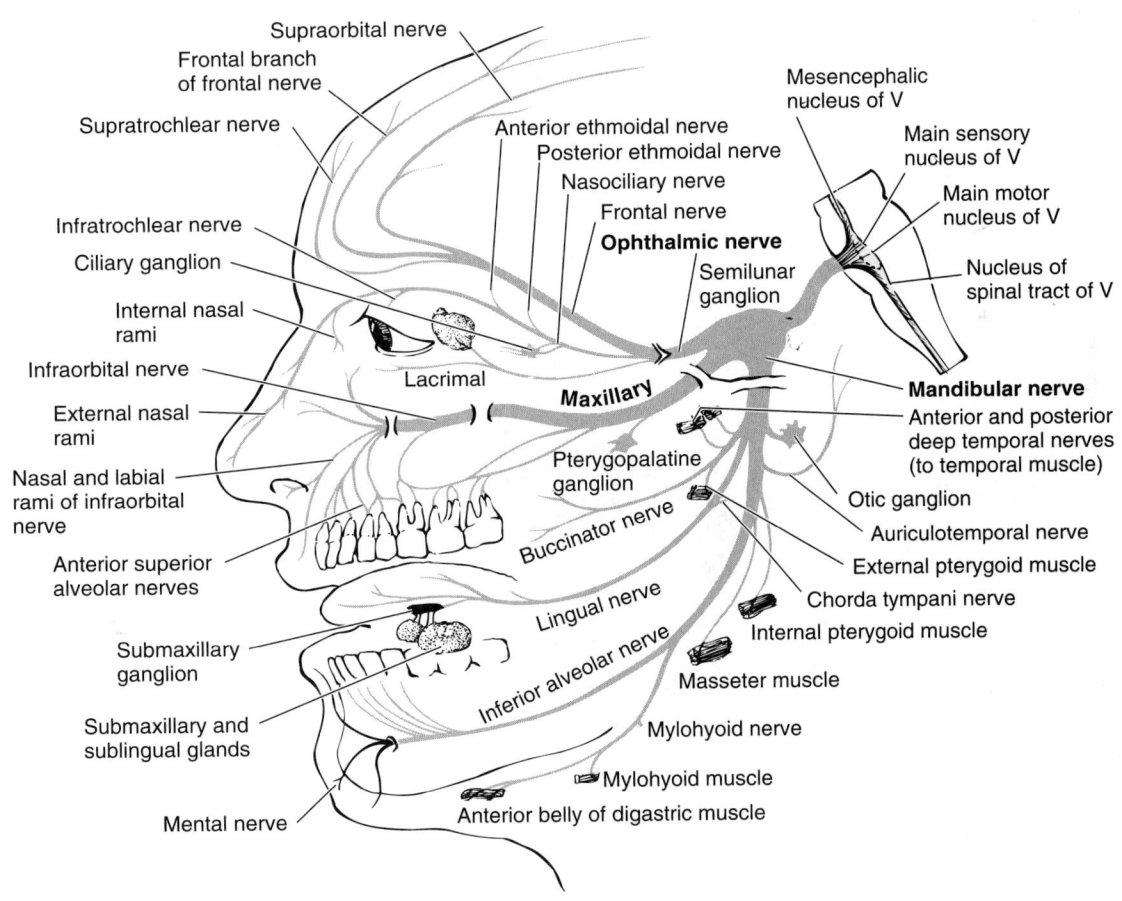

FIGURE 1-80. The trigeminal nerve and its branches.

Reproduced, with permission, from Waxman SG. *Clinical Neuroanatomy*, 25th ed. McGraw-Hill, 2003.

Division	Sensory	Motor
Ophthalmic (V1)	Upper eyelid, cornea, conjunctiva, frontal sinus, upper nasal mucosa, forehead	N/A
Maxillary (V2)	Lower eyelid, upper cheek, lip, gums, palate, nose, tonsils, hard palate, upper teeth	N/A
Mandibular (V3)	Tongue (general), temporoauricular skin, lower face, lower teeth	Muscles of mastication, tensor tympani, mylohyoid, anterior belly of digastric, tensor veli palatini

IMPORTANT BRANCHES OF V3

Nerve	Distribution
Lingual nerve	**General sensation:** Anterior 2/3 of tongue, floor of mouth, and mandibular lingual gingival. *Carries* [from chorda tympani (VII)]: **Taste sensation:** Anterior 2/3 tongue. **Preganglionic parasympathetics:** To submandibular ganglion.
Auriculotemporal nerve	**Sensory:** Front of ear, TMJ. **Postganglionic parasympathetic:** To parotid gland.
Inferior alveolar nerve	Gives off nerve to mylohyoid and inferior dental plexus; terminates as mental nerve. **Motor** to mylohyoid. **Sensory** to teeth, skin of chin, lower lip.
Mental nerve	Termination of inferior alveolar nerve. **Sensory** to skin of chin, skin and mucous membrane of lower lip.
Motor branches	**Motor to** muscles of mastication, anterior digastric, and so on.

INFERIOR ALVEOLAR NERVE BLOCK

- Anesthetize the mandibular teeth.
- Block this branch of V3 as it enters the mandibular foramen.

Needle Course

See Figure 1–81.

- Pierces:
    - Buccinator (between palatoglossal and palatopharyngeal folds).
    - Lies lateral to medial pterygoid at the mandibular foramen.
- If the needle penetrates too far posteriorly can hit parotid gland and CN VII:
    - Ipsilateral facial paralysis.

The lingual nerve is found in the pterygomandibular space with the inferior alveolar nerve, artery, and vein. The lingual artery does **not** run with the lingual nerve. The lingual artery is medial to the hyoglossus muscle, whereas the lingual vein and nerve are lateral to the hyoglossus (as is the submandibular duct and hypoglossal nerve [XII]).

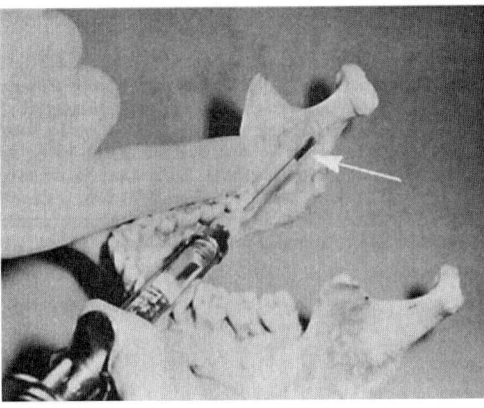

Figure 1–81. Needle Course.

Reproduced, with permission, from Montgomery RL. *Head and Neck Anatomy: With Clinical Correlations.* New York: McGraw-Hill, 1981.

The submandibular duct is crossed twice by the lingual nerve.

If the lingual nerve is cut after the chorda tympani joins, you lose **both** taste and tactile sensation.

Lingual Nerve

The lingual nerve can be damaged with third molar extraction because it lies close to the mandibular ramus in the vicinity of the third molar.

Course	Information	Chorda Tympani (VII) Component
Lies deep to the lateral pterygoid muscle, anteromedial to the inferior alveolar nerve (chorda tympani (from VII) joins here). Runs between the medial pterygoid and the mandibular ramus to enter the side of the tongue obliquely. Continues forward between the hyoglossus and deep part of the submandibular gland. Submandibular ganglion hangs from lingual nerve on top of hyoglossus muscle. Finally runs across the submandibular duct to lie at the tongue tip (beneath the mucous membrane).	**General sensation:** Anterior 2/3 of tongue, floor of mouth, and mandibular lingual gingiva.	Chorda tympani (of VII) contributes: - Preganglinic parasympathetic fibers to ganglion. submandibular - Taste fibers to anterior 2/3 of tongue.

TRIGEMINAL NUCLEI

- There are four paired nuclei (both motor and sensory).

Nuclei	Location	Comments
Motor (masticatory) nucleus	Lateral pons	Motor information originates in the motor (area 4) and premotor (area 6) cortices. This information is modulated by the basal ganglia and striatal motor systems then: Descends as corticobulbar tracts to the: Motor nucleus of the trigeminal where: LMNs then project past the trigeminal ganglion (without synapse) to the: Respective effector muscles.
Sensory nucleus	Pons	All sensory information from the face is relayed through **VPM nucleus of thalamus** (VPL for the body). From here information relays to the: **Somatosensory cortex** (areas 3, 1, 2) - The facial segment of the sensory homunculus comprises a large area of the lateral parietal lobe.
Spinal trigeminal nucleus	Midpons to cervical cord	Pain/temperature from the face travel to the spinal trigeminal nucleus (pain/temperature from body travel in the spinothalamic tract).
Mesencephalic nucleus	Upper pons, midbrain border	Proprioceptive inputs are **not** located within the trigeminal ganglia (all other afferent cell bodies are). Proprioceptive inputs synapse in the mesencephalic nucleus.

Proprioceptive fibers from muscles and TMJ are found only in the mandibular division (V-3).

Facial Sensation

CN V

- All sensory information from the face is relayed through VPM nucleus of thalamus; sensory info from the rest of the body is through the VPL.
- From the thalamic nuclei (VPM or VPL), information relays to the somatosensory cortex (areas 3, 1, 2); the facial segment of the sensory homunculus comprises a large area of the lateral parietal lobe.
- Remember, parts of CNs VII and IX travel with trigeminospinal tract.
- All CN V afferent cell bodies are located within trigeminal ganglion **except** proprioceptive inputs.
- Mesencephalic nucleus of CN V is the only case where primary sensory cell bodies are located within the CNS, rather than in ganglia.

Modality	Fiber Type	Tract	1st-Order Neuron	2nd-Order Neuron	3rd-Order Neuron
Touch and pressure	A-beta fibers	Dorsal trigeminothalamic tract (via Meissner's and Pacini's corpuscles)	Trigeminal ganglion, (principal sensory nucleus of CN V).	Principal sensory nucleus of CN V projects to ipsilateral VPM (doesn't cross over).	VPM projects through posterior internal capsule to the face area of somatosensory cortex.
Pain and temperature	A-delta C-fibers	Ventral trigeminothalamic tract	Trigeminal ganglion; then axons descend in the spinal trigeminal tract and synapse with the spinal trigeminal nucleus.	From the spinal trigeminal nucleus, ascend and **cross over** to the contralateral VPM.	From VPM, project via posterior limb of posterior capsule to the face area of somatosensory cortex
Proprioception	A-alpha fibers (stretch and tendon receptors in muscles of mastication)	Spinocerebellar tract	Afferents pass the trigeminal ganglia (without synapse).	Mesencephalic nucleus (within the CNS). Motor nucleus (many central fibers from mesencephalic nucleus synapse here to create reflex arc).	Cerebellum

Sensation in teeth can be misinterpreted in ear (because of the cross innervation).

Herpes zoster oft affects V1 division. Trigeminal neuralgia (tic douloureux) can affect V2, V3.

Sensory Information in the Face versus Body

	Face	Body
Touch and pressure	Trigeminal main sensory nucleus Dorsal trigeminothalamic tract VPM	Gracile and cuneate nuclei Dorsal columns Medial lemniscus VPL
Pain and temperature	Spinal trigeminal nucleus Ventral trigeminothalamic tract VPM, periaqueductal grey, reticular formation	Dorsal root ganglion Lissauers tract Spinothalamic tract VPL, periaqueductal grey, reticular formation
Proprioception	Mesencephalic nucleus Spinocerebellar tract Cerebellum	Clarke's nucleus Spinocerebellar tract Cerebellum

FACIAL SENSATION

See Figure 1–82 for areas of facial sensation.
See Figure 1–83 for cutaneous innervation of the face, scalp, and uricle.
See Figure 1–84 for innervation of the external ear.

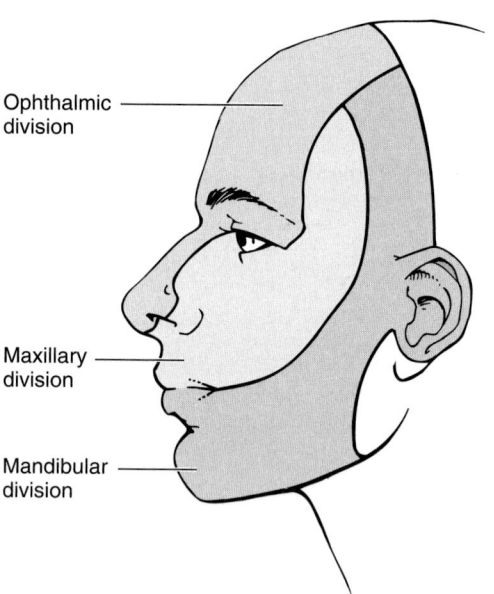

FIGURE 1-82. Sensory distribution of nerve V.

Reproduced, with permission, from Montgomery RL. *Head and Neck Anatomy: With Clinical Correlations.* New York: McGraw-Hill, 1981.

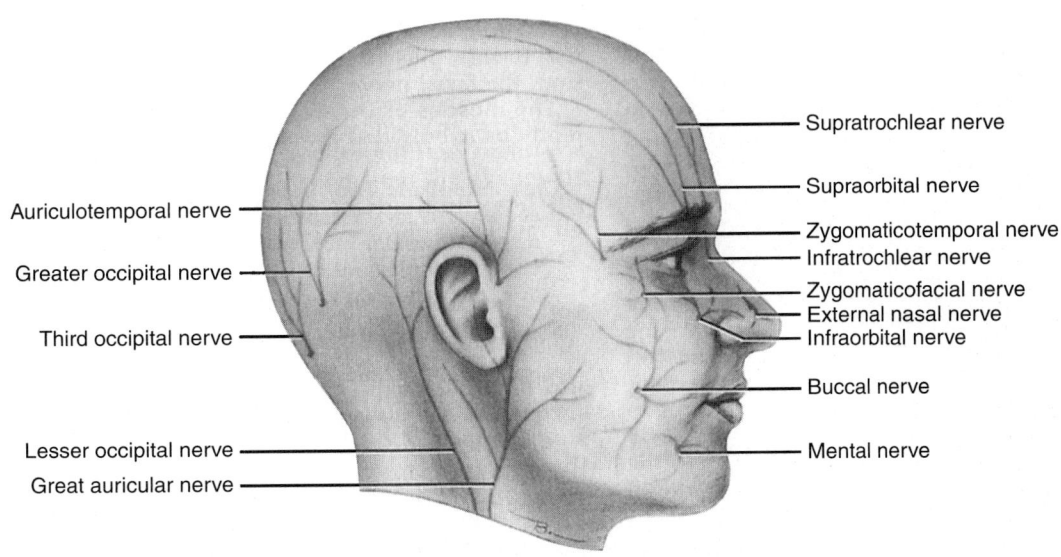

FIGURE 1-83. Cutaneous innervation of the face, scalp, and auricle.

Reproduced, with permission, from Montgomery RL. *Head and Neck Anatomy: With Clinical Correlations.* New York: McGraw-Hill, 1981.

Sensation of External Ear

Nerve	Distribution
Auriculotemporal nerve (V-3)	Anterior half of external ear canal and facial surface of upper part of auricle
Auricular branch of vagus (X)	Posterior half of external ear canal (so stimulation can cause reflex symptoms: e.g., fainting, coughing, gagging).
Greater auricular nerve (C2, C3)	Inferior auricle (anterior and posterior)
Lesser occipital nerve (C2, C3)	Cranial surface of upper auricle

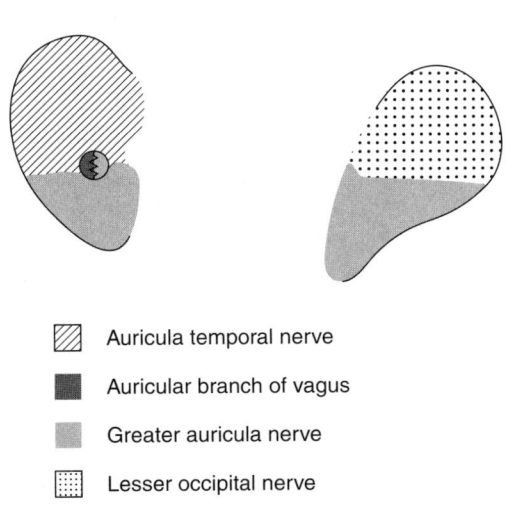

Auricula temporal nerve
Auricular branch of vagus
Greater auricula nerve
Lesser occipital nerve

FIGURE 1-84. Innervation of the external ear.

Corneal reflex: *If stimulating right eye:*
- Lesion R V1 neither eye blinks.
- Lesion L V1 bilateral blink.
- Lesion R VII only left eye blinks (indirect).
- Lesion L VII only right eye blinks (direct).

- Levator palpebrae superioris (CN III) keeps the eyelid open; lesion results in ptosis.
- Orbicularis oculi (CN VII) closes eyelid; lesion results in inability to close, no corneal reflex.

Trigeminal Lesions

Type	Location	Finding
Sensory	Division V1, 2, 3	Deficits along distribution (pain, temp, touch, pressure, proprioception)
Motor	Division V1 only	Temporalis and masseter muscles ■ Ipsilateral weakness of jaw closure ■ Ipsilateral open bite Pteygoid muscle ■ Weakness of jaw opening ■ Deviation to ipsilateral side on opening Diminished/loss of reflexes

Facial Reflexes (Involving CN V)

Reflex	Description	Afferent	Efferent	Comments
Corneal reflex	Touch cornea with cotton causes both eyes to close.	V1	CN VII (orbicularis oculi)	**Pathway** ■ Cornea (V1). ■ Main sensory nucleus of trigeminal. ■ Medial longitudinal fasciculus. ■ Main motor nucleus of facial nerve (CN VII). ■ Orbicularis oculi muscle). ■ Causes ipsilateral (**direct**) and contralaterl (**indirect**) eye blinking.
Jaw jerk reflex	Mouth open and relaxed; tap chin lightly to get contraction/mouth closure.	V3—proprioceptive	V3—motor	Reflex is lost only with bilateral CN V lesions (uncommon).

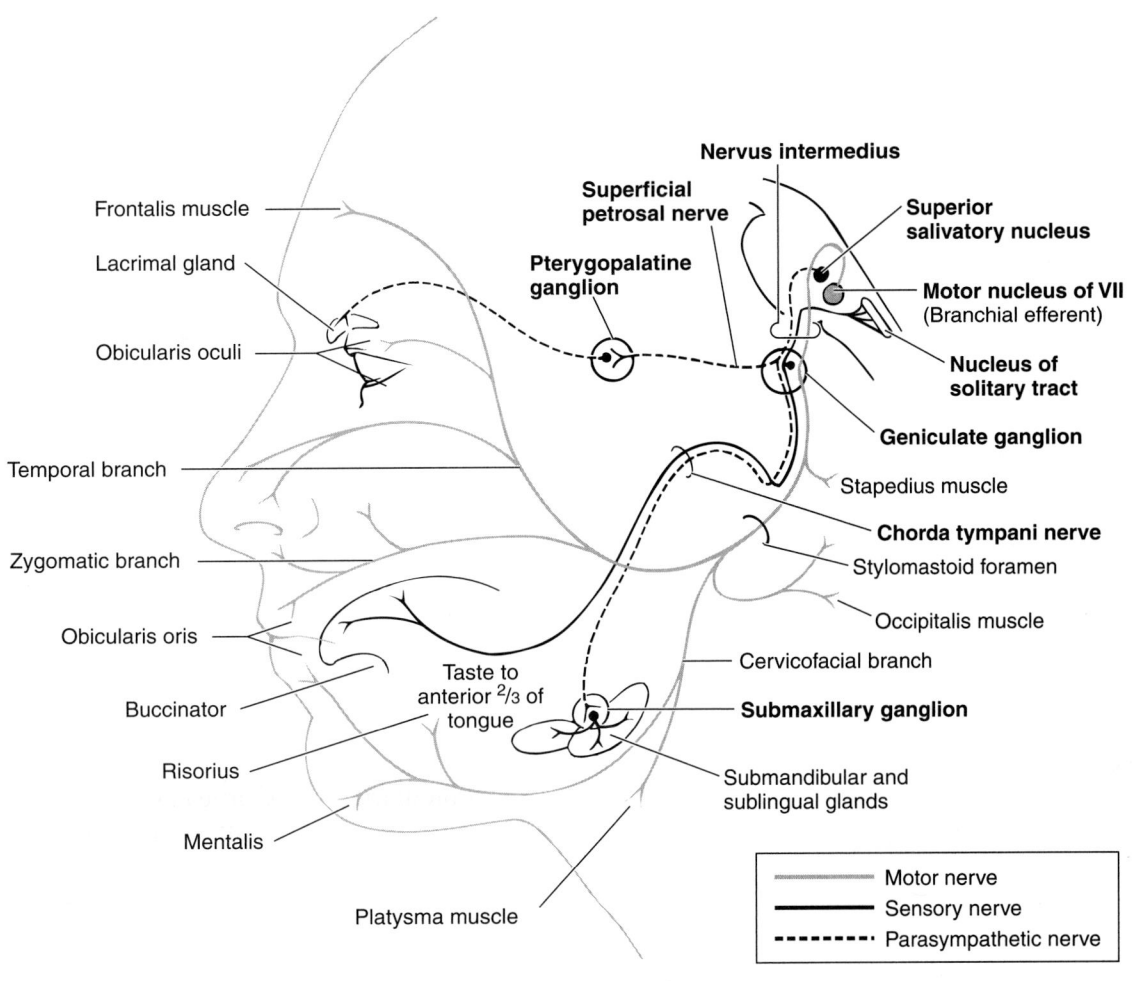

FIGURE 1-85. **The facial nerve.**

Reproduced, with permission, from Waxman SG. *Clinical Neuroanatomy*, 25th ed. McGraw-Hill, 2003.

CN VII–Facial Nerve

See Figure 1–85.

Course

- Originates in pons.
- Enters internal acoustic meatus.
- Passes through facial canal.
- Exits skull via stylomastoid foramen.
- Courses through the parotid gland (inadvertent deposition of anesthetic into parotid can result in facial paresis).
- Motor branches.

Components

- Motor
- Sensory
- Secretomotor (parasympathetic):
  - Lacrimal gland
  - Submandibular gland
  - Sublingual gland
- Special sense
  - Taste anterior two thirds of tongue, floor of mouth, palate

CN VII Nuclei

Nuclei	Comments
Main motor nucleus	Upper face receives bilateral innervation; lower face receives unilateral innervation. Muscles of facial expression, posterior belly of digastric, stylohoid muscle, stapedius.
Superior salivatory nucleus	Submandibular and sublingual glands
Nucleus of the solitary tract (gustatory nucleus)	Mediates taste.

Facial Expression

See Figure 1–86 for facial musculature.

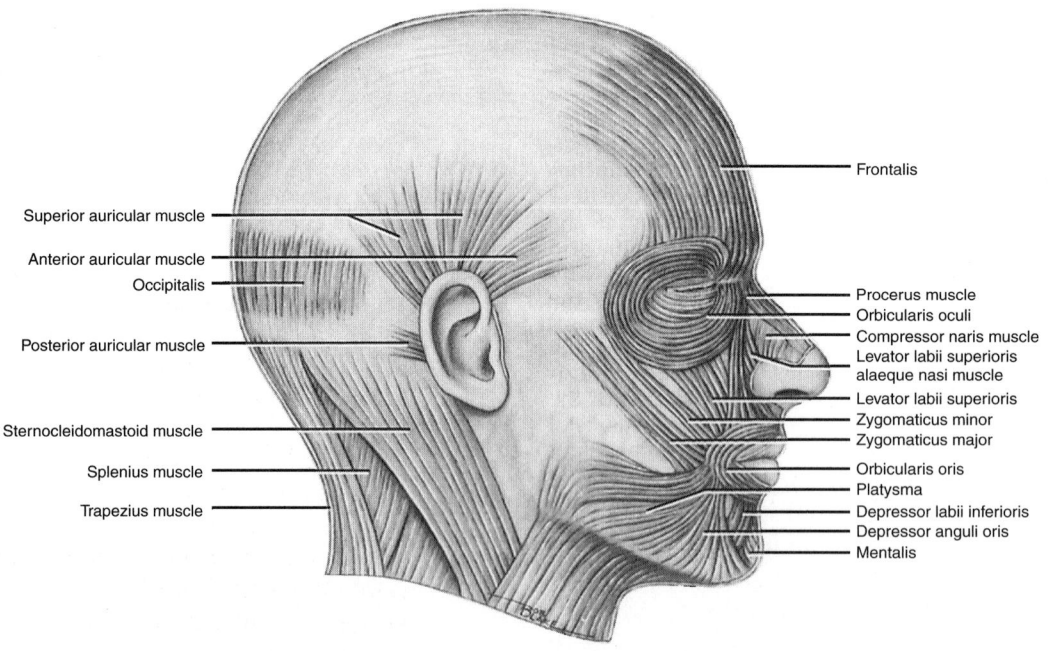

FIGURE 1-86. Facial musculature.

Reproduced, with permission, from Montgomery RL. *Head and Neck Anatomy: With Clinical Correlations*. New York: McGraw-Hill, 1981.

Important Muscles of Facial Expression (All Controlled by CN VII)

Muscle	Origin	Insertion	Action
Orbicularis oris	Circumoral muscles, maxilla, mandible	Lips and skin of lip.	**Whistle** Pulls lips against teeth, protrudes lips.
Depressor anguli oris	Mandibular oblique line	Angle of mouth.	**Frown** Pulls down angle of mouth.
Zygomaticus major	Zygomatic bone	Angle of mouth.	**Smile** Pulls angle of mouth up and back.
Risorius	Parotid and masseteric fascia	Angle of mouth.	**Smile** Pulls angle of mouth laterally.
Orbicularis oculi	Upper medial orbit, medial palpebral ligament, lacrimal bone	Encircle orbit; insert on medial palpebral, ligament medial side of lids, laterally in raphe.	**Closes eye.**

Other Muscles controlled by CN VII

Muscle	Origin	Insertion	Action	Paralysis
Buccinator	Alveolar process of maxilla and mandible Pterygomandibular raphe	Orbicularis oris	Holds food on occlusal table (accessory muscle of mastication); tenses cheek (blowing, whistling).	Food/saliva fall between teeth and cheek
Stapedius		Neck of stapes	Decreases vibration of the stapes (decreases perception of sound).	Hyperacusis

CN VII Lesions

Lesion	Clinical Finding	Comments
Lower motor neuron lesion	Ipsilateral paralysis/weakness of upper and lower face; loss of corneal reflex (efferent limb). (**Bell's palsy:** Acute 7th nerve palsy.)	If lesion proximal to greater petrosal and chorda tympani take off patient experiences: ■ Decreased taste (anterior 2/3). ■ Hyperacusis (due to stapedius muscle paralysis). ■ Decreased salivation on affected side (though not clinically apparent if other salivary glands intact).
Upper motor neuron lesion	Contralateral lower face weakness only	With a central lesion to the facial motor nucleus (e.g., stroke), can still raise eyebrows on affected side (the side opposite the central lesion) because of bilateral innervation to muscles of upper face.

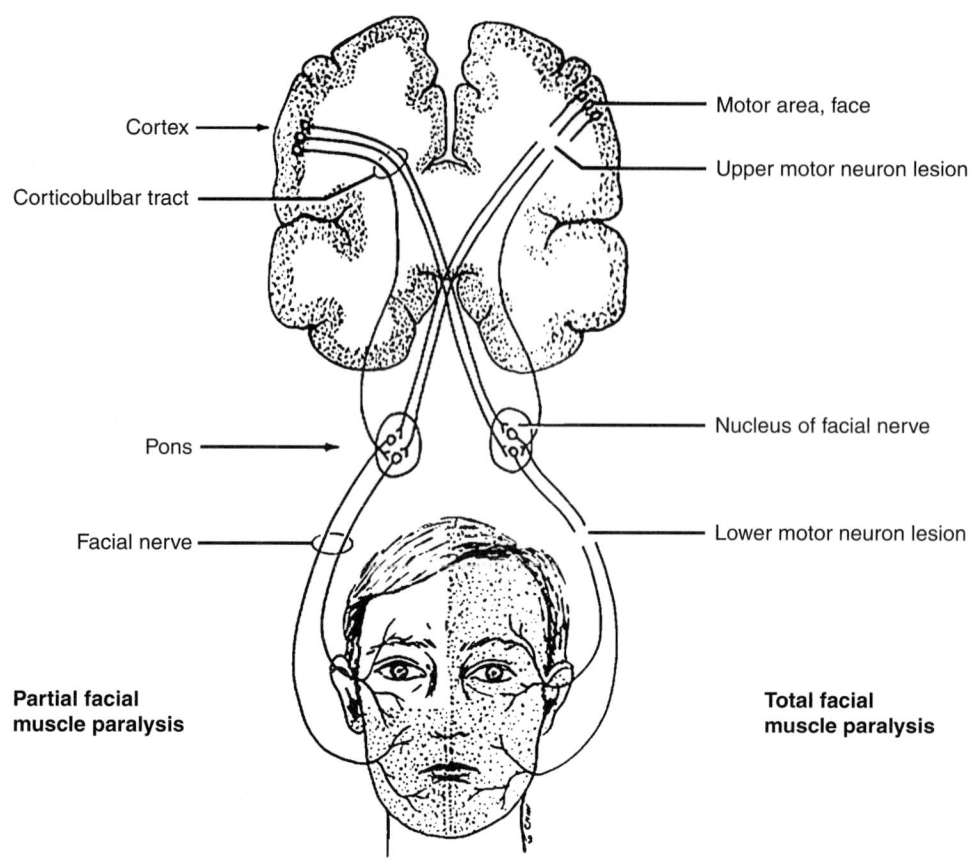

FIGURE 1–87. Total and partial facial paralysis.

Reproduced, with permission, from Montgomery RL. *Head and Neck Anatomy: With Clinical Correlations.* New York: McGraw-Hill, 1981.

See "Infrahyoid" section for posterior belly of digastric and stylohyoid, which are both innervated by CN VII.

Facial and maxillary arteries supply blood to the buccinator.

See Bell's Palsy.

See Figure 1–87 for total and partial facial paralysis.

GREATER PETROSAL NERVE

Course

- Cell body is at superior salivatory nucleus.
- Nerve arises at geniculate ganglion.
- Joins deep petrosal nerve (bringing sympathetic fibers from superior cervical ganglion).
- Exits cranium via foramen lacerum.
- Enters pterygoid canal (as nerve of the pterygoid canal).
- Nerve of pterygoid canal synapses in pterygopalatine ganglion (within the pterygopalatine fossa) (gives fibers to branches of V-1 or V-2 to supply structures).

Components

- Autonomic to:
  - Lacrimal gland.
  - Glands of mucous membrane of nasal cavity, pharynx, palate.
- **Parasympathetic** preganglionics
  - Synapse at geniculate ganglion (cell bodies in geniculate ganglion).

- **Sympathetics** (postganglionic)
  - Pass through geniculate without synapsing.
- **Taste**
  - From palate via palatine nerves.
  - Taste fibers pass through pterygopalatine ganglion and travel with nerve of pterygoid canal.
  - It reaches the greater petrosal nerve (the tractus solitarius and nucleus of solitary tract in pons).

Greater petrosal nerve is the parasympathetic root of the pterygopalatine ganglion.

CN VIII—Vestibulocochlear

See Figure 1–88.

Course

- Located within temporal bone, innervates:
  - Cochlea (hearing).
  - Semicircular canals and maculae (balance).
- Passes internal acoustic meatus.
- Into brainstem at the junction pons and medulla, fibers terminate in:
  - Cochlear nucleus.
  - Vestibular nuclear complex (near floor of fourth ventricle).

Ear Anatomy

See Figure 1–89.

- Parts of the ear
  - **External ear**—Receives sound waves
    - Auricle
    - External auditory canal
  - **Middle ear**—tympanic cavity
- Three ossicles:
  - Malleus (hammer)
  - Incus (anvil)
  - Stapes (stirrup)
- Two muscles:
  - Stapedius (VII)
  - Tensor tympani (V-3)

The stapedius is the smallest skeletal muscle in the body.

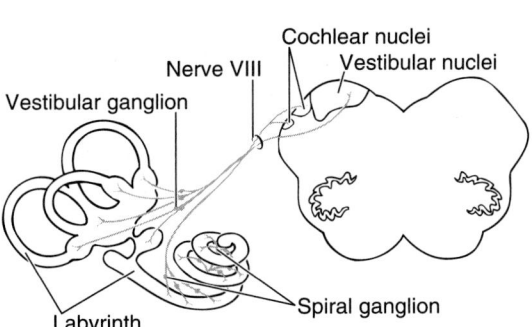

FIGURE 1-88. The vestibulocochlear nerve.

Reproduced, with permission, from Waxman SG. *Clinical Neuroanatomy*, 25th ed. McGraw-Hill, 2003.

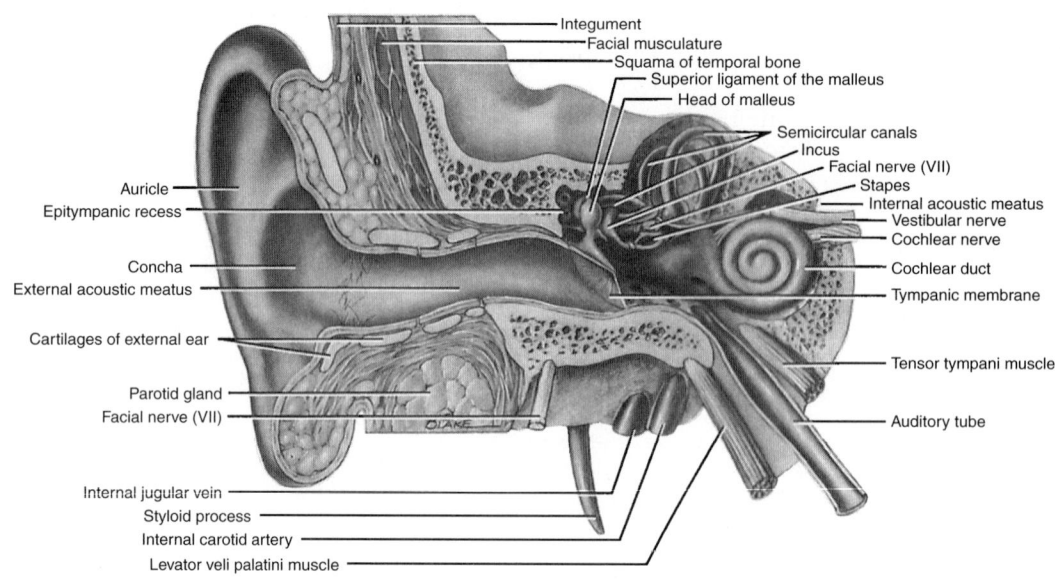

FIGURE 1-89. External, middle, and internal ear.

Reproduced, with permission, from Montgomery RL. *Head and Neck Anatomy: With Clinical Correlations.* New York: McGraw-Hill, 1981.

- **Inner ear**—composed of membranous and bony labyrinth
    - Acoustic apparatus
    - Vestibular apparatus
    - Semicircular canals

Muscles in Middle Ear

Middle ear communicates posteriorly with the mastoid cells and the mastoid antrum via the aditus ad antrum.

- The muscles in the middle dampen sounds; paralysis results in hyperacusis.

Muscle	Innervation
Tensor Tympani	V-3
Stapedius	VII

Otitis media: Middle ear infections; can extend to both mastoid and nasopharynx via eustachian tube.

Otitis externa: Infection of ear canal (past external auditory meatus).

Eustachian (Auditory) Tube

- Also called the pharyngotympanic tube.
- Connection between middle ear and pharynx.
- Equalizes air pressure between the tympanic cavity and nasopharynx.

CN VIII Lesions

Hearing Loss

Presbycusis

- Loss occurring gradually with aging because of changes in the inner or middle ear.

- **Conductive loss:** Thickening and stiffening of cochlear basilar membrane.
- **Sensorineural loss:** Loss of hair and/or nerve cells.

(See also hearing under special sense area.)

Nystagmus

- Involuntary rapid and repetitive movement of the eyes.
- Results from irritation to
  - Labyrinth.
  - Vestibular nerve or nuclei.
  - Cerebellum.
  - Visual system.
  - Cerebral cortex.
- Rhythmic oscillations are slow to one side rapid to the opposite side.
- Defined by the direction of the rapid reflex movement.
- Usually horizontal, occasionally vertical or rotatory.

Cold Caloric Test

- Instill water to the external auditory meatus stimulates nystagmus.
- Cool water fast component to side opposite.
- Warm water fast component toward stimulated side.

Central hearing connections are bilateral so a central lesion will not cause deafness in either ear.

Caloric test is testing the vestibulo-ocular reflex.

COWS

Cold
Opposite
Warm
Same

CN IX—Glossopharyngeal

See Figure 1–90.

Course

- Originates anterior surface of medulla oblongata (with X and XI).
- Passes laterally in the posterior cranial fossa.
- Leaves skull via jugular foramen.

Components

- **Motor:** Stylopharyngeus muscle
- **General sensory:** Sensory cell bodies are within superior and inferior ganglia of CN IX
- Mucosa of pharynx.
  - Posterior third of the tongue.
- **Visceral sensory**
  - Taste perceived on posterior third of the tongue.
  - Gag reflex (afferent limb) (fauces).
  - Chemo-, baroreception (afferent limb)—carotid body, carotid sinus.
- **Parasympathetic/secretomotor:** Parotid via otic ganglion
  - Preganglionics
    - Leave glossopharyngeal nerve as the tympanic nerve.
    - Enter middle ear cavity.
    - Contribute to tympanic plexus.
    - Re-form as the lesser petrosal nerve.
    - Leave cranial cavity via foramen ovale.
    - Enter otic ganglion.
  - Postganglionics
    - Carried by the auriculotemporal nerve (V3) to the parotid.

The gag reflex is mediated by CN IX (afferent-unilateral) and CN X (efferent-bilateral).

Chemoreception: *Carotid body; oxygen tension measurement.*
Baroreception: *Carotid sinus; blood pressure changes. Mediated CN IX (afferent) and CN X (efferent).*

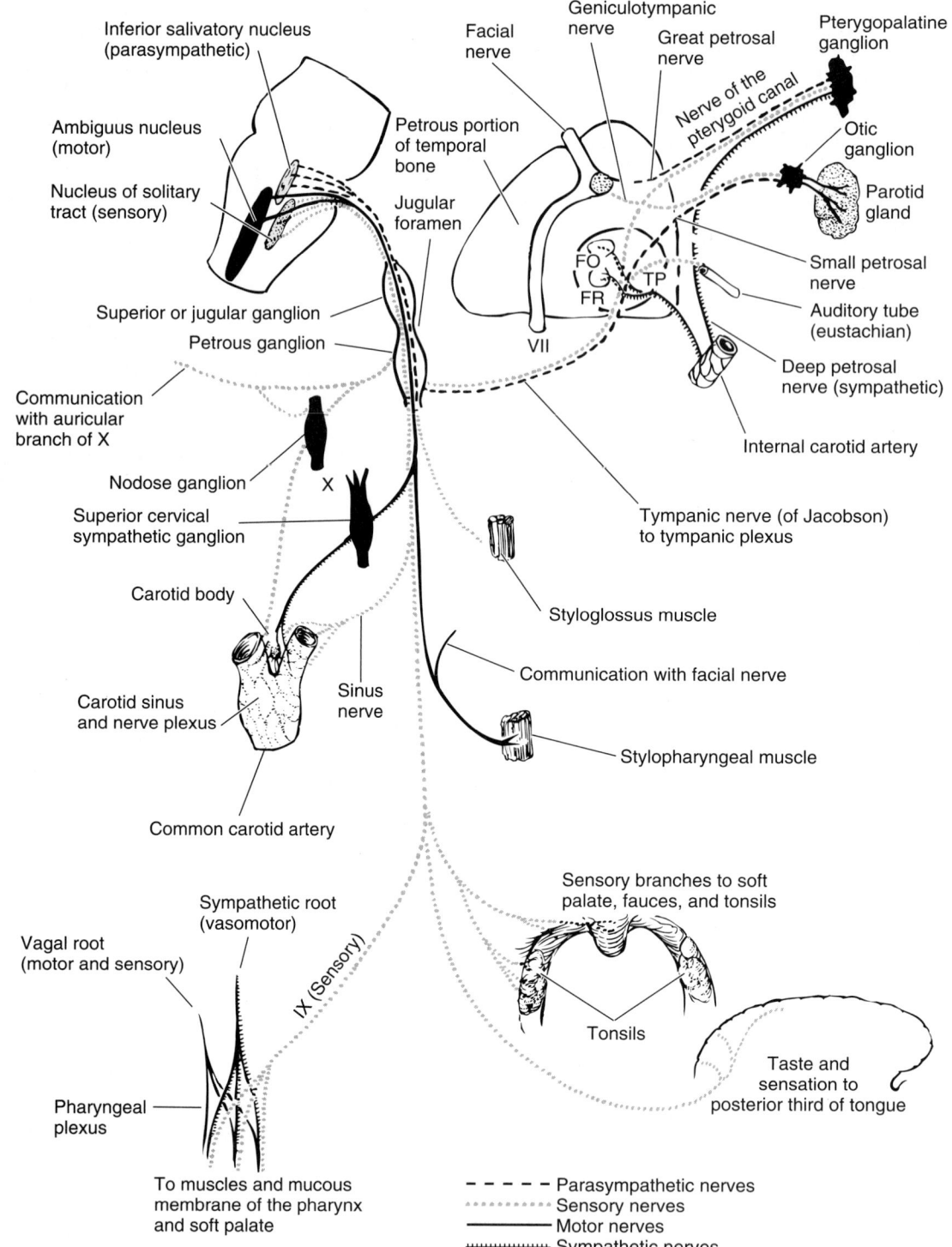

FIGURE 1-90. The glossopharyngeal nerve. TP, tympanum plexus; FR, foramen rotundum; FO, foramen ovale.

Reproduced, with permission, from Waxman SG. *Clinical Neuroanatomy*, 25th ed. McGraw-Hill, 2003.

CN X—Vagus

- Cranial nerve with the widest distribution.
- Supplies the viscera of neck, thorax, and abdomen to left colic flexure.
- Course:
  - Leaves the medulla.
  - Passes out jugular foramen.
  - Descends neck in carotid sheath (behind internal and common carotid arteries, and IJV).
  - Posterior mediastinum (travels on the esophagus).
  - Enters abdominal cavity with the esophagus.

Vagus nerves lose their identity in the esophageal plexus. The anterior gastric nerve can be cut (vagotomy) to reduce gastric secretion.

Right Vagus Nerve	Left Vagus Nerve
Crosses anterior surface of right subclavian artery. Enters the thorax posterolateral to the brachiocephalic trunk, lateral to the trachea, and medial to the azygos vein. Passes posterior to the root of the right lung (contributing to the pulmonary plexus). Travels with the esophagus (contributes to the esophageal plexus). Enters the abdomen behind the esophagus (via esophageal hiatus of diaphragm). Branches of esophageal plexus unite:	Enters thorax in front of left subclavian artery, behind left brachiocephalic vein. Crosses the left side of the aortic arch (and is itself crossed by left phrenic nerve). Passes behind left lung (contributing to the pulmonary plexus). Travels with the esophagus (contributes to esophageal plexus). Enters abdomen in front of esophagus (via the esophageal hiatus of the diaphragm). Branches of esophageal plexus unite:
Posterior vagal trunk (*posterior gastric nerve*—reaches posterior surface of stomach).	**Anterior vagal trunk** (*anterior gastric nerve*—reaches anterior surface of stomach).

BRANCHES OF THE VAGUS IN THE HEAD AND NECK

See Figure 1–91 and also Table 1–3.

Branch	Description
Meningeal	To dura.
Auricular	To auricle, external auditory meatus.
Pharyngeal	Forms pharyngeal plexus. Supplies: - Muscles of pharynx (except stylopharyngeus [innervated by CN IX]). - All the muscles of the soft palate (except tensor veli palatini, innervated by NC V-3).
Superior laryngeal - Internal laryngeal - External laryngeal	Travels with superior laryngeal artery. Pierces thyrohyoid membrane. Supplies mucous membranes of larynx above vocal fold. Travels with superior thyroid artery. Supplies cricothyroid muscle.

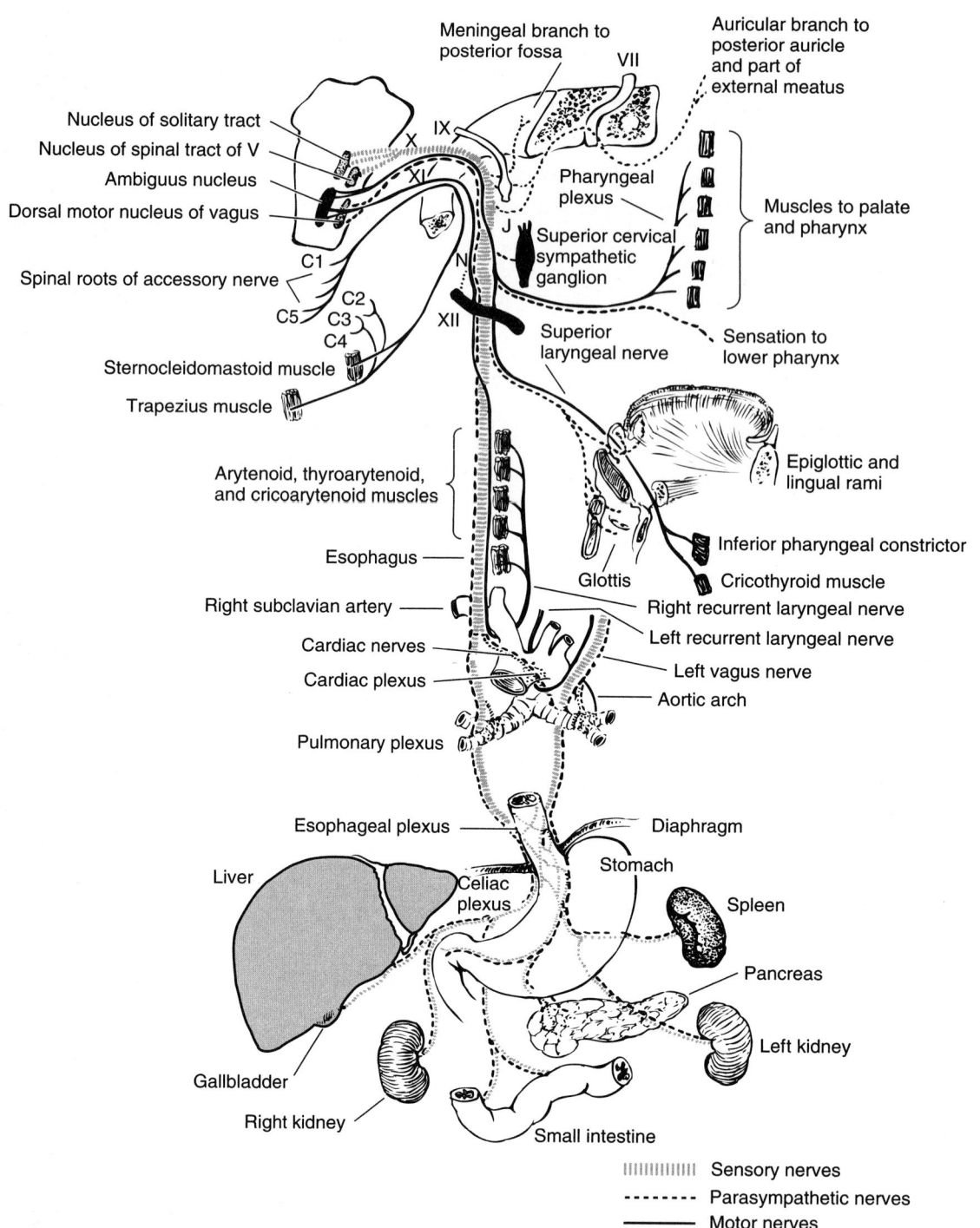

FIGURE 1-91. The vagus nerve. J, jugular (superior) ganglion; N, nodose (inferior) ganglion.

Reproduced, with permission, from Waxman SG. *Clinical Neuroanatomy*, 25th ed. McGraw-Hill, 2003.

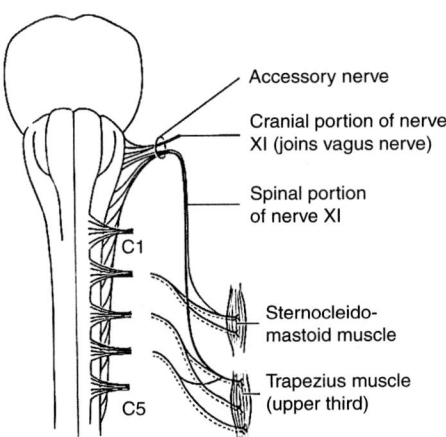

FIGURE 1-92. Schematic illustration of the accessory nerve, viewed from below.

Reproduced, with permission, from Waxman SG. *Clinical Neuroanatomy*, 25th ed. McGraw-Hill, 2003.

CN X Lesions

- Parasympathetic disturbances
- Loss of gag reflex
- Dysphagia
- Dysphonia

CN XI—Accessory

See Figure 1-92 for a schematic illustration of the accessory nerve.

CN XI Lesions

- Paralysis of SCM: difficulty turning head to contralateral side.
- Paralysis of trapezius: Shoulder droop.

CN XII—Hypoglossus

See Figure 1-93.

- The hypoglossal nerve is strictly a motor nerve.

Course

- Leaves skull through hypoglossal canal (of the occipital bone) (medial to carotid canal and jugular foramen).
- Joined by C1 fibers from the cervical plexus soon after it leaves skull.
- Passes above hyoid bone on the lateral surface of the hyoglossus muscle (deep to the mylohyoid).
- Loops around occipital artery.
- Passes between ECA and IJV.

The cardiac branches of the vagus (form the cardiac plexus) are preganglionic parasympathetic nerves that synapse with postganglionic parasympathetic nerves in the heart.

The abdominal viscera below the left colic flexure (and genitalia and pelvic viscera) are supplied by pelvic splanchnic nerves (parasympathetic preganglionics).

Also with CN XII paralysis, the tongue tends to fall back and obstruct the airway (genioglossus).

In addition to deviation to the affected side (with damage to CN XII and resultant denervation atrophy), dysarthria (inability to articulate) can be experienced by the patient.

CN XII Lesions

Lesion	Clinical Finding	Description
Lower motor neuron	Tongue deviates toward side of lesion.	Contralateral genioglossus pulls forward because there are ipsilateral fasciculations and atrophy.
Upper motor neuron	Tongue deviates toward side of lesion.	Paralysis without atrophy or fasciculations; (corticobulbar fibers are from contralateral hemisphere, so UMN lesion causes weakness of contralateral tongue; for example left cortical lesion causes deviation of tongue to right (affected side).

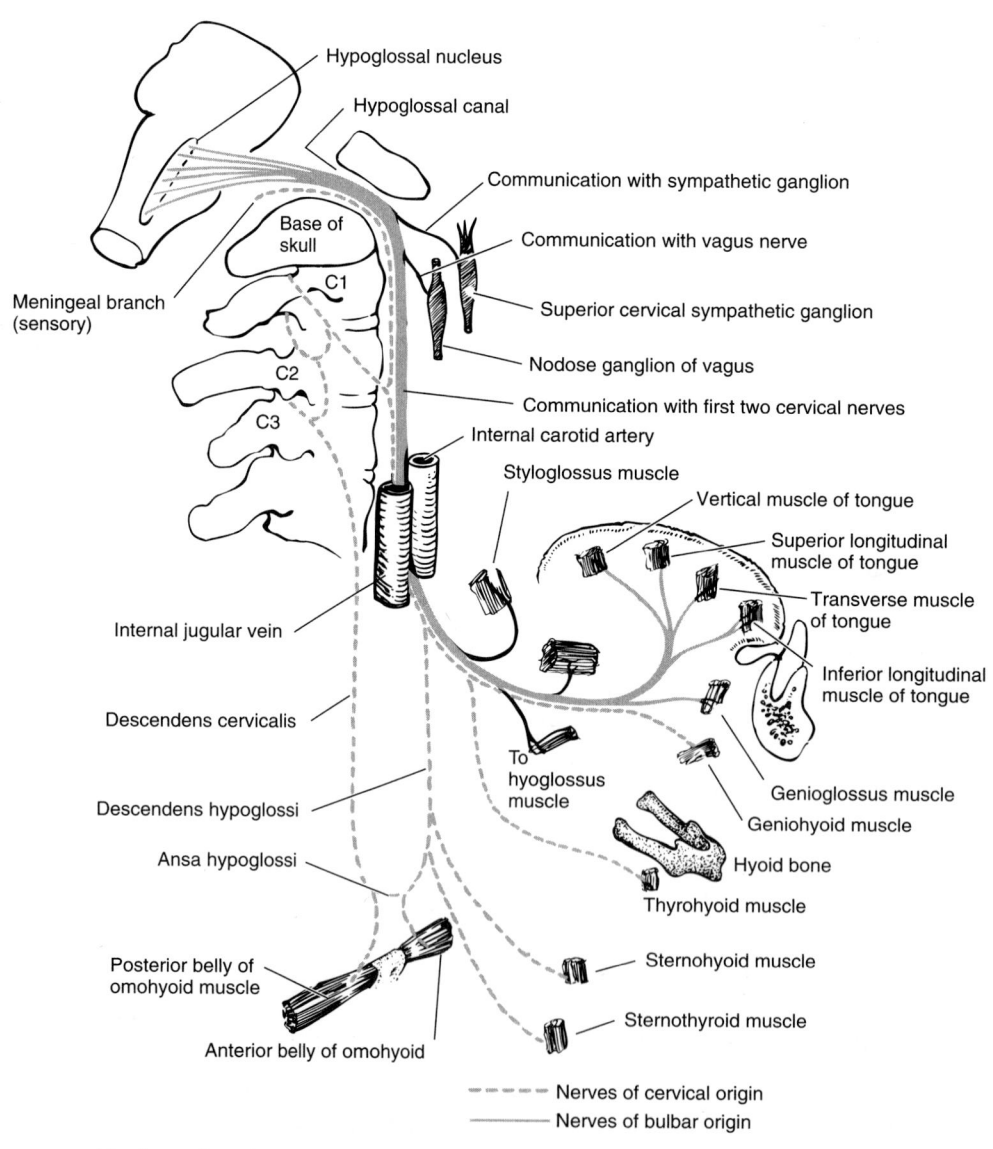

FIGURE 1-93. The hypoglossal nerve.

Reproduced, with permission, from Waxman SG. *Clinical Neuroanatomy*, 25th ed. McGraw-Hill, 2003.

Spinal Cord

- Located in the spinal canal.
- Is 40–45 cm long.
- Continuation of the medulla oblongata.
    - Exits foramen magnum.
- Extends to L1–2 (L3 in a child).
    - Occupies upper two thirds of the vertebral canal.
- **Conus medullaris**
    - Spinal cord tapers at L1.
- **Filum terminale**
    - Prolongation of pia matter at apex attaches to coccyx.
    - Where dura and arachnoid fuse at about S2.
- **Cauda equina** ("horse's tail")
    - Nerve roots extending down inferiorly below end of spinal cord.
    - These exit via lumbar and sacral foramina.
- **Meninges** (like brain)
    - Dura
    - Arachnoid (CSF in subarachnoid space)
    - Pia

CSF is located in the subarachnoid space. This space is entered during a lumbar "tap" or puncture.

SPINAL CORD CROSS SECTION

See Figures 1–94 and 1–95.

- Gray matter.
    - Located centrally; H-shaped.
    - Consists of unmeyelinated nerve cell bodies.
    - **Anterior/ventral horn**
        - Motor (efferent).
    - **Posterior/dorsal horn**
        - Sensory (afferent).
        - Dorsal root ganglion (cell bodies).
    - **Intermediolateral horn**
        - Autonomic.

In the spinal cord, white matter is peripheral and gray matter is central, the reverse of the cerebral cortex.

The spinal cord is protected by the bony and ligamentous walls of the vertebral canal and CSF.

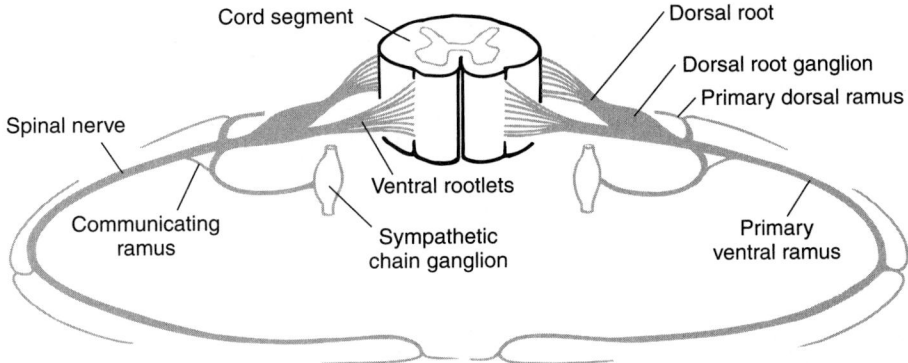

FIGURE 1-94. Schematic illustration of a cord segment with its roots, ganglia, and branches.

Reproduced, with permission, from Waxman SG. *Clinical Neuroanatomy*, 25th ed. McGraw-Hill, 2003.

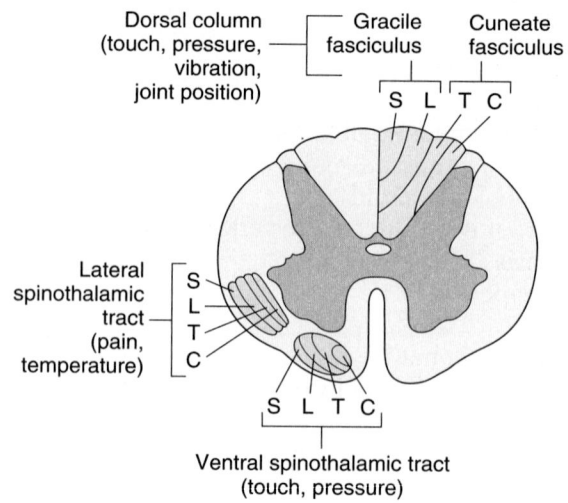

FIGURE 1-95. Spinal cord cross-section.

Reproduced, with permission, from Ganong, *Review of Medical Physiology*, 22nd ed. McGraw Hill, 2005.

- White matter.
  - Surrounds the gray matter peripherally.
  - Myelinated axons.
- Central canal.
  - Filled with CSF.

SPINAL CORD TRACTS

The cell bodies for afferent/sensory nerves are located in the dorsal root ganglion.

See also Chapter 10, "Neurophysiology."

Tract	Function
Ascending/sensory	
Anterior spinothalamic	Touch, pressure
Lateral spinothalamic	Pain, temperature
Posterior columns (gracilis and cuneatus)	Proprioception, position sense
Spinocerebellar	Motor coordination, proprioception
Descending/motor	
Corticospinal	Motor
Tectospinal	Movement of head
Rubrospinal	Muscle tone, posture, head, neck, upper extremities
Vestibulospinal	Equilibrium (interface with CN VIII)
Reticulospinal	Muscle tone, sweat gland function

Peripheral Nervous System

- Nerves outside the CNs.
- Consists of:
  - Cranial nerves (12): Leave the brain and pass out the skull foramina.
  - Spinal nerves (31): Leave the spinal cord and pass out via the intervertebral foramina.
    - 8 cervical spinal nerves (only 7 vertebrae).
    - 12 thoracic.
    - 5 lumbar.
    - 5 sacral.
    - 1 coccygeal
  - Associated plexi and ganglia.
- Divided into
  - Afferent and efferent.
  - Somatic and visceral.
- **Afferent** (sensory)
  - Somatic sensory (afferent).
    - From cutaneous and proprioceptive receptors.
  - Visceral sensory (afferent).
    - From viscera.
- **Efferent** (motor)
  - Somatic motor (efferent).
    - Motor neurons to skeletal muscle.
  - Visceral motor (efferent)
    - Autonomic (parasympathetic > sympathetic) to viscera (e.g., smooth and cardiac muscle, glands, GI tract).

SPINAL NERVES

- Comprise dorsal + ventral rami.
- Mixed nerves (motor + sensory).
- After they join as spinal nerve, they split into
  - Dorsal (posterior) rami.
  - Ventral (anterior) rami.
- Supplying both motor and sensory innervation to posterior and anterior body walls.

Spinal Nerve	Root	Location of Cell Body
Motor	Ventral (anterior)	Spinal cord (ventral horn-gray)
Sensory	Dorsal (posterior)	Dorsal root ganglion (outside of cord)

Remember histology: epinerium, perinerium, endoneurium.

A peripheral nerve may be a subsegment of a cranial nerve; for example, the lingual nerve is part of the third division of CN V (and it carries taste components from CN VII).

PERIPHERAL NERVE

- Bundle of nerve fibers.
- Formed from 1+ spinal nerve.
- **Example:** Musculocutaneous nerve
  - Formed from three spinal nerves (C5, C6, C7).

Nerve Fiber Types

Fiber	Conduction Velocity (m/s)	Diameter (μm)	Function	Myelin	Local Anesthetic Sensitivity
A Fiber					
A-α	70–120	12–20	Proprioception Motor	Y	Least
A-β	40–70	5–12	Sensory Touch Pressure	Y	
A-γ	10–50	2–5	Muscle spindle	Y	
A-δ	6–30	2–5	Sharp pain Temperature Touch	Y	
B Fiber	3–15	<3	Preganglionic autonomic	Y	
C Fiber	0.5–2	0.4–1.2	Dull pain Temperature Postganglionic autonomic	N	Most

Adapted in part from Waxman, *Clinical Neuroanatomy*, 24th ed. McGraw-Hill, 2003:26.

GANGLIA

- Collections of cell bodies.
- Sensory versus autonomic.
- **Sensory:** Dorsal root ganglia.
- **Autonomic:** Sympathetic.
    - Sympathetic chain ganglia.
        - Located on each sympathetic trunk, alongside vertebral column.
        - 3 cervical (superior, middle, inferior).
        - 12 thoracic.
        - 4 lumbar.
        - 4 sacral.

- Parasympathetic
  - Ciliary.
  - Pterygopalatine.
  - Submandibular.
  - Otic.
  - Celiac.
  - Superior mesenteric.
  - Inferior mesenteric.

Splanchnic nerves are sympathetic nerves to the viscera. They pass through the sympathetic chain ganglia without synapse (exceptions to short preganglionic and long post-ganglionic) and synapse in the effector.

PLEXUSES

- Interdigitations of nerves (nerves joining neighboring nerves).

Formed from anterior rami in cervical, brachial, lumbar, and sacral regions.

Four major plexuses:

- Cervical plexus (C1–4).
- Brachial plexus (C-5–T1).
- Lumbar plexus (L1–L4).
  - Formed in psoas muscle.
  - Supplies lower abdomen and parts of lower limb.
  - Main branches
    - Femoral nerve.
    - Obturator nerve.
- Sacral plexus (L4–L5 and S1–S4)
  - Posterior pelvic wall in front of piriformis.
  - Supplies lower back, pelvis, parts of thigh, leg, and foot.
  - Main branches
    - Sciatic nerve (largest nerve in body).
    - Gluteal nerve.
    - Pelvic splanchnic nerve.

AUTONOMIC NERVOUS SYSTEM

See Figures 1–96 and 1–97. See also Chapter 10, "Neurophysiology."

- **Sympathetic**
  - Thoracolumbar
  - "Fight or flight"
- **Parasympathetic**
  - Craniosacral
  - "Rest and digest"
  - All have afferent and efferent components.
  - Efferent is the major portion.
- **General visceral efferent motor system (GVE)**
  - Involuntary.
  - Controls and regulates smooth muscle, cardiac muscle, and glands.

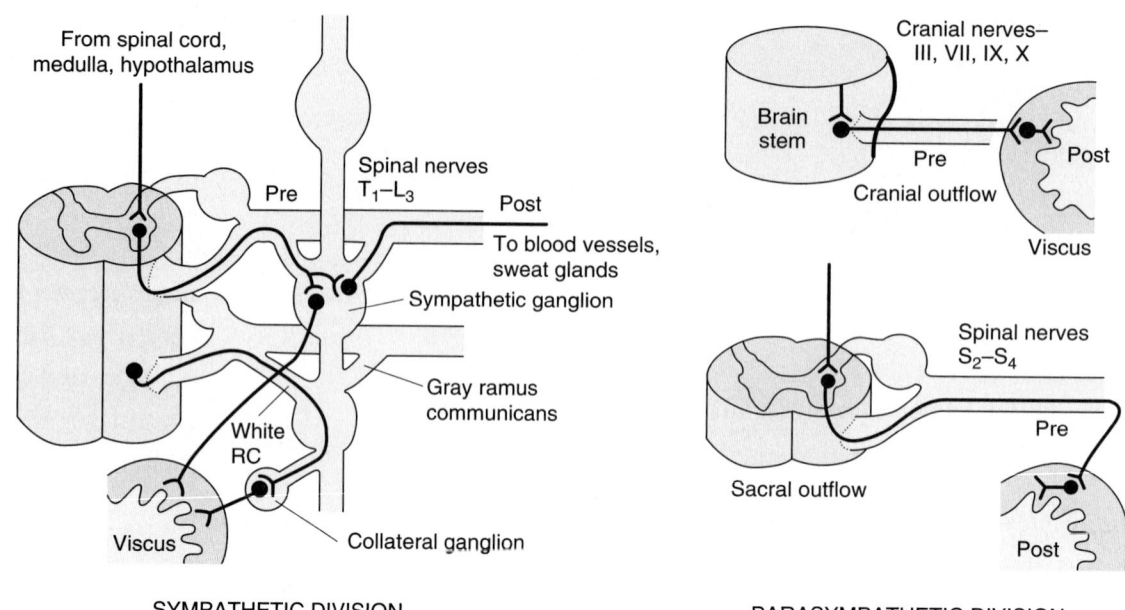

FIGURE 1-96. Autonomic nervous system.

Reproduced, with permission, from Ganong. *Review of Medical Physiology*, 22nd ed. McGraw-Hill, 2005.

Pathway

Hypothalamus, reticular formation
↓
Interomediolateral horn (cell body of preganglionic neuron)
↓
Preganglionic neuron (short in sympathetic; long in parasympathetic)
↓
Ganglion (outside of CNS)
↓
Postganglionic neuron (long in sympathetic; short in parasympathetic)
↓
Effector organ
↓

Postganglionic autonomic fibers are unmyelinated C-fibers.

Notes

- Gray rami connect sympathetic trunk to every spinal nerve.
- White rami are limited to spinal cord segments between T1 and L2.
- Cell bodies of the visceral efferent preganglionic fibers (visceral branches of sympathetic trunk) are located in the interomediolateral horn of the spinal cord.
- Cell bodies of visceral afferent fibers are located in the dorsal root ganglia.

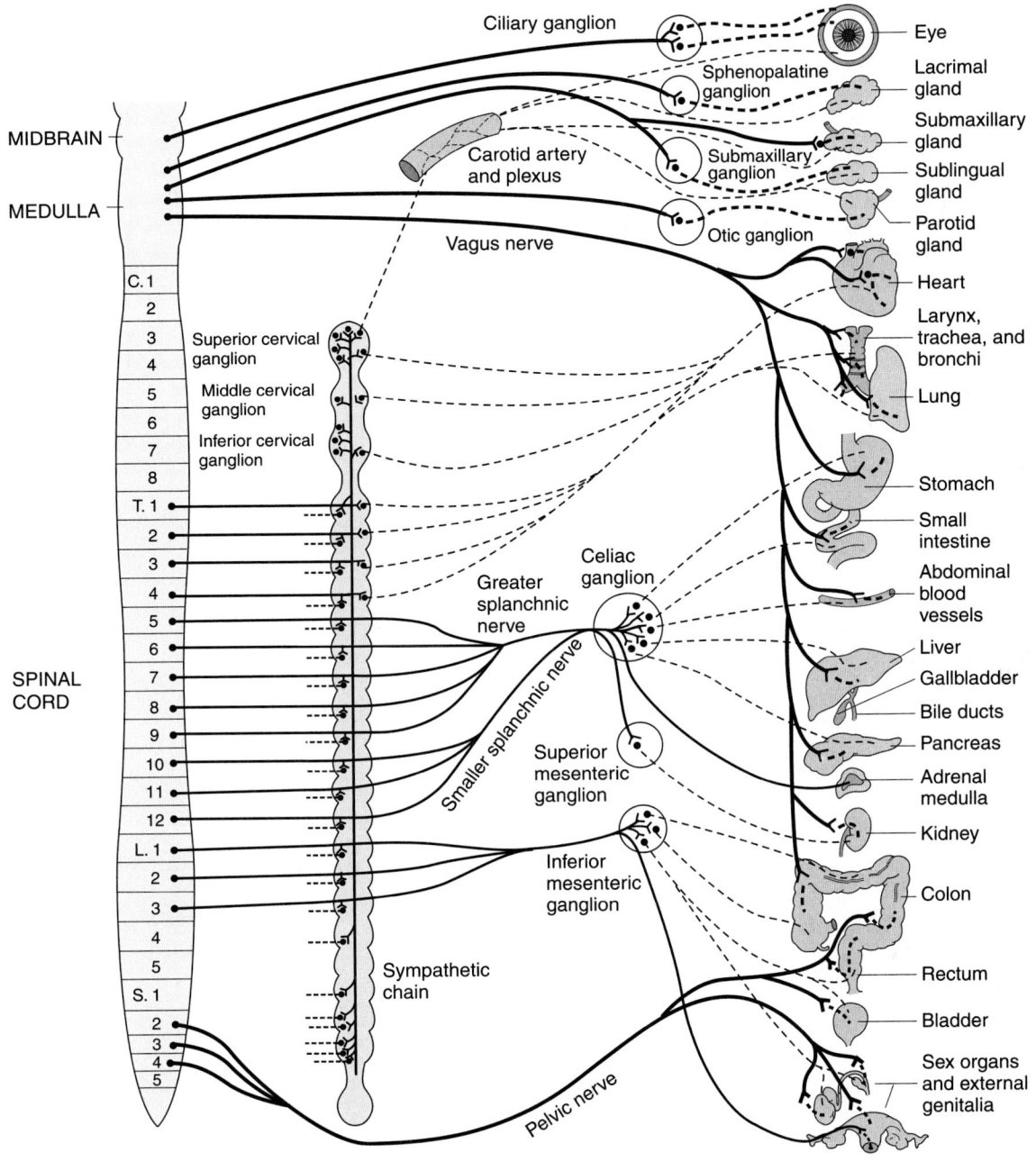

FIGURE 1-97. Autonomic nervous system.

Reproduced, with permission, from Ganong. *Review of Medical Physiology*, 22nd ed. McGraw-Hill, 2005.

Enteric Nervous System

See Chapter 15, "Gastrointestinal Physiology."

CHAPTER 2
General Histology

The Cell	160
PLASMA (CELL) MEMBRANE	160
CYTOPLASM	160
MEMBRANE-BOUND ORGANELLES	160
NON-MEMBRANE-BOUND ORGANELLES	161
NUCLEUS	161
CELL SURFACE APPENDAGES	161
THE CELL CYCLE	162
CELL-TO-CELL CONTACTS	162
Epithelium	164
CLASSIFICATION OF EPITHELIUM	164
Basement Membrane	165
COMPONENTS OF BASEMENT MEMBRANE	165
Connective Tissue	165
CLASSIFICATION OF CONNECTIVE TISSUE	165
CONNECTIVE TISSUE PROPER	165
CONNECTIVE TISSUE ATTACHMENTS	166
CELLS OF CT	166
Glandular Tissue	166
TYPES OF GLANDS	166
CLASSIFICATION OF EXOCRINE GLANDS	167
Cartilage	168
ECM OF CARTILAGE	168
SURFACE OF CARTILAGE	168
GROWTH OF CARTILAGE	168
Bone	169
FUNCTIONS OF BONE	169
BONE FORMATION	169
TYPES OF BONE	169
BONE SURFACES	169
BONE MARROW	170
BONE REMODELING	170
CALCIUM REGULATION	170

Joints	170
CLASSIFICATION OF JOINTS	170
SYNOVIAL JOINTS	170
Nervous Tissue	171
NEURONS	171
NEURON CLASSIFICATION	171
SYNAPSES	171
SUPPORTING CELLS	171
MYELINATION	172
Blood	172
FUNCTIONS	172
COMPONENTS	173
ERYTHROCYTES	174
LEUKOCYTES	174
HEMATOPOIESIS	175
Cardiovascular Tissue	175
ARRANGEMENT OF BLOOD VESSELS IN CIRCULATION	175
LAYERS OF BLOOD VESSEL WALLS	175
LAYERS OF THE HEART	176
CARDIAC CONDUCTION	176
Lymphatic System	176
FUNCTIONS OF THE LYMPHATIC SYSTEM	177
LYMPH DRAINAGE	177
Endocrine Glands	178
PITUITARY GLAND (HYPOPHYSIS)	178
THYROID GLAND	179
PARATHYROID GLANDS	179
ADRENAL (SUPRARENAL) GLANDS	179
Respiratory System	180
FUNCTIONS	180
DIVISIONS	180
ALVEOLI	181
Upper Digestive System	181
FUNCTIONS	181
LAYERS	182
ESOPHAGUS	182
STOMACH	182
SMALL INTESTINE	182
LARGE INTESTINE	184
GUT-ASSOCIATED LYMPHATIC TISSUE (GALT)	184
Lower Digestive System	184
LIVER	184
BILE	184
PORTAL TRIAD	185
LIVER LOBULES	185

HEPATOCYTES	185
SINUSOIDS	185
BILIARY TREE	185
BILE COMPOSITION	186
GALL BLADDER	186
PANCREAS	186
EXOCRINE PANCREAS	187
ENDOCRINE PANCREAS	187
Urinary System	187
COMPONENTS	187
FUNCTIONS OF KIDNEYS	188
COMPONENTS OF KIDNEYS	188
NEPHRON	188
URETHRA	189
Reproductive System	189
TESTIS	189
INTRA- AND EXTRA-TESTICULAR DUCT SYSTEM	189
PROSTATE GLAND	189
PENIS	189
OVARY	190
OVIDUCTS (FALLOPIAN TUBES)	190
UTERUS	190
VAGINA	190
MAMMARY GLANDS	190
Integument	190
FUNCTIONS OF SKIN	190
LAYERS OF SKIN	191
HAIR	191
SEBACEOUS GLANDS	192
Eye	192
LAYERS OF EYE	192
TEN LAYERS OF RETINA	193
OPTIC DISC	194
MACULA LUTEA	194

THE CELL

Plasma (Cell) Membrane

- See also the section "Membranes" in Chapter 9.
- A fluid, selectively permeable barrier consisting of an amphipathic phospholipid bilayer that contains integral and peripheral proteins.

Cytoplasm

- **Organelles** (See Figure 2–1)
- Cytoplasmic inclusions (metaplasm)
    - Glycogen
    - Pigment granules
    - Secretory granules
    - Lipid droplets
- Cytoplasmic matrix (cytosol)
    - Ground substance

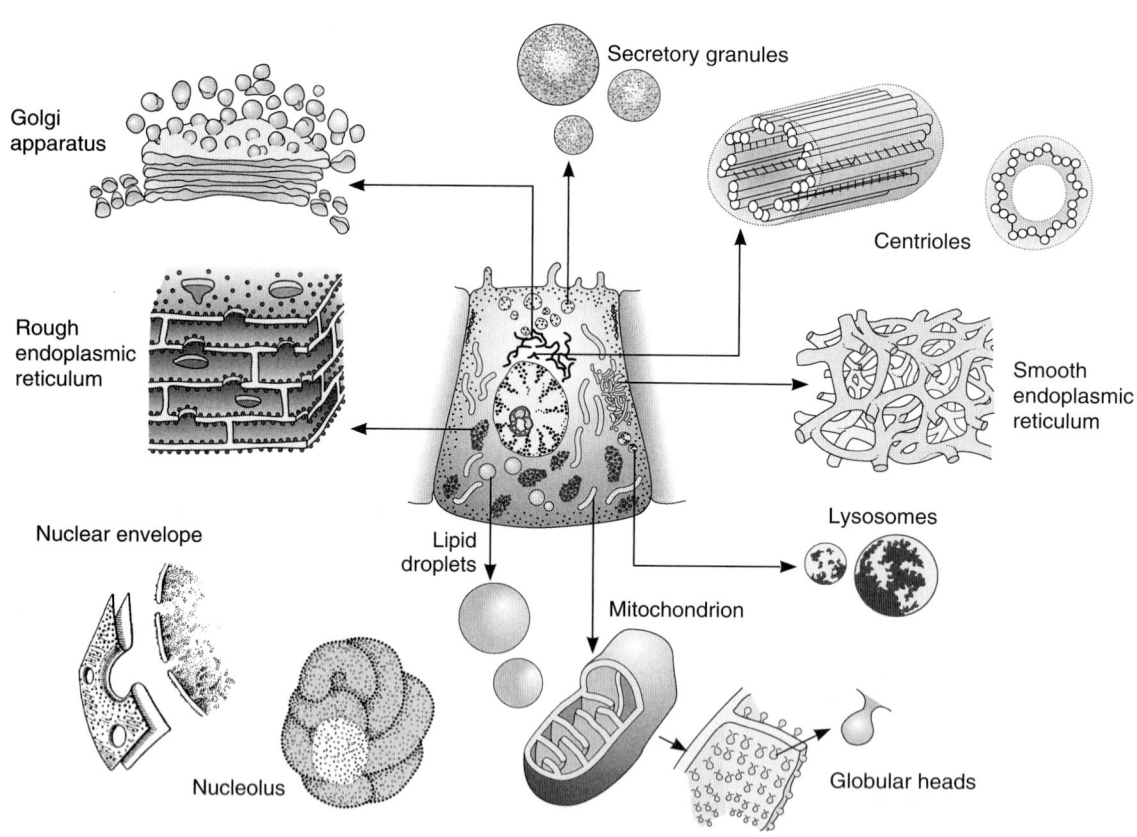

FIGURE 2–1. **Important cellular organelles.**

Reproduced, with permission, from Ganong. *Review of Medical Physiology*, 22nd ed. McGraw-Hill, 2005.

Membrane-Bound Organelles

- **Rough endoplasmic reticulum (rER):** Protein synthesis for *export* outside of the cell. Studded with ribosomes.
- **Smooth endoplasmic reticulum (sER):** Steroid synthesis (adrenal cortex and testes). Sequesters Ca^{2+} (skeletal and cardiac muscle). Lipid and glycogen metabolism (liver).
- **Golgi apparatus:** Posttranslational modification and packaging of proteins (adds oligosaccharides for glycoproteins, and sulfate groups for proteoglycans). Lysosome production.
- **Mitochondria:** ATP production via the Krebs cycle and oxidative phosphorylation. Have an inner and outer membrane. Contain their own cyclic DNA. Not present in erythrocytes.
- **Lysosomes:** Digestion of microorganisms or other cellular components by various hydrolytic enzymes. Produced by the Golgi apparatus.
- **Peroxisomes:** Elimination of H_2O_2 by various oxidative enzymes (catalase and peroxidase).
- **Endosomes:** Vesicles formed as a result of phagocytosis.

Non-Membrane-Bound Organelles

- **Microtubules:** Provide cytoskeletal support, intracellular transport, and cellular movement. Composed of *tubulin*.
    - **Axoneme:** Specialized group of microtubules found in cilia and flagella arranged in a "9 + 2" pattern.
- **Centrioles:** Provide microtubule organization. Form ends of mitotic spindle during mitosis.
- **Filaments**
    - **Microfilaments (actin, myosin, etc.):** Important for muscle contraction. Provide cellular movement or anchorage.
    - **Intermediate filaments (vimentin, desmin, cytokeratin, etc.):** Provide cytoskeletal support.
- **Ribosomes:** Protein synthesis for use *within* the cell. Composed of rRNA and protein.

Nucleus

- **Nuclear membrane:** Composed of inner and outer plasma membranes.
- **Nucleoplasm:** Ground substance of the nucleus.
- **Chromatin:** The complex of DNA and proteins (histones).
    - **Euchromatin:** Loosely arranged chromatin. Indicates nuclear activity.
    - **Heterochromatin:** Highly condensed chromatin.
- **Nucleolus:** Site of rRNA synthesis. Nonmembranous.
- **Barr body:** The repressed X chromosome found only in cells of *females*. Appears as a dense chromatin mass adjacent to the nuclear membrane. Its presence (or absence) is used in sex identification.

Cell Surface Appendages

- **Microvilli:** Fingerlike structures of various lengths located on the apical surface of most epithelial cells. Provide increased cell surface area for absorption and transport of fluids.
- **Stereocilia:** Unusually long microvilli located only in the *epididymis* and sensory cells of the *inner ear*.
- **Cilia:** Short, hairlike structures used for locomotion or movement of substances along the cell membrane. They wave in a synchronous pattern.
- **Flagella:** Long, whiplike structures used for locomotion. In humans, found only in *spermatozoa*.

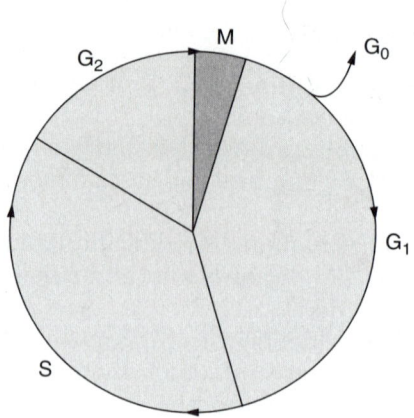

FIGURE 2-2. The cell cycle.

The turnover rate of cells varies among tissue types. Oral, epidermal, and gastrointestinal (GI) epithelial cells rapidly divide. Smooth muscle cells and vascular endothelial cells divide more slowly. Skeletal and cardiac muscle cells rarely divide. Neurons never divide.

The Cell Cycle

See Figure 2-2.

- **Mitosis:** Produces two daughter cells with the *same* chromosome number (diploid, $2n$) as the parent cell. All somatic cells except gametes undergo mitosis.
- **Interphase**
  - G_1: First variable period of cellular growth.
    - G_O: Period *outside* of the cell cycle of terminal differentiation.
  - S: Period of DNA synthesis. Takes about 7 hours.
  - G_2: Second variable period of cellular growth.
- **Mitosis (karyokinesis)**
  - **Prophase:** Chromatin coils within the nucleus. Mitotic spindle forms.
  - **Metaphase:** Nuclear membrane and nucleoli disappear. Chromosomes line up at the equatorial plate of the mitotic spindle.
  - **Anaphase:** Chromosomes split to opposite poles of the cell.
  - **Telophase:** Nuclear membrane forms around the chromosomes at each pole. The chromosomes uncoil and nucleoli reappear. The cytoplasm divides to form two daughter cells (cytokinesis).
- **Meiosis:** Produces four daughter cells with *half* the chromosome number (haploid, n) as the parent cell. Only gametes (spermatozoa and ova) undergo meiosis.

Cell-to-Cell Contacts

See Table 2-1.

- **Tight junction (zonula occludens):** A beltlike junction that completely seals off the intercellular space between adjacent cells.
- **Intermediate junction (zonula adherens):** A beltlike junction that leaves a 15–20 nm wide intercellular space between adjacent cells.
- **Desmosome (macula adherens):** Provides strong but localized adhesion sites between adjacent cells. Composed of an *attachment plaque* on the cytoplasmic side of each adjoining cell surface, to which intermediate filaments are anchored.
- **Hemidesmosome:** Provide strong but localized attachment of epithelial cells to connective tissue. Half of a desmosome (the attachment plaque is on the basal surface, facing the basement membrane).
- **Gap junction:** Localized areas of free communication between adjacent cells. Enables passage of fluids, ions, and small molecules.

*A **junctional complex** (See Figure 2-3.) is a specialized junction commonly found in epithelial tissues consisting of the following (from apical → upper regions):*

- *Tight junction*
- *Intermediate junction*
- *Desmosome*

TABLE 2-1. Comparison of Cell-to-Cell Contacts

Contact Type	Function	Area of Contact	Common Location
Tight junction	Occlusion	Entire cell	Various epithelium
Intermediate junction	Adhesion	Entire cell	Various epithelium
Desmosome	Adhesion	Focal	Epidermis and other epithelium
Hemidesmosome	Adhesion	Focal	Epithelium of oral mucosa, skin, esophagus, vagina, and cornea
Gap junction	Communication	Focal	Neurons. Smooth and cardiac muscle

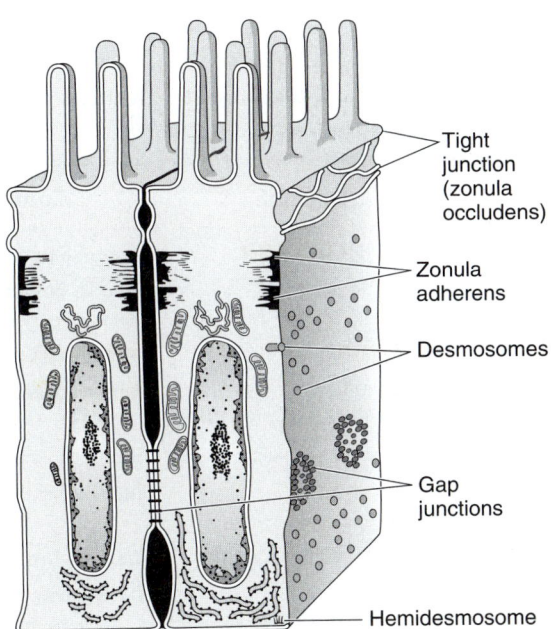

FIGURE 2-3. Epithelial intercellular junctions. Note the relative location of each junction within the cell.

Reproduced, with permission, from Ganong. *Review of Medical Physiology*, 22nd ed. McGraw-Hill, 2005.

▶ EPITHELIUM

Epithelium covers all body surfaces, lines all body cavities, makes up the secretory component of glands, and serves as the receptor in various sensory organs.

FUNCTIONS OF EPITHELIUM

- Barrier
- Diffusion
- Absorption
- Secretory
- Transport
- Sensory

Classification of Epithelium

- By number of cell layers.
    - **Simple:** One cell layer thick, all touching the basement membrane.
    - **Stratified:** Two or more cell layers thick, with only the deepest layer touching the basement membrane.
    - **Pesudostratified:** One cell layer thick, all touching the basement membrane, but not all reach the outer surface. Generally columnar.
- By cell morphology.
    - **Squamous:** Width > height.
    - **Cuboidal:** Width = height.

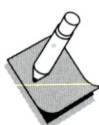

Epithelium is classified by cell morphology and arrangement, not by function. See Table 2-2.

TABLE 2-2. Comparison of Epithelial Types

EPITHELIUM TYPE	FUNCTION	COMMON LOCATION
Simple squamous	Barrier, diffusion	Endothelium, mesothelium, lung alveoli, Bowman's capsule
Simple cuboidal	Barrier, absorption, secretion	Small exocrine gland ducts (thyroid follicles), renal tubules
Simple columnar (often ciliated)	Absorption, secretion, transport	Stomach, small intestine, large intestine, gallbladder
Pseudostratified columnar (often ciliated)	Absorption, secretion, transport	Trachea, bronchi, nasopharynx, nasal cavity, paranasal sinuses
Stratified squamous	Barrier	Epidermis, oral cavity, oropharynx, laryngopharynx, esophagus, anus, vagina
Stratified cuboidal	Barrier, secretion	Medium exocrine gland ducts (sweat glands)
Stratified columnar (often ciliated)	Barrier, transport	Large exocrine gland ducts (salivary glands)
Transitional	Barrier, distension	Urinary bladder, urethra, ureters

- **Columnar:** Height > width.
- **Transitional:** Ranges from squamous to cuboidal. Distensible.
- By location (almost always simple squamous).
  - **Endothelium:** Lines all blood vessels.
  - **Mesothelium:** Lines all closed body cavities.

▶ BASEMENT MEMBRANE

- Connects the epithelial basal layer to underlying connective tissue.

FUNCTIONS OF BASEMENT MEMBRANE

- Attachment
- Separation
- Filtration
- Scaffolding

Components of Basement Membrane

From epithelium → connective tissue

- **Lamina lucida:** Electron-clear layer
- **Lamina densa (basal lamina):** Product of epithelium
  - *Type IV collagen*
  - Proteoglycans
  - Laminin
  - Fibronectin
  - Anchoring fibrils (type VII collagen)
- **Reticular lamina:** Product of CT
  - Reticular fibers (type III collagen)

▶ CONNECTIVE TISSUE

Classification of Connective Tissue

- Connective tissue proper
  - Loose CT
  - Dense CT
    - Regular
    - Irregular
- Specialized CT
  - Adipose tissue
  - Blood
  - Bone
  - Cartilage
  - Hematopoietic tissue
  - Lymphatic tissue
- Embryonic CT
  - Mesenchyme
  - Mucous CT

Almost all connective tissue (CT) originates from mesoderm; however, some CT of the head and neck region derives from neural crest ectoderm.

Connective Tissue Proper

- **Loose CT:** Abundant ground substance with sparse fibers and cells. Located under epithelial layers that cover body surfaces and line body cavities.

- **Dense CT:** Greater fiber concentration, which provides structural support.
  - **Irregular:** Irregular arrangement of fibers and cells. Makes up the majority of dense CT. Found in dermis, submucosa of the GI tract, and fibrous capsules.
  - **Regular:** Ordered arrangement of fibers and cells. Found in *tendons*, *ligaments*, and *aponeuroses*.

Connective Tissue Attachments

- **Ligament:** Connects bone to bone
- **Tendon:** Connects muscle to bone
- **Aponeurosis:** A sheetlike tendon
- **Sharpey's fiber:** The portion of a ligament or tendon that inserts into bone (or cementum)

Cells of CT

- Resident cell population
  - Fibroblasts
  - Myofibroblasts
  - Adipocytes
  - Macrophages (histiocytes)
  - Mast cells
  - Mesenchymal cells
- Transient cell population
  - Lymphocytes
  - Neutrophils
  - Monocytes
  - Plasma cells
  - Eosinophils
  - Basophils

▶ GLANDULAR TISSUE

Types of Glands

- There are three major types of glands.

Types of Glands

Gland Type	Function	Examples	Secretions
Exocrine	Secrete products through **ducts**	Sweat, salivary, sebaceous, von Ebner's glands	Sweat, saliva, sebum, digestive enzymes
Endocrine	Secrete products into the **bloodstream** (no ducts)	Pituitary, thyroid, parathyroid, adrenal, gonads, pineal glands	Various **hormones**
Paracrine	Secrete products into **exracellular spaces** that affect other cells within the same epithelium	Gastroenteropancreatic glands	Various peptides

Classification of Exocrine Glands

See Figure 2–4.

Classification	Type	Definition	Examples
Cellularity	Unicellular	Single secretory cells	Goblet cells
	Multicellular	Multiple secretory cells	Gastric pits
Secretion mechanism	Merocrine	Secretory product released from secretory granules	Major salivary glands, pancreatic acinar cells
	Apocrine	Secretory product is released with cytoplasm	Mammary glands, apocrine sweat glands
	Holocrine	Secretory product is released with portion of cell	Sebaceous glands
Duct structure	Simple	Unbranched	Sweat glands
	Compound	Branched	Major salivary glands, pancreas
Secretory unit	Tubular	Secretory portion shaped like a tube	Intestinal glands
	Coiled	Secretory portion shaped like a coiled tube	Eccrine sweat glands
	Acinar	Secretory portion shaped like a saclike dilation	Sebaceous glands, mammary glands, gastric cardiac glands, pancreas
	Tubuloacinar	Combination of tubular and acinar	Major salivary glands
Secretion type	Mucous	Viscous secretion	Sublingual salivary glands, goblet cells
	Serous	Watery secretion	Parotid salivary glands, paneth cells, gastric chief cells
	Mixed	Combination of mucous and serous	Submandibular salivary glands

 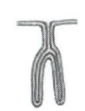 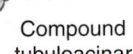

Simple tubular • Simple coiled tubular • Simple branched tubular • Simple branched acinar

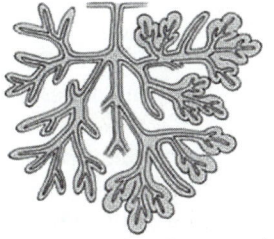 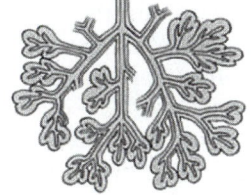

Compound tubular • Compound tubuloacinar • Compound acinar

FIGURE 2–4. Classification of exocrine glands.

Reproduced, with permission, from Ross MH. *Histology*, 3rd ed. Lippincott Williams & Wilkins, 1995. (Based on Weiss L. *Histology*, 4th ed. McGraw-Hill, 1977.)

Hyaline cartilage is essential for endochondral bone formation.

▶ CARTILAGE

- An **avascular** connective tissue.
- Composed of **chondrocytes,** which reside in **lacunae,** surrounded by their own specialized extracellular matrix (ECM).
- **Chondroblasts:** The initial cartilagenic cells (prior to extensive matrix formation).

ECM of Cartilage

- Type II collagen
- Ground substance: Extremely hydrophilic
    - Glycosaminoglycans (GAGs)
        - Hyaluronic acid
        - Chondroitin sulfate
        - Keratin sulfate
    - Proteoglycans

Surface of Cartilage

- Perichondrium
    - Inner *cellular* layer: Produces chondroblasts
    - Outer *fibrous* layer: Provides protection

Growth of Cartilage

- **Appositional growth:** New cartilage forms on the surface of existing cartilage. Fibroblastic cells from the inner perichondrium differentiate into chondroblasts, which secrete matrix.
- **Interstitial growth:** New cartilage forms within existing cartilage. Chondrocytes divide within their lacunae, enabling more matrix to be deposited.

Types of Cartilage

Cartilage	ECM Composition	Function	Ability to Calcify	Locations
Hyaline	Closely packed, thin collagen fibers.	Provides pliability and resilience. Precursor to endochondral bone formation.	Yes	Nose, trachea, bronchi, larynx, ribs (costal cartilage), articular surfaces of long bones
Elastic	Collagen and elastic fibers.	Provides elastic properties.	No	External ear, Eustachian tube, epiglottis
Fibrocartilage	Dense collagen fibers.	Withstands compression and tension.	No	Intervertebral discs, knee menisci, TMJ, symphysis pubis

BONE

- A yellowish, mineralized, vascular tissue of varying degrees of density.
- **Osteoblasts:** Produce **osteoid** (bone matrix), which is composed of collagen and ground substance. **Mature bone** forms when the osteoid calcifies.
- During the clacification process, osteoblasts become trapped in spaces within the mineralized matrix called **lacunae**. Here they differentiate into **osteocytes**, which are responsible for maintaining the bone matrix. They maintain nourishment via vascular tunnels within bone called **canaliculi**.

Functions of Bone

- Support
- Protection
- Movement
- Mineral storage
- Hematopoiesis

Bone Formation

- **Intramembranous ossification:** Mesenchymal cells differentiate into osteoblasts, which secrete bone matrix within an established locus of loosely arranged **collagen**. This new matrix calcifies, forming immature **woven bone**. Over time, osteoclastic resorption of woven bone occurs, and new osteoblastic matrix is deposited in a more tightly arranged manner. This matrix is then calcified, forming mature bone of a higher strength. The *maxilla* and the *body of the mandible* are formed by this method.
- **Endochondral ossification:** A subperiosteal bony cuff forms around an already established locus of **hyaline cartilage**, which grows larger and subsequently causes the hypertrophy and death of the chondrocytes. The cartilage matrix then becomes calcified. Over time, osteoclastic resorption of the calcified cartilage occurs, and new osteoblastic matrix is deposited, forming mature bone. The *mandibular condyles* are formed by this method.

Types of Bone

- **Cortical (compact):** Composed of **Haversian systems (osteons)**, which are composed of concentric bone matrix **lamellae** surrounding a central **Haversian canal** that contains neurovascular bundles. Canaliculi connect to the central canal, providing nourishment to osteocytes. Osteons are connected to each other by **Volkmann's canals**. The space between osteons is composed of previous osteonal lamellae, called **interstitial lamellae.**
- **Cancellous (spongy):** Similar to cortical bone in that it is lamellar, but their configuration and arrangement is less dense. Lamellae are arranged in thin spicules called **trabeculae**. If they are thick enough, they contain osteons. In between the trabeculae are *marrow spaces* of varyious sizes.

Bone Surfaces

- **Periosteum:** A fibrous connective tissue capsule that *surrounds* the outer surface of bone. Contains collagen, fibroblasts, and *osteoprogenitor cells.*
- **Endosteum:** A *one-cell thick layer* of mostly osteoprogenitor cells that *lines* the inner surface bone. *Contains bone marrow.*

Hydroxyapatite
$[Ca_{10}(PO_4)_6(OH)_3]$ is the predominant mineral found in bone.

Alkaline phosphatase increases the phosphate concentration, enhancing mineralization.

Intramembranous osteogenesis only forms by **appositional** *growth.*

Endochondral osteogenesis forms by both **appositional** and **interstitial** growth.

Bone Marrow

- **Yellow marrow:** Contains fat cells. The predominant marrow type in the maxilla and mandible.
- **Red marrow:** Contains hematopoietic cells. Found in the mandibular ramus and condyles.

Bone marrow is contained within the medullary spaces of spongy bone.

Bone Remodeling

- Bone constantly remodels, a process involving both osteoclasts (resorption) and osteoblasts (matrix deposition). **Osteoclasts** are multinucleated giant cells that reside in resorption bays known as **Howship's lacunae.** They produce a large number of hydrolytic enzymes from their characteristic ruffled border. The protons lower the pH at the site of resorption, subsequently dissolving the calcified bone matrix. Collagenases and other proteases then digest the decalcified bone matrix.

Mature bone grows only by appositional growth.

Calcium Regulation

- **Parathyroid hormone (PTH):** Stimulates osteoclastic bone resorption (↑ blood calcium). Secreted by the parathyroid gland.
- **Calcitonin:** Inhibits osteoclastic bone resorption (↓ blood calcium). Secreted by the parafollicular cells of the thyroid gland.

▶ JOINTS

Classification of Joints

- By motion
    - **Synarthrosis:** Immovable (cranial sutures)
    - **Amphiarthrosis:** Slightly movable (symphysis pubis)
    - **Diarthrosis:** Fully moveable (shoulder, hip, TMJ)
- By connective tissue type
    - **Fibrous:** Joined by fibrous CT
        - **Suture** (cranial sutures)
        - **Syndesmosis** (between radius and ulna)
        - **Gomphosis** (tooth socket)
    - **Cartilaginous:** Joined by cartilage
        - **Synchondrosis** (epiphyseal plates of long bones)
        - **Symphysis** (symphysis pubis)
    - **Synovial:** Lined by a synovial membrane
        - Majority of joints (shoulder, hip, TMJ)

*The TMJ is a synovial, diarthrosis joint. It contains an articular disc of fibrocartilage (**not** hyaline cartilage), which divides the synovial cavity into two compartments.*

Synovial Joints

- **Articular capsule (bursa):** Composed of fibrous connective tissue. Surrounds the joint. Lined by synovial membrane.
- **Articular cartilage (meniscus):** Layer of **hyaline** cartilage that covers the articular bone surfaces (**except** the TMJ, which is composed of fibrocartilage).
- **Synovial cavity:** Lies within the articular capsule and contains synovial fluid.
- **Synovial membrane:** Lines the articular capsule. Produces synovial fluid.
- **Synovial fluid:** Lubricates the articular cartilage.

NERVOUS TISSUE

Division	Origin	Location	Cell Body Clusters
CNS	Neural tube ectoderm	Brain and spinal cord	Nuclei
PNS	Neural crest ectoderm	Cranial and spinal nerves, ganglia, and nerve endings	Ganglia

Neurons

- Nerve cells that conduct electrical impulses.
    - **Perikaryon (cell body):** Contains plasma membrane, cytoplasm, nucleus, and **Nissl bodies (rER)**.
    - **Axon:** Conducts information *away* from cell body. Only one axon exists per cell body.
    - **Dendrites:** Conducts information *toward* the cell body. None to many dendrites may exist per cell body (depending on the neuron).
    - **Cytoskeleton**
        - Actin
        - Microubules (dendrites)
        - Neurofilaments (axons)

Neurons do not divide.

Neuron Classification

- By function
    - Motor (efferent)
    - Sensory (afferent)
    - Mixed (both)
- By number of processes
    - **Unipolar:** One process (axon only), sensory neurons
    - **Bipolar:** Two processes (one axon and one dendrite), retina and ganglia of CN VIII
    - **Multipolar:** Three or more processes (one axon and many dendrites), motor and mixed neurons

Synapses

- Junctions that transmit impulses from one neuron to another, or from one neuron to an effector cell.
- Two types of synapses:
    - Electrical: Synaptic cleft is a *gap junction*. Located in smooth and cardiac muscle.
    - Chemical: Synaptic cleft is a 20–30 nm intercellular space.

Supporting Cells

See Table 2–3.

- Non-conducting cells that insulate neurons.

TABLE 2-3. Supporting Cells of Nervous Tissue

Cell Type	Function
CNS (Glial Cells)	
Astrocytes	Regulation of metabolites
■ *Protoplasmic:* Gray matter	Scaffolding of BBB
■ *Fibrous:* White matter	
Oligodendrocytes	Myelination
Microglia	Phagocytosis
PNS	
Schwann cells	Myelination
	Surround nerve *processes*
Satellite cells	Support
	Surround nerve *ganglia*

TABLE 2-4. Myelin-Producing Cells of the Nervous System

Cell Type	Division	Cells/Neuron	Myelin Sheath
Oligodendrocyte	CNS	Multiple (as many as 50)	Composed of several internodal tongue-like processes that wrap around the axon
Schwann cell	PNS	1	Composed of multiple layers concentrically wrapped around the axon

Not all Schwann cells produce myelin:

A fibers: *Myelinated – have neurilemma and myelin.*

C fibers: *Unmyelinated – only have neurilemma.*

Myelination

See Table 2–4.

- **Myelin sheath:** Lipid-rich layer that surrounds and insulates myelinated axons.
- **Neurilemma:** Layer of myelin cell cytoplasm that is contiguous with the myelin sheath.
- **Node of Ranvier:** *Unmyelinated* junction between two myelin cells.
- Myelin formation begins before birth and during 1st year postnatally (see Babinski reflex).

▶ **BLOOD**

Functions

- Transportation
- Buffering
- Thermoregulation

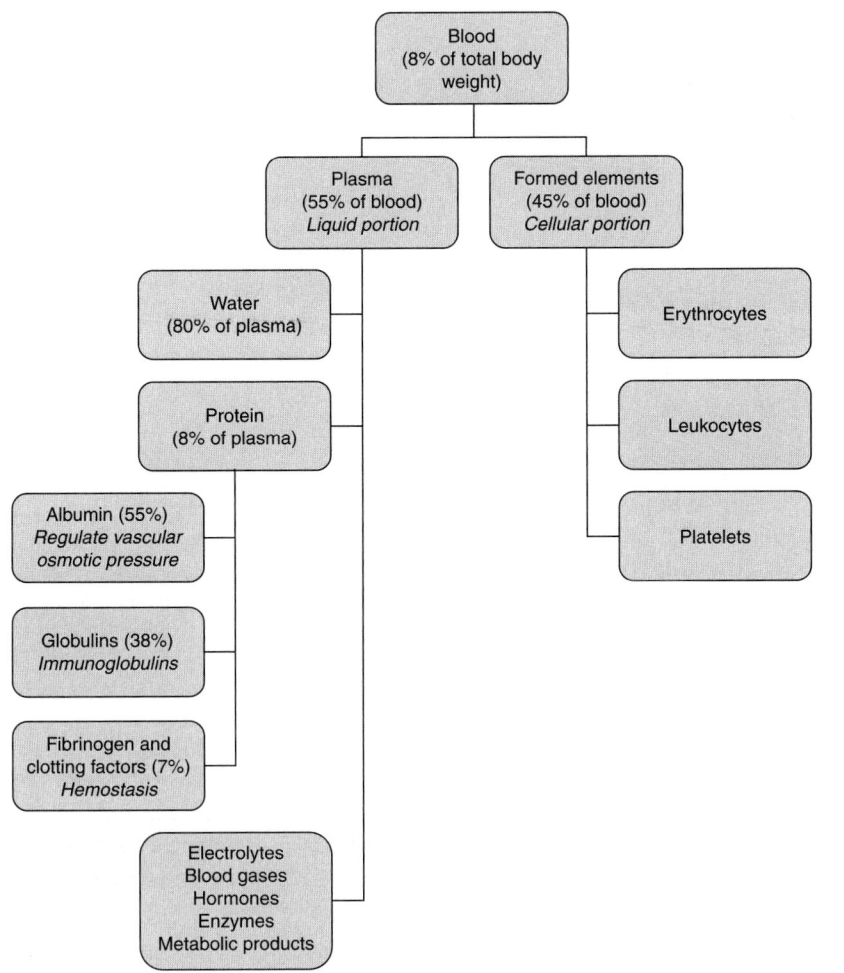

Serum is blood plasma minus fibrinogen and clotting factors.

Hematocrit is the percentage of erythrocytes in a blood sample. In males, the average hematocrit is 45%; in females it is 40%.

FIGURE 2-5. Components of blood.

Components

See Figure 2-5.

Formed Elements

Formed Element	Function	Characteristics	Average Lifespan	Normal Amount Per mm³ Blood
Erythrocytes	Transports O_2 (99%) Transports CO_2 (30%)	Biconcave discs No nucleus Elastic	120 days	4–5 million
Platelets	Hemostasis	Cytoplasmic fragments of **megakaryocytes** No nucleus	5–10 days	200,000–400,000
Leukocytes	Immunoregulation Inflammation Phagocytosis Hypersensitivity	Nucleated, but morphology is variable	Variable	6000–10,000

Erythrocytes

- Red blood cells.
- Biconcave discs (7–10 μm in diameter).
- Contain hemoglobin.
- Function: Transports O_2 (and CO_2).
- Lipid membrane contains lipoproteins and blood group surface markers (A, B, O).
- Amount of bile pigment excreted by liver estimates the amount of erythrocyte destruction per day.

Leukocytes

See Table 2–5.

*Monocytes transform into **macrophages** (histiocytes) once they leave the bloodstream and enter the surrounding connective tissue.*

- White blood cells.
- **Granulocytes:** Contain cytoplasmic granules.
    - Neutrophils (60%)
    - Eosinophils (5%)
    - Basophils (1%)
- **Agranulocytes:** Contain few cytoplasmic granules.
    - Lymphocytes (30%)
    - Monocytes (4%)

TABLE 2–5. Comparison of Leukocytes

Leukocyte	Nuclear Morphology	Cytoplasmic Granules	Function
Neutrophil	3–5 lobes	**Specific granules** (lysozyme, etc.) **Azurophilic granules** (peroxidases, etc.)	Phagocytosis Acute inflammation
Eosinophil	2 lobes	Peroxidase Histaminase Arylsulfatase	Phagocytosis (parasites) Chronic inflammation
Basophil	2–3 lobes, obscured by dense granules	Histamine Seratonin Heparin sulfate	Hypersensitivity (bind IgE)
Lymphocyte	Large, round	Few azurophilic granules	Immunoregulation Chronic inflammation
Monocyte	U-shaped	Few azurophilic granules	Phagocytosis Chronic inflammation

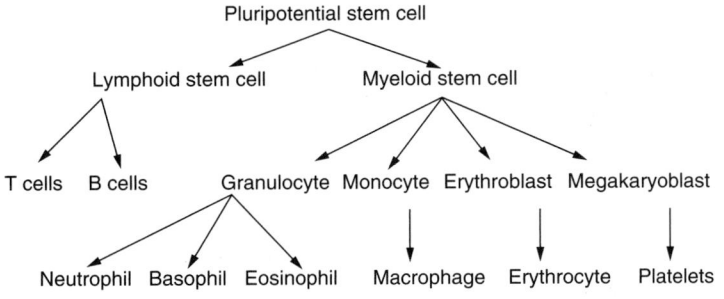

FIGURE 2-6. Hematopoiesis.

Hematopoiesis

See below figure.

- Blood cell formation.
- All blood cells derive from one **pluripotential stem cell.**
- Hormones (erythropoietin, thrombopoietin, etc.) and colony stimulating factors (CSFs) regulate hematopoiesis.
- Occurs primarily in **bone marrow,** although some lymphocytes also develop in lymphatic tissues.

▶ CARDIOVASCULAR TISSUE

Arrangement of Blood Vessels in Circulation

See figure below.

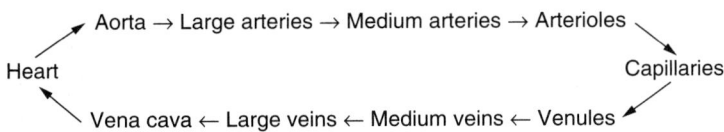

Arrangement of blood vessels in circulation.

Layers of Blood Vessel Walls

From lumen → outermost layer:

- **Tunica intima:** Contains *simple squamous epithelium* (**endothelium**) resting on a basement membrane and subendothelial connective tissue. Present in ALL blood vessels and heart wall. Only arteries have an additional elastic layer here called the **internal elastic membrane.**
- **Tunica media:** Contains *smooth muscle* and *elastic fibers*. Much thicker in arteries.
- **Tunica adventitia:** Connective tissue layer containing *collagen* and *elastic fibers*. Much thicker in veins. Large vessels contain **vasa vasora,** which supply the vessels themselves.

Sinusoids are fenestrated or discontinuous capillaries in the liver, spleen, and endocrine glands. They are larger and more irregularly shaped than capillaries to accommodate phagocytic cells of the reticuloendothelial system.

Major Histologic Differences among Blood Vessel Types

Blood Vessel	Distinguishing Characteristic
Elastic Arteries (aorta, pulmonary arteries, and their main branches)	Thickest tunica media. Elastic fibers > smooth muscle. Contain vasa vasora.
Muscular Arteries	Thick tunica media. Smooth muscle > elastic fibers. Some contain vasa vasora.
Arterioles	Thick tunica media. Smooth muscle > elastic fibers.
Capillaries	Endothelial layer only. One erythrocyte cell wide. Enable gas and metabolite exchange via **diffusion.**
Venules	Thick tunica adventitia.
Veins	Thickest tunica adventitia. Some contain valves. Some contain vasa vasora.

Layers of the Heart

From lumen → outermost layer.

- **Endocardium:** Same as tunica intima. Contains a simple squamous endothelium.
- **Myocardium:** Thickest portion of the heart. Contains *cardiac muscle.*
- **Pericardium:** Outer layer of *connective tissue* and *adipose tissue* surrounded by a simple squamous epithelium.

Cardiac Conduction

- Cardiac muscle maintains its *own* rhythmicity.
- The **sinoatrial (SA) node** is the "pacemaker" of the heart.
- Autonomic nerves only regulate the *rate* of cardiac impulses.
- SA node → AV node → Bundle of His → Purkinje fibers.

▶ LYMPHATIC SYSTEM

Lymph

- A yellowish, plasmalike liquid that contains mostly **lymphocytes.**
- Once absorbed in various tissues throughout the body, it is carried through a system of enclosed **lymphatic vessels** and ultimately drains into the venous circulation.
- Lymph is not pumped through its vessels, but relies on valves, gravity, and skeletal muscle contractions for its movement.

Functions of the Lymphatic System

- Transportation of tissue fluid (lymph) to the circulation
- Transportation of fat metabolites to the circulation
- Filtration of foreign agents in lymph nodes
- Provides immunological surveillance against pathogens

Lymph Drainage

- Thoracic duct (drains majority of the body) → left subclavian vein
- Right lymphatic duct (drains upper right body regions) → right subclavian vein

COMPONENTS OF THE LYMPHATIC SYSTEM

- Bone marrow
- Thymus
- Spleen
- Lymph
- Lymphatic vessels
- Lymph nodes
- Lymphatic nodules
    - Tonsils
    - Appendix
    - Peyer's patches of the ileum

LYMPH NODES

- Small, fibrous-encapsulated organs that filter lymph.
- **Macrophages** and **lymphocytes** process lymph in nodal **cortical and trabecular sinuses.**
- Nodes have fewer efferent vessels than afferent vessels.
- Widely distributed throughout the body, but concentrate in the axilla, groin, mesenteries, and neck.
- Consist of:
    - **Outer cortex:** Contains germinal nodes, which house **T-lymphocytes.**
    - **Inner medulla:** Contains medullary cords, which house **plasma cells.**

BONE MARROW

- Site of **B-cell maturation**
- Contains pluripotent stem cells capable of differentiating into lymphocytes or phagocytes

THYMUS

- Site of **T-cell maturation**
- Grows in size from birth until puberty, then is reduced and replaced with adipose tissue in adulthood
- Does *not* contain afferent lymphatic vessels
- Consists of:
    - **External capsule:** *Trabeculae* extend into cortex and medulla
    - **Outer cortex:** Contains high concentration of *lymphocytes*
    - **Inner medulla:** Contains *thymic corpuscles* (epithelioreticular cells)

Spleen

- Largest lymphatic organ.
- Site of lymphocyte proliferation, scavenging of large antigens and damaged erythrocytes, and fetal erythropoiesis.
- Consists of:
  - **White pulp:** Contains **lymphocytes** and splenic nodules.
  - **Red pulp:** Contains **erythrocytes**, macrophages, and lymphocytes.

▶ ENDOCRINE GLANDS

Pituitary Gland (Hypophysis)

See Table 2–6.

- Pea-shaped organ located in the sella turcica of the sphenoid bone.
- Attached to the hypothalamus.

GH is the most abundant of the pituitary hormones. ADH and oxytocin are synthesized in the hypothalamus and stored in the posterior pituitary.

Pituitary gland:
- *Vital to life*
- *"Master endocrine gland"*

TABLE 2–6. Functional Components of the Pituitary Gland

Functional Component	Embryonic Derivation	Components	Secretory Products	Function
Adenohypophysis (Anterior pituitary)	Rathke's pouch (oral ectoderm)	Pars distalis	**Somatotropes** Growth hormone (GH)	General growth ↑ AA uptake ↑ protein synthesis Carbohydrate and fat breakdown
			Lactotropes Prolactin (♀)	Mammary gland development Milk production
			Gonadotropes Follicle-stimulating hormone (FSH) Leutinizing hormone (LH)	Ovarian follicle maturation (♀) Spermatogenesis (♂) Stimulates sex steroid secretion Controls ovulation (♀)
			Corticotropes Adrenocorticotropic hormone (ACTH)	Stimulates glucocorticoid secretion
			Thyrotropes Thyroid-stimulating hormone (TSH)	Thyroxine secretion Uptake of iodine
		Pars intermedia	**Lipotropes** Lipotropic hormone (LPH)	No known human function
		Pars tuberalis	**Gonadotropes**	See above
Neurohypophysis (posterior pituitary): ■ Contains unmyelinated nerves	Infundibulum (neurectoderm)	Pars nervosa	Antidiuretic hormone (ADH)	Water reabsorption
			Oxytocin	Uterine contractions Milk ejection
		Infundibulum	None	
		Median eminence	None	

- Provides regulatory feedback to the hypothalamus.
- Contains its own *portal system*.
- Composed of two distinct functional compartments:
  - **Adenohypophysis**
  - **Neurohypophysis**

A portal system has two capillary beds. There are three portal systems in the body: hepatic, renal, pituitary.

Thyroid Gland

- Bilobed organ located anterolateral to the upper trachea.
- Surrounded by a connective tissue capsule.
- Composed of numerous **secretory follicles** surrounding a gel-like **colloid** (*inactive iodinated thyroglobulin*).
- Active cells stain basophilic; inactive cells stain acidophilic.
- The normal $T_4:T_3$ ratio is 20:1.

- Hypothyroidism
  - Cretinism (children)
  - Myxedema (adults)
  - Hashimoto's thyroiditis (autoimmune)
- Hyperthyroidism
  - Grave's disease (toxic goiter)

Major Cellular Components of Thyroid Follicles

Cell Type	Secretory Products	Function
Follicular cells	T_4 (thyroxine)	Regulate metabolism
	T_3	Regulate metabolism
Parafollicular cells	Calcitonin	↓ blood calcium levels

Parathyroid Glands

See Table 2–7.

- Small, ovoid organs arranged in pairs located in the thyroid connective tissue.
- Surrounded by their own connective tissue capsules.
- Derive from the third and fourth pharyngeal pouches.
- Regulate blood calcium and phosphate.

Effects of PTH

- ↑ blood calcium levels (*reciprocal action of calcitonin*)
- Stimulates bone resorption
- ↑ renal Ca^{2+} resorption (↓ Ca^{2+} excretion)
- ↓ renal PO_4^{3-} resorption (↑ PO_4^{3-} excretion)
- ↑ intestinal Ca^{2+} absorption

TABLE 2-7. Major Parathyroid Cells

Parathyroid Cell	Cytoplasm	Function
Chief (Principal) cell	Clear	Secretes PTH
Oxyphil cell	Granules	Unknown

Adrenal (Suprarenal) Glands

- Triangular organs located just superior to the kidneys.
- Surrounded by a thick connective tissue capsule.
- Provides regulatory feedback to the pituitary and hypothalamus
- Composed of two regions:
    - **Outer cortex**
    - **Inner medulla**

Zones of Adrenal Cortex: GFR = salt, sugar, sex.

Adrenal Region	Embryologic Derivation	Zones/Cells	Secretory Products	Examples
Outer cortex	Mesoderm	Zona glomerulosa - Thin layer just beneath the capsule	Mineralcorticoids	Aldosterone
		Zona fasiculata - Thick middle layer containing columns of cells	Glucocorticoids	Hydrocortisone Cortisone
		Zona reticularis - Innermost layer containing cells in a network of connected cords	Gonadocorticoids	Sex steroids
Inner medulla	Neural crest ectoderm	Chromaffin cells	Catecholamines	Epinephrine Norepinephrine

▶ RESPIRATORY SYSTEM

See Table 2–8.

Functions

- Air conduction
- Air filtration
- Gas exchange

Divisions

- Conduction: Warms air, moistens, removes particles
    - Nasal cavities
    - Nasopharynx and Oropharynx
    - Larynx
    - Trachea
    - Bronchi
- Respiration: Gas exchange
    - Bronchioles
    - Alveolar ducts
    - Alveolar sacs
    - Alveoli

TABLE 2-8. Major Respiratory Segments

Respiratory Segment	Components	Epithelium
Nasal cavities	Vestibule Respiratory segment Olfactory segment	Stratified squamous Psuedostratified ciliated columnar Olfactory
Pharynx	Nasopharynx Oropharynx	Pseudostratified ciliated columnar Pseudostratified ciliated columnar
Larynx	Vocal folds (true vocal cords) Ventricular folds (false vocal cords)	Stratified squamous Pseudostratified ciliated columnar
Trachea	C-shaped hyaline cartilage rings	Pseudostratified ciliated columnar
Bronchi	Primary Extrapulmonary	Pseudostratified columnar Pseudostratified columnar
Bronchioles	Terminal Respiratory	Simple columnar Simple cuboidal
Alveoli	Alveolar ducts Alveolar sacs Alveolar septa	Simple cuboidal Simple cuboidal Simple squamous

Alveoli

- Site of gas exchange
- **Alveolar septum:** Separates adjacent alveolar air spaces

Alveolar Epithelial Cell Types

Pneumocyte Type	Prevalence (%)	Function	Characteristic
Type I	9	Barrier	Joined by tight junctions
Type II	5	Secretion	Produce **surfactant**

Dust cells are alveolar macrophages.

▶ UPPER DIGESTIVE SYSTEM

Functions

- Barrier
- Absorption
- Secretion

Peristalsis is the waves of smooth muscle contraction of the muscularis externa that propels GI contents along.

Layers

From inner → outer

- Mucosa
    - Epithelium: Varies throughout the GI tract
    - Lamina propria: Underlying CT and lymphatic tissue
    - Muscularis mucosae: Smooth muscle
- Submucosa: Dense irregular CT, glands, submucosal plexus of unmyelinated nerves and ganglia
- Muscularis externa: Smooth muscle
    - Circular
    - Longitudinal
- Serosa
    - Mesothelium: Simple squamous epithelium
    - CT: Adipose tissue, vasculature, lymphatics
- Adventitia: Loose CT

Esophagus

- Function: Transports food from oropharynx → stomach
- Epithelium: Nonkeratinized stratified squamous
- Glands: Mucous
    - Esophageal glands proper: Upper portion
    - Esophageal cardiac glands: Lower portion
    - Innervation: CN X

Stomach

- Function: Mixing and partial digestion of food, producing **chyme**
- Epithelium: Simple columnar, renews every 3–5 days
- Lining
    - **Rugae:** Longitudinal folds along the lumen of the stomach that accommodate expansion
    - **Gastric pits:** Microscopic depressions of the mucosal surface into which the gastric glands empty
- Organization
    - Cardiac: Junction of esophagus
    - Fundic: Body of stomach
    - Pyloric: Junction of small intestine
- Glands: See Table 2–9
- Innervation: CN X (regulates emptying)

Small Intestine

See Table 2–10.

- Function: Digestion of chyme and absorption
- Epithelium: Simple columnar, renews every 5–6 days
- Lining
    - **Plicae circulares:** Transverse semilunar folds along the lumen of the small intestine, provide ↑ surface area
    - **Villi:** Fingerlike projections of the mucosa, provide movement of materials
    - **Microvilli:** Micro fingerlike projections of enterocytes, provide ↑ surface area

TABLE 2-9. Major Glands of the Stomach

GLAND	LOCATION	CELL TYPES	SECRETION	FUNCTION
Fundic (gastric)	Throughout gastric mucosa	Mucous neck cells	Soluble mucous	
		Chief cells	Pepsinogen	Converted to pepsin via gastric HCl
		Parietal cells	HCl	↓stomach pH
			Intrinsic factor	Required for vitamin B_{12} absorption
		Enteroendocrine (APUD) cells	Gastrin	Stimulates HCl secretion
Cardiac	Cardiac stomach	Cardiac mucosal cells	Mucous	
Pyloric	Pyloric stomach	Pyloric mucosal cells	Viscous mucous	

TABLE 2-10. Cells of the Small Intestine

CELL	LOCATION	SECRETION	FUNCTION
Enterocytes	*Epithelium* of small intestine	None	Absorption (contain microvilli)
		Glycoprotein enzymes	Digestion and absorption
Goblet cells	*Epithelium* of small intestine (most numerous in terminal ileum)	Mucous	
M cells	Peyer's patches (**ileum**)	None	Absorption of antigens to underlying lymphatic tissue
Paneth cells	Mucosal glands throughout small intestine	Lysozyme	Digestion of bacterial cell walls
Enteroendocrine cells	Intestinal crypt throughout small intestine (most numerous in duodenum)	CCK	↑ pancreatic secretion
		Secretin	↑ pancreatic HCO_3^- secretion
		Gastric inhibitory peptide (GIP)	↓ gastric acid secretion
Mucosal cells	*Submucosal* glands of Brunner (**duodenum**)	HCO_3^-	Neutralizes intestinal pH

- Organization
  - **Duodenum:** Shortest segment
  - **Jejunum:** Middle segment
  - **Ileum:** Longest segment
- Muscularis externa
  - **Myenteric (Auerbach's) plexus:** Located between two layers of smooth muscle
- Muscular Contractions
  - Peristalsis
  - Segmentation: Local contractions
- Glands
  - **Intestinal glands (crypts of Lieberkühn):** Throughout small intestine at base of villi
  - **Submucosal glands of Brunner:** Only in *duodenum*

Large Intestine

- Function: Reabsorption of water/electrolytes and elimination of waste
- Epithelium: Simple columnar, renews every 5–6 days
  - Goblet cells lubricate dehydrating fecal matter
  - Paneth cells *not* present
- Lining: Smooth surface (no plicae circulares or villi)
- Organization
  - Cecum
  - Ascending colon
  - Descending colon
  - Sigmoid colon
  - Rectum
  - Anal canal
- Muscularis externa
  - **Teniae coli:** Three longitudinal segments of muscle for peristalsis.
- Glands
  - Intestinal glands (crypts of Lieberkühn)

Gut-Associated Lymphatic Tissue (GALT)

- Lamina propria (GI tract)
- Peyer's patches (ileum)
- Lymphoid aggregates (large intestine and appendix)

▶ LOWER DIGESTIVE SYSTEM

Liver

- **Exocrine** (via ducts)

Bile

- **Endocrine** (via bloodstream)
  - Albumin
  - Lipoproteins
  - α and β globulins

- Prothrombin
- Fibronectin

Portal Triad

- Hepatic artery
- Portal vein
- Bile duct

Liver Lobules

- Hexagonal stacks of *hepatocyte cords* separated by anastamosing *sinusoids*
- Surround a *central vein* (into which sinusoids drain)
- *Portal triads* located at each corner

Hepatocytes

- Nuclei: Often bi-nucleate (tetraploid)
- Cytoplasm: Acidophilic
    - Mitochondria
    - Golgi bodies
    - rER
    - sER
    - **Peroxisomes**
        - Catalase
        - Alcohol degydrogenase
    - Lysosomes
        - Store iron
    - Glycogen deposits
    - Lipid droplets
- Life span: 5 months
- Capable of regeneration

Sinusoids

- Lined by a thin, discontinuous epithelium
    - Gaps: Between epithelial cells
    - Fenestrae: Within epithelial cells
- Cell types
    - Epithelial cells
    - **Kupffer cells:** Mononuclear macrophages
    - **Ito cells:** Adipocytes in the space of Disse—store *vitamin* A
- **Perisinusoidal space (space of Disse):** Site of exchange between blood and hepatocytes

Biliary Tree

See Figure 2–7.

- Ductal system that transports bile from hepatocytes → gall bladder (via cystic duct) and duodenum (via common bile duct).
- **Canaliculi:** Small canals formed by grooves in adjacent hepatocytes.
- Bile flow is *opposite* to that of blood flow (central vein → portal canal).
- **Ampulla of Vater:** Opening of common bile duct into the duodenum.
- Sphincters
    - **Sphincter of Boyden:** At common bile duct.
    - **Sphincter of Oddi:** At ampulla of Vater.

Elevated bilirubin levels result in jaundice.

Bile flow is increased by CCK, secretin, and gastrin.

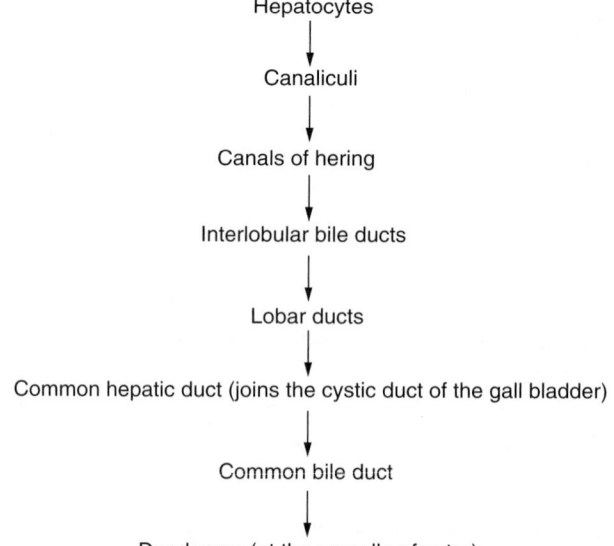

FIGURE 2-7. Biliary flow.

*Enzyme production is regulated by duodenal **secretin** (↑ bicarbonate secretion) and **CCK** (↑ proenzyme secretion).*

*Pancreatic digestive enzymes are activated only after they reach the **small intestine**, where trypsinogen is converted to trypsin via enterokinases. **Trypsin** then converts the other inactive digestive enzymes.*

Bile Composition

- Water
- Electrolytes
- Cholesterol
- Lecithin
- Bile salts
  - Glycocholic acid
  - Taurocholic acid
- Bile pigments
  - Bilirubin
  - Biliverdin
  - Glucuronide

Gall Bladder

- Function: Concentrates and stores bile
- Epithelium: Simple columnar
  - Contains microvilli
  - Has lateral plications
  - **Rokitansky-Aschoff sinuses:** Deep diverticula of the mucosa
- **No submucosa**
- Lamina propria: Does *not* contain lymphatic vessels
- Glands
  - Mucin-secreting glands

Pancreas

- **Exocrine** (via ducts)
  - Digestive enzymes

- **Endocrine** (via bloodstream)
  - Glucagon
  - Insulin
  - Somatostatin

Exocrine Pancreas

- Function: Produces digestive enzyme precursors (proenzymes)
  - Trypsinogen
  - Pepsinogen
  - Amylase
  - Lipase
  - Deoxyribonuclease
  - Ribonuclease
- Components: **Pancreatic acini**
- Cell types: **Centroacinar cells**

Endocrine Pancreas

- Function: Regulates blood glucose levels
- Components: **Islets of Langerhans**
- Cell types: See Table below

Major Cells of the Pancreatic Islets

Cell Type	Major Product	Function
Alpha	Glucagon	↑ blood glucose levels ↑ glycogenolysis, gluconeogenesis, and hepatic lipase
Beta	Insulin	↓ blood glucose levels ↑ cellular glucose uptake, utilization, and storage (as glycogen)
Delta	Somatostatin	Inhibits insulin and glucagon secretion

▶ URINARY SYSTEM

Components

- Kidneys
- Ureters
- Urinary bladder
- Urethra

Medullary rays are striations in the **cortex** (radiating from the medulla) composed of groups of cortical straight tubules and collecting ducts.

Pyramids are conical structures in the medulla composed of groups of medullary straight tubules, collecting ducts, and vasa recta. Usually 8–12 per kidney.

Functions of Kidneys

- Removes metabolic waste
- Conserves body fluids
- Synthesizes erythropoietin
- Synthesizes renin
- Hydroxylates vitamin D

Components of Kidneys

- **Capsule:** Tough, thin outer covering
- **Cortex:** Outer portion
    - Renal (Malpighian) corpuscles
        - **Glomerulus:** 10–20 capillary loops
        - **Bowman's capsule:** Double-layered epithelial covering
    - Proximal tubules
    - Distal tubules
    - Cortical collecting ducts
- **Medulla:** Inner portion
    - Medullary collecting ducts
    - Loop of Henle
    - Vasa recta

JG cells produce renin – regulates blood pressure.

Juxtaglomerular Apparatus (JGA)

- **Macula densa:** Part of distal convoluted tubule
- **Juxtaglomerular cells:** Modified smooth muscle cells

Nephron

- Functions
    - Filtration
    - Absorption
    - Secretion
    - Excretion
- Components
    - Glomerulus
    - Bowman's capsule
    - Proximal convoluted tubule
    - Loop of Henle (descending, ascending, thick, thin)
    - Distal convoluted tubule
    - Collecting duct

The nephron is the functional unit of the kidney. There are millions per kidney.

Types of Nephrons

Nephron	Location of Renal Corpuscles	Length of Loop of Henle
Cortical	Outer cortex	Short
Intermediate	Middle cortex	Medium
Juxtamedullary	Base of medullary pyramid	Long

Urethra

- The male urethra is long (20 cm) and has three segments:
    - **Prostatic urethra:** Travels from the urinary bladder through the prostate gland.
    - **Membranous urethra:** Travels from the end of the prostate through the body wall to the penis.
    - **Penile urethra:** Travels through the length of the penis within the corpus spongiosum.
- The female urethra is short (3–5 cm), and extends from the urinary bladder to the vaginal vestibule.

▶ REPRODUCTIVE SYSTEM

Testis

- Produces **sperm** and steroids (**testosterone**).
- Covered by a thick connective tissue capsule called the **tunica albuginea**.
- Composed of many lobules, each containing 1–4 **seminiferous tubules**, the site of **spermatogenesis**.
- The **epididymis** sits on the posterior aspect of the testis and contains the ductus epididymis.

Major Cellular Components of the Male Reproductive System

Cell	Location	Function
Leydig cell	Seminiferous tubules	Produces testosterone
Sertoli cell	Seminiferous tubules	Produces testicular fluid
Sperm cell	Produced in seminiferous tubules, but mature and are stored in the epididymis	Contains genetic code

Intra- and Extra-Testicular Duct System

- Seminiferous tubules (testis) → rete testis (testis) → efferent ductules (testis) → ductus epididymis (epididymis) → ductus (vas) deferens (spermatic cord) → ejaculatory duct (enters into urethra)

Prostate Gland

- Surrounds the proximal urethra
- Secretes acid phosphatase, fibrinolysin, and citric acid

Penis

- Composed of three major masses of tissue surrounded by a dense fibroelastic capsule (**tunica albuginea**):
    - **Corpora cavernosa:** Two *dorsal* sections of erectile tissue
    - **Corpus spongiosum:** One *ventral* section containing the urethra

Ovary

- Produces **ova** and steroids (**estrogen** and **progesterone**).
- Composed of two regions:
  - **Inner medulla:** Contains vasculature, nerves, and CT.
  - **Outer cortex:** Contains **ovarian follicles,** the site of **oogenesis.**

Oviducts (Fallopian Tubes)

- Extend bilaterally from the ovaries to the uterus.
- Divided into four sections (from ovary → uterus):
  - **Infundibulum:** Just adjacent to the ovary. Contains fingerlike extensions called **fimbriae.**
  - **Ampulla:** Longest section of the oviduct. Site of fertilization.
  - **Isthmus:** Just adjacent to the uterus.
  - **Uterine:** Opening into the uterus.

Uterus

- Site of embryonic and fetal development.
- Composed of three layers:
  - **Endometrium:** Mucosal layer shed during menstruation.
  - **Myometrium:** Thickest layer containing smooth muscle.
  - **Perimetrium:** External layer containing connective tissue.
- Contains uterine glands.
- The cervix is the lower section of the uterus, connecting it to the vagina. Its mucosa is *not* shed during menstruation.

Vagina

- Lined by nonkeratinized stratified squamous epithelium.
- Does *not* contain glands.

Mammary Glands

- Contain **tubuloalveolar glands** (produce milk), sebaceous glands, sweat glands, and glands of Montgomery.
- Milk is produced by both **merocrine** and **apocrine** secretion.
- Lactation is regulated by sex hormones produced during pregnancy, and is under the control of the pituitary and the hypothalamus.

Although both skin and oral mucosae have stratified squamous epithelial surfaces and subepithelial connective tissues, there are some important differences in terminology and structures.

▶ INTEGUMENT

Functions of Skin

- Protection: Against physical, chemical, and biological agents
- Sensory: Touch, pain, pressure, etc
- Homeostasis: Regulates body temperature and water loss
- Synthesis: Produces vitamin D from UV light
- Excretion: Via sweat glands

Layers of Skin

- **Epidermis:** Stratified squamous keratinized epithelium (from innermost → outermost).
    - **Stratum basale (germinativum):** Site of all epithelial mitotic activity (contains *melanocytes*, keratinocytes, and other specialized cells). Least cytodifferentiated. Cuboidal to low columnar in shape.
    - **Stratum spinosum:** Spinous (prickle cell) layer. Cells have peripheral cytoplasmic processes. *Langerhans cells* often extend into this layer.
    - **Stratum granulosum:** Cells appear flattened and may contain *keratohyalin granules*. Organelles are diminished.
    - **Stratum lucidum:** Clear cell layer found only in *thick skin*. Cells appear flattened with few (if any) organelles.
    - **Stratum corneum:** Keratinized cell layer. Cells appear flattened and pyknotic with few (if any) organelles.
- **Basement membrane:** Links the epidermis and dermis via hemidesmosomes.
- **Dermis:** Dense CT, vasculature, lymphatics, nerves, sweat glands, sebaceous glands, hair follicles.
    - **Papillary layer:** Thinner, cellular, less fibrous. Dermal papillae are the projections that interdigitate with the epidermal rete pegs (ridges), creating a variably tortuous epidermal-dermal interface.
    - **Reticular layer:** Thicker, fibrous, less cellular.
- **Hypodermis:** Loose CT, vasculature, lymphatics, *adipose tissue*.

> *Epidermal layers (from innermost to outermost):*
>
> **B**ad **S**printers **G**et **L**eg **C**ramps:
>
> **B**asale
> **S**pinosum
> **G**ranulosum
> **L**ucidum
> **C**orneum

SPECIALIZED EPIDERMAL CELLS

- Concentrated in the basal cell layer.
- **Melanocytes:** Produce melanin.
- **Keratinocytes:** Produce keratin.
- **Langerhans cells:** Antigen-presenting cells. Often extend into stratum spinosum.
- **Merkel cells:** Touch-sensory cells.

NEURONAL ENDINGS OF SKIN

- **Free nerve endings:** Most abundant nerve endings. Detect touch, temperature, pain. Extend into stratum granulosum.
- **Pacinian corpuscles:** Pressure receptors.
- **Meissner's corpuscles:** Touch receptors.
- **Ruffini endings:** Mechanoreceptors.

Hair

- Regulate body temperature
- Composed of keratinized cells
- Produced by hair follicles:
    - Bulb
    - Internal root sheath
    - External root sheath
    - Arrector pili muscle

Sweat Glands

Type	Function	Cells	Secretion	Location	Innervation
Eccrine	Regulates body temperature	Clear Dark Myoepithelial Duct	Sweat	Entire body except lips and parts of external genitalia	SNS (cholinergic)
Apocrine	Produces pheromones	Myoepithelial Duct	Secretes serous	Axilla, areola, nipple, circumanal region, external genitalia	SNS (adrenergic)

Sebaceous Glands

- Secrete **sebum,** an oily substance that coats skin and hair.
- Outgrowths of external root sheaths of hair follicles.

▶ EYE

Layers of Eye

See Figure 2–8.
From outermost → innermost:

- **Corneoscleral coat**
- **Cornea:** Transparent portion (anterior 1/6) of eye.
    - **Limbus:** Transitional zone between cornea and sclera.
    - **Sclera:** "White" portion (posterior 5/6) of eye.

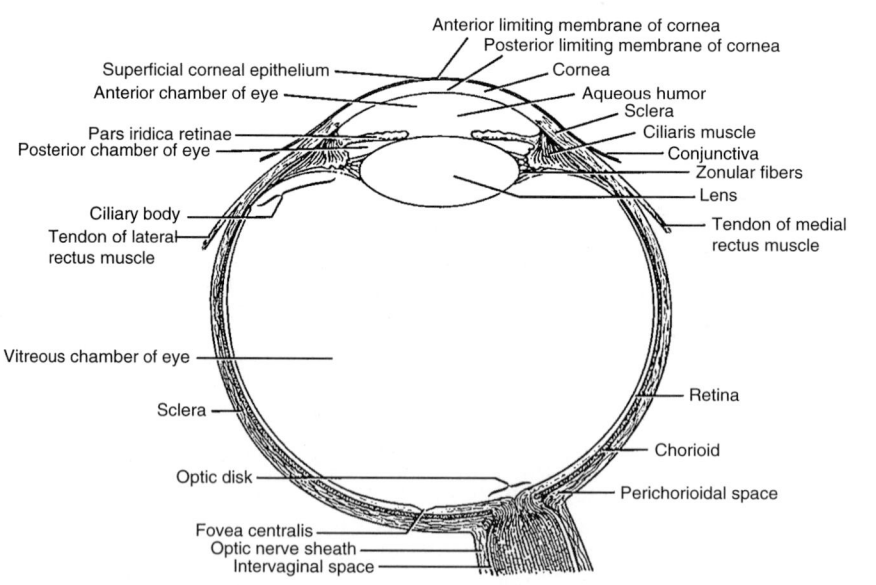

FIGURE 2–8. General structure of the eye.

Reproduced, with permission, from Montgomery, RL. *Head and Neck Anatomy: With Clinical considerations.* McGraw-Hill, 1981.

- **Uvea**
  - **Choroid:** Vascular layer. Dark brown color.
  - **Ciliary body:** Smooth muscle—lens accommodation. See Figure 2–9.
  - **Iris:** Smooth-muscle—changes pupil diameter. Pigmented portion of eye.
    - **Pupil:** Central aperture of iris.
- **Retina**
- **Pigment epithelium:** Melanin-containing cells.
  - **Neural retina:** Rods and cones.

Chambers

- Anterior chamber: From cornea → iris
- Posterior chamber: From iris → lens
- Vitreous chamber: From lens → neural retina

Ten Layers of Retina

From outermost → innermost:

- Pigment epithelium
- Photoreceptor cells
  - **Rods:** Sensitive to **light**; contain **rhodopsin**
  - **Cones:** Sensitive to **color**; contain **iodopsin**
- External limiting membrane
- Outer nuclear layer
  - Nuclei of rods and cones
  - Outer plexiform layer
  - Inner nuclear layer
  - Nuclei of horizontal, amacrine, bipolar, and Müller's cells
- Inner plexiform layer
- Ganglion cell layer
- Optic nerve fibers
- Internal limiting membrane

Aqueous humor *is the watery fluid within the anterior and posterior chambers.*

Vitreous humor *is the transparent watery gel within the vitreous chamber.*

Vitamin A *is a source of retinal, an essential component of rods. Dietary deficiency of vitamin A results in the inability to see in dim light ("night blindness").*

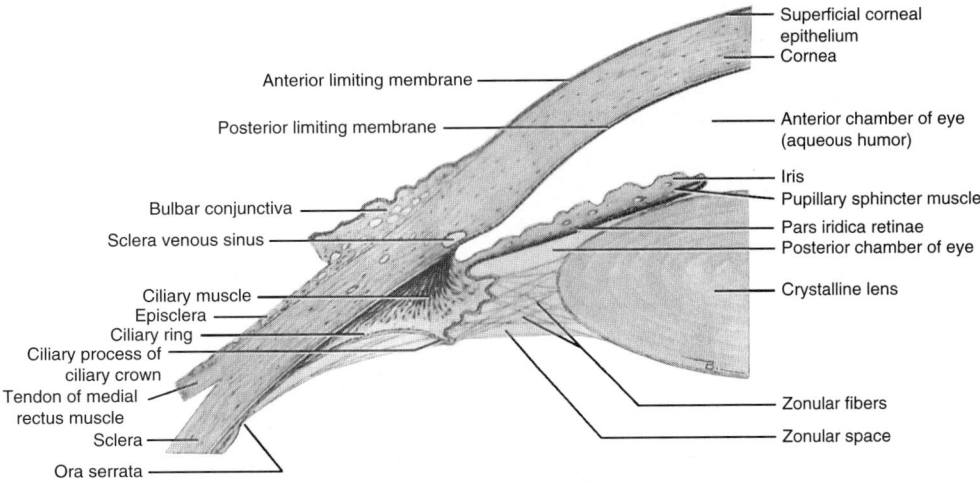

FIGURE 2–9. Ciliary Zone.

Reproduced, with permission, from Montgomery, RL. *Head and Neck Anatomy: With Clinical Considerations.* McGraw-Hill, 1981.

Optic Disc

- Collection of retinal ganglion cell nerve fibers (axons) leaving eye as optic nerve (central artery and vein of the retina also exit here; artery is in center of disc and fans out).
- Small blind spot on the retina; 3 mm to nasal side of macula.
- Only part of retina without rods or cones.

Macula Lutea

- Just temporal to optic disc
- Responsible for detailed central vision (e.g., reading)
- **Fovea:** Very center of macula—no blood vessels, very high concentration of cones, area of sharpest vision

CHAPTER 3
Oral Histology

Soft Oral Tissues	196
ORAL MUCOSA	196
GINGIVA	196
DENTOGINGIVAL JUNCTION	198
Tooth and Supporting Tissues	200
DENTIN	200
PULP	204
CEMENTUM	205
ALVEOLAR BONE	207
ORIGIN	207
PERIODONTAL LIGAMENT (PDL)	208

SOFT ORAL TISSUES

Oral Mucosa

LAYERS OF ORAL MUCOSA

From outermost → innermost:

- **Stratified squamous epithelium:** Keratinized or nonkeratinized.
    - **Stratum corneum:** Keratinized cell layer. Cells appear flattened and pyknotic with few (if any) organelles.
    - **Stratum granulosum:** Cells appear flattened and may contain *keratohyalin* granules. Organelles are diminished.
    - **Stratum spinosum:** Spinous (prickle cell) layer. Cells have peripheral cytoplasmic processes. Langerhans cells often extend into this layer.
    - **Stratum basale (germinativum):** Site of all epithelial mitotic activity. Least cytodifferentiated. Cuboidal to low columnar in shape.
- **Basement membrane:** Contains **type IV collagen** and **laminin.** Epithelial attachment to the basement membrane is mediated by *hemidesmosomes*.
- **Subepithelial connective tissue:** Contains collagen and elastic fibers, ground substance, blood vessels, nerves, and inflammatory cells.
    - **Lamina propria**
        - **Papillary layer:** Connective tissue **papillae** are the projections that interdigitate with the epithelial **rete pegs (ridges),** creating a variably tortuous epithelial–connective tissue interface.
        - **Reticular layer:** Constitutes the remainder of the lamina propria.
- **Submucosa.** Present in areas of high compression. Often indistinguishable with the lamina propria.

*Most specialized epithelial cells concentrate in the basal cell layer; however, **Langerhans cells** may extend into the stratum spinosum.*

SPECIALIZED EPITHELIAL CELLS

- **Melanocytes:** Produce melanin.
- **Keratinocytes:** Produce keratin. Not present in all oral mucosa.
- **Langerhans cells:** Antigen-presenting cells.
- **Merkel cells:** Touch-sensory cells.

TYPES OF ORAL MUCOSA

See Table 3–1.

- ***All*** oral mucosa contains **stratified squamous epithelium.**

Gingiva

See Figures 3–1 and 3–2.

- The fibrous, keratinized tissue that surrounds a tooth and is contiguous with the periodontal ligament and oral mucosa.
- Contains a stratified squamous **keratinized** epithelium with rete pegs.
- Extends from the **gingival margin** (the most coronal portion of the gingiva) to the **mucogingival junction (MGJ).** The MGJ separates the gingiva from the alveolar mucosa.
- Color ranges from pink to brown, depending on the amount of melanin expression, which is correlated with cutaneous pigmentation.

TABLE 3-1. The Three Major Types of Oral Epithelium

Mucosa Type	Location	Epithelium	Characteristics
Masticatory	Gingiva Hard palate	*Thick* stratified squamous **keratinized** (75% parakeratinized).	*Thin* submucosa
Lining	Alveolar mucosa Vestibule Buccal mucosa Floor of the mouth Soft palate Ventral surface of tongue Vestibular aspect of lips	*Thin* stratified squamous **nonkeratinized**.	*Thick* submucosa
Specialized	Dorsal surface of tongue	*Both* stratified squamous keratinized and nonkeratinized.	Taste buds

Zones of Gingiva

- **Attached gingiva:** Firmly bound to periosteum and cementum. About 40% of the adult population exhibits **stippling** of the attached gingiva, which is an orange-peel-like surface characteristic caused by the intersection of epithelial rete pegs.
- **Free (unattached, marginal) gingiva:** Located coronal to the attached gingiva and is separated from the tooth surface by the **gingival sulcus**.

*The two zones are separated by the **free gingival groove.***

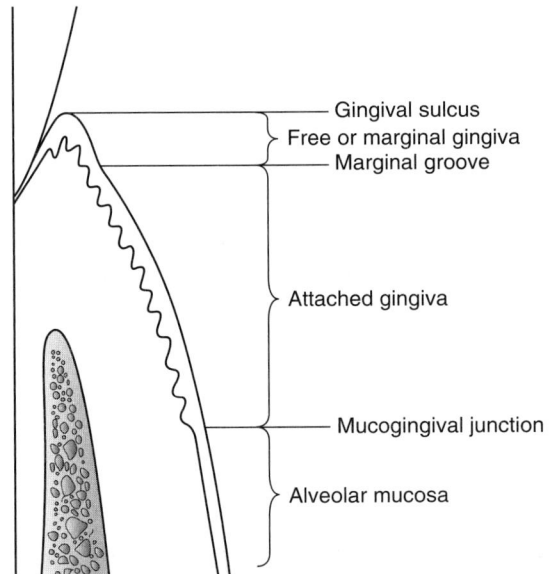

*Chronic **mouth breathing** often manifests as pronounced gingival erythema, especially in the anterior regions.*

FIGURE 3-1. Gingival anatomy.

Reproduced, with permission, from Elsevier. Carranza FA. *Clinical Periodontology*, 8th ed. Saunders, 1996:130.

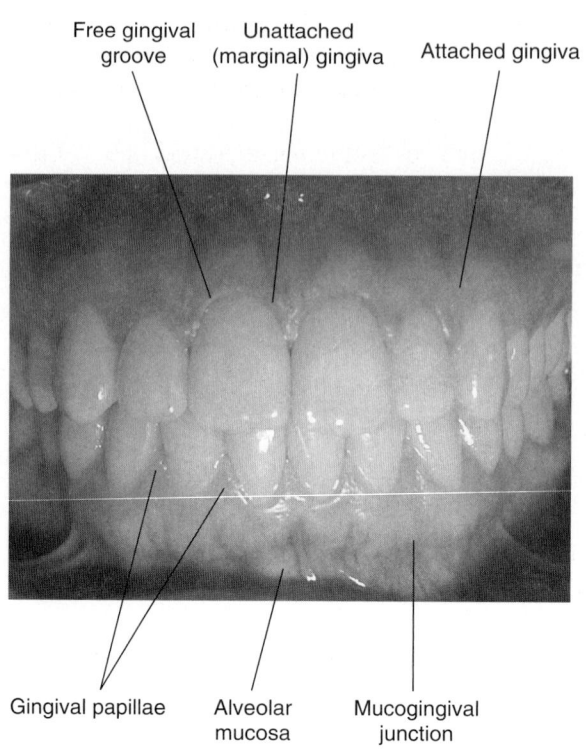

FIGURE 3-2. **Healthy gingival anatomy.**

Note the gingival stippling in the maxillary anterior region.

- **Interdental papilla:** The triangular portion of the free gingiva located in the interproximal embrasures between teeth just apical to their contact areas.
- **Gingival col:** The depression in the interdental gingiva connecting the buccal and lingual papilla immediately apical to the contact areas of adjacent teeth. Its epithelium is generally **nonkeratinized,** and its presence is based solely on the presence of an interdental contact.

Dentogingival Junction

Biologic width is defined as the length of the dentogingival junction. In humans, the average width of epithelial attachment is 0.97 mm and 1.07 mm for the connective tissue attachment, creating a mean biologic width of 2.04 mm.

- The attachment of the gingiva to the tooth.
- Consists of epithelial (**epithelial attachment**) and connective tissue (**connective tissue attachment**) components.
- Forms as the oral epithelium fuses with the reduced enamel epithelium (REE) during tooth eruption. As the tooth reaches its fully erupted position, cells of the junctional epithelium replace those of the REE.

DENTOGINGIVAL EPITHELIUM

- **Sulcular epithelium:** Stratified squamous **non-keratinized** epithelium without rete pegs that extends from the gingival margin to the junctional epithelium. It lines the gingival sulcus.
- **Junctional epithelium:** Stratified to single-layer (at its apical extent) **nonkeratinized** epithelium without rete pegs that adheres to the tooth

surface at the base of the sulcus. It provides the epithelial attachment to the tooth. Junctional epithelial cells have higher turnover rates and larger intercellular spaces than sulcular and gingival epithelia. It consists of two basal laminae:
- **External basal lamina:** Attaches to underlying connective tissue as elsewhere in the body.
- **Internal basal lamina:** Attaches to the cementum via *hemidesmosomes*. It is unlike other basal laminae in that it does not contain type IV collagen.

DENTOGINGIVAL CONNECTIVE TISSUE

- **Type I collagen** makes up the bulk of the connective tissue.
- Other major components include fibroblasts, leukocytes, mast cells, elastic fibers, proteoglycans, and glycoproteins.

GINGIVAL FIBER GROUPS

See Figure 3-3.

- Support the gingiva and aid in its attachment to alveolar bone and teeth.
- They are continuous with the PDL.
- Do not confuse these with PDL fibers!
  - **Dentogingival fibers:** Fan laterally from cementum into the adjacent CT.
  - **Alveologingival fibers:** Fan coronally from the alveolar crest into the adjacent CT.
  - **Dentoperiosteal fibers:** Extend from cementum over the alveolar crest, and turn apically to insert into the periosteum of the buccal side of the alveolar bone.
  - **Circumferential fibers:** Surround the tooth in a circular fashion. Help prevent rotational forces.

The subepithelial connective tissue provides the cellular signaling that determines epithelial expression.

The connective tissue adjacent to the sulcular and junctional epithelia generally contains an **increased inflammatory infiltrate** compared to that adjacent to the oral epithelium. PMNs and other leukocytes continually migrate between these epithelial cells into the sulcus, and account for a significant portion of **gingival crevicular fluid (GCF)** along with plasma proteins, epithelial cells, and bacteria.

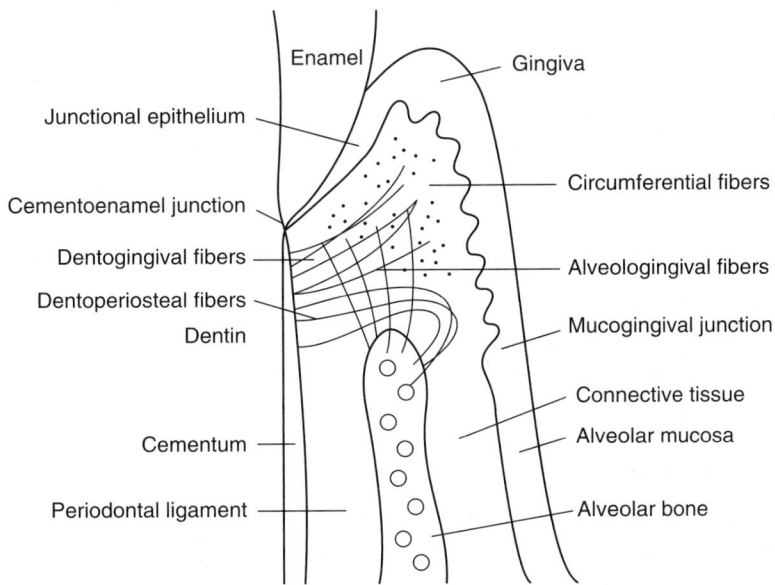

FIGURE 3-3. **The gingival fibers.**

Comparison of the Major Tissues of Teeth and the Periodontium

	Enamel	Dentin	Cementum	Alveolar Bone	Pulp
Mineral composition	96%	70%	55%	50%	<5%
Organic composition	4%	30%	45%	50%	>95%
Embryologic origin	Ectoderm	Ectomesenchyme (neural crest)	Ectomesenchyme (neural crest)	Ectomesenchyme (neural crest)	Ectomesenchyme (neural crest)
Formative cell	Ameloblast	Odontoblast	Cementoblast	Osteoblast	Fibroblast, Mesenchymal
Formative cells differentiated from	IEE	Dental papilla	Dental follicle	Dental follicle	Dental papilla
Tissue type	Epithelial	Connective	Connective	Connective	Connective
Viability	No	Repair	Repair	Remodeling	Yes
Incremental lines	Neonatal Retzius (daily)	Neonatal Owen von Ebner (daily)	Resting	Resting Reversal	None
Sensitivity	No	Yes	No	Yes	Yes (pain)
Nutritive supply	None	Pulp	PDL (diffusion)	Vessels (diffusion)	Vessels

Dentin

- An elastic, avascular, mineralized tissue that is harder than bone but softer than enamel.
- Color is generally yellowish.

Origin

- Differentiated ectomesenchymal cells of the dental papilla.

Dentinogenesis

- Organization
    - The odontoblasts become elongated and the organelles become polarized by ameloblastic induction.

- **Mantle dentin formation**
  - The dentin matrix formed by odontoblasts starts at the DEJ and progresses inward toward the eventual pulp. The dentin matrix first produced by the odontoblasts consists largely of type I collagen and ground substance, known as **predentin**.
  - As the odontoblasts retreat inward, they leave cytoplasmic extensions called **odontoblastic processes** (Tomes' fibers) at the DEJ. These processes are housed in **dentinal tubules**, which form channels from the DEJ/DCJ to the pulp.
  - The odontoblastic processes release **matrix vesicles** containing calcium, which crystallize and rupture. These crystals act as a nidus for the formation of more **hydroxyapatite** (HA) crystals in and around the organic dentin matrix.
  - This initial 150 μm of dentin in known as **mantle dentin**.
- **Circumpulpal dentin formation**
  - Once mantle dentin is formed, odontoblasts (with well-developed rough ER and Golgi bodies) begin to secrete collagen fibrils perpendicularly to the odontoblastic processes, as well as other organic substances such as lipids, phospholipids, and phosphoproteins.
  - Mineralization occurs by globular calcification by which globules of HA fuse to form a calcified mass. Occasionally, the globules fail to fuse, leaving hypomineralized **interglobular dentin** in between.
  - The odontoblastic processes shrink in width, providing a space for a hypermineralized **peritubular dentin** to form. If several adjacent dentinal tubules become occluded with this peritubular dentin, it takes on a glassy appearance and is called **sclerotic dentin**.
  - Most of the circumpulpal dentin produced is between the tubules, known as **intertubular dentin**.
  - **Dead tracts** are groups of necrotic odontoblastic processes within the dentinal tubules (often caused by trauma).
- **Reparative dentin formation**
  - **Reparative dentin** is formed only at specific sites of injury.
  - The types I and III collagens in its matrix are produced by differentiated odontoblast-like cells from the pulp. The tubular pattern is often distorted due to an increased rate of its formation.

Coronal dentinal tubules follow an S-shape (primary curvature); radicular tubules are generally straight. There are more tubules concentrated near the pulp than the DEJ.

CLASSIFICATIONS OF DENTIN

- By time of formation
  - **Mantle:** The first 150 μm of dentin formed. Located closest to enamel (CEJ) and cementum (CDJ).
  - **Circumpulpal:** All dentin formed thereafter until tooth formation is complete.
  - **Reparative:** Formed in response to trauma (e.g., caries, restorations, attrition, erosion, abrasion, etc.).
  - **Sclerotic:** Results from calcification of the dentinal tubules as one ages over time. Helps prevent pulpal irritation.
- By root completion
  - **Primary:** Formed before root completion. Tubules are most regular.
  - **Secondary:** Formed after root completion, but not in response to trauma.
  - **Tertiary:** Formed in response to trauma (e.g., caries, restorations, attrition, erosion, abrasion, etc.). Tubules are least regular.

- By proximity to dentinal tubules
  - **Peritubular:** *Hyper*mineralized dentin formed within the perimeter of dentinal tubules as odontoblastic processes shrink.
  - **Intertubular:** *Hypo*mineralized dentin located between the dentinal tubules. Makes up the bulk of the dentin formed.
  - **Interglobular:** *Hypo*mineralized dentin located between improperly fused HA globules.
- By location
  - **Coronal**
    - May contain hypomineralized **interglobular dentin.**
    - May contain **dead tracts.**
  - **Radicular**
    - May contain hypomineralized **Tomes granular layer.**

CROSS STRIATIONS AND INCREMENTAL LINES

- **Daily imbrication line of von Ebner:** Daily periodoic bands.
- **Contour lines of Owen:** Wide rings produced by metabolic disturbances during odontogenesis that run perpendicular to dentinal tubules.
- **Neonatal line:** A more pronounced contour line of Owen formed during the physiologic trauma at birth.

Odontoblasts move at a rate of 4–8 μm/day.

EFFECTS OF AGING ON DENTIN

- ↑ sclerotic dentin (↓ dentinal tubule diameter due to continued deposition of peritubular dentin).
- ↑ reparative dentin formation.
- ↑ dead tracts.

CLINICAL IMPLICATIONS

- **Dentinal hypersensitivity:** Can occur for several reasons:
  - Myelinated nerve fibers have been found in dentinal tubules which can be directly stimulated.
  - Changes in dentinal tubule fluid pressures may affect pulpal nerve fibers directly or may cause damage to odontoblasts, releasing inflammatory mediators in the pulp.

DEFORMITIES OF DENTIN

- **Dentinogenesis imperfecta:** Generally *autosomal dominant* defects in dentin formation. Teeth exhibit an opalescent color and have bulb-shaped crowns. The dentin is abnormally soft (allowing enamel to easily chip) and pulp chambers are often obliterated.
  - **Type I:** Often occurs with osteogenesis imperfecta (**blue sclera** is a common finding).
  - **Type II:** Not associated with osteogenesis imperfecta.
  - **Type III:** Very rare form which exhibits multiple pulp exposures of the primary dentition.
- **Dentin dysplasia:** *Autosomal dominant* defects in dentin formation and pulp morphology. Tooth color is usually normal. Often called "**rootless teeth**" because root dentin is usually affected more often than coronal dentin. Roots are short, blunt, or absent.

ENAMEL

- The most calcified and brittle substance in the human body.
- Color ranges from yellowish to grayish-white.
- Semitranslucent.

ORIGIN

- Differentiated ectodermal cells of the inner enamel epithelium.

AMELOGENESIS

- **Organization**
  - The ameloblasts become elongated and the organelles become polarized *before* the same occurs to odontoblasts.
- **Formation**
  - The enamel matrix produced by ameloblasts starts virtually perpendicularly to the DEJ and progresses outward toward the eventual tooth surface.
  - Ameloblastic activity starts immediately *after* mantle dentin formation.
  - As ameloblasts retreat, **Tomes' processes** are formed around which enamel matrix proteins are secreted, most of which are almost instantly partially mineralized to form enamel matrix.
- **Maturation**
  - Final mineralization occurs with inorganic ion influx and removal of protein and water by cyclic ameloblastic activity, forming **hydroxyapatite (HA)** crystals.
  - As the HA crystals accumulate, they are tightly stacked in elongated units called **enamel rods (prisms).** The rods are surrounded by a **rod sheath** and separated by an **inter-rod substance** that consists of HA crystals aligned in a different direction than the rods themselves.
  - Each keyhole-shaped enamel rod is formed by **four** ameloblasts (one for the head and three for the tail).
  - At cusp tips, the enamel rods appear twisted and intertwined in a formation known as **gnarled enamel.**
- **Protection**
  - When enamel maturation is complete, the outer enamel epithelium, stratum intermedium, and stellate reticulum collapse onto the ameloblastic layer, forming the **reduced enamel epithelium (Nasmyth's membrane).** This is worn away soon after tooth eruption and quickly replaced by the **salivary pellicle.** Hemidesmosomes are also produced, which are critical in providing epithelial attachment to the tooth.

Amelogenin constitutes about 90% of the enamel matrix protein secreted. Others proteins include enamelin and tuftelin.

CROSS STRIATIONS AND INCREMENTAL LINES

- **Daily imbrication lines:** Daily periodic bands.
- **Striae of Retzius:** More pronounced weekly periodic bands.
  - Shallow depressions, called **perikymata,** are formed on the enamel surface where these lines reach the tooth surface. Perikymata disappear with age due to attrition of the raised areas between them.
- **Neonatal line:** A more apparent stria of Retzius formed during the physiologic trauma at birth.
- **Hunter–Schreger bands:** Alternating light and dark zones produced only as an *optical phenomenon* during light microscopy of longitudinal ground sections.

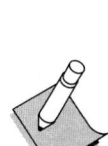

Enamel matrix is produced at a rate of **4 μm per day.**

THE DENTINO–ENAMEL JUNCTION (DEJ)

- **Enamel tufts:** *Hypo*calcified, fan-shaped enamel protein projecting a short distance into the enamel.

The DEJ is scalloped, which provides more surface area for enamel–dentin adhesion.

- **Enamel lamellae:** *Hypo*calcified enamel defects that can extend all the way to the enamel surface. They generally consist of enamel protein or oral debris.
- **Enamel spindles:** Trapped odontoblastic processes in the enamel.

EFFECTS OF AGING ON ENAMEL

- Attrition: Enamel wear by masticatory forces.
- Discoloration: Becomes darker as more dentin becomes visible.
- ↓ permeability: Enamel crystals have accepted more ions, especially fluoride.

CLINICAL IMPLICATIONS

- Since enamel is **translucent,** its color depends on its thickness. The more translucent, the more yellow it appears because the underlying dentin becomes more visible.
- **Tetracycline** antibiotics can be incorporated into mineralizing tissues by chelation to divalent cations. This leads to a **brownish-gray banding** within the enamel. Drugs from this family should not be given until about age 8 (about the time the second molar completes calcification).

DEFORMITIES OF ENAMEL

- **Amelogenesis imperfecta:** Autosomal dominant or recessive enamel defects of three basic types:
    - **Hypoplastic:** Enamel has abnormal thickness or pitting, but normal hardness. Defect in enamel *matrix formation.*
    - **Hypocalcified:** Enamel has normal thickness, but is soft and chalky. Defect in enamel *mineralization.*
    - **Hypomaturation:** Enamel has normal thickness, but abnormal hardness. Mild forms exhibit "snow-capped" incisal edges, while severe forms lose their translucency. Defect in enamel *maturation.*
- **Enamel hypoplasia:** Enamel is hard, but deficient in amount. Caused by defective or altered enamel *matrix formation.* Can be acquired or developmentally-induced.
    - **Fluorosis:** Enamel is *selectively permeable* to water and certain ions. This allows fluoride (in drinking water and topical applications) to concentrate in enamel apatite, forming fluorapatite, which is highly resistant to acid dissolution. Fluoride concentrations greater than 5 parts per million, however, affect ameloblastic enamel matrix secretion, leading to the appearance of **enamel mottling** and a **brownish pigmentation.**
    - **Nutritional deficiencies:** Deficiencies of vitamins A, C, and D and calcium often lead to enamel pitting.
    - **Infections:** Febrile diseases at the time of amelogenesis can halt enamel formation, leaving bands of malformed surface enamel.
- **Congenital syphilis:** Often causes incisors to look screwdriver-shaped **(Hutchinson incisors)** and molars to look globular **(mulberry molars).**

Pulp

- The soft connective tissue that supports the dentin and is contained inside the **pulp chamber** of the tooth.
- Communicates to the periodontal tissues via the **apical foramen** and **accessory canals.**

ORIGIN

- Ectomesenchymal cells of the dental papilla.

CLASSIFICATIONS OF PULP

- By location
  - Coronal: Found in the pulp horns.
  - Radicular: Found in pulp canals.

FUNCTIONS OF PULP

- Formative: Has mesenchymal cells that ultimately form dentin.
- Nutritive: Nourishes the avascular dentin.
- Sensory: Free nerve endings provide pain sensation.
- Protective: Produces reparative dentin as needed.

ZONES OF PULP

From outer → inner:

- Odontoblastic zone: A single layer of odontoblasts lining the pulp chamber.
- **Cell free zone of Weil:** Devoid of cells (except during dentinogenesis). Contains the parietal plexus of nerves (Raschkow's plexus) and a plexus of blood vessels (including arteriovenous anastamoses).
- **Cell rich zone:** Contains **fibroblasts** and undifferentiated mesenchymal cells.
- **Pulp core:** Contains fibroblasts, macrophages, leukocytes, blood and lymph vessels, myelinated (mostly Aδ) and unmyelinated (C) sympathetic nerve fibers, collagen types I and III (55:45 ratio), and ground substance. There are no elastic fibers.

*Virtually all of the nerve bundles of the pulp terminate as **free nerve endings** that are specific for **pain**, regardless of the type of stimulation.*

PULP CALCIFICATIONS

- **Denticles (pulp stones):** Concentric layers of mineralized tissue.
  - **True:** Surround dentinal tubules or odontoblastic processes.
  - **False:** Surround dead cells or collagen fibers.
  - **Free:** Located freely (unattached) in the pulp chamber.
  - **Attached:** Attached to the pulp chamber wall.
  - **Interstitial:** Embedded in the pulp chamber wall.
- **Dystrophic calcifications:** Calcifications of collagen bundles or collagen fibers surrounding blood vessels and nerves.

EFFECTS OF AGING ON PULP

- ↑ collagen fibers and calcifications.
- ↓ pulp chamber volume (due to continued dentin deposition), apical foramen size, cellularity, vascularity, and sensitivity.

Cementum

- An avascular tissue about 10 μm thick that covers the radicular dentin.
- Composition most closely resembles bone.

Origin

- Differentiated ectomesenchymal cells of the dental follicle.

Functions of Cementum

- Support: Provides attachment for teeth (Sharpey's fibers).
- Protection: Helps prevent root resorption during tooth movement.
- Formative: Continual apical cementum deposition accounts for continual tooth eruption and movement.

Cementogenesis

- During root formation, ectomesenchymal cells of the dental follicle migrate through gaps in Hertwig's epithelial root sheath and orient themselves along radicular dentin. Here, they differentiate to **cementoblasts** and secrete **cementoid** (cementum matrix).
- As the cementoblasts retreat away from the dentin, the matrix is calcified and a new layer of cementum matrix is secreted. These layers form **resting lines**, which can be seen microscopically.
- Cementoblasts may be trapped in their own matrix. When this occurs, they are known as **cementocytes**, which reside in **lacunae**. They receive nutrients via **canaliculi** that extend to the periodontal ligament.
- Cementum is constantly produced at the apical portion of the root to account for the continual eruption of teeth. Deposition of excessive cementum is known as **hypercementosis**.

Classifications of Cementum

- By formation
    - **Primary**: First formed cementum. Covers coronal cementum, is acellular, and consists of extrinsic collagen fibers.
    - **Secondary**: Overlies primary cementum. Covers apical cementum, may be either acellular or cellular, and consists of mixed collagen fibers.
- By cellularity
    - **Cellular**: Contains cementocytes, cementoblasts, and cementoclasts. Most commonly found in apical areas of cementum.
    - **Acellular**: Devoid of cells. Most commonly found in coronal areas of cementum.
- By collagen fibers
    - **Intrinic fibers**: Produced by cementoblasts. Arranged parallel to the tooth surface.
    - **Extrinsic fibers**: Produced by the PDL. Arranged perpendicular to the tooth surface. As they become trapped in the cementum, they are known as Sharpey's fibers.
    - **Mixed fibers**: Combination of intrinsic and extrinsic fibers.

Approximation with Enamel at the CEJ

See Figure 3–4.

Effects of Aging on Cementum

- ↑ cementum deposition.

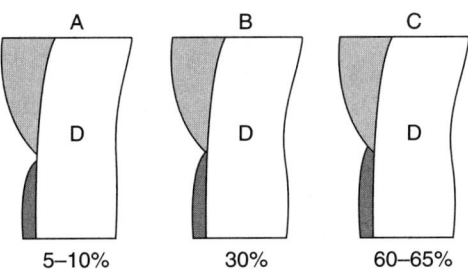

FIGURE 3-4. Cementum morphology at the CEJ.

Reproduced, with permission, from Elsevier. Carranza FA. *Clinical Periodontology*, 8th ed. Saunders, 1996:38.

CLINICAL IMPLICATIONS

- Cementum enables orthodontic tooth movement because it is more resistant to resorption than alveolar bone.

Alveolar Bone

- **Alveolar bone:** A general term to describe the bone in the maxilla and mandible which houses the teeth.
- **Interalveolar septum:** The bony projection separating two alveoli.
- **Interradicular septum:** Alveolar bone between the roots of multirooted teeth.

Origin

- Differentiated ectomesenchymal cells of the dental follicle.

COMPONENTS OF ALVEOLAR BONE

- **Alveolar bone proper:** The thin layer of **cortical bone** that immediately surrounds the teeth and into which PDL fibers (Sharpey's fibers) are embedded. It is also called **bundle bone, lamina dura,** or **cribriform plate.**
- **Supporting alveolar bone:** The part of the alveolus that surrounds the alveolar bone proper. It consists of the following:
  - **Cortical bone (cortical plate):** Forms the buccal and lingual outer surfaces of the maxilla and mandible. It is generally thicker in the mandible and in posterior (molar) regions.
  - **Cancellous bone (spongy bone, trabecular bone):** Fills the area between the cortical plates. It makes up the majority of alveolar bone.

The only function of alveolar bone is to support teeth. During tooth development, it grows in all dimensions to accommodate the new dentition. When a tooth is lost, it continually resorbs until complete alveolar ridge atrophy occurs.

CLINICAL IMPLICATIONS

- The radiographic appearance of the **lamina dura** is determined as much by the x-ray beam angulation as it is by its integrity.
- The radiographic presence (or absence) of the **crestal lamina dura** has no correlation with periodontal attachment loss.

The **periodontium** is the attachment apparatus of the tooth. It consists of:

- Cementum
- Alveolar bone proper
- Periodontal ligament (PDL)

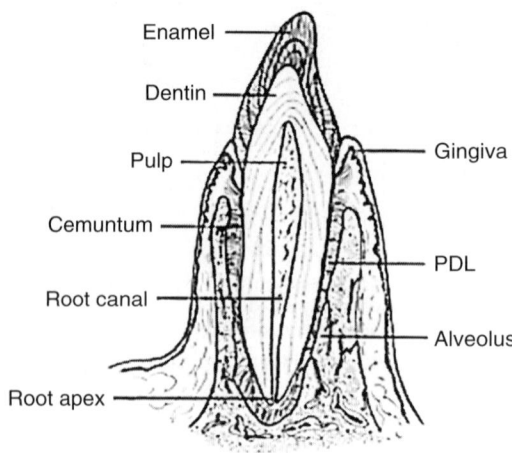

FIGURE 3-5. The tooth and its periodontium.

(Reproduced, with permission, from Liebgott B. *The Anatomical Basis of Dentistry*. Toronto: BC Decker, 1986.)

Periodontal Ligament (PDL)

See Figure 3–5.

- A soft connective tissue located between the tooth and alveolar bone. Approximately **0.2 mm wide** but varies with tooth function and age.

ORIGIN

- Differentiated ectomesenchymal cells of the dental follicle.

FUNCTIONS OF THE PDL

- Support: Provides attachment of the tooth to the alveolar bone.
- Formative: Contains cells responsible for formation of the periodontium.
- Nutritive: Contains a vascular network providing nutrients to its cells.
- Sensory: Contains afferent nerve fibers responsible for pain, pressure, and proprioception.
- Remodeling: Contains cells responsible for remodeling of the periodontium.

CONTENTS OF THE PDL

- Cells and cellular elements
  - **Fibroblasts:** Most common cell of the PDL.
  - Cementoblasts and cementoclasts.
  - Osteoblasts and oseoclasts.
  - Macrophages, mast cells, and eosinophils.
  - Undifferentiated mesenchymal cells.
  - Ground substance: proteoglycans, glycosaminoglycans, glycoproteins, and water (70%).

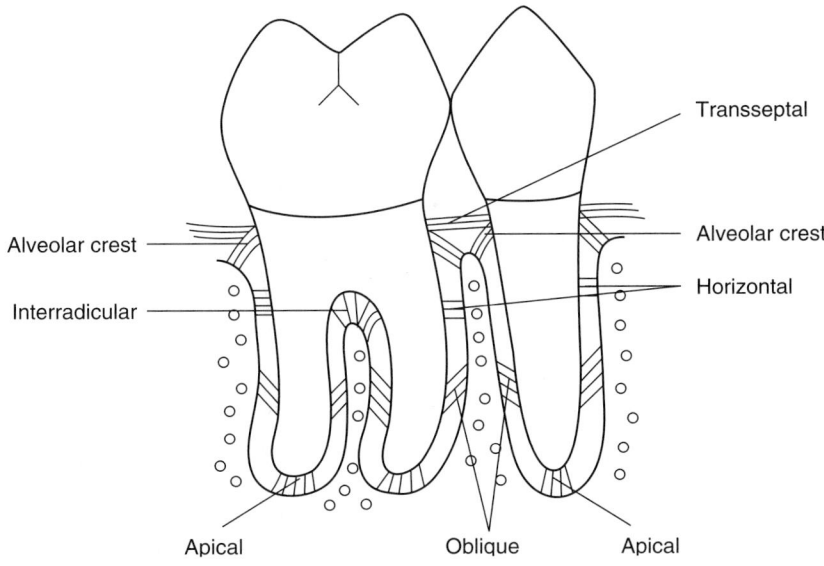

FIGURE 3-6. The principal PDL fibers.

- **Epithelial rests of Malassez:** Found closer to cementum than alveolar bone.
  - **Cementicles:** Calcified masses either attached or unattached to root surfaces.
- Fibers (See Figure 3–6.)
  - **Principal collagen fibers:** Composed mostly of type I collagen, but also type III collagen.
    - **Transseptal:** Extend interproximally over the alveolar crest from the cementum of one tooth to that of an adjacent tooth.
    - **Alveolar crest:** Extend obliquely from cementum just apical to the junctional epithelium to the alveolar crest.
    - **Horizontal:** Extend at right angles from cementum to alveolar bone.
    - **Oblique:** Extend obliquely from cementum to alveolar bone. They are the *most abundant* principal fibers.
    - **Apical:** Extend from cementum to alveolar bone at root apices.
    - **Interradicular:** Extend from radicular cementum to interradicular alveolar bone. Only present in multirooted teeth.
  - **Oxytalan fibers:** Elastic-like fibers that run parallel to the tooth surface and bend to attach to cementum. They are largely associated with blood vessels.
- Blood vessels
  - The vasculature of the PDL arises from the **maxillary artery**. Vessels can reach the PDL from various sources:
    - **Periosteal vessels:** Branches from the periosteum. This is the *primary source* of PDL vasculature.
    - **Apical vessels:** Branches of the dental vessels that supply the apical regions of the PDL.
    - **Transalveolar vessels:** Branches of transseptal vessels that perforate the alveolar bone proper.
    - **Anastomosing vessels** of the gingiva.

Sharpey's fibers are the portions of the principal fibers that insert into cementum or alveolar bone proper. They are thicker on the alveolar bone side.

- Nerve fibers
    - Arise from branches of the **trigeminal nerve (CN V).**
        - Free nerve endings: *Most abundant.*
        - Ruffini corpuscles: Provide mechanoreception.
        - Coiled endings.
        - Spindle endings.
- Lymphatics
    - Drain to the **submandibular lymph nodes.**

EFFECTS OF AGING ON THE PDL

- ↓ PDL width.
- ↓ cellularity and fiber content.

CLINICAL IMPLICATIONS

- Teeth in **hypofunction** have a decreased PDL width with fibers arranged parallel to the root.
- Teeth in **hyperfunction** have an increased PDL width.

CHAPTER 4
Developmental Biology

Tooth Development	212
ODONTOGENESIS	212
General Embryology	215
GAMETOGENESIS	215
EMBRYOLOGY OF THE CENTRAL NERVOUS SYSTEM	225
EMBRYOLOGY OF THE CARDIAC SYSTEM	228
EMBRYOLOGY OF THE GASTROINTESTINAL SYSTEM	229
EMBRYOLOGY OF THE RENAL SYSTEM	231
Embryology of the Face and Phayrngeal Arches	233
BRANCHIAL ARCHES	233
PHARYNGEAL POUCHES	236
FORMATION OF THE FACE	237
MOUTH AND ORAL CAVITY	237

TOOTH DEVELOPMENT

Odontogenesis

INITIATION

See Figure 4–1(a).

- Starts at week 6 in utero.
- Underlying ectomesenchymal cells induce the overlying ectoderm (oral epithelium) to proliferate, forming a localized thickening at the site of each tooth called the **dental lamina.**

BUD STAGE

See Figure 4–1(b).

- Starts at week 8 in utero.
- Both ectodermal and ectomesenchymal cells **proliferate**, creating the round shape of each tooth bud.

CAP STAGE

See Figure 4–1(c).

- Starts at week 9 in utero.
- The **enamel organ** begins to form, which is composed of a single layer of cells at the convex region (**outer enamel epithelium, OEE**) and the concave region (**inner enamel epithelium, IEE**). Between the two epithelial layers is the loosely-arranged **stellate reticulum.** Some cells of the stellate reticulum become densely packed near the IEE and are known as the **enamel knot.**

It is the underlying ectomesenchyme that determines the type of tooth to be formed.

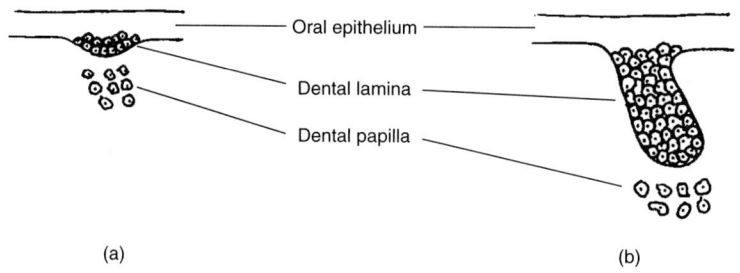

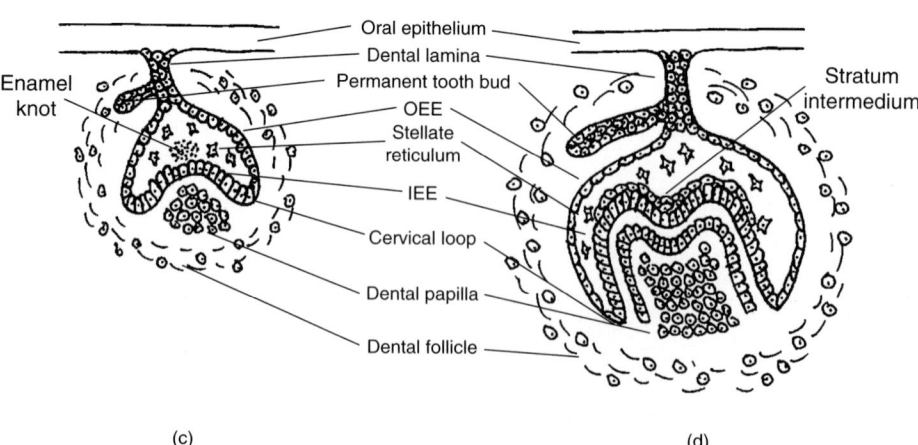

FIGURE 4-1. (A) Initiation stage. (B) Bud stage. (C) Cap stage. (D) Bell stage.

- The **dental papilla** is composed of condensed ectomesenchymal cells located within the concavity of the enamel organ.
- The **dental follicle (dental sac)** is the capsulelike encasing of mesenchyme surrounding the enamel organ.
- The **succedaneous dental lamina** begins to form adjacent to the primary enamel organ.

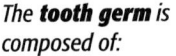

The **tooth germ** is composed of:
- Enamel organ
- Dental papilla
- Dental follicle

Bell Stage

See Figure 4–1(d).

- Starts at week 11 in utero.
- Morphodifferentiation and histodifferentiation of specific cells occurs.
- The **enamel organ** is now well-defined and composed of the following:
  - **OEE:** Outermost layer of the enamel organ.
  - **IEE:** Innermost layer of the enamel organ.
  - **Stratum intermedium:** Forms directly lateral to the IEE.
  - **Stellate reticulum:** Becomes more sparsely arranged due to increased proteoglycan synthesis.
- The enamel knot disappears.
- The cells of the IEE become tall and columnar (now called **preameloblasts**) *first*.
- The cells of the dental papilla closest to the IEE become tall and columnar (now called **preodontoblasts**) *after* the preameloblasts are formed.
- The dental lamina disintegrates. Its remnants are known as **epithelial rests of Serres.**

The differentiation of the IEE cells to preameloblasts induces the differentiation of preodontoblasts from mesenchymal cells of the dental papilla.

Appositional Stage

- The **reduced enamel epithelium (REE)** forms when the stellate reticulum collapses, merging the OEE with the IEE.
- Odontoblasts secrete dentin matrix *first*.
- Ameloblasts secrete enamel matrix *after* dentin is first formed.
- Root formation (see below) begins.
- The dental papilla forms pulp tissue.
- The dental follicle forms cementum, alveolar bone, and PDL.

Remember the chronological order of enamel and dentin formation. Root, pulp, and periodontium formation occurs after these events.
- Differentiation of ameloblasts.
- Differentiation of odontoblasts.
- Deposition of dentin matrix.
- Deposition of enamel matrix.

Mineralization Stage

- Starts at the **DEJ** (where odontoblasts and ameloblasts first secrete matrix).
- Takes about 2 years to complete.

Root Formation

See Figure 4–2.

- Begins at the **cervical loop** (where the IEE and OEE join) *after* enamel is first formed.
- As the cervical loop elongates, **Hertwig's epithelial root sheath (HERS)** is formed, which shapes the root(s) and ultimately surrounds the majority of the dental papilla. Its most apical segment, the **epithelial diaphragm,** turns medially, ensuring that the root tapers as odontogenesis proceeds.
- As root formation continues, the tooth erupts, leaving the epithelial diaphragm always at the same location. This eventually forms the **apical foramen.**

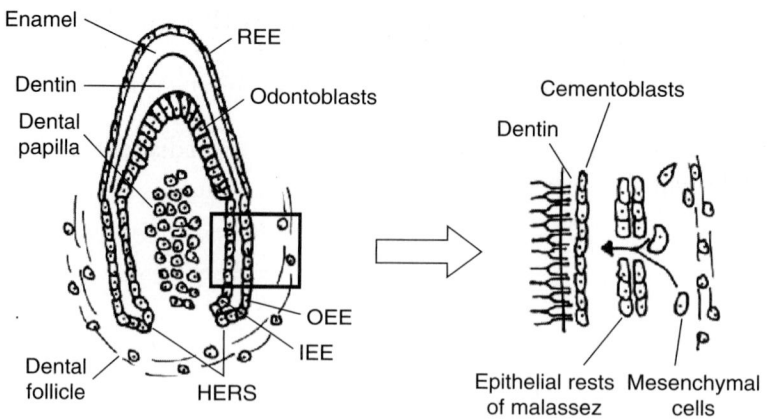

FIGURE 4-2. Root formation.

- As radicular dentin is formed, HERS begins to disintegrate, leaving behind patches of epithelial cells called **epithelial rests of Malassez**. The collapse of HERS enables ectomesenchymal cells of the dental follicle to contact dentin and differentiate into the formative cells of the periodontium: cementoblasts (forming cementum), osteoblasts (forming alveolar bone proper), and fibroblasts (forming the PDL).

ERUPTION

See Figure 4–3.

- As the tooth erupts into the oral cavity, the REE fuses with the oral epithelium, forming the **dentogingival junction (epithelial attachment)**.
- This later migrates apically along the tooth to its normal position. A delay in this apical migration is known as **delayed (altered) passive eruption**.

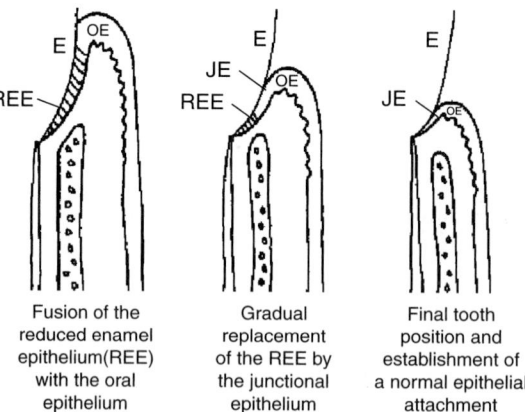

FIGURE 4-3. Tooth eruption.

GENERAL EMBRYOLOGY

Gametogenesis

- See Figure 4–4 for stages of meiosis in sperm and egg.
- See Figure 4–5 for sperm development.
- See Figure 4–6 for mature sperm.
- See Figure 4–7 for oocyte maturation.

FERTILIZATION

- Capacitation and acrosomal reaction of sperm.
- Entry of spermatozoon.
    - Inhibition of polyspermy.
        - Cortical reaction.
        - Zona reaction.

Fertilization usually occurs in the uterine tube. Implantation normally occurs in the uterus; if not, it is ectopic.

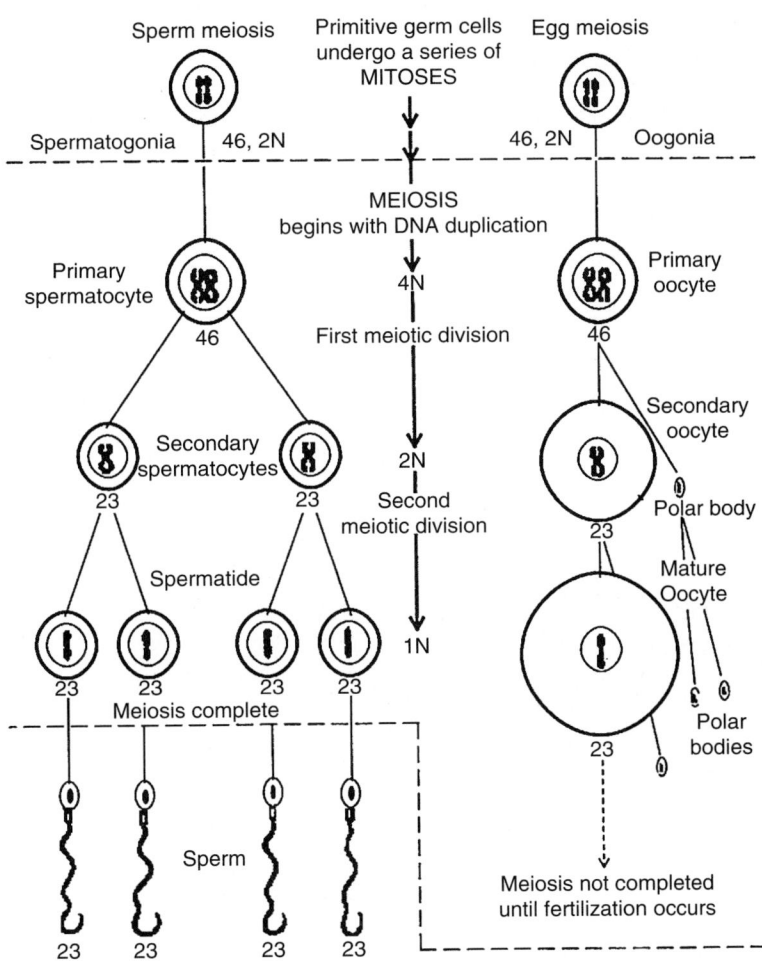

23, 46 = number of chromosomes; 1N, 2N, 4N = number of chromatid copies (N = 23)

FIGURE 4–4. Stages of meiosis in sperm and egg.

Reproduced, with permission, from Sweeney LJ. *Basic Concepts in Embryology.* New York, McGraw-Hill, 1998.

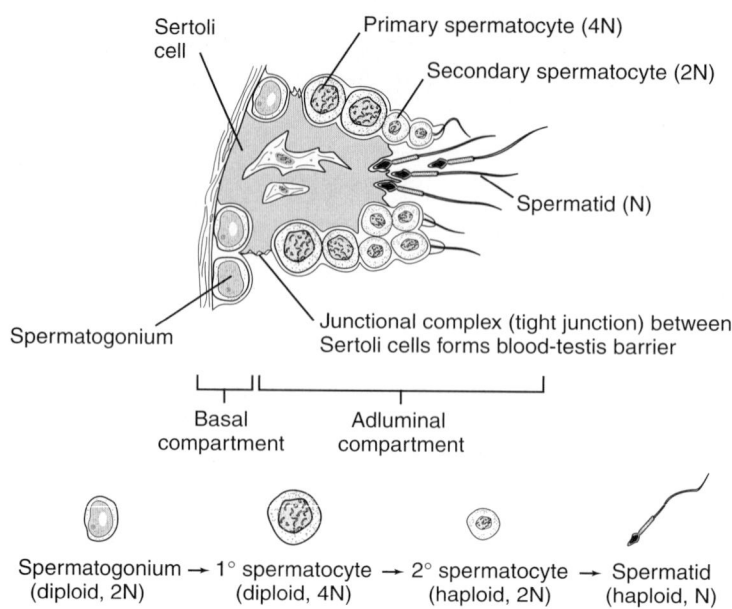

FIGURE 4-5. Sperm development.

Reproduced, with permission, from Bhushan V, Le T, Amin C. *First Aid for the USMLE Step-1.* New York, McGraw-Hill, 2003.

Acrosome contains a packet of enzymes to penetrate and fertilize the egg-acrosome reaction.

Acrosome is derived from Golgi; the middle piece contains numerous mitochondria; the tail is flagellum (9 x 2 + 2).

Sperm become motile in the epididymis.

Meiosis II occurs only if fertilization occurs.

- Meiosis II occurs in oocyte.
  - Barr body (second polar body).
- Fusion of male and female pronuclei.
  - = Zygote.
  - Restores diploid (46).

IMPLANTATION

See Figure 4–8.

- Occurs by the end of the first week.
- Trophoblast cells invade endometrial epithelium.
- Trophoblast produces hCG.
- See Figure 4–9 for cleavage stages.

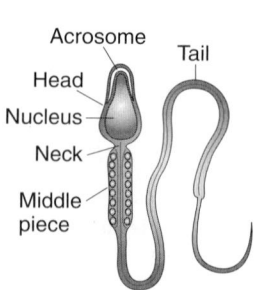

FIGURE 4-6. Mature sperm.

Reproduced, with permission, from Bhushan V, Le T, Amin C. *First Aid of the USMLE Step-1.* New York, McGraw-Hill, 2003.

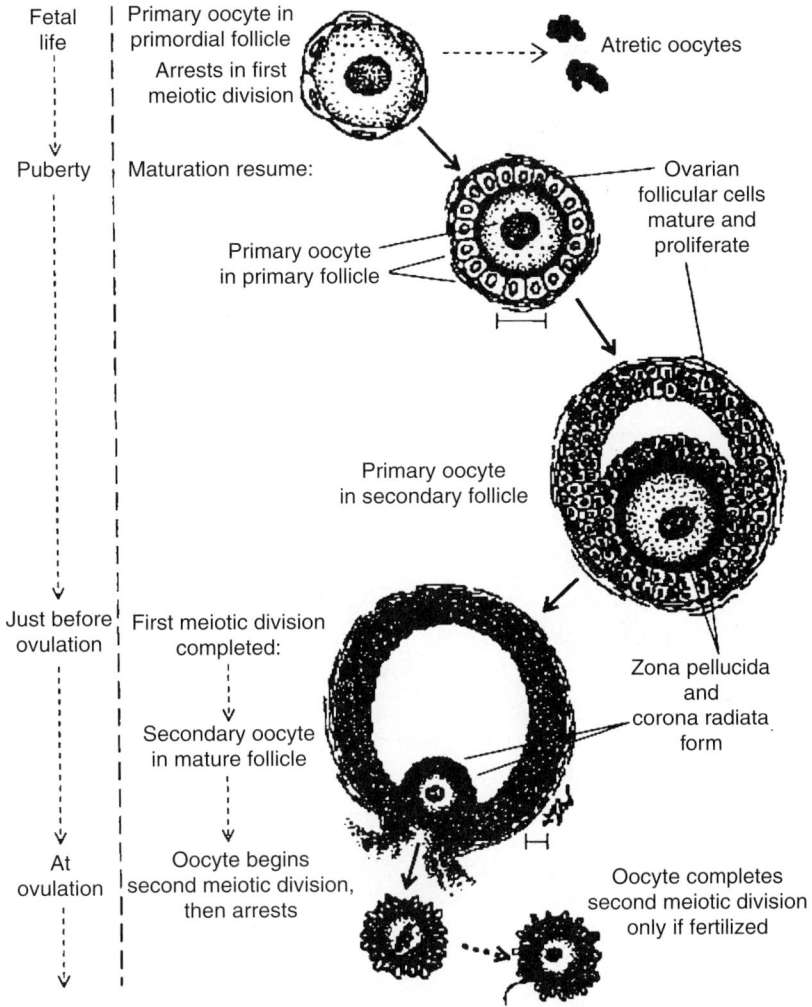

FIGURE 4-7. Maturation of the oocyte and its ovarian follicle.

Reproduced, with permission, from Sweeney LJ. *Basic Concepts in Embryology*. New York, McGraw-Hill, 1998.

BILAMINAR DISC

- Occurs in the second week.
- Epiblast (primary ectoderm).
    - Amniotic cavity.
    - Ultimately gives rise to:
        - Ectoderm.
        - Mesoderm.
- Hypoblast (primary endoderm).
    - Lining of yolk sac.

See Figure 4–10 for placentation.
See Figure 4–11 for twinning.

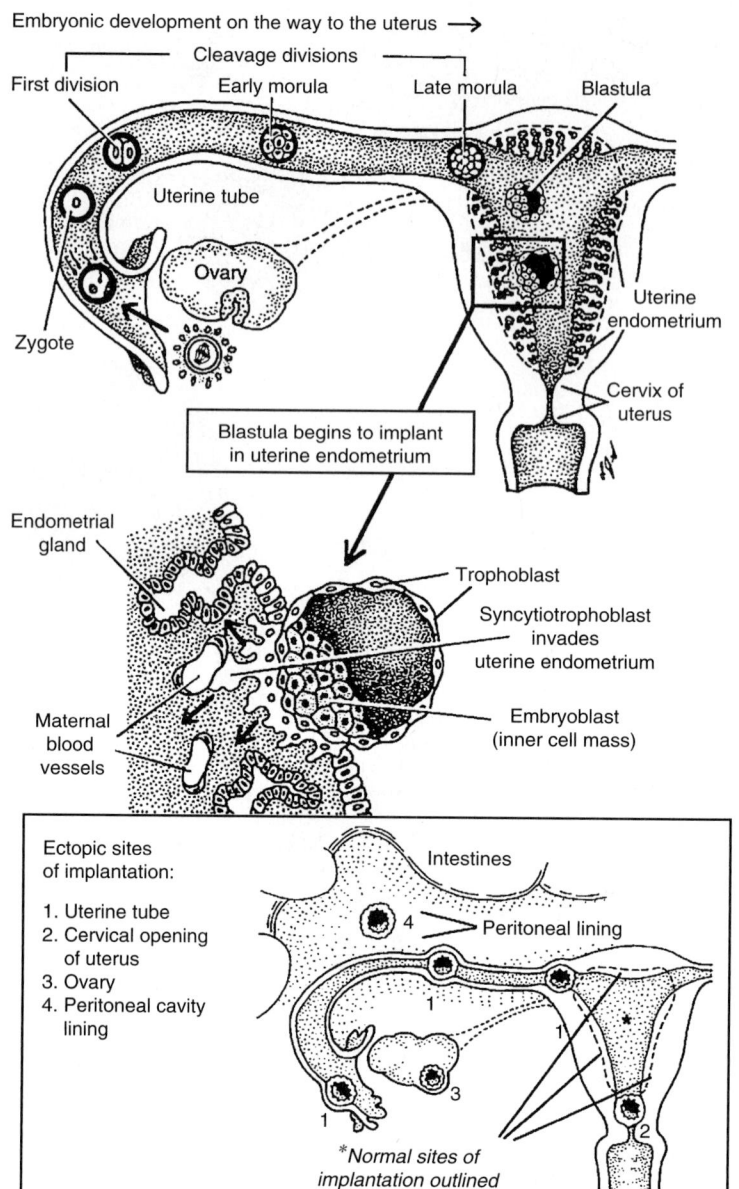

FIGURE 4-8. Development of the embryo and its travels during week 1.

Reproduced, with permission, from Sweeney LJ. *Basic Concepts in Embryology*. New York, McGraw-Hill, 1998.

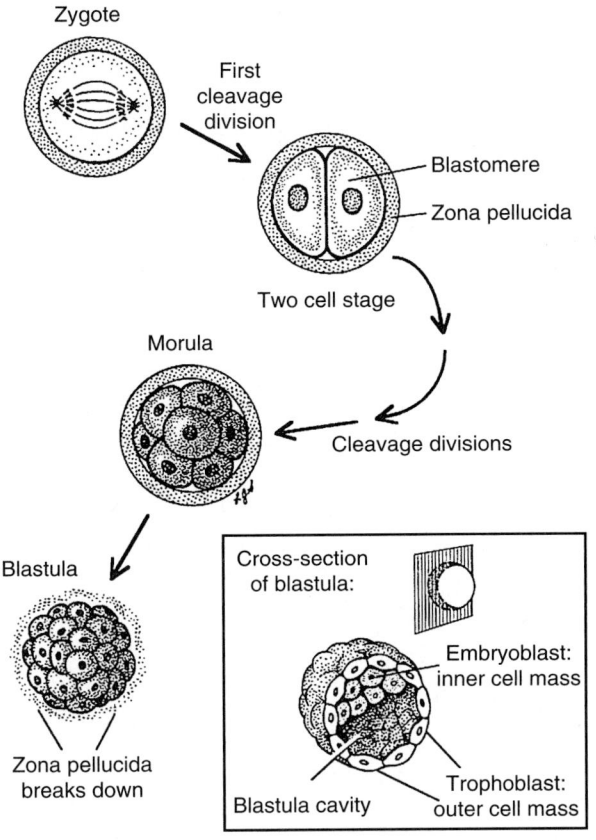

FIGURE 4-9. Cleavage stages: morula and blastula.

Reproduced, with permission, from Sweeney LJ. *Basic Concepts in Embryology*. New York, McGraw-Hill, 1998.

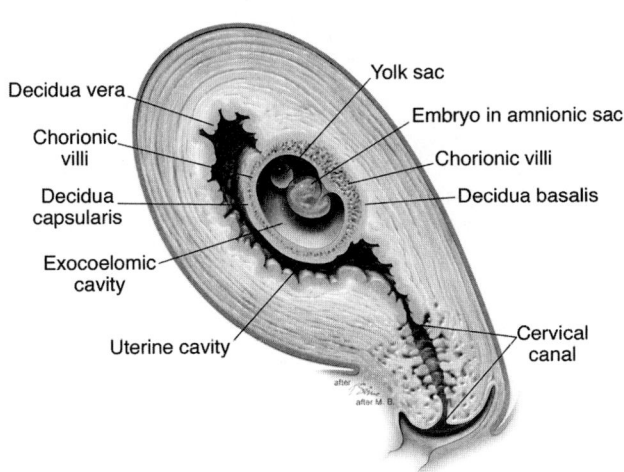

FIGURE 4-10. Placentation.

Reproduced, with permission, from Cunningham FG, et al. (eds). *Williams Obstetrics*. 21st ed. New York, McGraw-Hill, 2001.

Decidual reaction occurs during week 2. Pregnant endometrium enlarges, accumulates lipid and glycogen.

Allantois forms on day 16.

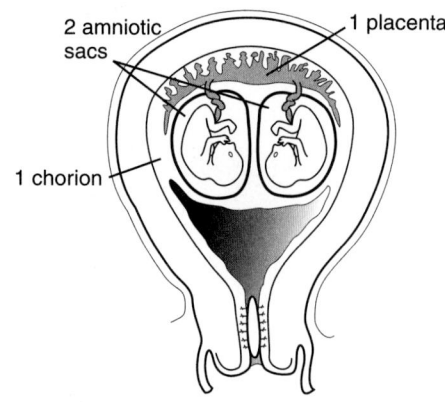
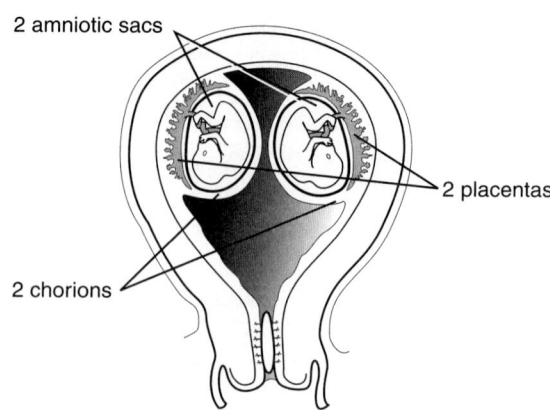

FIGURE 4-11. Twinning.

Reproduced, with permission, from Bhushan V, Le T, Amin C. *First Aid for the USMLE Step-1*. New York, McGraw-Hill, 2003.

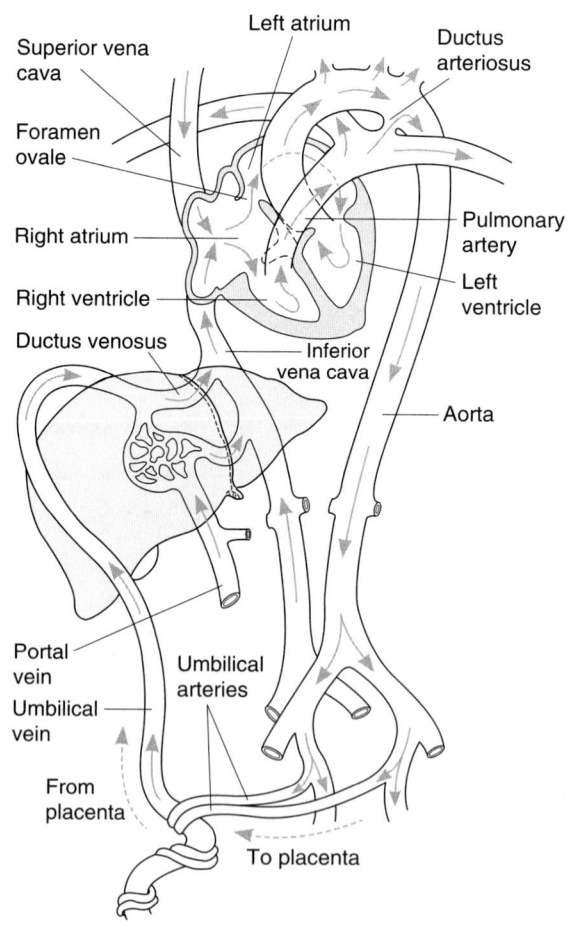

FIGURE 4-12. Fetal circulation.

Reproduced, with permission, from Hay WW, Hayward AR, Levin MJ, Sondheimer JM. (eds). *Current Pediatric Diagnosis & Treatment*, 16th ed. New York, Lange/McGraw-Hill, 2003.

FETAL CIRCULATION

See Figure 4–12.
- Oxygenated blood to heart via
  - Umbilical vein.
  - Inferior vena cava.
- Foramen ovale
  - Allows most of the oxygenated blood to bypass the pulmonary circuit.
  - Pumps out the aorta to the head.
- Deoxygenated blood returned via
  - Superior vena cava.
  - Mostly pumped through the pulmonary artery and ductus arteriosus to the:
    - Feet.
    - Umbilical arteries.

Primitive blood formation occurs in the allantois, yolk sac, liver, spleen, and bone.

Foramen Ovale
- In fetal heart allows blood to flow from RA to LA.
- Bypass pulmonary circuit.
  - Because oxygenated blood comes from the mother/placenta.
- Closes with fibrous connective tissue to become fossa ovalis in the adult.

EMBRYOLOGIC BODY AXES

See Figure 4–13 for anatomic orientation of the embryo.
See Table 4–1 for germ layer derivatives.
See Figure 4–14 for germ layer derivatives.
See Figure 4–15 for stages of fetal life.

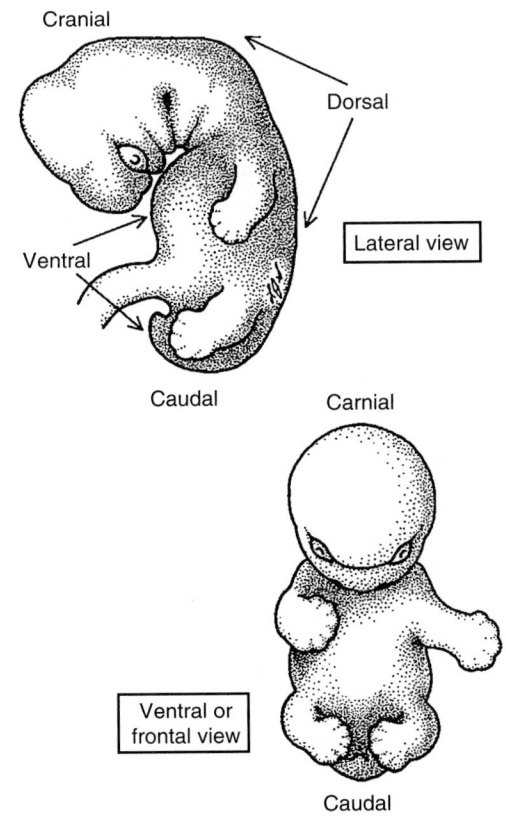

FIGURE 4–13. Embryonic body axes.

Reproduced, with permission, from Sweeney LJ. *Basic Concepts in Embryology.* New York, McGraw-Hill, 1998.

TABLE 4-1. **Germ Layer Derivatives**

ECTODERM DERIVATIVES	
Epithelium of skin (superficial epidermis layer)	All nervous tissue: formed by neuroectoderm: Brain and spinal cord (neural tube) All peripheral nerve tissue (neural crest)

ENDODERM DERIVATIVES	
EPITHELIAL LININGS OF:	
The gastrointestinal tract Organs that form as buds from the endoderm tube: Pharyngeal gland derivatives* Respiratory system Digestive organs (liver, pancreas) Terminal part of urogenital systems	Hypoblast endoderm: Gametes migrate to gonads

MESODERM DERIVATIVES		
ALL CONNECTIVE TISSUES**	**ALL MUSCLE TYPES:**	**EPITHELIAL LININGS OF:**
General connective tissues Cartilage and bone Blood cells (red and white)	Cardiac, skeletal, smooth	Body cavities Some organs: Cardiovascular system Reproductive and urinary systems (most parts)

*Pharyngeal derivatives: palatine tonsils, thymus, thyroid, parathyroids
**Some connective tissues in the head are derived from neural crest

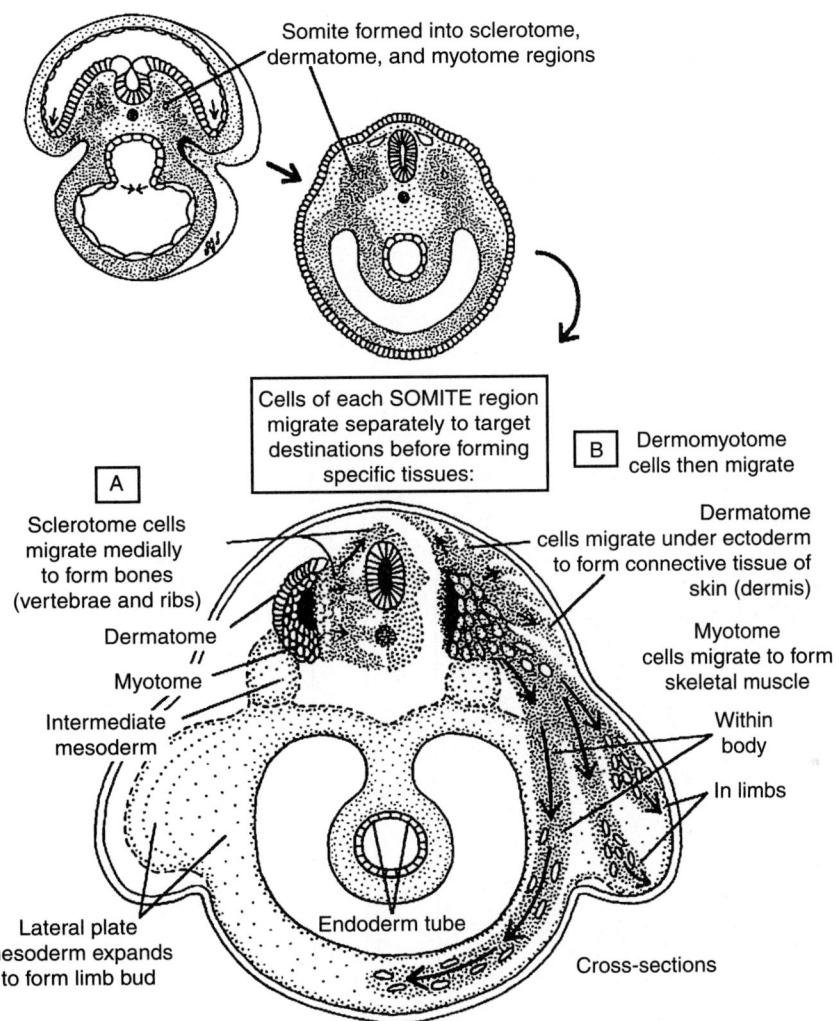

FIGURE 4–14. Dermatome, myotome, and sclerotome derivatives.

Reproduced, with permission, from Sweeney LJ. *Basic Concepts in Embryology.* New York, McGraw-Hill, 1998.

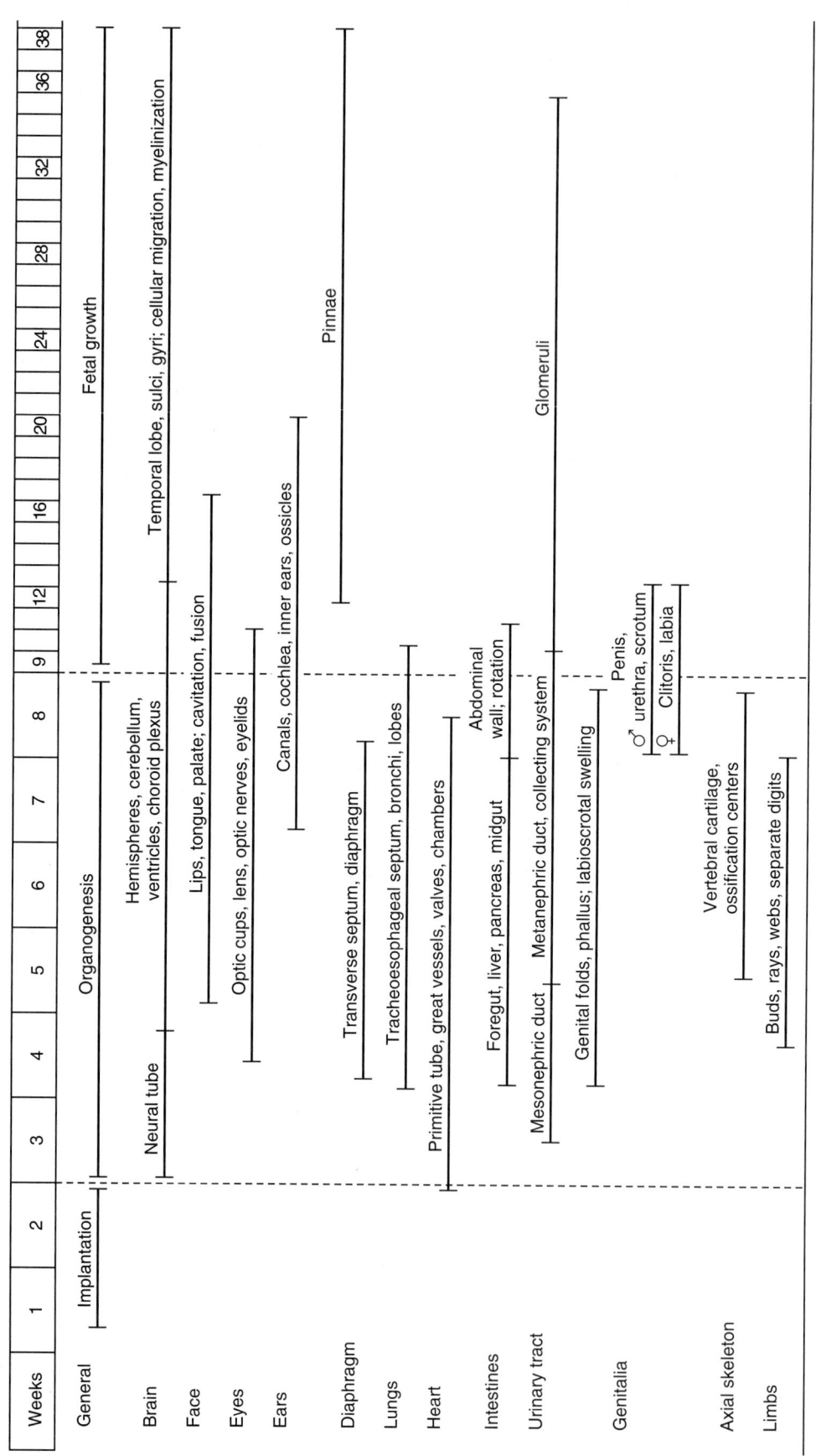

FIGURE 4-15. Stages of fetal life.

Reproduced, with permission, from Hay WW, Hayward AR, Levin MJ, Sondheimer JM. (eds). *Current Pediatric Diagnosis & Treatment*, 16th ed. New York, Lange/McGraw-Hill, 2003.

Embryology of the Central Nervous System

See Figure 4–16.

- Neural plate.
- Neural Tube.
- Alar plate: Alar = sensory (posterior, dorsal).
- Basal plate: Basal = motor (anterior, ventral).
- See Figure 4–17 for formation of the nervous system.

Organogenesis occurs from week 3 to 8.

The neural plate invaginates to form neural groove with neural folds on each side on day 18 of embryonic life (two neural folds fuse forming the neural tube). Neuroectoderm (ectoderm of neural plate) gives rise to CNS (brain and spinal cord).

Week 4 of embryologic development:

- Neural tube is closed.
- Four pairs of branchial arches are visible externally.
- Characteristic C-shaped curvature of embryo is appreciated due to folding.
- Upper and lower limb buds appear.

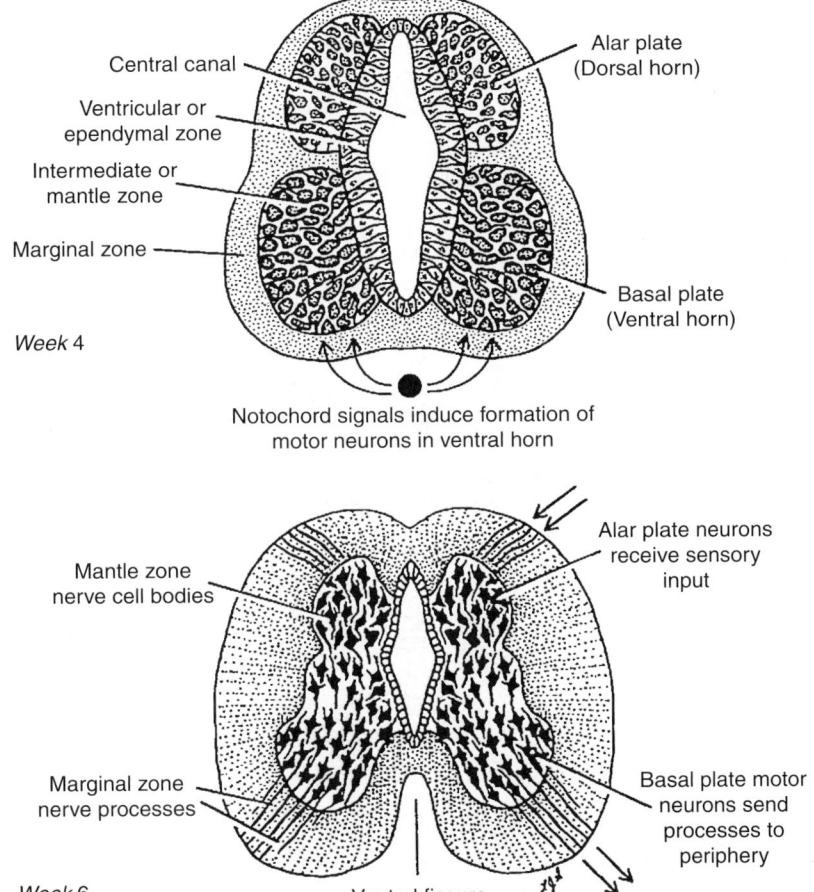

Figure 4–16. Development of regional specialization across the neural tube.

Reproduced, with permission, from Sweeney LJ. *Basic Concepts in Embryology.* New York, McGraw-Hill, 1998.

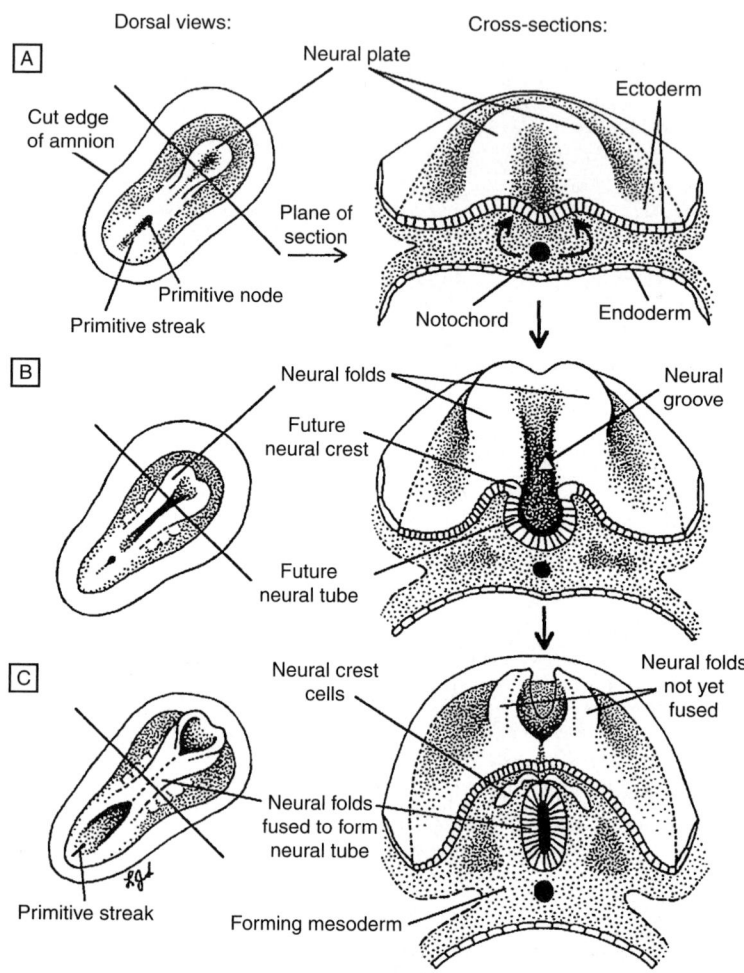

FIGURE 4-17. Neuroectoderm forms the neural tube and neural crest in late week 3 (A and B) and early week 4 (C).

Reproduced, with permission, from Sweeney LJ. *Basic Concepts in Embryology*. New York, McGraw-Hill, 1998.

EMBRYOLOGY OF THE BRAIN

Embyologic Division	Subset	Second Subset	Adult Derivative
Forebrain	Prosencephalon	Telencephalon	Cerebrum, basal ganglia
		Diencephalon	Thalamus Hypothalamus Epithalamus Subthalamus Posterior pituitary (neurohypophysis)
Midbrain	Mesencephalon		Midbrain
Hindbrain	Metencephalon Myelencephalon		Pons Medulla oblongata

Brainstem = midbrain + hindbrain

Brainstem = midbrain + pons + medulla.

NEURAL TUBE CELLS

Neural Tube Cells	Give Rise To
Neural crest	Sensory ganglia (CNs V, VII, IX, X) Dorsal root ganglia (in peripheral nervous system) Schwann cells (peripheral) Melanocytes and odontoblasts Enterochromaffin cells Neurons in parasympathetic and sympathetic ganglia (adrenal medulla) Leptomeninges (pia and arachnoid) Parafollicular cells (C-cells) of parathyroid
Neuroepithelial	Neuroblasts → neurons Ependymal cells (lining ventricles, central canal) Glioblasts-astrocytes, oligodenrocytes (myelin in CNS)
Mesenchymal (mesoderm)	Microglia

The cardiovascular system is derived from mesoderm.

Atrial Septal Defect

- Results from incomplete fusion of septum primum and septum secundum.
- Often asymptomatic until middle age.
- Located near the foramen ovale.

Patent Foramen Ovale

- Failure of complete fusion of foramen ovale.
- Usually of no hemodynamic significance.

Embryology of the Cardiac System

AORTIC ARCH DERIVATIVES

See Figure 4–18.

- Aortic arch arteries
- Form during week 4.
- Arise from distal truncus arteriosus (aortic sac).
- Associated with corresponding pharyngeal arch.
- Connect to the paired dorsal aortae.
    - Dorsal aortae fuse in week 5 to form:
        - Descending thoracic aorta.
        - Abdominal aorta.

Aortic Arch	Adult Analogue
1	Maxillary artery
2	Hyoid artery Stapedial artery
3	Common carotid artery ICA (first part)
4	Aortic arch Right subclavian (proximal)
5	Involutes
6	Pulmonary arteries (proximal) Ductus arteriosus

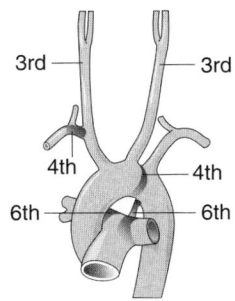

FIGURE 4-18. Aortic arch derivatives.

Reproduced, with permission, from Bhushan V, Le T, Amin C. *First Aid for the USMLE Step-1*. New York, McGraw-Hill, 2003.

Embryology of the Gastrointestinal System

Segment	Artery	Innervation	Derivatives
Foregut	Celiac trunk	Vagus nerve (parasympathetic) Splanchnic nerve (sympathetic) Thoracic nerve	Esophagus Stomach Duodenum (1st part) Liver Gallbladder Pancreas
Midgut	SMA	Vagus nerve (parasympathetic) Splanchnic nerve (sympathetic)	Duodenum (2nd–4th parts) Jejunum Ileum Appendix Colon (to L colic / splenic flexure)
Hindgut	IMA	Pelvic splanchnic (S2-4) nerve (parasympathetic) Lumbar splanchnic nerve (sympathetic)	Colon (distal to splenic flexure) Sigmoid Rectum

Ectodermal derivatives to GI tract:

- Oropharynx (mucosa, tongue, lips, parotid, enamel)
- Rectum (distal to pectinate line)
- Anus

See Figure 4–19 for cardiac development.
See Figure 4–20 for heart embryology.

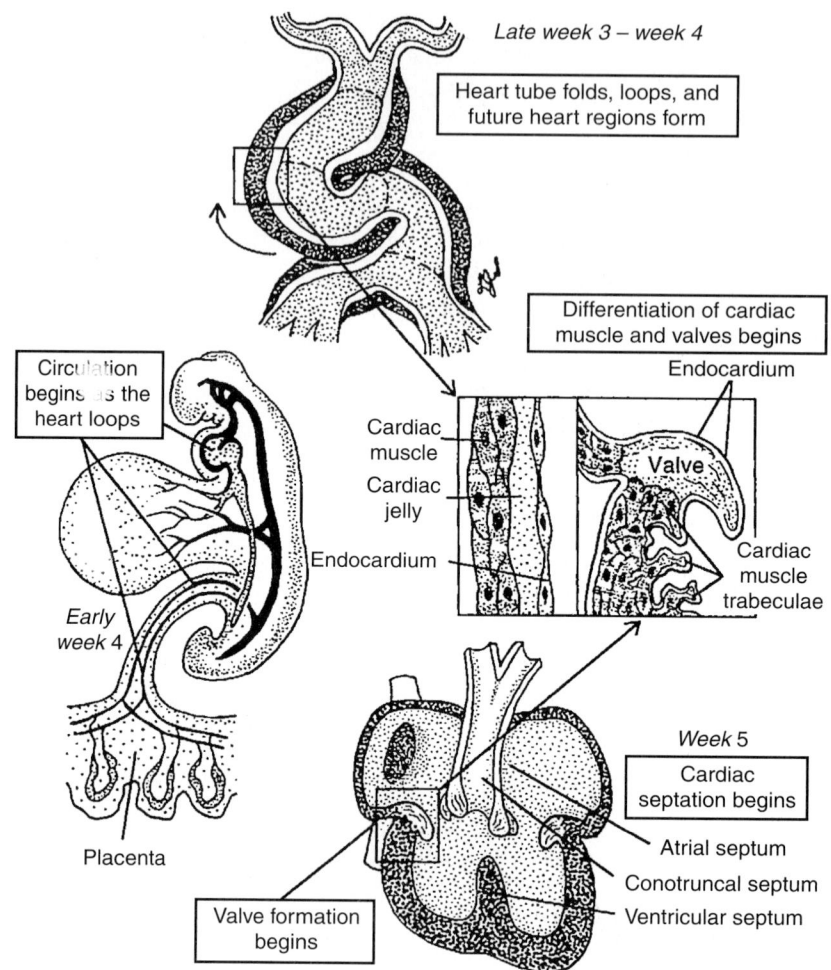

FIGURE 4–19. **Overview of cardiac development.**

Reproduced, with permission, from Sweeney LJ. *Basic Concepts in Embryology.* New York, McGraw-Hill, 1998.

Heart embryology

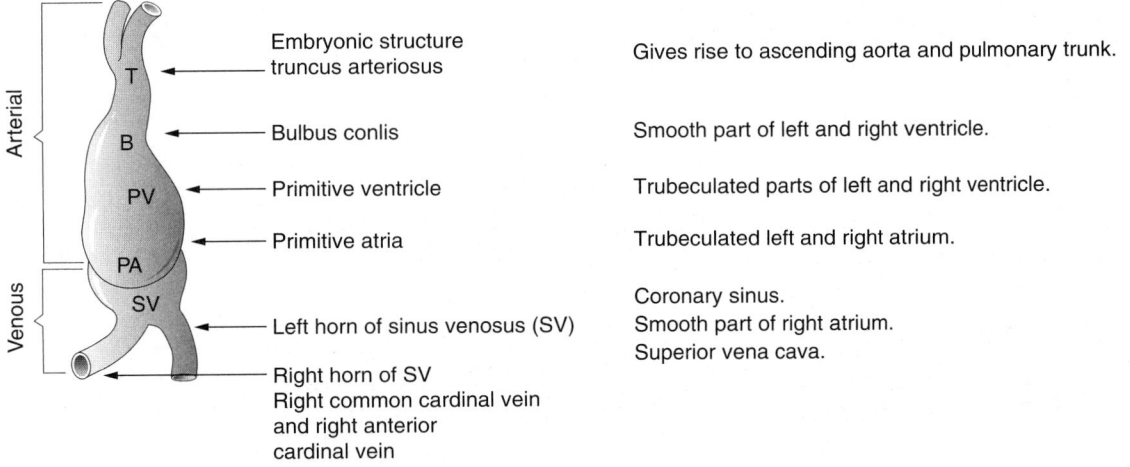

	Embryonic structure	
T	truncus arteriosus	Gives rise to ascending aorta and pulmonary trunk.
B	Bulbus cordis	Smooth part of left and right ventricle.
PV	Primitive ventricle	Trubeculated parts of left and right ventricle.
PA	Primitive atria	Trubeculated left and right atrium.
SV	Left horn of sinus venosus (SV)	Coronary sinus.
		Smooth part of right atrium.
		Superior vena cava.
	Right horn of SV	
	Right common cardinal vein and right anterior cardinal vein	

FIGURE 4–20. Heart embryology.

Reproduced, with permission, from Bhushan V, Le T, Amin C. *First Aid for the USMLE Step-1*. New York, McGraw-Hill, 2003.

Embryology of the Renal System

Structure	Week of Development	Structures Formed
Pronephros	4	Regresses
Mesonephros	4	Mesonephric duct (gives rise to): Ductus deferens, Epididymis, Ejaculatory duct, Seminal vesicle. Ureteric bud (forms): Ureter, Renal pelvis, Calyces, Collecting tubules
Metanephros	5	Adult kidney (from): Ureteric bud, Metanephric Mass. Kidney forms in pelvis but "ascends" to abdomen with fetal growth. Ureters lengthen

Wolffian duct (mesonephric duct). Embryonic duct develops into deferent duct, etc. in males; obliterated in females.

Embryology of the Renal System

See Figure 4–21 for the three stages of kidney development.

- From intermediate mesoderm
  - Nephrogenic cord gives rise to:
    - Pronephros.
    - Mesonephros.
    - Metanephros.

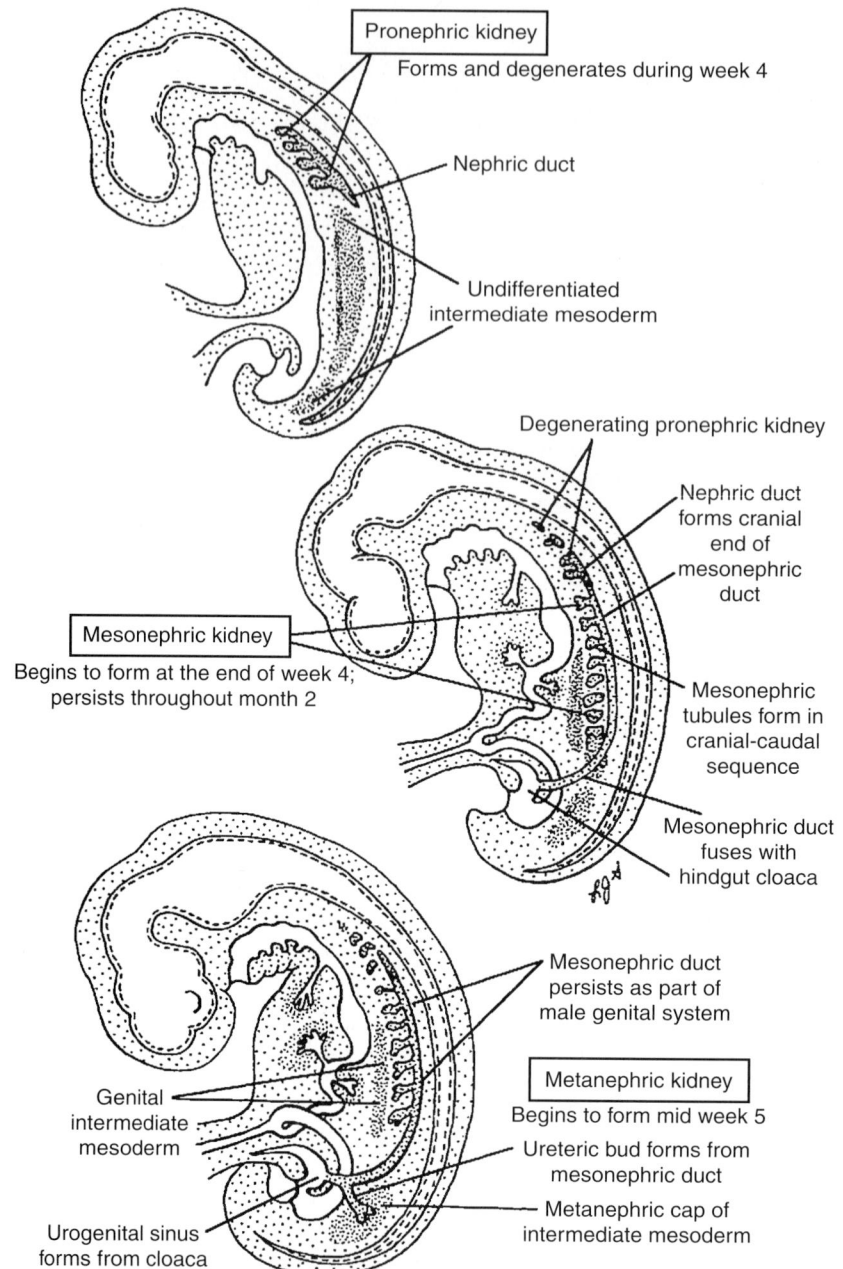

FIGURE 4-21. The three stages of kidney development.

Reproduced, with permission, from Sweeney LJ. *Basic Concepts in Embryology*. New York, McGraw-Hill, 1998.

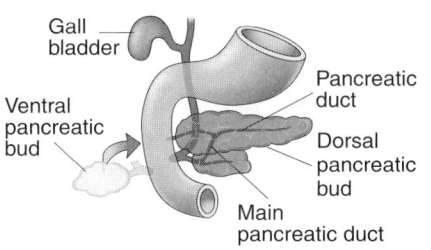

FIGURE 4-22. Embryology of the pancreas.

Reproduced, with permission, from Bhushan V, Le T, Amin C. *First Aid for the USMLE Step-1.* New York, McGraw-Hill, 2003.

See Figure 4-22 for embryology of the pancreas.

▶ **EMBRYOLOGY OF THE FACE AND PHAYRNGEAL ARCHES**

See Figure 4-23 for formation of the neurocranium and viscerocranium.

First arch

- See Figure 4-25.
- Meckel's cartilage
  - Model for the mandible.
- Dissolutes with only minor contribution to ossification.
- Mandibular process (forms mandible).
- Maxillary process (forms maxilla, zygoma, squamous temporal).
- Tongue formation (anterior two thirds).
  - Tuberculum impar (median tongue bud).
  - Lateral lingual swellings (2) (distal tongue buds).

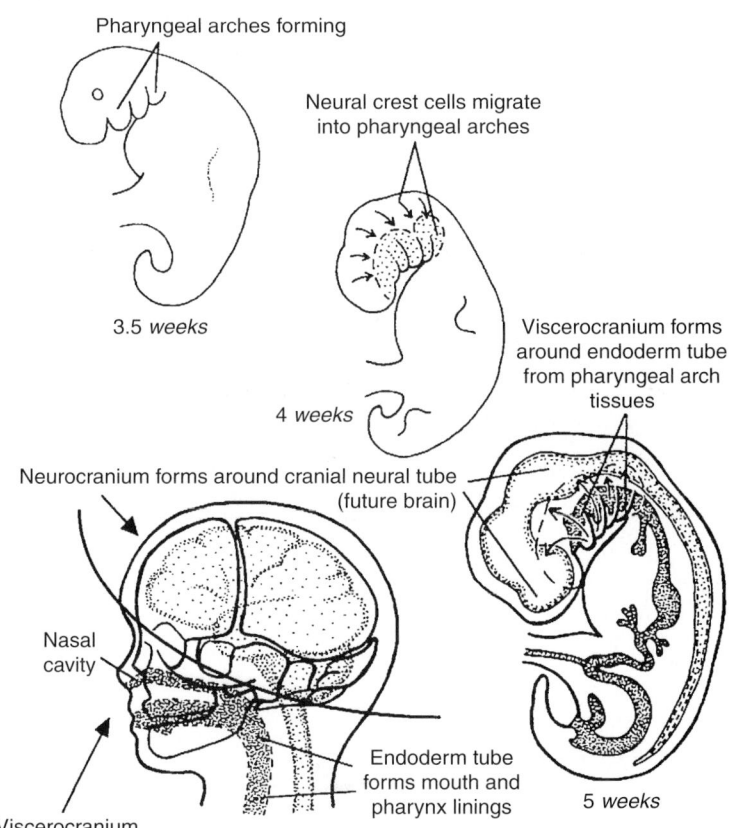

FIGURE 4-23. Formation of neurocranial and viscerocranial regions of the head.

Reproduced, with permission, from Sweeney LJ. *Basic Concepts in Embryology.* New York, McGraw-Hill, 1998.

Branchial Arches

- Rounded, mesodermal ridges (neural crest cells).
- Form from proliferative activity of neural crest cells.
- Each arch contains nerve, artery, muscle, and cartilaginous bar.
    - Nerves (V, VII, IX, X) are **branchiomeric** because they originate from the branchial arches.
        - Not from somites.
        - Develop about week 4 of life.
- End of week 4 the arches are well-defined and visible externally.
- During week 4 the first branchial arch divides into:
    - Mandibular process.
    - Maxillary process.
    - Weeks 5–6, arches are smaller, not seen on surface.
    - Arches 1–3 play role in forming face and oral cavity.
- Arch 1
    - Mandible
    - Maxilla (most)
- Arches 2 and 3
    - Tongue

See Figure 4–24 for derivatives in the pharyngeal region.

Third arch

- Hyoid bone
- Tongue formation (root-posterior third)
- Hypobranchial eminence

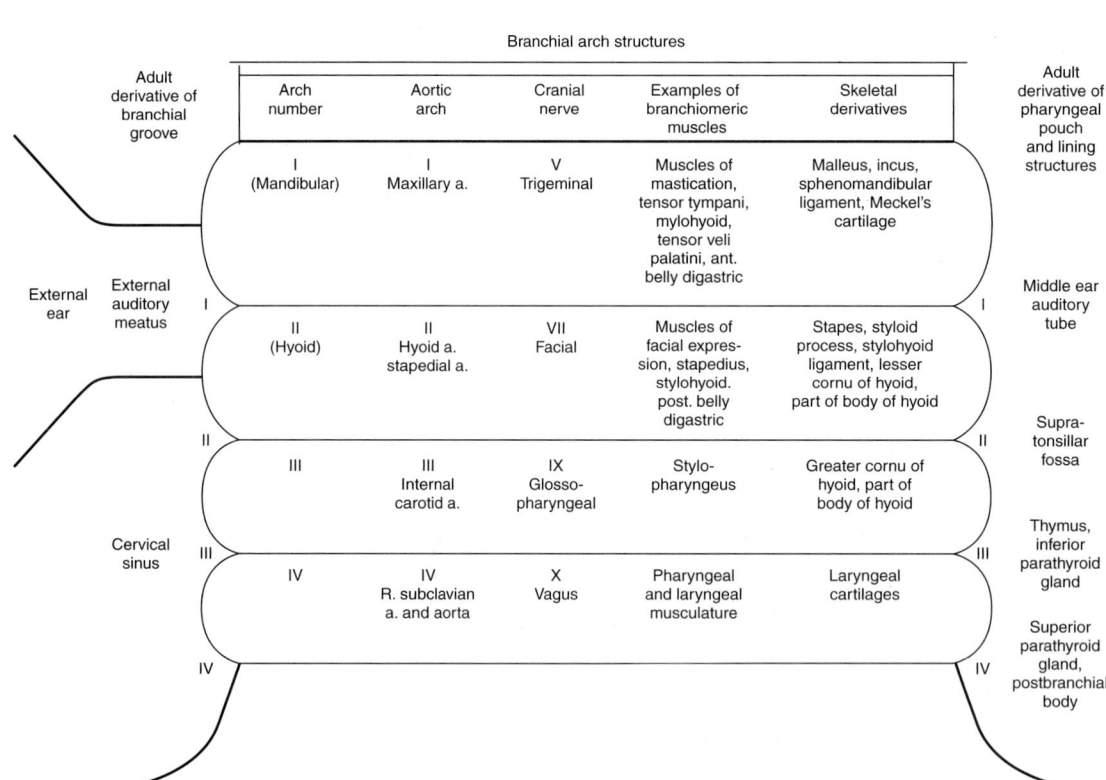

FIGURE 4-24. Diagram of derivatives in the pharyngeal region.

Reproduced, with permission, from Carlson BM. *Patten's Foundations of Embryology.* 5th ed. New York: McGraw-Hill, 1988.

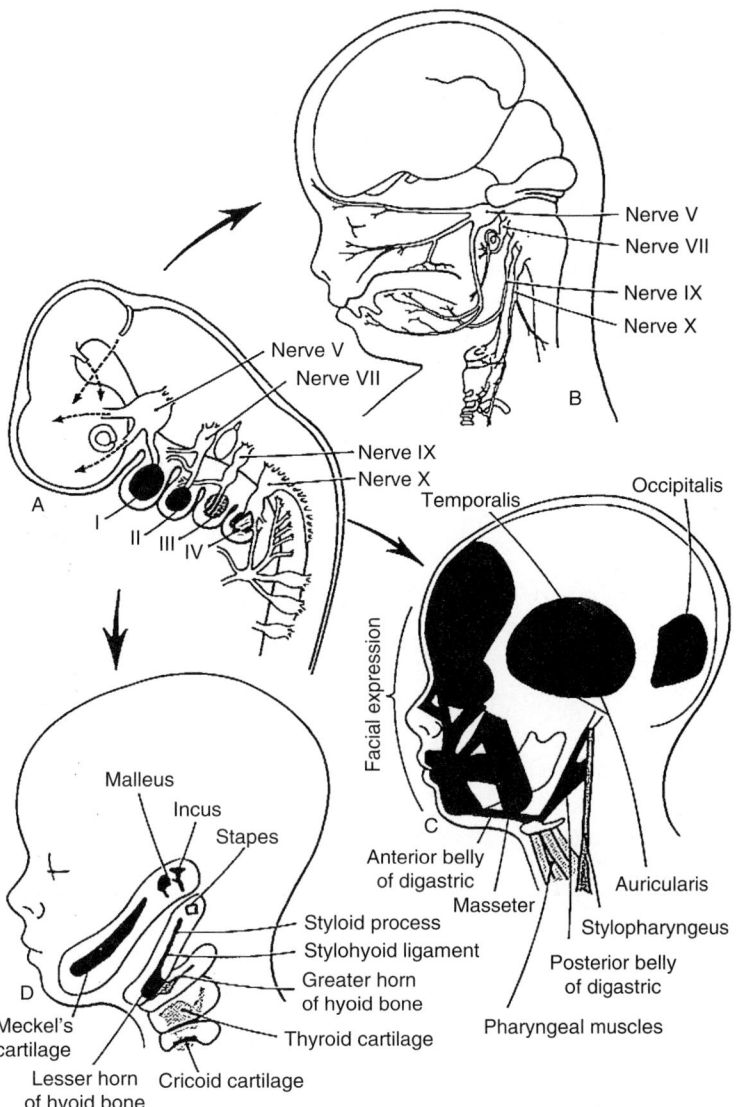

FIGURE 4-25. Schematic diagram showing major derivatives of structures that constitute the branchial arches. (A) 5-week embryo; (B–D) 4- to 5-month fetuses. The gray tones of structures in C and D correspond to those of the branchial arches depicted in A.

Reproduced, with permission, from Carlson BM. *Patten's Foundations of Embryology.* 5th ed. New York. McGraw-Hill, 1988.

Pharyngeal Pouches

See Figure 4–26.

- Paired evaginations of pharyngeal endoderm that lines inner aspects of branchial arches

Pouch	Structures
1	Tympanic membrane Auditory tube Middle ear cavity
2	Lymphatic nodule Palatine tonsil
3	Inferior parathyroid gland Thymus
4	Superior parathyroid gland Ultimobranchial body 　■ Gives rise to thyroid parafollicular/C-cells 　■ Calcitonin
5	Rudimentary structure (becomes part of pouch 4)

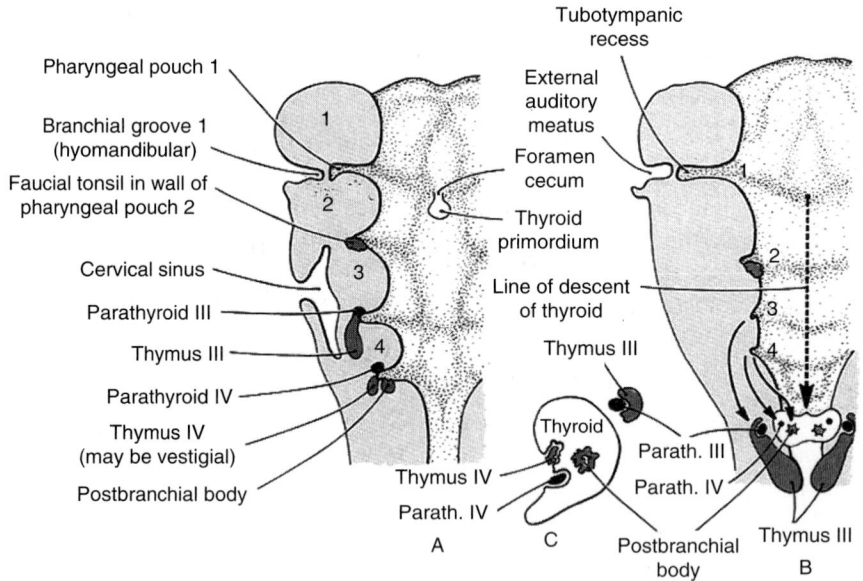

FIGURE 4–26. Diagrams showing the origin of the pharyngeal derivatives. **(A)** The primary relationships of the several primordial to the pharyngeal pouches. **(B)** Course of migration of some of the primordial from their place of origin. **(C)** Definitive relations of parathyroids, postbranchial body, thymus, and thyroid as they appear in a transverse section of the right lobe of the thyroid taken above the level of the isthmus. Abbreviation: *Parath.*, parathyroid.

Reproduced, with permission, from Carlson BM. *Patten's Foundations of Embryology.* 5th ed. New York. McGraw-Hill, 1988.

Formation of the Face

MANDIBLE

- Two mandibular processes (branchial arch 1) merge.
- Medial ends merge at week 4.
- Mandibular processes → merge to form lower lip.

MAXILLA

- Two maxillary processes (branchial arch 1) merge.
  - Form upper cheek regions and most of upper lip.

FRONTAL NASAL PROCESSES

- Form with growth of forebrain.
- Develop into forehead and nose.
- Two medial nasal processes merge.
- Form philtrum of upper lip.

NASAL PLACODES

- Thickened areas of specialized ectoderm.
- Located on either side of the frontal nasal process.
- Give off elevations at their margins.
- Lateral nasal processes (2).
  - Form sides/alae of nose.
- Medial nasal processes (2).
  - Form bridge of nose.
  - Nostrils.
  - Upper lip philtrum.

Mouth and Oral Cavity

See Figure 4–27(a) and (b).

- Begins as a slight depression on the stomodeum.
- Located between branchial arch 1 and the forebrain.
- **Buccopharyngeal membrane** (oropharyngeal membrane)
  - Thin bilaminar membrane.
  - Composed of ectoderm externally and endoderm internally.
  - Separates the stomodeum from the primitive pharynx (until rupture).
  - Ruptures around week $3\frac{1}{2}$ (~24 days).
  - Connecting the primitive mouth and primitive pharynx.

See Figure 4–28 for formation of the nasal cavities and the teeth.

FORMATION OF THE PALATE

See Figure 4–29.

PRIMARY PALATE

- Forms from merging of the **two median nasal processes.**
- Becomes the premaxillary part of the maxilla.
  - Maxilla anterior to incisive foramen in adults.
  - Contains central and lateral incisors.

The mandible and maxilla, except the mandibular condyles, are formed by intramembranous ossification.

Most of the upper lip is formed by the maxillary processes.

The corner of the mouth is formed by the fusion of the maxillary and mandibular processes.

The vestibular lamina separates the lips and cheeks externally and jaw structures internally in the developing embryo.

The stomodeum is the primitive mouth; lined by ectoderm.

The plane passing through the right and left anterior pillars marks the separation between the oral cavity and oropharynx in the adult.

Nasal processes are proliferations of mesenchyme at the margins of the nasal placodes. The nasal placodes develop on the lower part of the frontonasal process, on each side.

Secondary Palate

- Forms from the two maxillary processes (lateral palatine processes).
- Forms hard and soft palates.
- Extends from incisive foramen posteriorly.

Lateral cleft lip occurs because the maxillary and medial nasal processes fail to fuse. Cleft lip can be unilateral or bilateral.

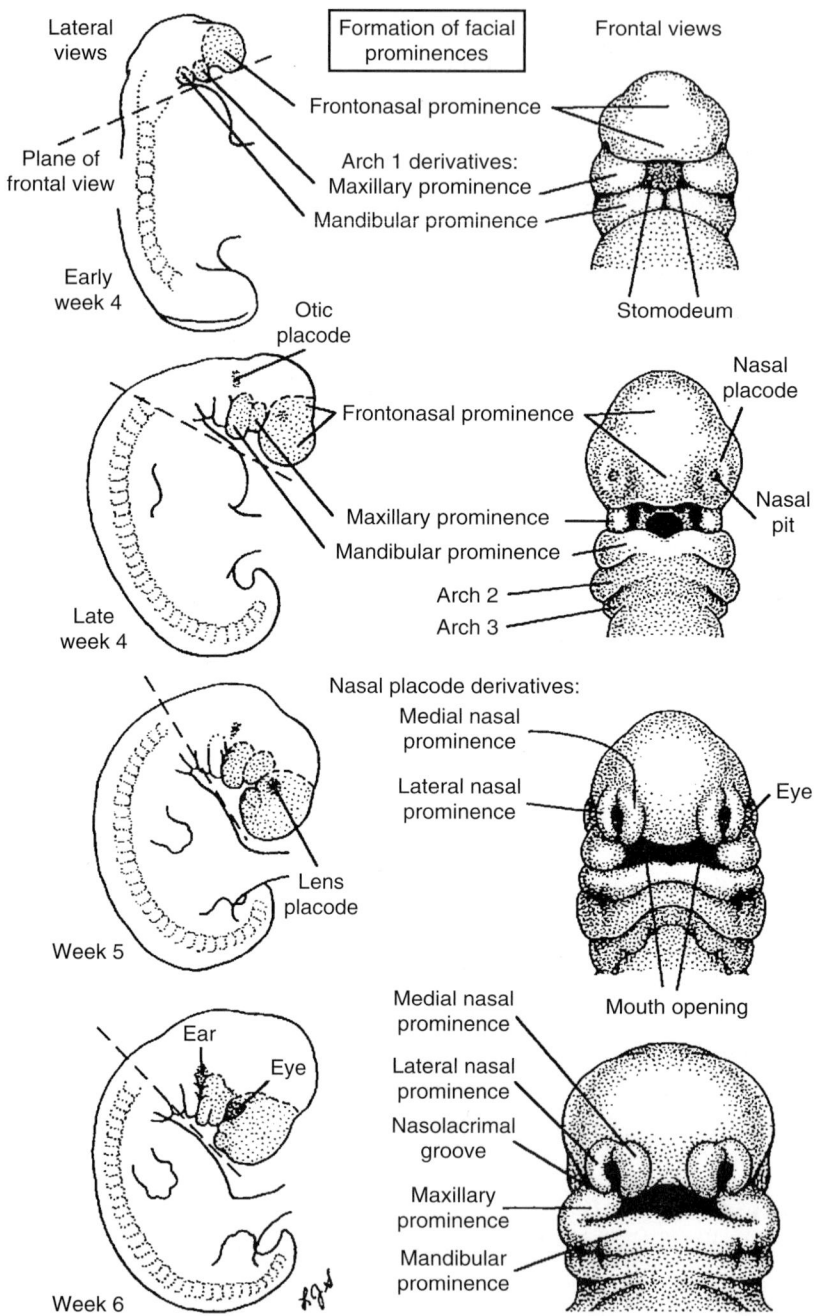

FIGURE 4–27. (A) Development of the face from facial prominences. (B) Development of the mature face and formation of cleft lip defects.

Reproduced, with permission, from Sweeney LJ. *Basic Concepts in Embryology.* New York, McGraw-Hill, 1998.

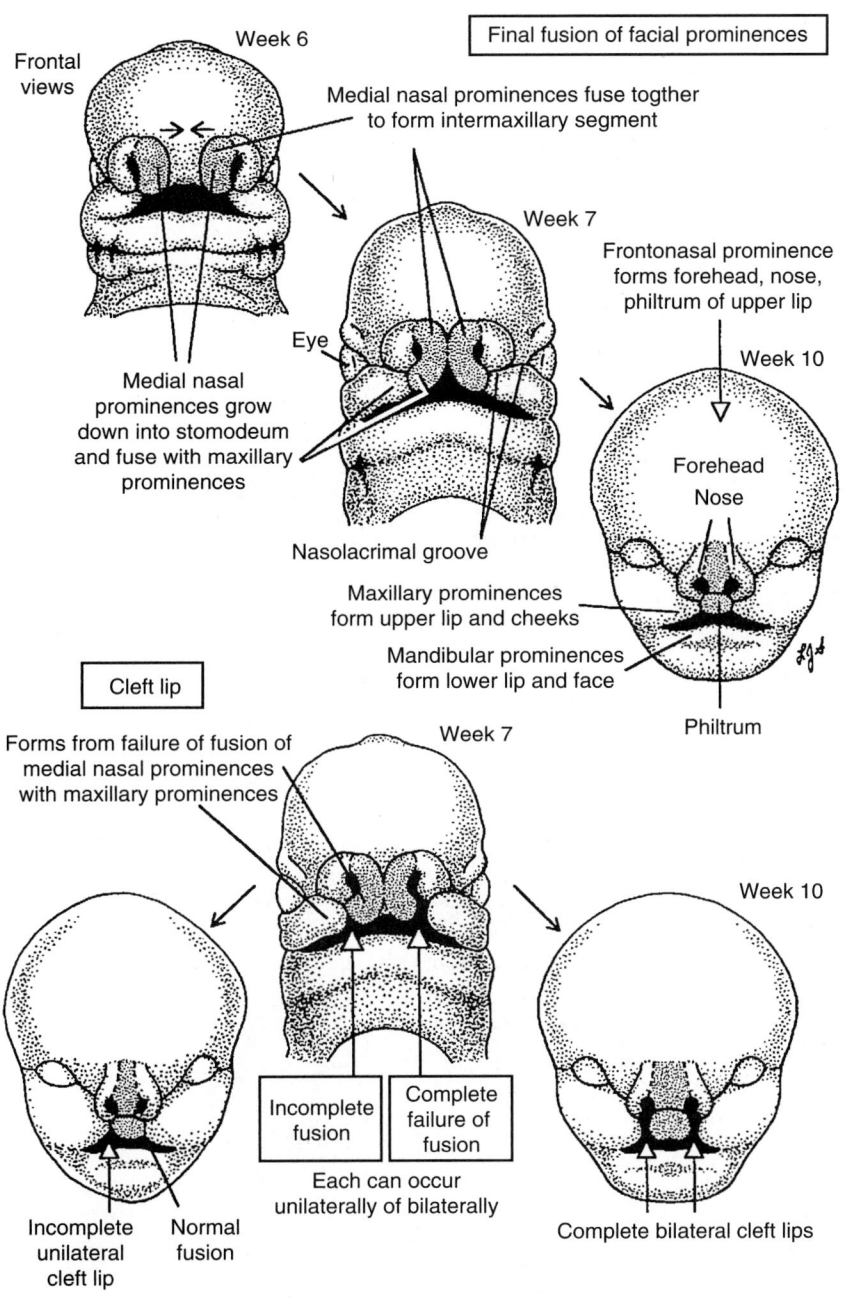

FIGURE 4-27. (Continued)

CLEFT PALATE

- Occurs with failure to fuse >1 of the following:
  - Lateral palatine processes (palatal shelves).
  - Nasal septum.
  - Primary palate.

VARIATIONS OF CLEFT LIP AND PALATE

- May involve uvula only, or extend through hard and soft portions of palate.
- Cleft uvula only.

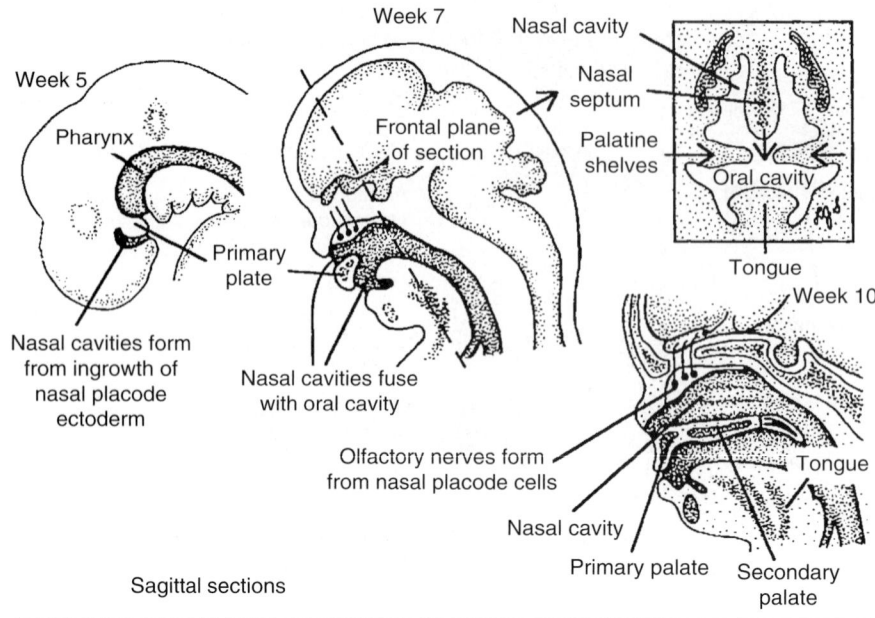
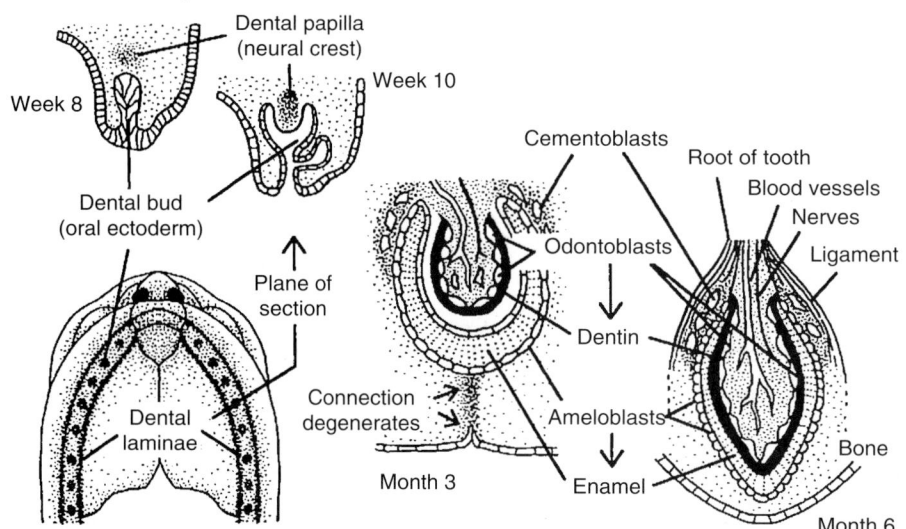

FIGURE 4-28. Formation of (A) the nasal cavities and (B) the teeth.

Reproduced, with permission, from Sweeney LJ. *Basic Concepts in Embryology.* New York, McGraw-Hill, 1998.

- Unilateral cleft of secondary palate.
- Bilateral cleft of secondary palate.
- Complete unilateral cleft.
  - Lip.
  - Alveolar process (of maxilla).
  - Primary palate.
- Complete bilateral cleft (except secondary palate).
  - Lip.
  - Alveolar process (of maxilla).
  - Anterior palate.
  - Secondary palate (unilateral).

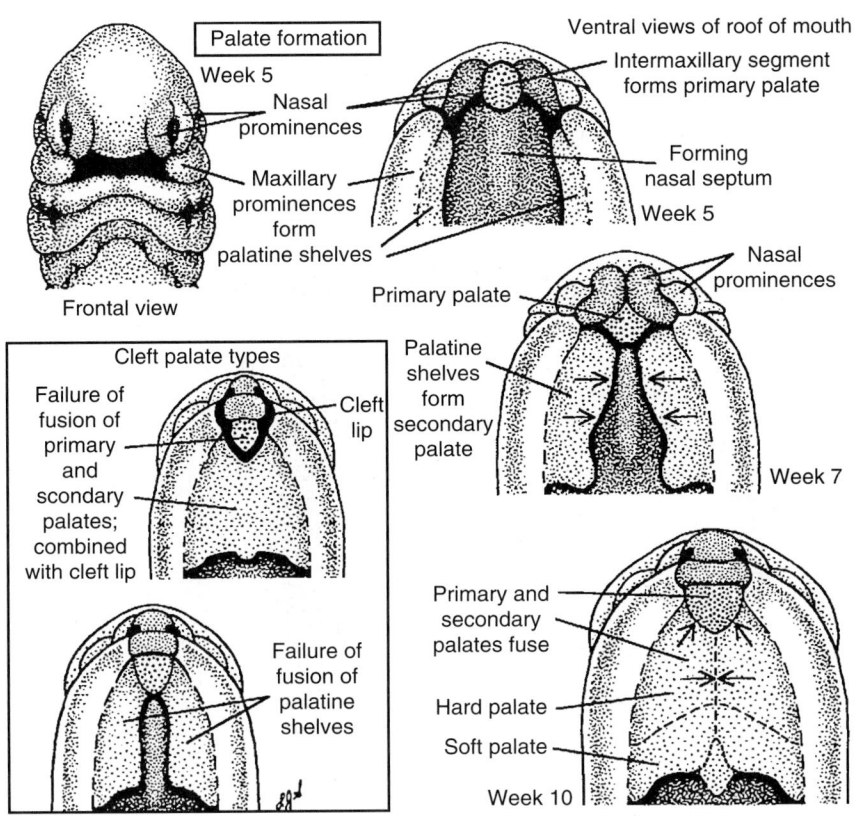

FIGURE 4-29. Normal formation of the mouth and palate and defects in palate formation.

Reproduced, with permission, from Sweeney LJ. *Basic Concepts in Embryology.* New York, McGraw-Hill, 1998.

- Complete bilateral cleft.
  - Lip.
  - Alveolar process.
  - Anterior (primary) palate.
  - Posterior (secondary) palate.

TONGUE DEVELOPMENT

See Figure 4–30.

- Begins in the first week with the formation of the tuberculum impar.
- Tuberculum impar.
  - Median, triangular elevation.
  - Appears on floor of pharynx, just in front of foramen cecum.

Anterior Two Thirds of Tongue

- Lateral lingual swellings (distal tongue buds [2]).
- Form on each side of the tuberculum impar.
- From the proliferation of mesenchyme (arches 1, 2, 3).
- Swellings fuse to form the anterior two thirds of tongue.

Embryologically, the tongue is derived from the first four pharyngeal arches; and innervation comes from associated nerves of those arches (arch 1, V; arch 2 VII; arch 3 IX; arch 4, X).

Bifid tongue occurs because of lack of fusion of distal tongue buds (lateral swellings).

Posterior Third of Tongue:
- Formed by two elevations.
  - Copula (arch 2).
  - Hypobranchial eminence (arch 3).

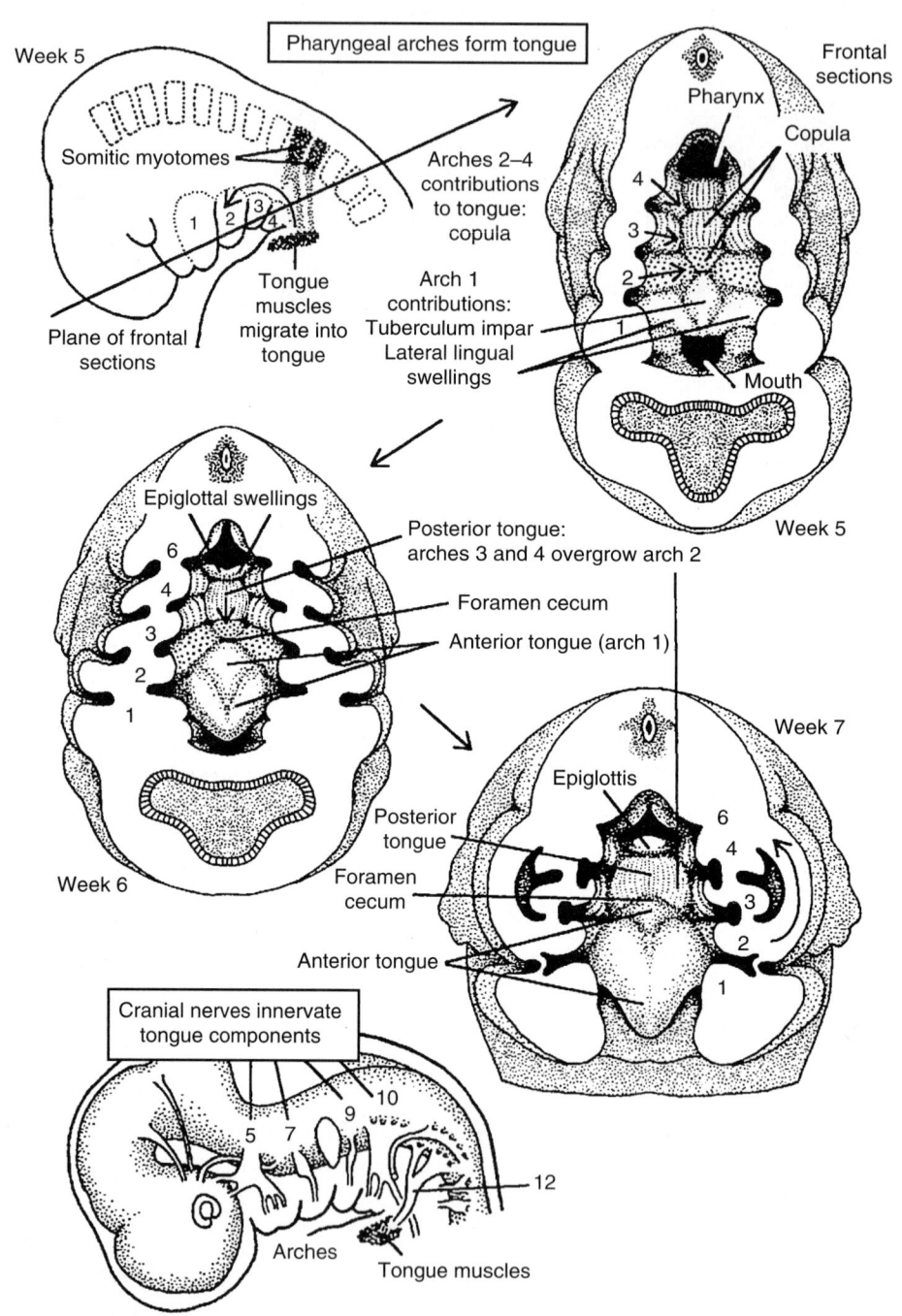

FIGURE 4-30. Development of the tongue.

Reproduced, with permission, from Sweeney LJ. *Basic Concepts in Embryology.* New York, McGraw-Hill, 1998.

SECTION 2
Biochemistry-Physiology

- Physical-Chemical Principles
- Biological Compounds
- Metabolism
- Molecular Biology
- Membranes
- Neurophysiology
- Muscle Physiology
- Circulatory and Cardiac Physiology
- Respiratory Physiology
- Renal, Fluid, and Acid-Base Physiology
- Gastrointestinal Physiology
- Nutrition
- Endocrine Physiology

CHAPTER 5
Physical-Chemical Principles

Molecular Bonds	246
Water	246
CARBONIC ANHYDRASE	**246**
Laws of Thermodynamics	246
Calorimetry	246

▶ MOLECULAR BONDS

- **Covalent bonds:** *Strong* molecular interactions mediated by shared electrons.
- **Noncovalent bonds:** *Weak, reversible* molecular interactions.
  - **Ionic bonds:** Mediated by opposite electrostatic charges.
  - **Hydrogen bonds:** Mediated by a shared hydrogen atom.
  - **Van der Waals bonds:** A nonspecific attraction (occurs when any two atoms are 3–4 Å apart).

▶ WATER

- Polar.
- Triangular.
- Highly cohesive.
- Excellent solvent for polar molecules.
- Weakens ionic and H-bonds.

Carbonic Anhydrase

See Figure 5–1.

- Catalyzes the reaction between CO_2 and H_2O.
- Extremely *fast* enzyme.
- Located largely in **erythrocytes** and **kidneys.**

▶ LAWS OF THERMODYNAMICS

Enthalpy is the heat content of a system.

Entropy is the degree of disorder of a system.

- **First law:** The total energy of a *closed* system is conserved.
- **Second law:** The entropy of a *closed* system always increases.

▶ CALORIMETRY

- **Direct calorimetry:** Direct measurement of the amount of heat produced in a given system.
- **Indirect calorimetry:** Measurement of the amount of heat produced in terms of inhaled O_2 and exhaled CO_2.

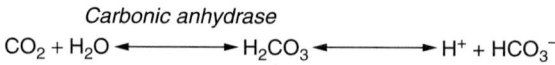

$$CO_2 + H_2O \xrightleftharpoons{\text{Carbonic anhydrase}} H_2CO_3 \rightleftharpoons H^+ + HCO_3^-$$

FIGURE 5–1. Carbonic anhydrase reaction.

CHAPTER 6
Biological Compounds

Carbohydrates	248
CARBOHYDRATE STRUCTURE	248
STORAGE OF POLYSACCHARIDES	249
STRUCTURAL POLYSACCHARIDES	250
BACTERIAL POLYSACCHARIDES	251
COMPLEX CARBOHYDRATES	251
SALIVA	252
Proteins	252
AMINO ACIDS	253
PROTEIN STRUCTURE	255
PHYSIOLOGICALLY RELEVANT PROTEINS	256
Lipids	259
LIPID TRANSPORT	262
LIPID STORAGE	264

▶ **CARBOHYDRATES**

Carbohydrate Structure

GLUCOSE

- The most fundamental carbohydrate; required for carbohydrate metabolism, storage, and cellular structure.
- If carbohydrates are not absorbed by dietary intake, they are generally converted to glucose in the *liver*.

CARBOHYDRATE CLASSIFICATION

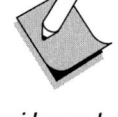

- **Monosaccharides:** The simplest carbohydrates.
  - Further classified by:
    - Number of carbon atoms: Trioses, tetroses, pentoses, hexoses, heptoses.
    - Functional group: Aldoses (aldehyde) or ketoses (ketone).
    - See Figure 6–1 for important aldoses.
    - See Figure 6–2 for important keratoses.
- **Disaccharides:** Glycosidic condensation of two monosaccharides.
  - Maltose → glucose + glucose; via maltase.
  - Sucrose → glucose + fructose; via sucrase.
  - Lactose → glucose + galactose; via lactase.
- **Oligosaccharides:** Glycosidic condensation of 2–10 monosaccharides.
- **Polysaccharides:** Glycosidic condensation of >10 monosaccharides.
  - Mostly used as storage molecules or cellular structural components.
  - Can be linear or branched.

Disaccharides are hydrolyzed mostly in the small intestine.

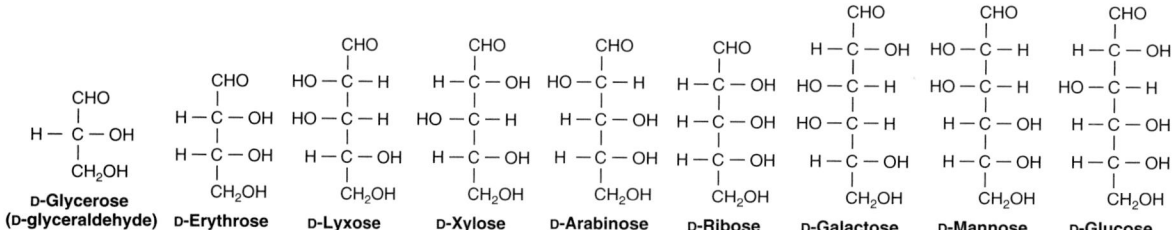

FIGURE 6–1. Important aldoses.

Reproduced, with permission, from Murray RK. *Harper's Illustrated Biochemistry*, 26th ed. McGraw-Hill, 2003.

FIGURE 6–2. Important keratoses.

Reproduced, with permission, from Murray RK. *Harper's Illustrated Biochemistry*, 26th ed. McGraw-Hill, 2003.

Storage of Polysaccharides

STARCH

- A homopolymer of glucose linked by α–1, 4 glycosidic bonds.
- The major glucose storage molecule in *plants*.
- Contains unbranched helical *amylose* (15–20%) and branched (α–1, 6) *amylopectin* (80–85%).
- **Amylases** are the key enzymes in starch catabolism. (See Table below.)

Isomaltase cleaves α-1, 6 branch points.

Major Amylases Important for Starch Hydrolysis

Amylase	Hydrolysis Products
α-amylase	Maltose + dextrins
β-amylase	Maltose
Glucamylase	Glucose

α-amylase is secreted by both the pancreas and the parotid gland.

GLYCOGEN

- A homopolymer of glucose linked by α-1, 4 glycosidic bonds.
- The major glucose storage molecule in *animals*.
- Contains numerous branch points via α-1, 6 glycosidic linkages.

Glycogen is stored in the liver.

Glycogen Storage Diseases

Disease	Enzyme Deficiency	Clinical Features	Inheritance
von Gierke disease (type I glycogenosis)	Glucose-6-phosphatase	Hepatomegaly Renomegaly Platelet dysfunction Stunted growth	Autosomal recessive
Pompe disease (type II glycogenosis)	Lysosomal glucosidase	Hepatomegaly Cardiomegaly Muscle hypotonia	Autosomal recessive
McArdle syndrome (type V glycogenosis)	Muscle glycogen phosphorylase	Muscle cramping Myoglobinuria	Autosomal recessive

INULIN

- A homopolymer of *fructose*.
- Highly water soluble.
- Used to determine glomerular filtration rate (GFR).

Structural Polysaccharides

GLYCOSAMINOGLYCANS (GAGs)

See Table 6–1.

Proteoglycans are complex carbohydrates that have a central protein molecule to which many GAGs are attached in a radial (brushlike) pattern. Located mostly in the ECM.

- Heteropolymer chains containing *repeating disaccharide units* of an **amino sugar** and an **uronic acid.**
- The major structural polysaccharides of extracellular matrix (ECM), connective tissue (CT), and outer cell membrane surfaces.
- Because they contain sulfate and carboxyl groups, GAGs are *highly negatively charged* and *easily attract water*, enabling them to cushion their surrounding structures.
- Accumulation of various GAGs (due to enzyme deficiencies) results in several syndromic diseases.

TABLE 6–1. Major Glycosaminoglycans

GAG	PROMINENT LOCATION	COMPONENTS
Chondroitin sulfate - *Most abundant* GAG.	Cartilage Bone Tendon Ligament	N-acetylgalactosamine + D-glucuronic acid
Hyaluronic acid - *Most unique* GAG. - Does not form a proteoglycan. - Does not contain sulfur.	ECM Synovial fluid Vitreous humor	N-acetylglucosamine + D-glucuronic acid
Heparan sulfate	Basement membranes	N-acetylglucosamine + L-glucuronic acid (or L-iduronic acid)
Heparin - More sulfated than heparan sulfates.	Mast cell granules	N-acetylglucosamine + L-glucuronic acid (or L-iduronic acid)
Dermatan sulfate	Skin Vasculature	N-acetylgalactosamine + L-iduronic acid
Keratan sulfate	Cornea Cartilage Bone	N-acetylglucosamine + galactose

Mucopolysaccharide Storage Diseases

Disease	Enzyme Deficiency	Accumulation of	Clinical Features	Inheritance
Hurler's syndrome	α-L-iduronidase	Heparan sulfate Dermatan sulfate	Mental retardation. Corneal clouding. Gargoylism.	Autosomal recessive.
Hunter's syndrome	L-iduronate sulfatase	Heparan sulfate Dermatan sulfate	Mental retardation. Gargoylism.	X-linked recessive.

CELLULOSE

- A homopolymer of β-D-glucopyranose linked by β-1, 4 bonds.
- Major component of **plants.**
- Cannot be digested by humans.

CHITIN

- A homopolymer of N-acetyl-D-glucosamine linked by β-1, 4 glycosidic bonds.
- Major component of insect and crustacean **exoskeletons.**

Bacterial Polysaccharides

DEXTRAN

- A homopolymer of **glucose** formed by the hydrolysis of sucrose.
- Produced by *Streptococcus mutans*.

LEVAN

- A homopolymer of **fructose** formed by the hydrolysis of sucrose.

Cariogenic bacteria synthesize glucans (dextrans) and fructans (levans) from their metabolism of dietary sucrose, which aid in their adherence to teeth.

Complex Carbohydrates

GLYCOPROTEINS

- Proteins with covalently linked oligosaccharide (glycan) chains.
- Function: Structural components, transport molecules, enzymes, receptors, and hormones.
- Examples: Collagens, proteoglycans, immunoglobulins, selectins, fibronectin, laminin, thyroid-stimulating hormone (TSH), and alkaline phosphatase.

GLYCOLIPIDS

- Sphingolipids with attached carbohydrates.
- Commonly found on outer cell membrane surfaces, especially in brain and other nervous tissues.
- Examples: Gangliosides, galactosylceramide, and glucosylceramide.

Saliva

- A *hypotonic* fluid with an average pH ranging from 6 to 7.
- Contains mostly water, electrolytes, and organic factors.

Major Components of Saliva

Function	Major Salivary Component	Purpose
Antimicrobial	Secretory IgA Lysozyme Lactoperoxidase	Opsonization. Hydrolyzes bacterial cell wall. ↓ lysine/glutamic acid accumulation.
Buffering	Bicarbonate	Maintains pH.
Cleansing	Water	Washes away debris.
Digesting	α-amylase	Hydrolyzes starch.
Lubricating	Mucins	Coats food for swallowing.
Dental integrity	Calcium, phosphate Glycoproteins	Enamel mineralization. Pellicle formation.

SALIVARY SECRETIONS

- **Serous** (watery) → contain α-amylase.
- **Mucous** (viscous) → contain mucins.

Salivary Glands and Their Primary Secretions

Salivary Gland	Primary Secretion
Parotid	Serous
Submandibular	Mixed
Sublingual	Mucous
Minor (except von Ebner)	Mucous

SALIVARY CONTROL

- Controlled by the autonomic nervous system.
- **Parasympathetic** action → *serous* secretions.
- **Sympathetic** action → *mucous* secretions.

Vagotomy inhibits salivary production.

▶ PROTEINS

- Consist of chains of amino acids (*polypeptides*), which are arranged in specific three-dimensional conformations.

Amino Acids

See Tables 6–2 through 6–4.

- Building blocks of polypeptides.
- Basic structure consists of a central α-carbon atom surrounded by four groups: a hydrogen atom, carboxyl group, amino group, and an R-group specific to each amino acid.
- All amino acids found in proteins are stereoisomers in the *L-configuration*.

TABLE 6-2. Classification of Amino Acids by R-Group

R-GROUP	AMINO ACIDS
Polar	Asparagine, Cysteine, Glutamine, Methionine, Serine, Threonine.
Nonpolar	Alanine, Isoleucine, Leucine, Glycine, Proline, Valine.
Acidic	Aspartate, Glutamate.
Basic	Arginine, Histidine, Lysine.
Aromatic	Phenylalanine, Tryptophan, Tyrosine.
Thiol	Cysteine, Methionine.

TABLE 6-3. Classification of Amino Acids by Dietary Necessity

DIETARY NECESSITY	CHARACTERISTIC	AMINO ACIDS
Essential (9)	Must be obtained from dietary intake.	Phenylalanine, Valine, Threonine, Tryptophan, Isoleucine, Methionine, Histidine, Lysine, Leucine
Nonessential (11)	All synthesized from **glucose** (from α-ketoacids, α-amino acids, transaminases, vitamin B_6), *except tyrosine*.	Arginine, Aspartate, Asparagine, Alanine, Cysteine, Glycine, Glutamate, Glutamine, Proline, Serine, Tyrosine

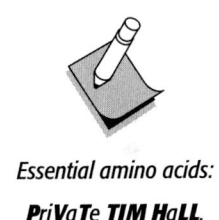

Essential amino acids:
PriVaTe TIM HaLL.

TABLE 6-4. **Classification of Amino Acids by Metabolic End Product**

METABOLIC CATEGORY	AMINO ACIDS
Ketogenic ■ Yields *acetyl-CoA*.	Leucine, lysine.
Glucogenic ■ Yields *pyruvate*.	Arginine, aspartate, asparagine, alanine, cysteine, histidine, methionine, glycine, glutamate, glutamine, proline, serine, threonine, valine.
Both	Isoleucine, phenylalanine, tryptophan, tyrosine.

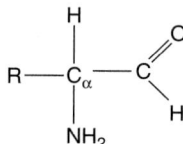

Amino acid structure.

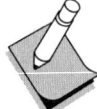

Glycine is the only amino acid that has two of the same group (hydrogen atoms) bonded to the α-carbon.

PEPTIDE BONDS

- Amino acids are *covalently* linked by peptide bonds at their amino (N-terminus) and carboxyl (C-terminus) groups.
- Generally short and polar, they allow the α-carbon to rotate freely about its axis.
- Generally a *trans* (not *cis*) bond.
- Very stable; generally require proteolytic enzymes to break them.

CLASSIFICATION

- By R-group. (See Table 6–2.)
- By dietary necessity. (See Table 6–3.)
- By metabolic end product. (See Table 6–4.)

Nitric oxide is released largely by vascular endothelium, causing vasodilation.

AMINO ACID DERIVATIVES

- Phenylalanine. See Figure below.
- **Tryptophan** → 5-hydroxytryptamine (seratonin).
- **Histidine** → Histamine.
- **Arginine** → Nitric oxide.
- **Glycine** → Porphyrin → heme.

Epinephrine and norepinephrine are produced by the adrenal medulla. They cause potent vasoconstriction and bronchodilation.

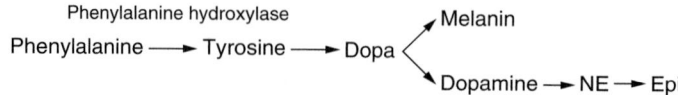

Derivatives of Phenylaline.

Defects of Amino Acid Metabolism

Disorders of Amino Acid Metabolism

Disease	Affected AA	Cause	Effects
Phenylketonuria (PKU)	Phenylalanine	Deficiency of *phenylalanine hydroxylase*.	Severe mental retardation, ↓ skin/hair pigmentation.
Albinism	Tyrosine	Deficiency of *tyrosinase*.	Lack of melanin pigmentation.
Alkaptonuria	Tyrosine	Deficiency of *homogentisic acid oxidase*.	Excessive urinary excretion of homogentisic acid, causing **black urine.**
Cystinuria	Cysteine	Impaired renal reabsorption of cysteine.	Excessive urinary excretion of cysteine.

Histamine is released largely by basophils and mast cells, causing vasodilation and bronchoconstriction.

H1 *receptors mediate type I hypersensitivity.*
H2 *receptors mediate gastric acid and pepsin secretion.*

Protein Structure

- **Primary structure:** The specific sequence of amino acids in a polypeptide chain. Each amino acid in the polypeptide chain is called a **residue**.
- **Secondary structure:** The folding of portions of a polypeptide chain.
    - α-Helix: Coiled configuration.
    - β-Pleated sheet: Zigzag or pleated configuration.
    - β-Turn: Reverse turns that link two sides of a β-pleated sheet.
- **Tertiary structure:** The overall three-dimensional conformation of a polypeptide. Each portion of the polypeptide that can perform a biochemical or physical function is called a **domain**.
- **Quaternary structure:** The spatial arrangement of two or more polypeptides. Each polypeptide is known as a **subunit**.

Heme is a major component of hemoglobin and myoglobin.

*Protein structures are determined by **x-ray diffraction** analysis.*

Physiologically Relevant Proteins

Collagen

See Figure 6–3 for collage structure and Figure 6–4 for collagen synthesis.

- Consists of three polypeptide α-chains wound around one another to form a **triple helix.**
- Produced by many cells: *fibroblasts*, epithelial cells, odontoblasts, osteoblasts, and chondrocytes.
- Fibers have high tensile strength.
- Collagen synthesis:
    - Intracellular events
        - Synthesis of α-chains in rER. The typical amino acid sequence of each α-chain is **glycine-x-y.**
        - Hydroxylation of proline and lysine residues in rER.
        - Glycosylation of α-chains in Golgi. The **procollagen** triple helix contains N- and C-terminal propeptides.
    - Extracellular events
        - Endopeptidases cleave the N- and C-terminal propeptides of procollagen, forming **tropocollagen.**
        - Tropocollagen molecules aggregate at specific intervals, forming **collagen fibrils.**

Elastin

- Fibers are extremely elastic.
- Synthesized similarly to collagen.
    - The amino acid sequence of the proelastin polypeptide chain is typically **glycine-x-y.** Other residues include proline, lysine, alanine, and hydroxyproline (to a lesser extent).
    - Endopeptidases cleave the N- and C-terminal propeptides of proelastin, forming tropoelastin.
    - Tropoelastin molecules cross-link via *desmosine*, forming elastin fibers.

*Elastin does **not** contain **hydroxylysine**, which makes it much more elastic than collagen.*

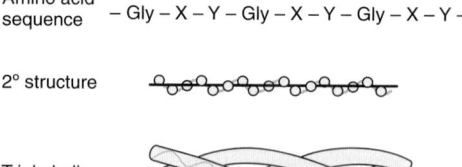

FIGURE 6-3. Collagen structure.

Reproduced, with permission, from Murray RK. *Harper's Illustrated Biochemistry*, 26th ed. McGraw-Hill, 2003.

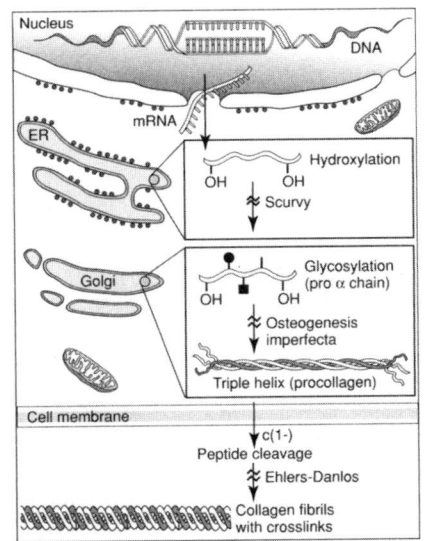

*Vitamin C is required for the hydroxylation of **proline** and **lysine** during collagen synthesis.*

FIGURE 6–4. Collagen synthesis.

Reproduced, with permission, from Bhushan V. *First Aid for the USMLE Step 1.* McGraw-Hill, 2006:85.

Plasma Proteins

- Most plasma proteins are synthesized in the liver.

Major Plasma Proteins

Plasma Protein	Examples	Function
Albumin	Albumin	Maintains plasma osmotic pressure. Transports various molecules (calcium, copper, free fatty acids, bilirubin, steroid hormones, drugs). *Most abundant* plasma protein (60%).
Fibrinogen (Factor I)	Fibrinogen	Hemostasis.
Alpha globulins	Lipoproteins (HDL) Prothrombin Erythropoietin Angiotensinogen α_2-macroglobulin	Transports cholesterol esters. Hemostasis. Erythrocyte synthesis. Regulates blood pressure. Protease inhibition.
Beta globulins	Lipoproteins (LDL) Transferrin	Transports cholesterol. Transports copper and iron.
Gamma globulins	Immunoglobulins	Antibodies.
Complement proteins	C3, C5, etc.	Bacterial cell lysis. Inflammation.

IMMUNOGLOBULINS

See also Chapter 21, "Immunology and Immunopathology."

HEMOGLOBIN

See Tables 6–5 and 6–6 and Figure 6–5.

- Transports O_2 in erythrocytes.
- Contains one globin and *four* hemes.
- Each globin contains two α-chains and two β-chains.
- Each heme reversibly binds one molecule of O_2 when the iron is in a reduced ferrous (Fe_2^+) state.
- Heme binds carbon monoxide (CO) with a greater affinity than O_2.
- Hb binds ~15% of the CO_2 carried in venous blood (the majority is carried by bicarbonate).
- Mutations of α and β subunits result in numerous hemoglobin types.

Methemoglobinemia is a condition in which Fe_2^+ (ferrous) is oxidized to Fe_3^+ (ferric), which cannot bind oxygen. Methemoglobin is formed due to decreased activity of methemoglobin reductase—a side effect of drugs (e.g., sulfonamides) or a hereditary phenotype of increased hemoglobin M.

TABLE 6–5. The Major Types of Hemoglobin

HB TYPE	CHARACTERISTIC	CAUSE OF ABNORMALITY
Hb A	Normal Hb	N/A.
Hb F	Fetal Hb	N/A.
Hb C	Chronic anemia	Lysine replaces glutamate.
Hb H	α-Thalassemia	Defect of α chain genes (composed of four β chains).
Hb M	Methemoglobinemia	Tyrosine replaces histidine.
Hb S	Sickle-cell anemia	Valine replaces glutamate.

TABLE 6–6. Comparison of Hemoglobin and Myglobin

GLOBIN	LOCATION	HEMES (NO.)	O_2 USAGE	O_2 AFFINITY
Hemoglobin	Erythrocyte	4	Transport	+
Myoglobin	Muscle	1	Storage	++++

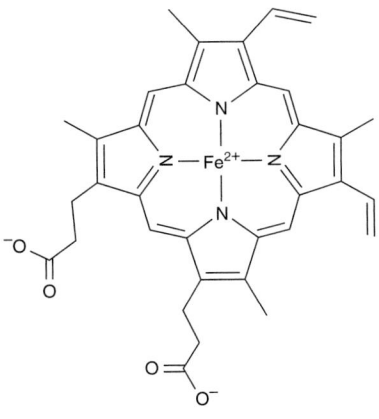

Heme is a cyclic structure composed of four pyrrole rings with a central **iron** atom.

FIGURE 6–5. **Heme.**

Reproduced, with permission, from Murray RK. *Harper's Illustrated Biochemistry*, 26th ed. McGraw-Hill, 2003.

Myoglobin

- Stores O_2 in muscle.
- Similar structure to hemoglobin.
- Contains only *one* heme.

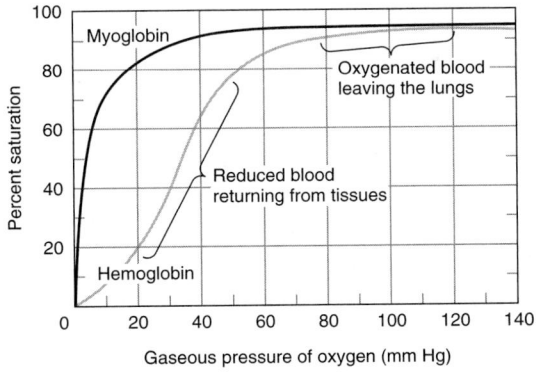

Oxygen-binding curves of hemoglobin and myoglobin.

Reproduced, with permission, from Murray RK. *Harper's Illustrated Biochemistry*, 26th ed. McGraw-Hill, 2003. (Modified, with permission, from Scriver CR, et al. [ed.]. *The Molecular and Metabolic Basis of Inherited Disease*, 7th ed., McGraw-Hill, 1995).

▶ LIPIDS

Structure

- Highly *hydrophobic* molecules.
- Soluble in *nonpolar* solvents such as chloroform, ether, and other organic solvents.
- Functions:
    - Cellular structure
    - Metabolism
    - Transportation
    - Storage

FATTY ACIDS

- Basic building blocks of most lipids.
- All are aliphatic carboxylic acids.
- Most are esters, although some exist as unesterified free fatty acids.
- The carbon chain can be *saturated* or *unsaturated*.
- Most are nonessential (can be synthesized).
- Only a few are essential:
  - Linoleic acid
  - Linolenic acid

$$C_\omega H_3 - (CH_2)_n - C_\beta H_2 - C_\alpha H_2 - C\begin{smallmatrix}O\\\\OH\end{smallmatrix}$$

Basic fatty acid structure.

CLASSIFICATION

- By number of double bonds.
  - **Saturated:** No double bonds.
  - **Monounsaturated:** One double bond.
  - **Polyunsaturated:** Multiple double bonds.

LIPID TYPES

- Triacylglycerols
- Phospholipids
- Steroids
- Eicosanoids

Triglycerides are not found in cell membranes.

TRIACYLGLYCEROLS (TRIGLYCERIDES)

- Consists of three fatty acids acylated to a glycerol molecule.
- Important source of energy.
- Stored in *adipose tissue*.
- Transported in the plasma by *lipoproteins*.

$$\begin{array}{c} {}^{1}CH_2 - O - \overset{O}{\underset{\|}{C}} - R_1 \\ R_2 - \overset{O}{\underset{\|}{C}} - O - {}^{2}CH \\ {}^{3}CH_2 - O - \overset{O}{\underset{\|}{C}} - R_2 \end{array}$$

Basic triglyceride structure.

Reproduced, with permission, from Murray RK. *Harper's Illustrated Biochemistry*, 26th ed. McGraw-Hill, 2003.

PHOSPHOLIPIDS

- Consists of two fatty acids acylated to two carbons of a glycerol molecule and a phosphate group esterified to the third carbon.
- Derive from *phosphatate*.
- Major constituents of cell and mitochondrial membranes.
- Precursors for second messengers and metabolic intermediates.

Three Major Types of Phospholipids

Phospholipid	Function	Formed From
Lecithins (phosphatidycholines)	Water soluble emulsifiers.	Choline
Cephalins (phosphatidylethanolamines)	Nerve tissue components.	Ethanolamine
Sphingomyelins	Plasma membrane components.	Ceramide

Phosphatidic acid

Basic phospholipid structure.

Reproduced, with permission, from Murray RK. *Harper's Illustrated Biochemistry*, 26th ed. McGraw-Hill, 2003.

STEROIDS

- **Cholesterol** is the most basic steroid.
- Major constituent of cell membranes and lipoproteins.
- Commonly present as a cholesterol ester.
- Conversion of HMG-CoA → mevalonate via HMG-CoA reductase is the *rate-limiting step*.
- Precursor molecule for other steroids:
    - Bile salts
    - Sex hormones
    - Adrenocortical hormones
    - Vitamin D

Corticosteroids inhibit phospholipase A_2 (PLA_2).

EICOSANOIDS

- 20-carbon long polyunsaturated fatty acids.
- Derivatives of **arachidonic acid.**
- **Phospholipase A_2 (PLA_2)** releases arachidonic acid from plasma membrane phospholipids upon hormone or cytokine stimulation or cellular damage.

Aspirin and nonsteroidal anti-inflammatory drugs (NSAIDs) inhibit cyclooxygenase (COX).

Eicosanoids

Eicosanoid	Formative Pathway	Examples
Prostanoids	Cyclooxygenase (COX)	Prostaglandins Prostacyclins Thromboxanes
Leukotrienes	Lipoxygenase (LOX)	Various leukotrienes
Lipoxins	Lipoxygenase (LOX)	Various lipoxins

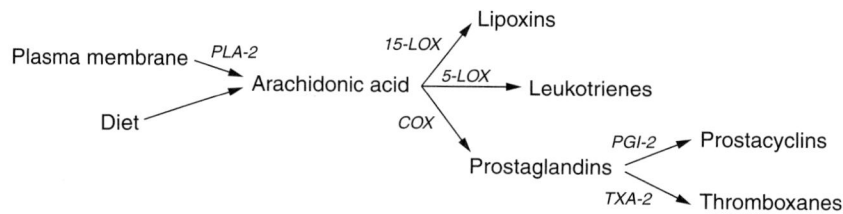

Eicosanoid formation pathways.

__Familial hypercholesterolemia__ is caused by an autosomal dominant defect of the low-density lipoprotein (LDL) receptor, leading to increased plasma LDL cholesterol and atherosclerosis.

Lipid Transport

LIPOPROTEINS

- Transport lipids in blood plasma.
- Composed of a nonpolar lipid core surrounded by a single layer of amphipathic phospholipids and cholesterol.
- Characterized by the protein moiety embedded in their outer layer (**apoprotein**).
- Contain triglycerides (16%), phospholipids (30%), cholesterol (14%), cholesterol esters (36%), and free fatty acids (4%).
- **Choline** is essential for the secretion of lipoproteins from hepatocytes, especially very low density lipoproteins (VLDL).

The Major Lipoproteins

Lipoprotein	Density	Protein (%)	Major Lipid Content	Carries Lipid From	Carries Lipid To
Chylomicron	+	1	TG	Small intestine	Extrahepatic tissues
Chylomicron remnants	++	7	TG Cholesterol	Chylomicrons of extrahepatic tissues.	Liver
VLDL	++	10	TG Cholesterol	Liver	Extrahepatic tissues
IDL (VLDL remnant)	+++	11	TG Cholesterol	VLDL of extrahepatic tissues.	Liver
LDL	+++	20	Cholesterol	VLDL of eExtrahepatic tissues.	Liver
HDL	++++	30–55	Cholesterol esters	Extrahepatic tissues	Liver

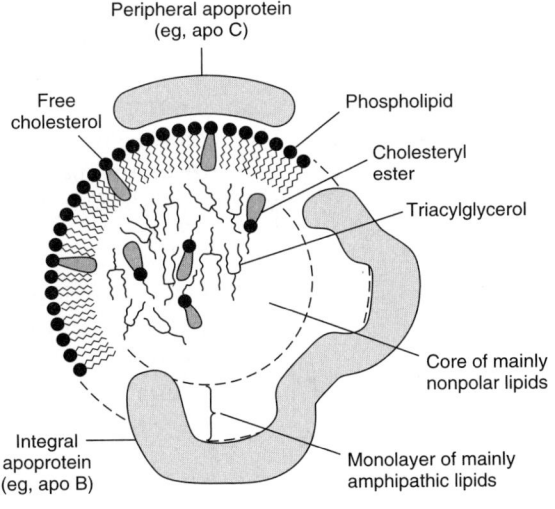

Lipoprotein structure.

Reproduced, with permission, from Murray RK. *Harper's Illustrated Biochemistry*, 26th ed. McGraw-Hill, 2003.

BILE SALTS

- Aid in lipid absorption (emulsification and solubilization).
- Formed from cholesterol in the liver.
- Almost exclusively absorbed in the *ileum* and returned to the liver via the **enterohepatic circulation.**
- Those that are not reabsorbed are excreted.
- Surplus bile salts are stored in the **gall bladder.**
- Two major bile salts:
  - **Glycocholic acid.**
  - **Taurocholic acid.**

Lipid Storage

- Most lipid triglycerides are stored in **adipose tissue**.

LIPID STORAGE DISEASES

- Inherited disorders of the **reticuloendothelial system**.
- Caused by incomplete lysosomal breakdown of sphinoglipids and mucopolysaccharides within phagocytes, leading to their accumulation.
- Most are common to Ashkenazi Jewish ancestry.

Lipid Storage Diseases

Disease	Deficient Enzyme	Accumulated Lipid	Clinical Features	Inheritance
Gaucher's disease	β-glucocerebrosidase	Glucocerebrosides	Splenomegaly Hepatomegaly Anemia Skin pigmentation *Most common*	Autosomal recessive
Niemann-Pick disease	Sphingomyelinase	Sphingomyelin	Splenomegaly Hepatomegaly Anemia CNS degeneration *Rapidly fatal*	Autosomal recessive
Tay-Sachs disease	Hexosaminidase A	Gangliosides	CNS degeneration Mental retardation Cherry red spot on retina *Rapidly fatal*	Autosomal recessive
Fabry's disease	α-galactosidase	Ceramide trihexoside	Skin lesions (angiokeratomas) Renal failure Cardiovascular Peripheral neuropathy	X-linked recessive

CHAPTER 7
Metabolism

Enzymes	266
CLASSIFICATION	266
ENZYME MECHANICS	266
ENZYME KINETICS	267
ENZYME INHIBITION	268
ENZYME REGULATION	269
Metabolic Pathways	271
SUMMARY	271
ATP PRODUCTION	272
CARBOHYDRATE METABOLISM	272
LIPID METABOLISM	276
PROTEIN METABOLISM	278
BACTERIAL METABOLISM	281

Isozymes *are enzymes with subtle molecular differences that catalyze the same reaction.*

Enzyme Classification:
Over **T**he **HILL**

Metals* and *B-complex vitamins *serve as the majority of nonprotein enzyme components.*

▶ ENZYMES

- Highly specific catalysts for biochemical reactions.
- Classified according to their mechanism of action.
- Mostly *proteins*.
- Nonprotein components aid in enzymatic function.
  - Coenzymes
  - Cofactors
  - Prosthetic groups

Classification

Oxidoreductases: Catalyze redox reactions.
Transferases: Catalyze the transfer of functional groups.
Hydrolases: Catalyze bond cleavage by hydrolysis.
Isomerases: Catalyze a change in molecular structure.
Lyases: Catalyze bond cleavage by elimination.
Ligases: Catalyze the union of two molecules.

Enzyme Mechanics

INDUCED-FIT MODEL

See Figure 7–1.

- Substrate-binding induces a conformational change in an enzyme.
- The energy produced by these changes enables the reactions to progress.

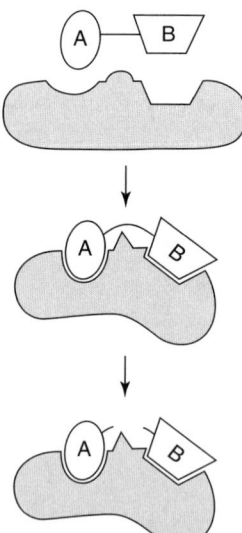

FIGURE 7–1. The induced-fit model of enzyme biomechanics.

Reproduced, with permission, from Murray RK. *Harper's Illustrated Biochemistry*, 26th ed. McGraw-Hill, 2003.

$$V_i = \frac{V_{max} \cdot [S]}{K_m + [S]}$$

FIGURE 7-2. Michaelis–Menten equation.

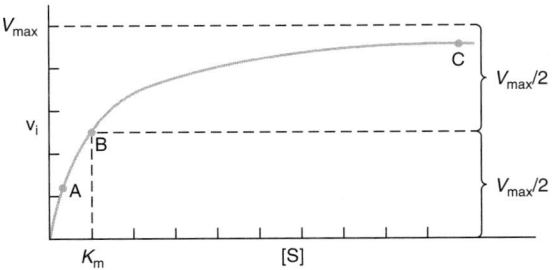

FIGURE 7-3. The effect of substrate concentration on reaction kinetics.

Reproduced, with permission, from Murray RK. *Harper's Illustrated Biochemistry*, 26th ed. McGraw-Hill, 2003.

Enzyme Kinetics

Substrate Concentration

See Figures 7–2 and 7–3.

- Increasing substrate concentration increases reaction rate only until the enzyme-binding sites are saturated.
- Maximum reaction velocity (V_{max}) is achieved when any further increase in substrate concentration does not increase reaction rate.
- The Michaelis constant (K_m) is the substrate concentration when the initial reaction velocity (v_i) is *half* of the maximum reaction velocity (V_{max}).
- Illustrated mathematically by the **Michaelis–Menten equation.**

Gibbs Free Energy Change (ΔG)

See Table 7–1 and Figure 7–4.

- Determines reaction *direction*.
- If $\Delta G_S > \Delta G_P$, then ΔG will be *negative* and the reaction will proceed spontaneously toward equilibrium.
- Equilibrium is attained when ΔG = 0.
- Reactions are based on their ΔG.
  - Exergonic
  - Endergonic

ΔG provides no information about the reaction rate and is independent of the path of the reaction.

TABLE 7-1. Classification of Reactions Based on ΔG

Reaction Type	ΔG	Energy Flow
Exergonic	Negative	Released
Endergonic	Positive	Required

$$\Delta G = \Delta G_P - \Delta G_S$$

FIGURE 7-4. Gibbs free energy change.

REACTION DIRECTION

The reaction direction is determined by the ΔG.

REACTION EQUILIBRIUM

See figure below.

- Enzymes have *no effect* on reaction equilibrium.

A. $\quad A + B + Enz \rightleftharpoons C + D + Enz$

B. $\quad K_{eq} = \dfrac{[C][D][Enz]}{[A][B][Enz]}$

Reaction equilibrium.

A. Any reaction with enzyme present; B. Equilibrium constant of the reaction.

REACTION RATE

Activation energy is the energy needed to initiate a reaction.

- Determined by the **activation energy.**
- Attaining activation energy requires an increase in reactant **kinetic energy.**
- Kinetic energy is largely influenced by *temperature* and *substrate concentration*.
- Enzymes *lower* the activation energy of a reaction, accelerating the rate.
- Influenced by five major factors. (See Table 7–2.)

TABLE 7-2. Factors Influencing Reaction Rate

CONTRIBUTING FACTOR	CHANGE IN FACTOR	CHARACTERISTICS
pH	Extreme changes can alter the charged state of the enzyme or substrate.	Enzymes function within an optimal pH range.
Temperature	An increase in temperature increases the reaction rate.	Extreme increase in temperature can cause enzyme denaturation.
Enzyme concentration	An increase in enzyme concentration increases the reaction rate.	
Inhibitor concentration	An increase in inhibitor concentration decreases the reaction rate.	
Substrate concentration	An increase in substrate concentration increases reaction rate *only until* the enzyme-binding sites are saturated.	Enzymes have a limited number of active sites.

Enzyme Inhibition

COMPETITIVE INHIBITION

See Figure 7–5.

- Inhibitor and substrate compete for the same enzyme binding site.
- Inhibition is reversed with increased substrate concentration.
- No effect on V_{max}.
- K_m is *increased*.

NONCOMPETITIVE INHIBITION

See Figure 7–6.

- Inhibitor and substrate simultaneously bind to the enzyme.
- Inhibition cannot be reversed with increased substrate concentration.
- V_{max} is *decreased*.
- No *effect* on K_m.

Kompetitive inhibition: K_m increases; V_{max} does not change.

Non-**K**ompetitive inhibition: K_m does **Not** change; V_{max} decreases.

A noncompetitive inhibitor is also called an **allosteric** inhibitor.

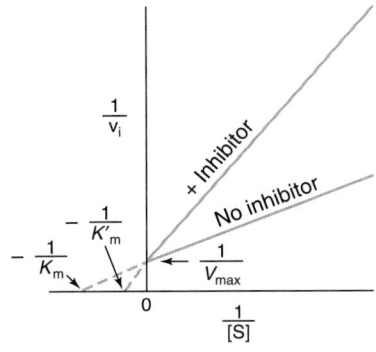

FIGURE 7-5. Competitive inhibition.

Reproduced, with permission, from Murray RK. *Harper's Illustrated Biochemistry*, 26th ed. McGraw-Hill, 2003.

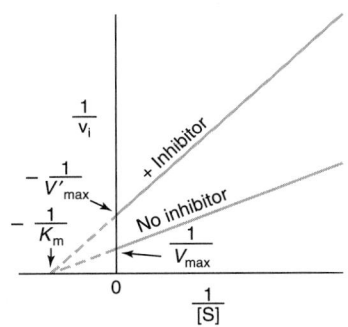

FIGURE 7-6. Noncompetitive inhibition.

Reproduced, with permission, from Murray RK. *Harper's Illustrated Biochemistry*, 26th ed. McGraw-Hill, 2003.

IRREVERSIBLE INHIBITION

Inhibitor alters the molecular structure of an enzyme, prohibiting its continued activity.

Aspirin irreversibly inhibits cyclooxygenase.

Enzyme Regulation

COVALENT MODIFICATION

- Reversible or irreversible enzymatic modification alters enzyme activity.
- Examples:
    - Phosphorylation (kinases)
    - Dephosphorylation (phosphatases)
    - Methylation (methyltransferases)

PROTEASE FUNCTION

See Figure 7–7.

- Proteases cleave proenzyme (**zymogen**) propeptides, activating the enzyme.

Zymogens are enzymatically inactive precursors of proteolytic enzymes.

ALLOSTERIC REGULATION

- An allosteric modifier (either a substrate or an inhibitor) binds to a site (allosteric site) on an enzyme other than the active site, eliciting a *conformational change* and subsequent change in enzymatic activity.
- A form of **feedback regulation** in which an enzyme of a metabolic pathway is controlled by the end product of that same pathway. (See Figure 7–8.)
- Simple Michaelis–Menten kinetics are *not* followed.

$$\text{Trypsinogen} \xrightarrow{\text{Enteropeptidase}} \text{Trypsin}$$

$$\text{Fibrinogen} \xrightarrow{\text{Thrombin}} \text{Fibrin}$$

FIGURE 7–7. Examples of protease function.

$$A \xrightarrow{Enz_1} B \xrightarrow{Enz_2} C \xrightarrow{Enz_3} D$$

FIGURE 7–8. Feedback regulation.

► METABOLIC PATHWAYS

Summary

See Figure 7–9 for summary of metabolic pathways.

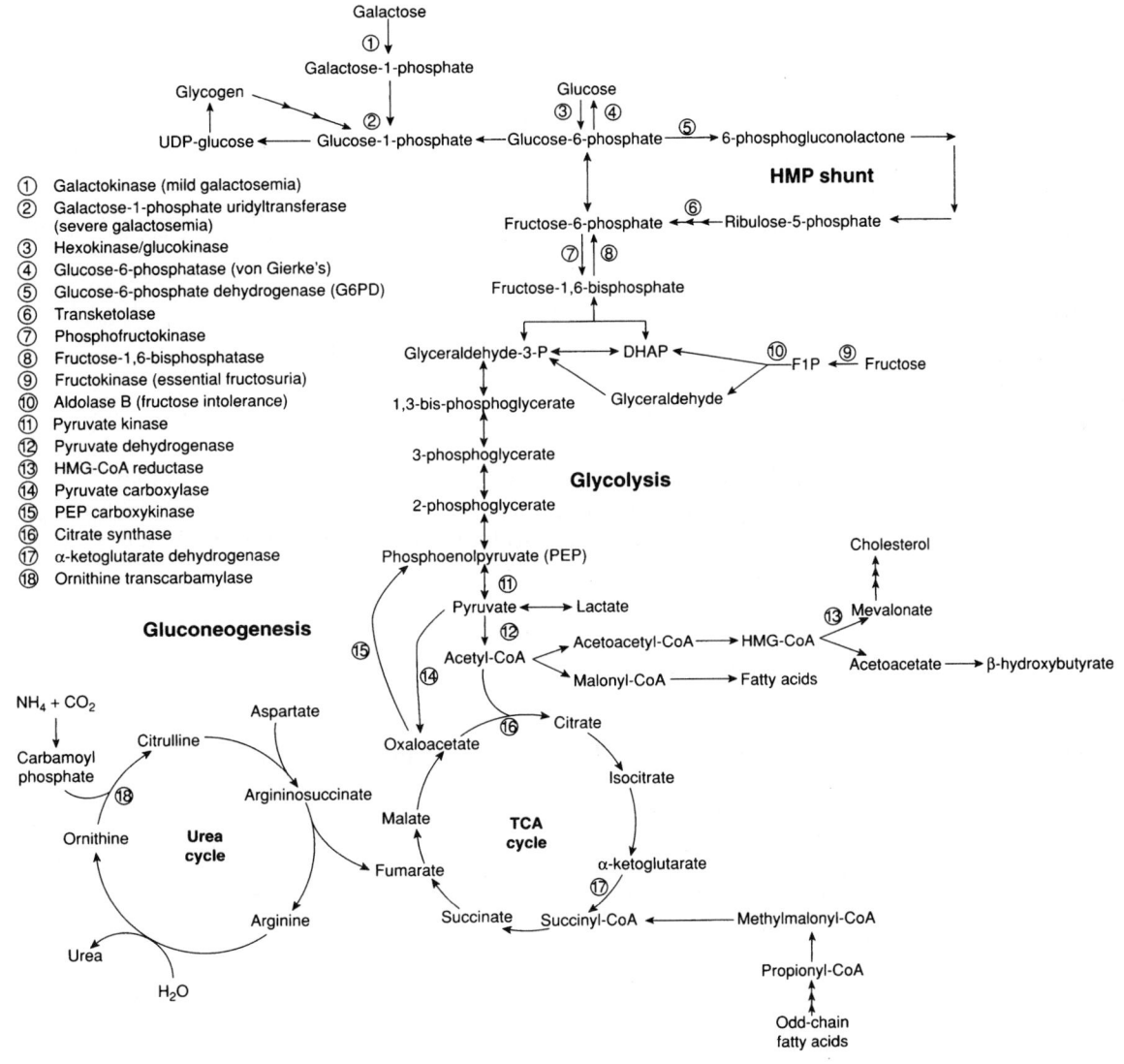

FIGURE 7-9. Summary of metabolic pathways.

Reproduced, with permission, from Bhushan V. *First Aid for the USMLE Step 1*. McGraw-Hill, 2006.

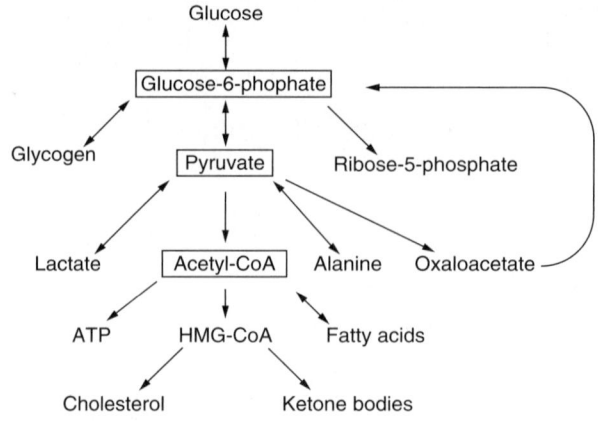

FIGURE 7–10. Common metabolic intermediates.

KEY INTERMEDIATES

See Figure 7–10.

- Glucose-6-phosphate
- Pyruvate
- Acetyl-CoA

ATP Production

- **Substrate-level phosphorylation:** ADP + P_i → ATP.
  - **Glycolysis:** 2 ATP per glucose.
  - **TCA cycle:** 2 ATP per glucose (as GTP).
- **Oxidative phosphorylation:** Major source of ATP (*aerobic*).
  - **Inner mitochondrial membrane (ETC):** 32–34 ATP per glucose.

Carbohydrate Metabolism

- Determines the fate of *glucose*.
- **ATP production per molecule of glucose.** It is assumed that the NADH produced in glycolysis is carried into mitochondria via the malate–aspartate shuttle. If the glycerol–phosphate shuttle is used, the net ATP production would be 36.

Metabolic Pathway	ATP Produced
Glycolysis (cytosol)	
2 ATP consumed (by hexokinase and PFK)	−2
4 ATP formed	+4
2 NADH formed	
TCA cycle (mitochondrial matrix)	
2 GTP formed	+2
8 NADH formed	
2 $FADH_2$ formed	
ETC (inner mitochondrial membrane)	
10 NADH oxidized	+30
2 $FADH_2$ oxidized	+4
	+38

GLYCOLYSIS

- Also called the Embden–Meyerhof Pathway. (See Figures 7–11 and 7–12.)
- Occurs in the *cytosol*.
- Converts glucose (as glucose-6-phosphate) → two molecules of pyruvate.
- Conversion of fructose-6-phosphate → fructose-1, 6-biphosphate via **phosphofructokinase (PFK)** is the *rate-limiting step*.

Fluoride inhibits *enolase*, the enzyme that converts 2-phosphoglycerate → phosphoenolpyruvate.

Metabolic Fates of Pyruvate

Type of Reaction	Enzyme	Product	Function
Oxidation	Pyruvate dehydrogenase	Acetyl-CoA	ATP production; Fatty acid synthesis
Reduction	Lactate dehydrogenase	Lactate	*Anaerobic* glycolysis
Carboxylation	Pyruvate carboxylase	Oxaloacetate	Gluconeogenesis; Replenishes TCA cycle
Transamination	Alanine aminotransferase	Alanine	Amino acid synthesis

Because erythrocytes do not have mitochondria, glycolysis always ends in lactate. The lactic acid is converted back to glucose via the Cori cycle.

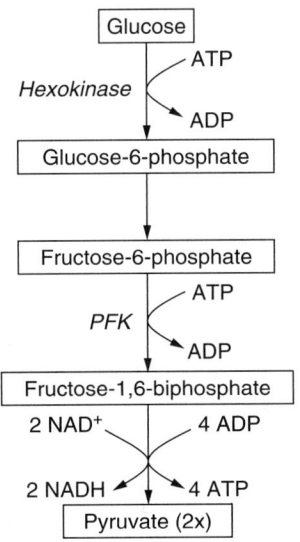

FIGURE 7–11. Major reactions of glycolysis.

Glucose + 2 P_i + 2 ADP + 2 NAD^+ → 2 Pyruvate + 2 ATP + 2 NADH + 2 H^+ + 2 H_2O

FIGURE 7–12. Stoichiometry of glycolysis.

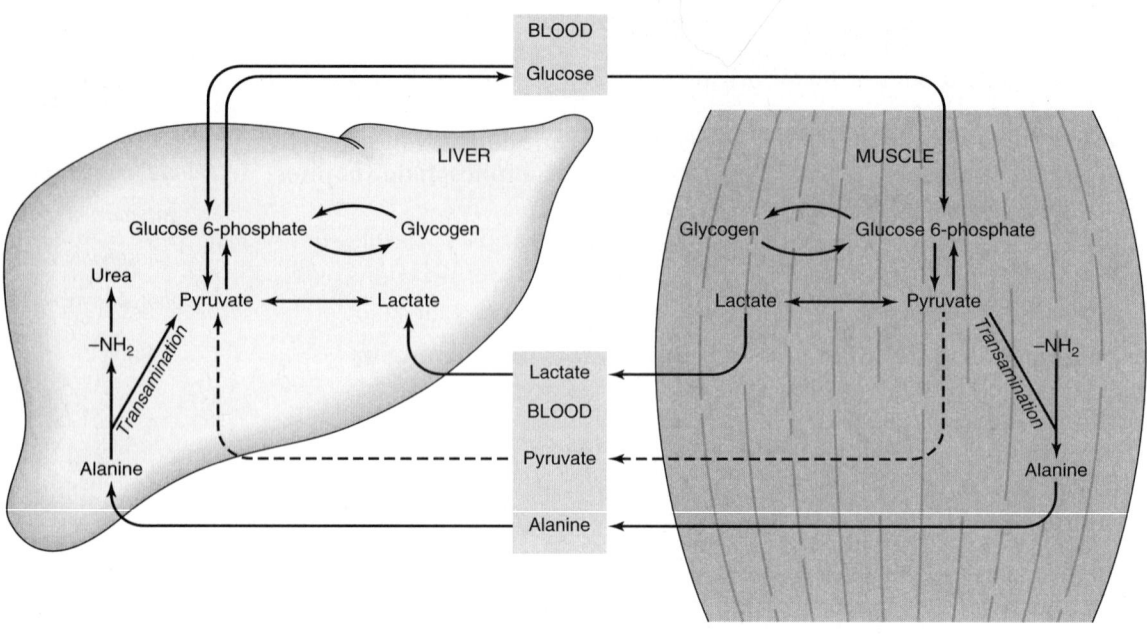

FIGURE 7-13. **The Cori cycle.**

Reproduced, with permission, from Murray RK. *Harper's Illustrated Biochemistry*, 26th ed. McGraw-Hill, 2003.

THE LACTIC ACID CYCLE

- Also called the Cori cycle. (See Figure 7–13.)
- Occurs in the *liver*.
- Converts lactate → glucose, which is then reoxidized via glycolysis.
- Provides quick ATP production during *anaerobic* glycolysis in muscle and erythrocytes.

THE CITRIC ACID CYCLE

- Also called the Krebs' cycle and the tricarboxylic acid cycle.
- Occurs in the *mitochondrial matrix*.
- Oxidizes acetyl-CoA.
- Reduces NAD^+ and FAD → NADH and $FADH_2$, which are reoxidized in the ETC to produce ATP.
- Tightly regulated by both *ATP* and *NAD^+*.

Photophosphorylation *occurs in plants as a result of photosynthesis. Also involves an ETC.*

THE ELECTRON TRANSPORT CHAIN

- Also called the respiratory chain. (See Figure 7–14.)
- Occurs in the *inner mitochondrial membrane*.
- Produces ATP via **oxidative phosphorylation** of ADP.
- Reoxidizes NADH and $FADH_2$ back → NAD^+ and FAD as electrons flow through a series of *four* cytochrome complexes of increasing redox potential (along a proton gradient).
- **Cytochromes** contain a central iron atom (similar to hemoglobin), which can exist in an oxidized ferric (Fe^{3+}) state or a reduced ferrous (Fe^{2+}) state.
- Cytochromes carry electrons as flavins, iron-sulfur groups, hemes, and copper ions.

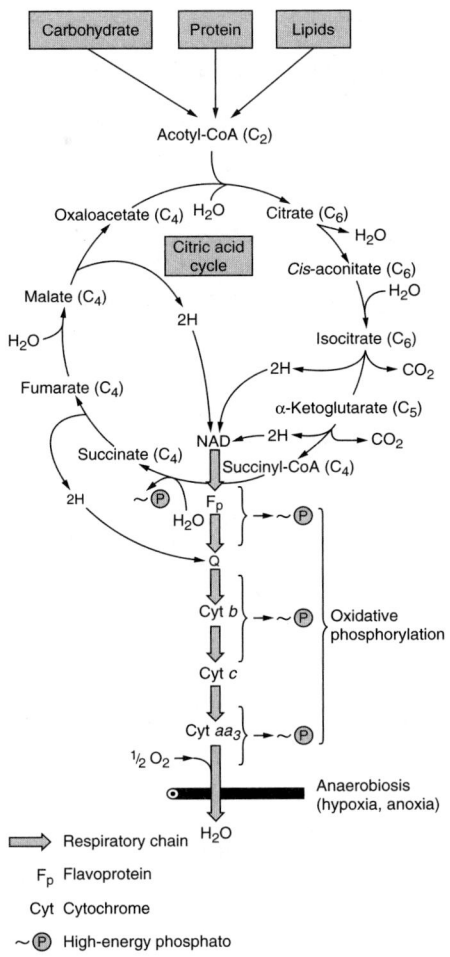

FIGURE 7–14. The citric acid cycle and electron transport chain.

Reproduced, with permission, from Murray RK. *Harper's Illustrated Biochemistry*, 26th ed. McGraw-Hill, 2003.

Cytochrome Complexes

Complex	Enzyme	Comments
Complex I	NADH-Q reductase	
Complex II	Succinate-Q reductase	Does not pump protons.
Complex III	Cytochrome reductase	
Complex IV	**Cytochrome oxidase**	Protons + **O_2** (final e-receptor) → H_2O.

Acetyl-CoA + 3 NAD$^+$ + FAD + P$_i$ + GDP + 2 H$_2$O → 2 CO$_2$ + 3 NADH + FADH$_2$ + GTP + 2 H$^+$ + CoA

FIGURE 7–15. Stoichiometry of TCA cycle.

*Coenzyme Q is also known as **ubiquinone**.*

Each NADH yields ~3 ATP.
Each FADH$_2$ yields ~2 ATP.

THE PENTOSE PHOSPHATE PATHWAY

No ATP is produced from the PPP.

- Also call the hexose monophosphate shunt.
- See Figure 7–16 for the stoichiometry of the pentose phosphate pathway (PPP).
- Occurs in the *cytosol*.
- An alternative to glycolysis in the metabolism of glucose.
- Coverts glucose-6-phosphate → ribose-5-phosphate.
- Conversion of glucose-6-phosphate → 6-phosphogluconolactone via **glucose-6-phosphate dehydrogenase (G6PD)** is the *rate-limiting step*.
- Produces **ribose** (for nucleotide synthesis) and **NADPH** (for fatty acid and steroid synthesis).
- Not all cells use the PPP (most active in liver, adipose tissue, adrenal cortex, thyroid, mammary gland, testis, and erythrocytes).

The NADPH produced from the PPP helps to rid erythrocytes of free radicals and H_2O_2. G6PD deficiency causes hemolytic anemia due to a ↓ in NADPH production, and subsequent ↑ of oxidizing agents in RBCs.

GLUCONEOGENESIS

See Figure 7–17 for the stoichiometry of gluconeogenesis.

- Occurs mostly in the *liver* and kidneys.
- *Not* a direct reversal of the glycolysis.
- Converts *amino acids* → glucose or glycogen in states of carbohydrate need.
- Clears *lactic acid* (from anaerobic glycolysis) and *glycerol* (from fatty acid metabolism).
- Under strict hormonal regulation.

GLYCOGEN SYNTHESIS AND CATABOLISM

See Figure 7–18 for the enzymatic regulation of glycogen metabolism.

- **Glycogen synthase** is the key regulatory enzyme in its synthesis.
- **Glycogen phosphorylase** is the key regulatory enzyme in its catabolism.
- Under strict hormonal regulation.

Glycogen is a branched polymer of glucose residues.

Lipid Metabolism

FATTY ACID SYNTHESIS

See Figure 7–19.

- Occurs in the *cytosol* of mostly hepatocytes.
- Conversion of acetyl-CoA → **malonyl-CoA** is the *rate-limiting step*.
- **Citrate–malate shuttle** transports acetyl groups from mitochondria to the cytosol.

Glucagon and epinephrine stimulate glycogenolysis and gluconeogenesis, whereas insulin triggers glycogen formation and cellular glucose uptake.

TRIGLYCERIDE LIPOLYSIS

See Figure 7–20.

- Occurs in *adipocytes*.
- The glycerol is phosphorylated and ultimately oxidized in glycolysis.
- The free fatty acids are transported to the *liver* for β-oxidation.
- **Triacyglycerol lipase** is under strict hormone regulation.

β-OXIDATION

See Figure 7–21.

- Occurs in the *mitochondrial matrix* of **hepatocytes**.
- Converts acyl-CoA → **acetyl-CoA.**

In humans, fatty acids can not be converted to glucose.

$$\text{Glucose-6-phosphate} + 2\ NADP^+ + H_2O \rightarrow \text{Ribose-5-phosphate} + 2\ NADPH + 2\ H^+ + CO_2$$

FIGURE 7-16. Stoichiometry of the PPP.

$$\text{Pyruvate} + 2\ ATP + GTP + NADH + 2\ H_2O \rightarrow \text{Glucose-6-phosphate} + 2\ ADP + GDP + 3\ P_i + NAD^+ + H^+$$

FIGURE 7-17. Stoichiometry of gluconeogeneis.

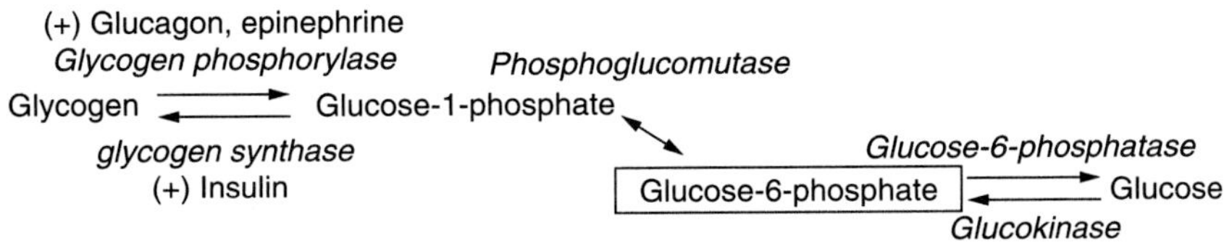

(+) Glucagon, epinephrine
Glycogen phosphorylase
Glycogen
Glucose-1-phosphate
glycogen synthase
(+) Insulin
Phosphoglucomutase
Glucose-6-phosphate
Glucose-6-phosphatase
Glucose
Glucokinase

FIGURE 7-18. Enzymatic regulation of glycogen metabolism.

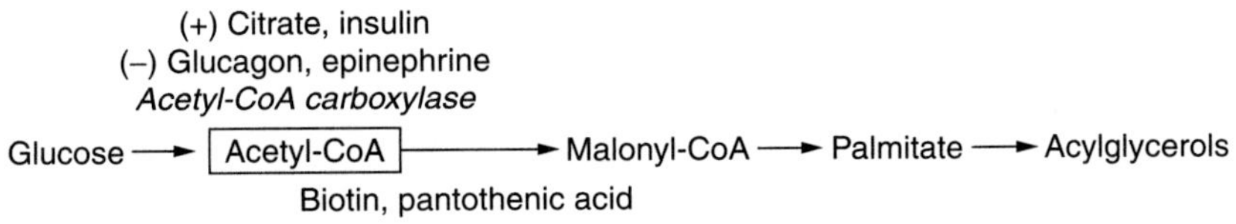

(+) Citrate, insulin
(–) Glucagon, epinephrine
Acetyl-CoA carboxylase
Glucose
Acetyl-CoA
Malonyl-CoA
Palmitate
Acylglycerols
Biotin, pantothenic acid

FIGURE 7-19. Overview of fatty acid synthesis.

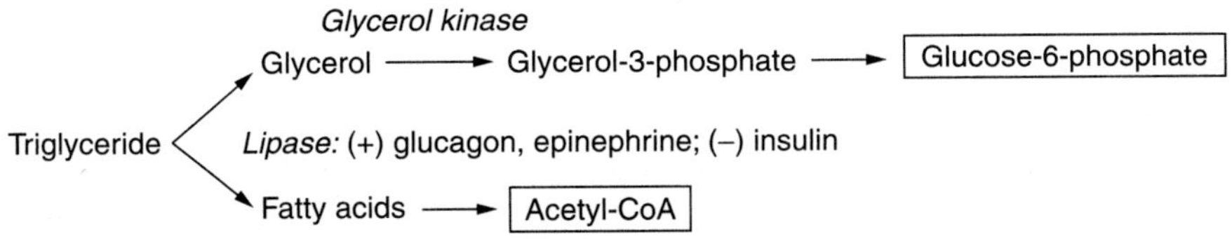

Glycerol kinase
Glycerol
Glycerol-3-phosphate
Glucose-6-phosphate
Triglyceride
Lipase: (+) glucagon, epinephrine; (–) insulin
Fatty acids
Acetyl-CoA

FIGURE 7-20. Overview of triglyceride lipolysis.

Acyl-CoA synthetase
Fatty acid
Acyl-CoA
Carnitine
β-Oxidation
Acetyl-CoA
Re-esterification
TCA cycle
HMG-CoA
Ketone bodies
Cholesterol

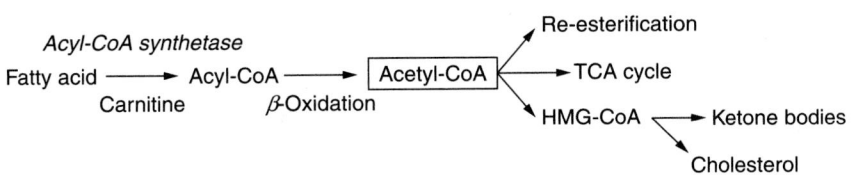

FIGURE 7-21. Overview of β-oxidation.

*Of the three ketone bodies, **acetone** is not used for energy production. Its accumulation can cause breath with a fruity odor.*

- Fatty acids are carried into the mitochondrial matrix by a **carnitine**-mediated enzyme system.
- Under certain metabolic states (starvation, diabetes mellitus), much of the acetyl-CoA is converted to **ketone bodies**:
  - Acetoacetate
  - β-Hydroxybutyrate
  - Acetone
- Ketone bodies are a source of fuel in extrahepatic tissues such as muscle.
- **Ketosis** is the accumulation of ketone bodies leading to ketoacidosis and diabetic coma.

Metabolic Fates of Acetyl-CoA

Fate	Pathway
ATP production	Via TCA cycle and the ETC
Cholesterol synthesis	Via HMG-CoA lyase
Ketone body synthesis	Via HMG-CoA reductase
Fatty acid synthesis	Via malonyl-CoA

Protein Metabolism

Both dietary and structural proteins are degraded daily to their amino acid constituents by various proteases and peptidases.

TRANSAMINATION

Only lysine, serine, and threonine are not transaminated.

- Amino acids are used to synthesize other *amino acids* (and proteins) or *metabolic intermediates* (pyruvate, acetyl-CoA, oxaloacetate, succinyl CoA, and α-ketoacids).
- **Aminotransferases (transaminases)** cleave the α-amino nitrogen of most amino acids, leaving hydrocarbon skeletons, which are degraded to the various glucogenic and ketogenic intermediates.
- Requires either *pyridoxal phosphate or pyridoxamine phosphate*, forms of pyridoxine (**vitamin B_6**), as a coenzyme.
- The transamination of pyruvate to alanine yields either α-ketoglutarate or oxaloacetate.

- See Figure 7–22 for Key metabolic intermediates formed from the carbon skeletons of amino acids.
- See Figure 7–23 for Transamination of pyruvate to alanine and Table 7–3 for Medically relevant transaminases.

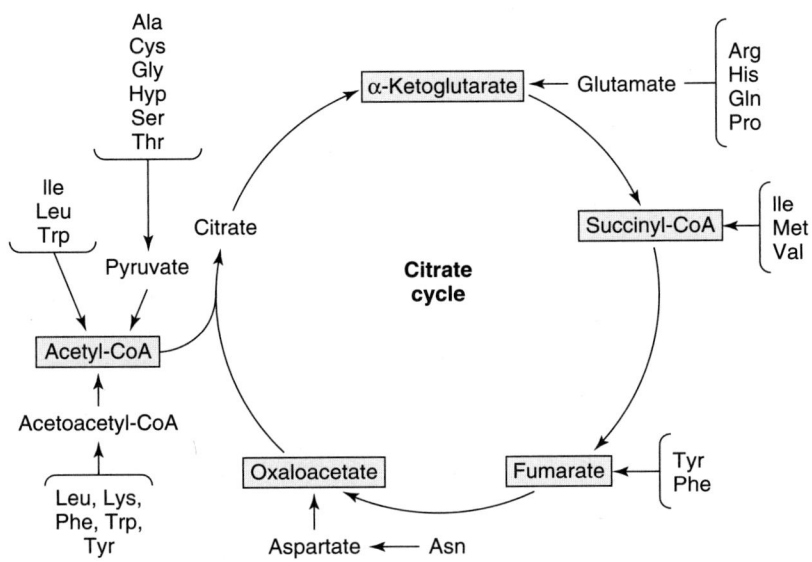

FIGURE 7-22. **Key metabolic intermediates formed from the carbon skeletons of amino acids.**

Reproduced, with permission, from Murray RK. *Harper's Illustrated Biochemistry*, 26th ed. McGraw-Hill, 2003.

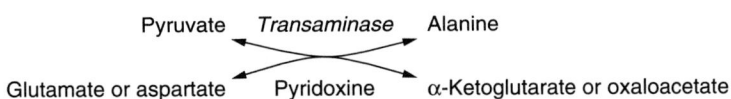

FIGURE 7-23. **Transamination of pyruvate to alanine.**

TABLE 7-3. **Medically Relevant Transaminases**

Transaminase	Location	Elevated Levels Suggest
Aspartate aminotransferase (AST)	Many tissues, including cardiac muscle.	Tissue necrosis (myocardial infarction).
Alanine aminotransferase (ALT)	Mostly **hepatic** tissue.	Tissue necrosis (cirrhosis).

$$\text{L-Glutamate} + \text{NAD(P)}^+ + H_2O \xrightleftharpoons[]{\text{Glutamate dehydrogenase}} \alpha\text{-Ketoglutarate} + \text{NAD(P)H} + NH_4^+ + H^+$$

FIGURE 7-24. Oxidative deamination of glutamate.

The reaction is reversible but favors the formation of glutamate.

OXIDATIVE DEAMINATION

See Figure 7–24 for oxidative deamination of glutamate.

- An alternative to transamination in the metabolism of amino acids.
- Results in the formation of **α-ketoacids** (for energy) and **ammonia** (for urea formation).
- In humans, the vast majority of oxidative deamination derives from **glutamate**; the major enzyme responsible is **glutamate dehydrogenase**.
- Other amino acids that can undergo oxidative deamination are asparagine, histidine, serine, and threonine.

THE UREA CYCLE

The urea cycle requires 3 ATP.

- See Figure 7–25.
- See Figure 7–26 for the stoichiometry of the urea cycle.
- Occurs in the *cytosol* and *mitochondrial matrix* of **hepatocytes**.
- Eliminates the **ammonia** produced by oxidative deamination in the form of **urea**.

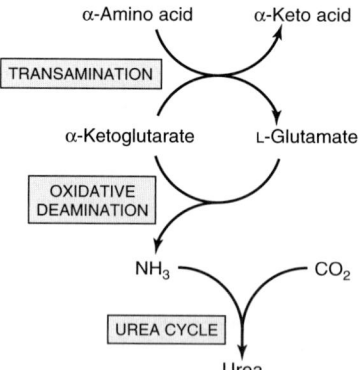

FIGURE 7-25. Key reactions and intermediates in the formation of urea.

Reproduced, with permission, from Murray RK. *Harper's Illustrated Biochemistry*, 26th ed. McGraw Hill, 2003.

$CO_2 + NH_4^+ + 3\ ATP + Aspartate + 2\ H_2O \rightarrow Urea + 2\ ADP + 2\ P_i + AMP + PP_i + Fumarate$

FIGURE 7-26. Stoichiometry of the urea cycle.

Bacterial Metabolism

ENTNER–DOUDOROFF PATHWAY

- **Glycolytic** pathway in *aerobic* bacteria.
- Converts glucose → pyruvate + glyceraldehydes-3-phosphate.
- Produces 1 ATP per glucose via substrate-level phosporylation.

CHAPTER 8
Molecular Biology

Nucleotides	284
Base Pairing	284
ORGANIZATION	284
BIOSYNTHESIS	284
Nucleic Acids	285
DNA	286
RNA	286
TYPES OF RNA	286
DNA Organization	287
NUCLEOSOMES	287
CHROMATIN	287
DNA Synthesis	289
Transcription and Translation	289
RNA SYNTHESIS (TRANSCRIPTION)	289
PROTEIN SYNTHESIS (TRANSLATION)	290
Mutations	290
POINT MUTATIONS	290
FRAMESHIFT MUTATIONS	291
REPEAT MUTATIONS	291
Clinical Considerations	291
REVERSE TRANSCRIPTASE	291
RECOMBINANT DNA TECHNOLOGY	291

NUCLEOTIDES

*A **nucleoside** is a nucleotide without esterified phosphate groups.*

- Building blocks of DNA and RNA.
- Functions:
    - Protein synthesis
    - Nucleic acid synthesis
    - Signal transduction pathways
- Composed of three basic compounds:
    - **Nitrogenous base**
        - Purine
        - Pyrimidine
    - **Pentose sugar**
        - Deoxyribose
        - Ribose
    - **Phosphate group(s)**

BASE PAIRING

See Figure 8–1 for base pairing in DNA.

Purines:

Pure **Ag** (silver)
Purines are **A**denine and **G**uanine

Pyrimidines:

CUT the **PY** (pie)
Cytosine, **U**racil, **T**hymine are the **Py**rimidines

Organization

- Purines pair with pyrimidines.
- Held together via **hydrogen bonds.**
    - Adenine—Thymine/Uracil (**two** H-bonds).
    - Guanine—Cytosine (**three** H-bonds).

Comparison of Purines and Pyrimidines

Nucleotide	DNA Bases	RNA Bases	Metabolic Defects	Catabolize to	Catabolic Defects
Purines	Adenine (A) Guanine (G)	Adenine (A) Guanine (G)	Antifolate drugs Anticancer drugs	Uric acid	Gout Hyperuricemia G-6-P Deficiency
Pyrimidines	Thymine (T) Cytosine (C)	Uracil (U) Cytosine (C)	UV light Methotrexate Other anticancer drugs	β-Alanine β-Amino-isobutyrate	Rare (highly water soluble)

*The strongest bonds (three hydrogen bonds) are between **C**ytosine and **G**uanine, like **C**razy **G**lue. Adenine and Thymine/Uracil are held by two hydrogen bonds.*

Biosynthesis

See Figure 8–2 for biosynthesis of nucleotides.
See Figure 8–3 for uric acid synthesis.

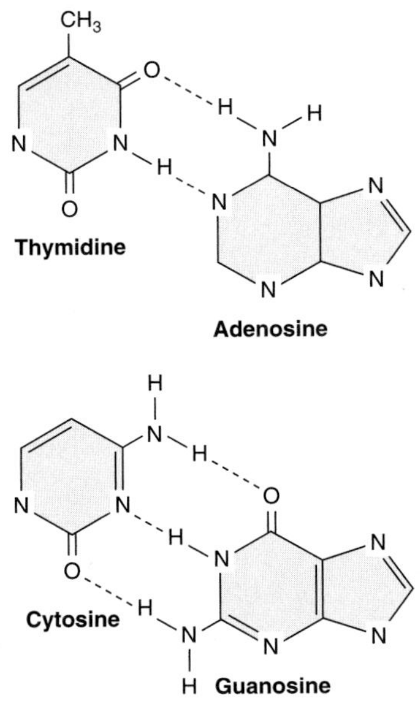

FIGURE 8–1. Base pairing in DNA.

Reproduced, with permission, from Murray, RK. *Harper's Illustrated Biochemistry*, 26th ed. McGraw-Hill, 2003.

$$\text{Ribose 5-phosphate} \xrightarrow{\text{ATP}} \text{5-phosphoribosyl-1-pyrophosphate} \to \text{Purines}$$
$$\text{(PRPP)}$$
$$\downarrow$$
$$\text{Orotic acid} \to \text{Orotate monophosphate} \to \text{Pyrimidines}$$

FIGURE 8–2. Biosynthesis of nucleotides.

$$\text{Purines} \to \text{Xanthine} \to \text{Uric acid}$$
$$\text{Xanthine oxidase}$$

FIGURE 8–3. Uric acid synthesis.

▶ NUCLEIC ACIDS

- Extremely *polar* and *hydrophilic*.
- The "backbone" consists of pentose sugars linked by **phosphodiester bonds** at the third and fifth carbon atoms.
- The two polynucleotide chains are considered **antiparallel** and **complementary** (one chain runs in the $5' \to 3'$ direction; the other runs in the $3' \to 5'$ direction).

Comparison of DNA and RNA

Nucleic Acid	Strands	Sugar	Bases
DNA	Double	Deoxyribose	A-T, G-C
RNA	Single	Ribose	A-U, G-C

*DNA and RNA are differentiated in the laboratory by the **Feulgen reaction**, which is specific for deoxyribose.*

DNA

See Figure 8–4 for the backbone structure of a single DNA strand.

RNA

See Figure 8–5 for the backbone structure of a single RNA strand.

Types of RNA

The Three Major Types of RNA

RNA	Site of Synthesis	Function	Note
Ribosomal (rRNA)	Nucleolus	Major component of ribosomes.	*Most prevalent* RNA.
Transfer (tRNA)	Nucleus	Carries amino acids from cytosol to ribosomes.	Contains an **anticodon** (complementary to mRNA codons).
Messenger (mRNA)	Nucleus	Carries genetic code from DNA to ribosomes.	*Least prevalent* RNA. Contains **codons** (complementary to DNA template and tRNA anticodon).

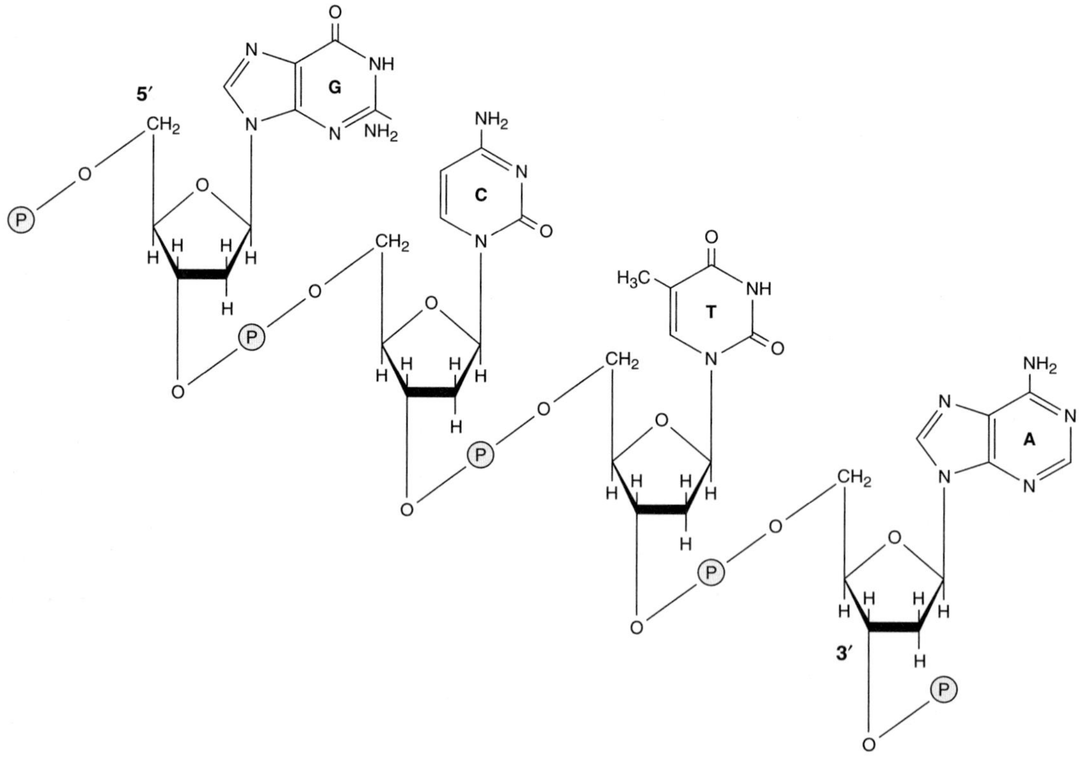

FIGURE 8-4. The backbone structure of a single DNA strand.

Reproduced, with permission, from Murray RK. *Harper's Illustrated Biochemistry*, 26th ed. McGraw-Hill, 2003.

FIGURE 8–5. The backbone structure of a single RNA strand.

Reproduced, with permission, from Murray RK. *Harper's Illustrated Biochemistry*, 26th ed. McGraw-Hill, 2003.

▶ DNA ORGANIZATION

Nucleosomes

See Figures 8–6 and 8–7.

- Consists of DNA wrapped around a **histone** octomer.
- Held by *ionic bonds*.

*Histones are composed largely of **arginine** and **lysine**.*

Chromatin

- Consists of nucleosomes, enzymes, gene regulatory proteins, and small amounts of RNA.

Chromatin looks like beads of nucleosomes on a string of DNA.

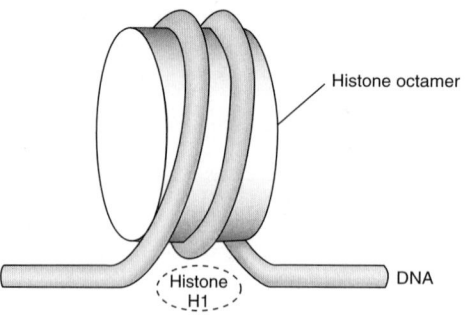

FIGURE 8–6. Nucleosome structure.

Reproduced, with permission, from Murray RK. *Harper's Illustrated Biochemistry*, 26th ed. McGraw-Hill, 2003.

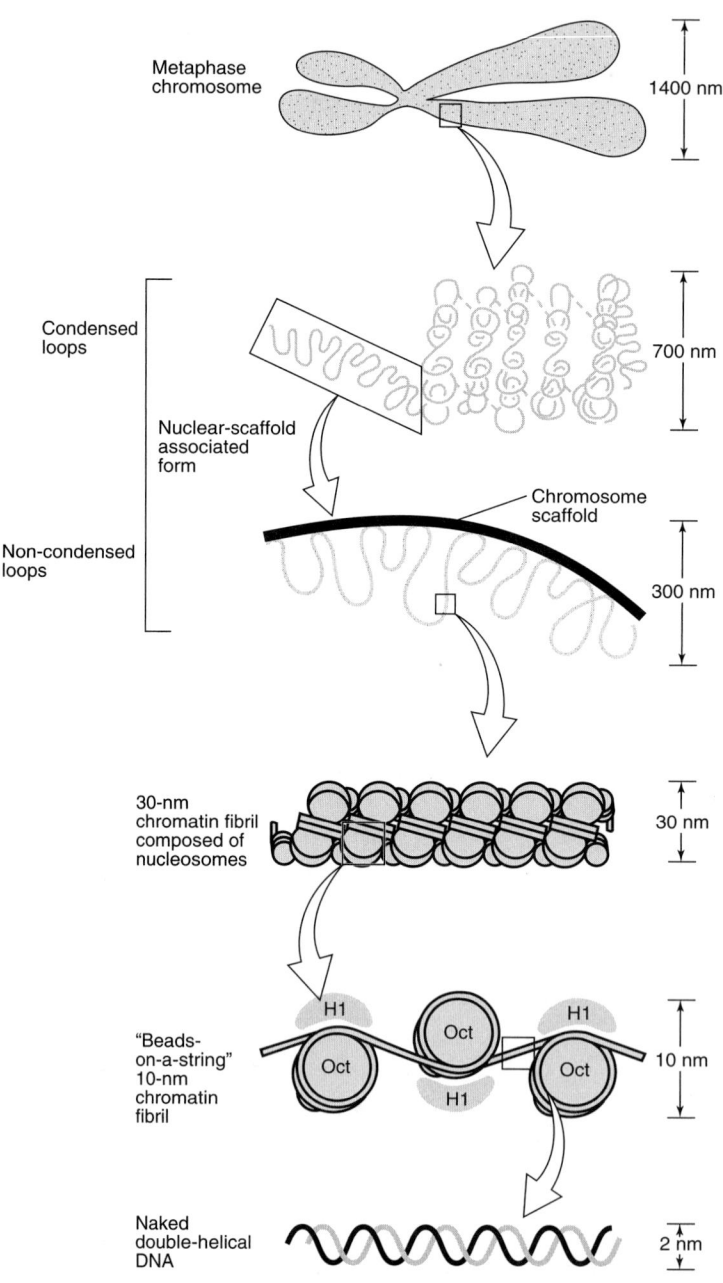

FIGURE 8–7. DNA organization.

Reproduced, with permission, from Murray RK. *Harper's Illustrated Biochemistry*, 26th ed. McGraw-Hill, 2003.

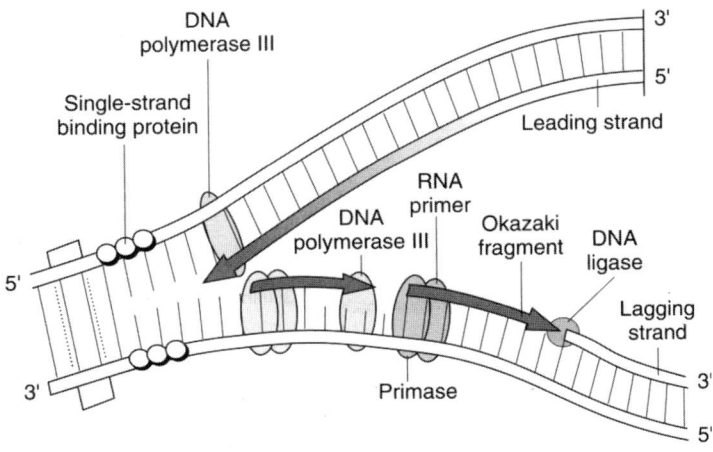

FIGURE 8-8. DNA synthesis.

Reproduced, with permission, from Bhushan V. *First Aid for the USMLE Step 1*. McGraw-Hill, 2006.

DNA SYNTHESIS

See Figure 8–8.

- **Helicase:** Unwinds the DNA molecule.
- **Topoisomerase:** Secures the replication fork, where the two DNA strands are separated into leading and lagging strands.
- **DNA polymerase:** Forms new complementary strands in the 5′ → 3′ direction.
    - **Leading strand:** Runs in the 3′ → 5′ direction. Forms a continuous complementary strand.
    - **Lagging strand:** Runs in the 5′ → 3′ direction. Forms a series of segments (**Okazaki fragments**).
- **DNA ligase:** Joins Okazaki fragments.
- **Exonuclease:** Removes the nucluetide primer.

TRANSCRIPTION AND TRANSLATION

See Figure 8–9.

RNA Synthesis (Transcription)

- DNA is used as a template to form RNA.
- Occurs in the *nucleus*.
- DNA is unwound and the replication fork is exposed.
- **RNA polymerase** binds to a promoter site on the DNA strand.
- Synthesis occurs in the 5′ → 3′ direction.
- Post-transcriptional modifications:
    - Addition of a **5′ cap** and a **3′ poly(A) tail**.
    - RNA splicing:
        - Removal of **introns** (noncoding segments).
        - Subsequent joining of **exons** (coding segements).

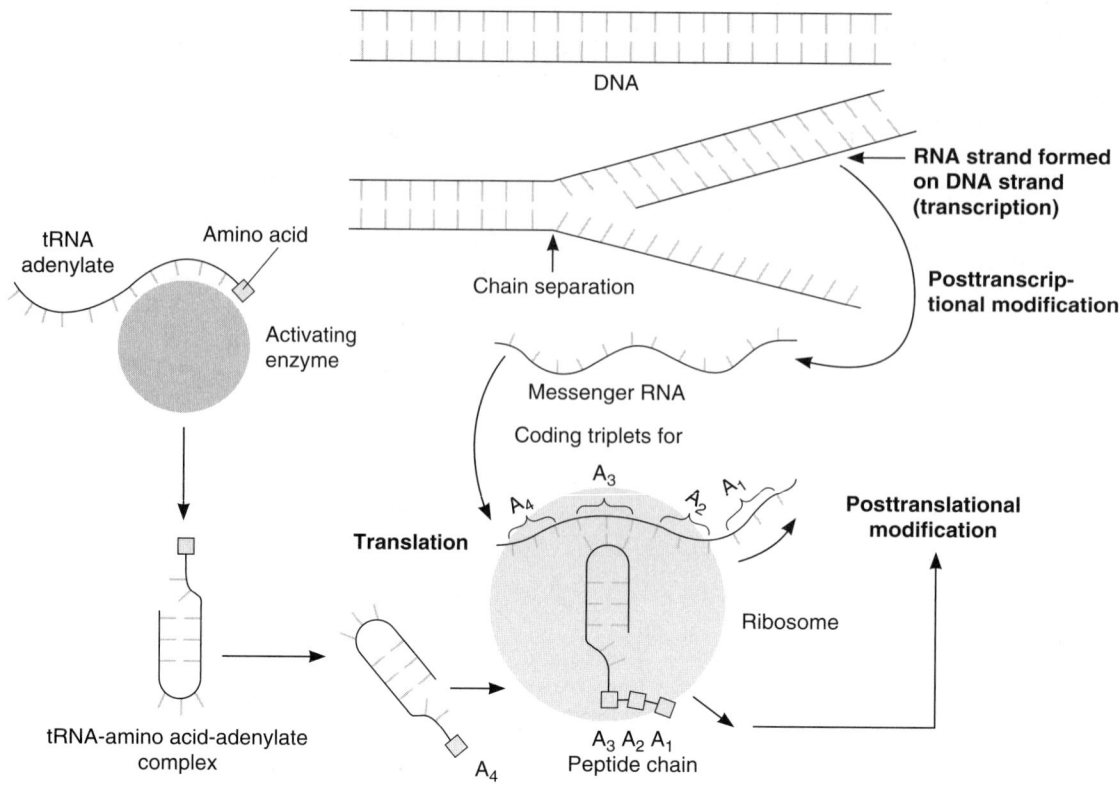

FIGURE 8-9. **Transcription and translation.**

Reproduced, with permission, from Ganong. *Review of Medical Physiology.* McGraw-Hill, 2003.

Protein Synthesis (Translation)

- An mRNA template is used to determine the specific amino acid sequence for polypeptide synthesis.
- Occurs in the *cytoplasm* (in ribosomes).
- A *small* ribosomal subunit binds to mRNA.
- **Aminoacyl-tRNA synthetase:** Adds each amino acid to tRNA.
- The complementary *anticodon* of tRNA (carrying the first amino acid) binds to the mRNA start codon.
- A *large* ribosomal subunit attaches, forming a complete ribosome.
- Synthesis occurs in the 5′ → 3′ direction until a stop codon is reached.

70s ribosomes are found in prokaryotic cells.

80s ribosomes are found in eukaryotic cells.

▶ MUTATIONS

- Caused by mutagenic chemicals, radiation, UV light, and some viruses.

Point Mutations

- Substitution of one base with another.
    - **Missense mutation:** Results in a codon that causes an altered amino acid sequence (e.g., valine replaces glutamate causing sickle cell anemia).
    - **Nonsense mutation:** Results in a *stop codon* that causes polypeptide chain termination.
    - **Transverse mutation:** A purine is replaced with a pyrimidine, or vice versa (the purine–pyrimidine orientation is changed).

- **Transition mutation:** A purine is replaced with another purine, or a pyrimidine is replaced with another pyrimidine (the purine–pyrimidine orientation is not changed).

Frameshift Mutations

- Deletion or insertion of one or two base pairs, changing the reading frame of the DNA template and the amino acid sequence.

Repeat Mutations

- Amplification of the sequence of three nucleotides.

▶ **CLINICAL CONSIDERATIONS**

Reverse Transcriptase

- Forms a complementary strand of DNA from the original RNA.
- HIV contains only a single-stranded RNA molecule and its own reverse transcriptase.

AZT inhibits reverse transcriptase function.

Recombinant DNA Technology

- **Restriction endonucleases:** Cleave DNA at various points to allow addition of various vectors, plasmids, or bacteriophages.
- **DNA ligases:** Join DNA fragments.
- **DNA polymerase:** Adds nucleotides.
- **Exonucleases:** Remove nucleotides.

CHAPTER 9
Membranes

Plasma Membranes	294
Fluid Mosaic Model	294
Membrane Components	294
LIPIDS	294
PROTEINS	295
CARBOHYDRATES	295
Movement Through Membranes	295
MEMBRANE TRANSPORT	295
TRANSPORT PROTEINS	295

▶ PLASMA MEMBRANES

- Function as barriers, separating the contents of cells and organelles.
- **Asymmetric** sheetlike structures consisting of an outer and an inner surface.
- **Selectively permeable,** enabling only certain molecules (**water** and **small, nonpolar**) to easily pass.
- Contains lipids, proteins, and carbohydrates in varying ratios.
- Lipids and integral proteins generally interact *noncovalently*, allowing molecules to move freely within the membrane.

▶ FLUID MOSAIC MODEL

See Figure 9–1 for the fluid mosaic model of plasma membrane structure.

▶ MEMBRANE COMPONENTS

Lipids

- Form an **amphipathic lipid bilayer** suspended in water with *hydrophilic head groups* (on the outer and inner surfaces) and *hydrophobic tail groups* (on the inside of the bilayer).
- Types of plasma membrane lipids:
    - **Phospholipids**
        - Phosphoglycerides
        - Sphingomyelin
    - **Glycosphingolipids**
    - **Cholesterol**
- See Figure 9–2 for membrane phospholipids.

Phospholipids constitute the majority of membrane lipids.

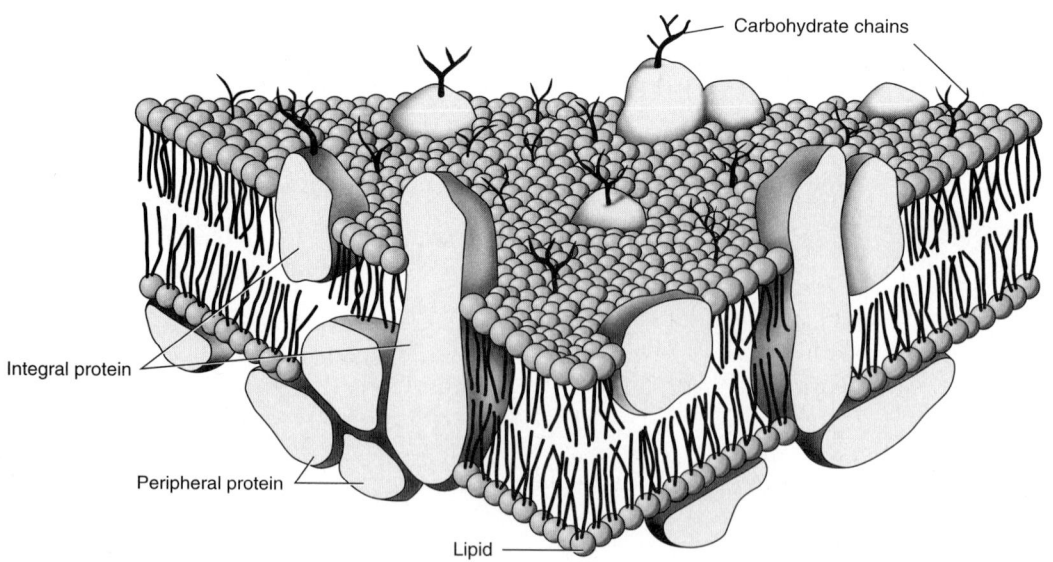

FIGURE 9–1. The fluid mosaic model of plasma membrane structure.

Reproduced, with permission, from Murray RK. *Harper's Illustrated Biochemistry*, 26th ed. McGraw-Hill, 2003.

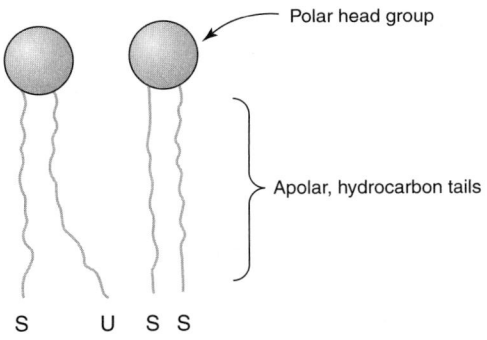

FIGURE 9-2. **Membrane phospholipids.**

Reproduced, with permission, from Murray RK. *Harper's Illustrated Biochemistry*, 26th ed. McGraw-Hill, 2003.

Proteins

- Function as receptors, transport channels, enzymes, antigens, and other structural components.
- Two types of plasma membrane protein:
    - **Integral:** Amphipathic proteins that are embedded within either one or both (traverse the entire membrane) portions of the lipid bilayer.
    - **Peripheral:** Proteins that weakly bind to hydrophilic head groups on the inner or outer membrane surfaces.

Carbohydrates

- Attach to proteins and lipids *only* on the *external surface* of cell membranes.

▶ MOVEMENT THROUGH MEMBRANES

Membrane Transport

See Figure 9–3 for the types of movement of substances through membranes.

Transport Proteins

- **Uniport:** Transport of a single molecule in both directions.
- **Coupled:** Transport of one molecule depends on the presence of another (different) molecule.
    - **Symport:** Transports molecules in the *same* direction.
    - **Antiport:** Transports molecules in *opposite* directions.

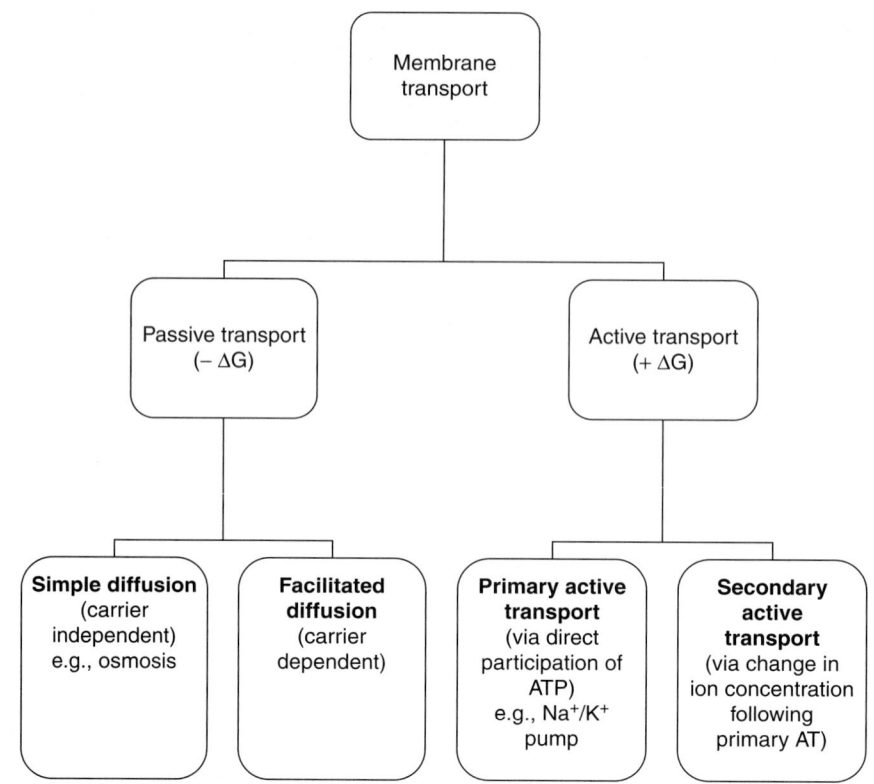

FIGURE 9-3. Outline of the types of movement of substances through membranes.

CHAPTER 10

Neurophysiology

Central Nervous System	299
Peripheral Nervous System	299
Autonomic Nervous System	299
BRAIN	299
DIENCEPHALON	299
HYPOTHALAMUS	300
HEAT REGULATION	300
LIMBIC SYSTEM	301
Motor Control and Coordination	301
BASAL GANGLIA	301
CEREBELLUM	302
Brainstem	302
MIDBRAIN (MESENCEPHALON)	302
PONS	302
MEDULLA OBLONGATA	302
Peripheral Nervous System	303
Autonomic Nervous System	303
AUTONOMIC GANGLIA	303
PARASYMPATHETIC NERVOUS SYSTEM	304
SYMPATHETIC NERVOUS SYSTEM	304
Spinal Tracts	306
Somatosensory Pathways	308
SENSORY TRACTS (ASCENDING)	308
DESCENDING MOTOR TRACTS (EFFERENT OR DESCENDING PATHWAYS)	310
UPPER MOTOR NEURONS	311
CORTICOSPIANL TRACT (PYRAMIDAL SYSTEM)	311
EXTRAPYRAMIDAL SYSTEM	311
Spinal Cord Lesions	312
Neurophysiology	312
RESTING MEMBRANE POTENTIAL	312
ACTION POTENTIAL	313

REPOLARIZATION	**313**
HYPERPOLARIZATION	**314**
Local Anesthetics	**314**
LOCAL ANESTHETICS	**314**
Neurotransmitters	**315**
EXCITATORY	**315**
INHIBITORY	**315**
Summation	**315**
SPATIAL SUMMATION	**315**
TEMPORAL SUMMATION	**315**
Nerve Conduction	**315**
SALTATORY CONDUCTION	**315**
PROBLEMS WITH NERVE CONDUCTION	**316**
Synapse	**317**
NEURONAL EXCITABILITY	**317**
TYPES OF SYNAPSE	**317**
Neuromuscular Junction (NMJ)	**318**
ACETYLCHOLINE METABOLISM	**319**
Special Senses	**319**
VISION	**319**
Hearing	**323**
ANATOMY OF THE EAR	**323**
HEARING	**324**
Taste	**325**
Taste Buds	**325**
Smell	**326**
SMELL PATHWAY	**326**

▶ CENTRAL NERVOUS SYSTEM

CNS = Brain + spinal cord

▶ PERIPHERAL NERVOUS SYSTEM

- All nerves outside the brain and spinal cord:
  - Cranial nerves.
  - Spinal nerves.
  - Nerve plexuses.
  - Associated spinal and autonomic ganglia.

▶ AUTONOMIC NERVOUS SYSTEM

- ANS = nervous system involved in controlling involuntary functions.
  - Sympathetic.
  - Parasympathetic.

Brain

See embryology of the nervous system, Chapter 4—forebrain, midbrain, hindbrain.

CEREBRAL CORTEX

TWO CEREBRAL HEMISPHERES

- Right and left.
- Connected by corpus callosum.
  - Thick white matter tract; nerve fibers.

FOUR LOBES PER HEMISPHERE

- Frontal lobes.
  - Control skilled motor behavior.
- Parietal lobes.
  - Interpret somatosensory input.
- Occipital lobes.
  - Interpret visual input.
- Temporal lobes.
  - Interpret auditory input.

Note: Beyond the primary function of each lobe, much of the cerebral cortex works together for associative and higher order functions (including ideation, language, and thought).

Diencephalon

Thalamus + hypothalamus

THALAMUS

- Ovoid mass of gray matter.
- Ascending input (all sensory stimuli **except** olfactory) is relayed through the thalamus to the cerebral cortex.
- Descending output (from cortex) can also pass through/synapse within thalamus.

Hypothalamus

- Collection of nerve cells (nuclei).
- Lies subcortical (at base of cerebrum).
- Controls homeostatic processes.
    - Often associated with autonomic nervous system.
- Regulates:
    - Body temperature
    - Appetite
    - Water balance
    - Sexual activity
    - Sleep
    - Emotions
    - Pituitary secretions: Releasing hormones to the pituitary gland (endocrine system)
    - Autonomic functions: GI and cardiac activity, etc.

Heat Regulation

- Controlled by the posterior hypothalamus.
    - Both heat generation and heat loss.
- Goal is to keep human body temperature constant.
    - Heat gained = heat loss.

SHIVERING

- Potent mechanism for heat production.
- When body core temperature drops the shivering reflex is triggered,
    - Causes fibrillation of muscle for heat production.

HEAT LOSS

- When environmental temperature < body temperature,
    - Want to produce more heat.
- When exercise or warm environment,
    - Want to give off excess heat:
        - Vasodilation of skin vessels.
        - ↑sympathetic outflow to sweat glands.

Heat Transfer

Heat transfer	Conduction	Convection	Evaporation
Emission of heat in the form of infrared rays.	Flow of heat energy from warmer to cooler environment (down gradient).	Movement of heat by currents in the medium, e.g., wind.	Conversion of a liquid into vapor. Heat is lost when water evaporates from body surfaces.[a]
Body is continually exchanging heat by radiation with objects in the environment.[b]	Usually, transfer of thermal energy with direct contact between two objects.	Air molecules exchange heat with body surface and continue to breeze past (replaced by other molecules).	Two ways evaporation occurs on body surfaces: ■ Insensible water loss 　■ Respiratory 　■ Skin ■ Sweating ■ Active fluid secretion by sweat glands

[a.] For sweat to produce cooling effects, it must evaporate. It is a more effective means of cooling in low humidity environments than high humidity environments because of the gradient.

[b.] The body surface temperature is higher than the surface temperature of most objects in the environment.

Limbic System

- Primitive brain area.
- Located deep in the temporal lobe.
- Communicates with the cerebral cortex.
- Initiates basic drives:
  - Hunger
  - Aggression
  - Emotional feelings
  - Sexual arousal
- Consists of:
  - **Hippocampus**
    - Functions in learning and memory.
  - **Amygdala**
    - Center of emotions.
    - Communicates with autonomic system (fight or flight).
    - Oxytocin and ADH receptors.

▶ MOTOR CONTROL AND COORDINATION

Basal Ganglia

- Located deep to cerebral cortex.
- Controls complex patterns of voluntary motor behavior.
- Includes:
  - Caudate nucleus.
  - Putamen.
  - Globus pallidus.
  - Substantia nigra.
  - Subthalamic nucleus.

Motor pathway:

Motor Cortex (precentral gyrus)
↓
Upper motor neuron
↓
Internal capsule
↓
Corticospinal tract
↓
(Cerebral peduncles – midbrain)
↓
(Pyramids – medulla – fibers cross)
↓
Ventral horn (spinal cord)
↓
Lower motor neuron
↓
Muscle

Cerebellum

- Lies posteroinferior to cerebrum, superoposterior to brainstem.
- Morphologically divided:
  - Two lateral hemispheres.
  - Middle portion (Vermis).
- Functions:
  - Maintain muscle tone.
  - Coordinate muscle movement.
  - Control balance.

Note: The basal ganglia and cerebellum modify movement on a minute to minute basis. The output of the cerebellum is excitatory, whereas that of the basal ganglia is inhibitory.

These two systems work together to achieve smooth, coordinated movement. Movement disorders result from aberration to each of these systems (e.g., Parkinson's, Huntington's, dysmetria, ataxia [see pathology]).

▶ BRAINSTEM

Lies immediately inferior to cerebrum, just anterior to cerebellum.

Midbrain (Mesencephalon)

- Connects dorsally with the cerebellum.
- Large voluntary motor nerve tracts pass through.
- Location of:
  - CN III, IV nuclei.
  - Substantia nigra. (See also "Parkinson's Disease" in Neuropathology)

Pons

- Between the midbrain and medulla.
- Connects to the cerebellum posteriorly.
- Location of:
  - CN V and VI nuclei.
  - Motor nuclei of CN VII.
  - Exit points for CNs V, VI, VII.

Medulla Oblongata

- Most inferior segment of vertebrate brain.
- Continues with the spinal cord below.
- Joins the spinal cord at foramen magnum.
- Contains:
  - Important regulatory centers:
    - Swallowing.
    - Cardiac.
    - Vasomotor.
    - Respiratory.
  - Nuclei of CNs VIII, IX, X, XI, XII.

▶ PERIPHERAL NERVOUS SYSTEM

PNS is composed of:

- **Afferent neurons:** From sensory receptors to CNS.
- **Efferent neurons:** From CNS to muscles, organs, and glands (and their associated ganglia and plexuses.

Subdivisions of the Peripheral Nervous System

Somatic Nervous System	Autonomic Nervous System

12 pairs of cranial nerves.
31 pairs of spinal nerves.
Both sensory and motor neurons.
Innervates skeletal muscle (voluntary).
Motor:
No synapse in peripheral ganglion.
  ■ Uses 1 efferent neuron from the CNS to end-organ.
Sensory:
Synapse within dorsal root ganglion (peripheral) prior to CNS.
Modalities:
  ■ Touch.
  ■ Movement (position sense).
  ■ Temperature.
  ■ Pain.
	2 subdivisions:
	  ■ Sympathetic.
	  ■ Parasympathetic.
	Action is largely involuntary.
	Controls:
	Glands (exocrine and endocrine).
	Cardiac muscle.
	Smooth muscle.
	Visceral organs.
	Not skeletal muscle.
	Motor:
	Synapses within autonomic ganglion.
	  ■ Uses 2 efferent neurons from CNS to effector.

▶ AUTONOMIC NERVOUS SYSTEM

See the illustrations of the neuroanatomy section.

BASIC ANATOMIC PATHWAY

Preganglionic neuron (within CNS).

↓

Ganglion (cell bodies of postganglionic neurons; outside of the CNS).

↓

Postganglionic neuron (outside of the CNS).

↓

Effector organ.

Autonomic Ganglia

- Collections of cell bodies of the postganglionic neurons.
- **Sympathetic:** Sympathetic chain ganglia (near spinal cord):
    - Short preganglionic neuron.
    - Long postganglionic neuron.
- **Parasympathetic:** Ganglia at, within organ (e.g., celiac ganglion):
    - Long preganglionic neuron.
    - Short postganglionic neuron.

Remember: Both parasympathetic and sympathetic preganglionic neurons are cholinergic (release Ach). However, parasympathetic postganglionic neurons are cholinergic (muscarinic receptors); sympathetic postganglionic neurons are largely adrenergic (release norepinephrine, which binds to sympathetic receptors). The exception is in sweat glands and blood vessels in skeletal muscle. Here the postganglionic sympathetic neurons are cholinergic (release Ach at muscarinic receptors).

Parasympathetic Nervous System

- Craniosacral: Composed of:
  - CN nuclei.
  - S2–4.
- Major nerve is the Vagus nerve (CN X): Originates in medulla.
- **Preganglionic neuron**
  - Cholinergic (releases Ach).
  - Binds nicotinic cholinergic receptors on postganglionic neurons (ganglia within effector).
  - Each preganglionic parasympathetic neuron synapses on only a few postganglionic parasympathetic neurons.
- **Postganglionic neuron**
  - Cholinergic (releases Ach).
  - Bind muscarinic cholinergic receptors in the tissue.

Postganglionic Receptors

	Nicotinic		Muscarinic
	N1 (N_N)	N2 (N_M)	M
Principal location	Autonomic ganglia	Motor endplate (NMJ)	Effector organs (including sweat glands under sympathetic control)
Effect(s)	Excitatory - Nerve transmission - Postganglionics are activated	Excitatory - Muscle contraction	Excitatory or inhibitory

Notes

- All preganglionic autonomic neurons (both sympathetic and parasympathetic) and all postganglionic parasympathetic neurons are cholinergic (use Ach as NT).
- Cholinergic effects of preganglionic autonomic systems (at ganglia of sympathetic and parasympathetic systems) are excitatory.
- Cholinergic effects of postganglionic parasympathetic fibers are either excitatory or inhibitory, depending on the end-organ (e.g., parasympathetic fibers innervating heart ↓ HR).

Sympathetic Nervous System

- Thoracolumbar.
  - Composed of: Spinal segments T1–L3.
- Exerts widespread effect because of high ratio of postganglionic to preganglionic fibers.
  - Each sympathetic preganglionic neuron branches extensively and synapses with numerous postganglionic neurons.
- **Preganglionic neuron**
  - Cholinergic (releases Ach).
  - Binds nicotinic cholinergic receptors on postganglionic neurons (ganglia within effector).

- Each preganglionic parasympathetic neuron synapses on only a few postganglionic parasympathetic neurons.
- **Postganglionic neuron**
  - Adrenergic (releases NE).
  - Binds adrenergic receptors in the tissue **except** sweat glands and skeletal muscle blood vessels.

Note: Three cervical sympathetic ganglia supply the head and neck.

Adrenergic Receptors

- Membrane receptor proteins.
- G-protein coupled receptors.
- Located on autonomic effector organs.
- Bound by catecholamine ligands (epinephrine, norepinephrine).
- Norepinephrine (NE) stimulates mainly alpha receptors.
- Epinephrine stimulates both alpha and beta equally.

Alpha- and Beta-Adrenergic Receptors

	Alpha-1 (α-1)	Alpha-2 (α-2)	Beta-1 (β-1)	Beta-2 (β-2)
Principal location	Vascular smooth muscle: - Skin - Mucosa - GI	Presynaptic nerve terminals Platelets Fat cells GI tract wall	Heart	Skeletal muscle Bronchial smooth muscle
Effect(s)	Vasoconstriction	Inhibition (relaxation or dilation)	↑ Heart rate ↑ Contractility	Vasodilation Bronchodilation

Note: Monoamine oxidase (MAO) is an enzyme that catalyzes oxidative deamination of monoamines (including NE, serotonin, and epinephrine). The deamination process ↑ breakdown (metabolism) of excess NTs that accumulate at postsynaptic terminals.

Summary of Autonomic Effects

	Sympathetic	Parasympathetic
	Adrenergic	Cholinergic
Pupils	Mydriasis (dilate)	Miosis (constrict)
Salivation	Thick	Watery (ready to eat)
Bronchi	Bronchodilation	Bronchoconstriction
Heart rate	↑	↓
Adrenal medulla	Causes epi and NE release	No effect

▶ SPINAL TRACTS

- See also the "Neuroanatomy" section.
- Spinal cord is part of the CNS.
- White matter tracts:
  - Composed of myelinated nerve fibers bundles.
  - Surround gray matter horns.
- Form ascending and descending tracts.
- Axons of a tract have the same origin, termination, and function.
- Tracts are often named for origin and termination (e.g., spinothalamic tract).
- Tracts are sensory or motor (see the following chart).

Tracts can be:

- **Ipsilateral:** Axons run on same side as cell bodies.
- **Contralateral:** Axons run on opposite side (have crossed over).

Spinal Tracts

Sensory (Ascending)	Motor (Descending)
Spinothalamic • Pain • Temperature	Corticospinal (pyramidal) Extrapyramidal
Dorsal column, medial lemniscus • Touch • Pressure • Vibration • Proprioception (position)	

Spinal cord anatomy:
- Dorsal horn
  - Sensory.
  - Receives fibers from the dorsal root ganglia.
- Ventral (anterior) root
  - Motor.

SENSORY PATHWAY

Receptor
↓
Peripheral nerve (sensory fibers)
↓
Dorsal root ganglion (synapse)
↓
Spinal cord
↓
Spinal tracts (spinothalamic or dorsal column, medial lemniscus)
↓
Brainstem nuclei
↓
Thalamus
↓
Cortex

Receptors

- Receive information from internal or external environment.
- Send nerve impulses to CNS.
- Two broad types: According to location of stimuli.
- **Exteroreceptors:** Receive external stimuli (from body surface):
  - Touch.
  - Pressure.
  - Pain.
  - Temperature.
  - Light.
  - Sound.
- **Interoreceptors** (visceroreceptors): Receive input from internal environment of body:
  - Pressure.
  - Pain.
  - Chemical changes.

Proprioreceptors

- Type of interoceptor.
- Relays information concerning position of body parts (in space).
- Separate from visual input.
  - *Kinesthetic sense*
- Located in muscles, tendons, joints.
- Communicate with the vestibular apparatus.

> *There are many types of joint receptors:*
> - Nonencapsulated
>   - Free nerve endings: Pain.
> - Encapsulated
>   - Pacinian: Vibration, pressure.
>   - Ruffini: Stretch.
> - Neuromuscular spindles
>   - Stretch.
> - Neurotendons
>   - Tension.

Nonencapsulated Versus Capsulated Receptors

Nonencapsulated	Encapsulated Receptors
Free nerve endings Pain primarily, touch, pressure, tickle, hot/cold. Terminal ends have no myelin. In epithelial cells, skin, cornea, alimentary tract, connective tissue, haversian system of bone, dental pulp.	**Meissner's corpuscles** Mechanoreceptors, allow 2-point discrimination. In dermal papilla of skin. Ovoid stack of Schwann cells.
Merkel's disc Tactile (touch, pressure). In hairless skin—fingertips, pressure.	**Pacinian corpuscles** Vibration, pressure. In dermis, subcutaneous tissue, ligaments, joints. Concentric lamellae of flattened cells.
Hair follicle receptors Mechanoreception—bending hair stimulates touch. Fiber winds around hair.	**Ruffini's corpuscles** Stretch. In dermis of hairy skin. Large unmyelinated nerve fibers ending within bundles of collagen fibers.

Receptors Classified by Stimulus Type

	Mechanoreceptor	Thermoreceptor	Nocioreceptor	Chemoreceptor	Photoreceptor
Stimulus	Pressure or stretch	Temperature	Pain	Chemicals (inhaled, ingested, or in blood)	Light
Examples	Pacinian corpuscles Muscle spindles (Golgi tendon organs) Meissner's corpuscles Hair cells	Free nerve endings	Free nerve endings	Taste receptors Smell receptors Osmoreceptors Carotid body O_2 receptors	Retina ■ Rods ■ Cones

Hair cells transduce senses of hearing and balance.

Osmoreceptors and carotid body O_2 receptors monitor pH and gas levels.

▶ SOMATOSENSORY PATHWAYS

Sensory Tracts (Ascending)

See Figure 10–1 for somatosensory pathways.

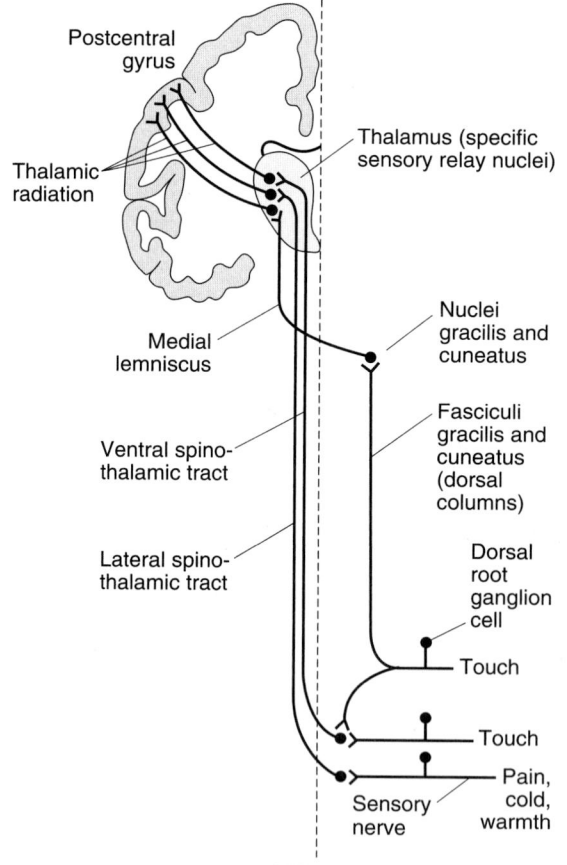

FIGURE 10–1. Somatosensory pathways.

Reproduced, with permission, from Ganong. *Review of Medical Physiology*, 22nd ed. McGraw-Hill, 2005.

Spinothalamic Tract (Anterolateral System)

- **Lateral spinothalamic tract:** Transmits pain and temperature.
- **Anterior spinothalamic tract:** Transmits light touch.

Pathway

Sensory nerve
↓
Dorsal horn of spinal cord gray matter
↓
Cross to opposite side of cord (decussate)
↓
Ascend contralateral spinal cord (through anterior and lateral white matter columns/tracts)
↓
Thalamus
↓
Somatosensory cortex

Dorsal Column, Medial Lemniscus System

- Conveys touch, pressure, and vibration.

Pathway

Sensory nerve
↓
Dorsal horn of spinal cord gray matter
↓
Ascend ipsilateral spinal cord
↓
Posterior columns: Fasciculus gracilis (fibers from lower extremities) and Fasciculus cuneatis (fibers from upper extremities)
↓
Synapse in medulla (nucleus gracilis and cuneatis)
↓
Decussate and ascend contralateral brainstem in medial lemniscus
↓
Thalamus
↓
Somatosensory cortex

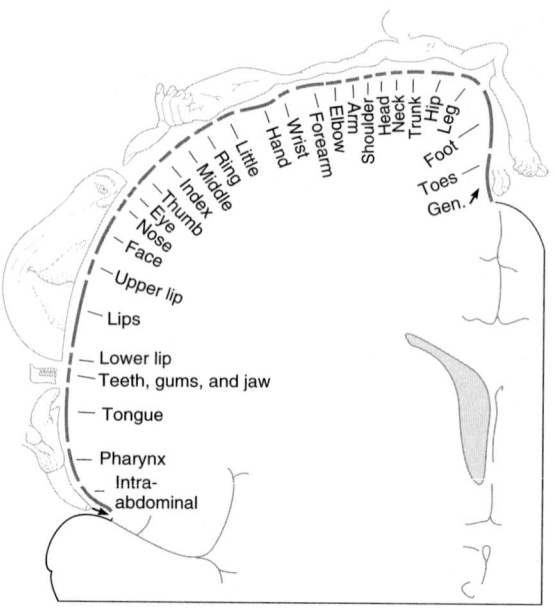

FIGURE 10-2. Somatosensory cortex.

Reproduced, with permission, from Ganong. *Review of Medical Physiology*, 22nd ed. McGraw-Hill, 2005.

SOMATOSENSORY CORTEX (POSTCENTRAL GYRUS)

See Figures 10–2 and 10–3 for somatosensory cortex.

- Representation is homunculus.

Descending Motor Tracts (Efferent or Descending Pathways)

- The upper motor neuron tracts sending signals from the brain muscles.

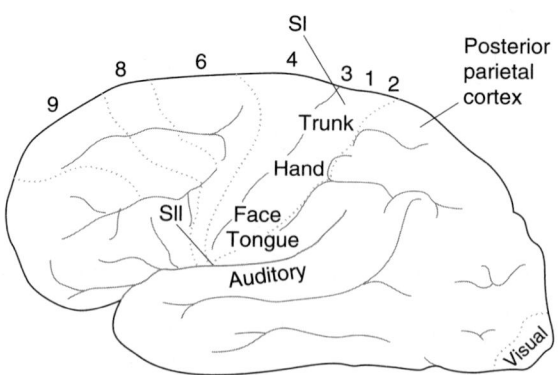

FIGURE 10-3. Somatosensory cortex.

Reproduced, with permission, from Ganong. *Review of Medical Physiology*, 22nd ed. McGraw-Hill, 2005.

MOTOR PATHWAY

Motor area of brain (precentral gyrus of frontal lobe)
↓
Upper motor neurons (= descending motor tracts, e.g., corticospinal tract)
↓
Lower motor neurons
↓
Skeletal muscle.

Upper Motor Neurons

- Originate in white matter of brain.
- Form two major systems:
  - Corticospinal tract (pyramidal system).
  - Extrapyramidal system.

Corticospianl Tract (Pyramidal System)

See Figure 10–4 for corticospinal tract (pyramid system).

- Two components:
  - **Lateral** (70–90%).
  - **Anterior/ventral** (10–30%).
- Travel via primary motor cortex through internal capsule to medulla.
  - **Decussate in medulla.**
  - Continue down opposite side of spinal cord →
  - Anterior horn → lower motor neurons → muscles.
  - Right brain controls left somatic muscles.
- Control fine, skilled movements of skeletal muscle.

Note: This tract is called pyramidal system because fibers of the corticospinal tract form the pyramids in the medulla.

Extrapyramidal System

- Collection of smaller tracts:
  - **Rubrospinal.**
  - **Reticulospinal.**
  - **Olivospinal.**
  - **Vestibulospinal.**
  - **Tectospinal.**
- Travel from premotor area of frontal lobe (and other areas) to pons.
  - **Decussate in pons.**
  - Continue down opposite side of spinal cord →
  - Anterior horn → lower motor neurons → muscles.
  - Right brain controls left lower motor neuron.
- Controls gross motor movement, posture, and balance.

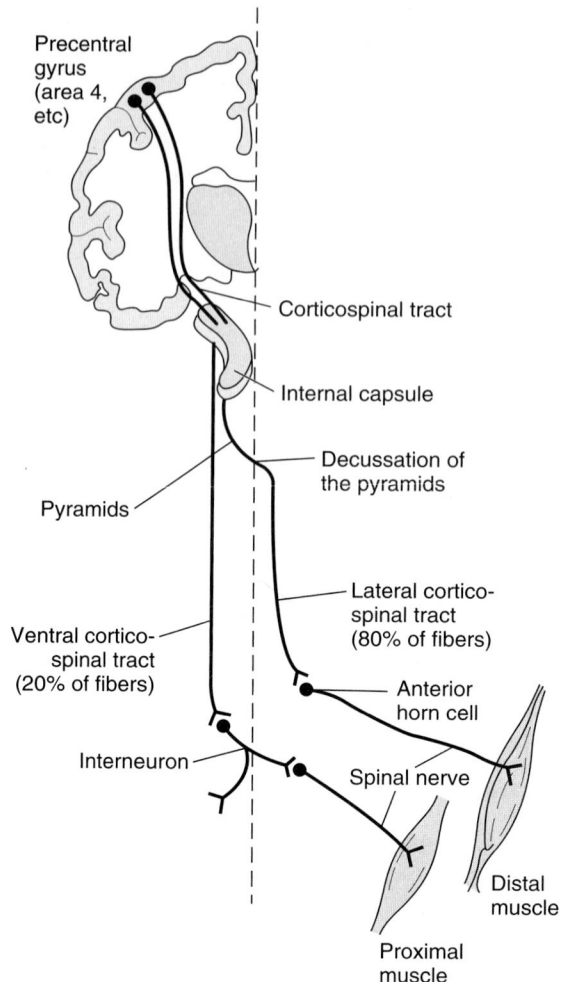

FIGURE 10-4.   Corticospinal tract (pyramid system).

Reproduced, with permission, from Ganong. *Review of Medical Physiology*, 22nd ed. McGraw-Hill, 2005.

► SPINAL CORD LESIONS

Lesion on one side causes:

- Ipsilateral motor loss (corticospinal).
- Contralateral pain and temperature loss (spinothalamic).
- Example: If you hemitransect the right side of the spinal cord, you lose right-sided (ipsilateral) motor control (corticospinal) and left-sided (contralateral) pain and temperature sense (spinothalamic).

► NEUROPHYSIOLOGY

Resting Membrane Potential

- Charge differential or voltage set up across the resting nerve membrane.
  - Due to separation of charged particles (ions and proteins) between extracellular and intracellular fluids.

- *Polarized membrane*
  - More positive ions (cations) outside (extracellular).
  - More negative (anions) inside (intracellular).
- Charge separation occurs because:
  - **K^+ leak** (resting K^+ conductance)
    - + charges leave cell down electrochemical gradient.
    - *Most important determinant of RMP.*
  - **Na^+/K^+ pump**
    - Using ATP, establishes the Na^+ and K^+ gradient; creates gradient to allow K^+ leak to occur.
    - Pump is electrogenic: 2 K^+ in for every 3 Na^+ pumped out = net loss of + charges from the cell.
- RMP: ranges between –40 and –85 mV.

Note: Visceral smooth muscle and cardiac pacemaker cells lack a stable RMP.

Action Potential

- Initiated by depolarizing stimulus (depolarization).
- RMP becomes more positive (less negative).
  - Ion channels open.
  - Positive ions move from outside to in.
  - As positive ions go intracellularly, RMP becomes positive.
- Na^+ (sodium)
  - Na+ entry initially causes more Na^+ channels to open.
  - Membrane potential approaches that of sodium equilibrium potential.
  - Once threshold reached, the action potential (AP) will fire.
  - Threshold = 20 mV+.
- All or none phenomenon.
  - If don't reach threshold, don't get AP.
  - AP is same with supra threshold and threshold stimuli.

REFRACTORY PERIOD

- Period of time after an AP that the membrane cannot again be stimulated, i.e., another AP cannot be initiated.

ABSOLUTE REFRACTORY PERIOD

- No stimulus, no matter how large, will stimulate an AP.

RELATIVE REFRACTORY PERIOD

- A larger than usual stimulus will stimulate an AP, i.e., the threshold is increased.

Repolarization

- Membrane potential returns to normal following an AP.
- ↓ **Na^+ permeability** (rapid).
- Block Na^+ entry.
- ↑ **K^+ permeability** (in to out)(slower).
- K^+ leaks out of the cell.

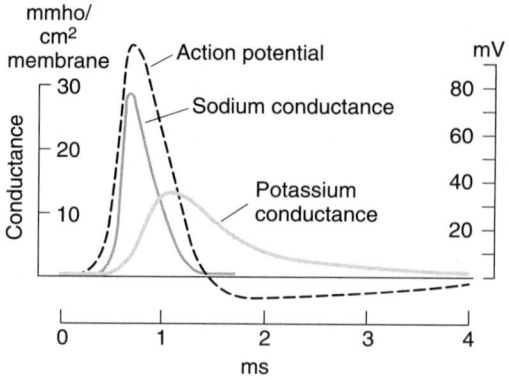

FIGURE 10-5. Repolarization.

Reproduced, with permission, from Ganong. *Review of Medical Physiology*, 22nd ed. McGraw-Hill, 2005.

See Figure 10–5 for repolarization.

Hyperpolarization

- During repolarization there is an overshoot in the more negative direction.
- Membrane potential briefly becomes more negative than RMP before returning to RMP.
- This is because of ↑ **K conductance**.
  - K⁺ channels stay open.
  - K efflux is greater than in resting.

Note: Hyperpolarization is responsible for the relative refractory period (cell remains hypoexcitable). Influx of Cl- will also hyperpolarize and make AP more difficult to generate.

Remember:
Excitable cells
- Neurons
- Muscle cells
- Cardiac pacemaker

▶ LOCAL ANESTHETICS

- Block sodium channels (↓ Na⁺ permeability).
  - Bind to inactivation gates of fast, voltage gated Na⁺ channels,
    - keeping them closed and
    - prolonging absolute refractory period.
- ↓ Membrane excitability → cannot generate AP → no nerve impulse conduction.
- Reversible.
- K, Cl, Ca conductances are *unchanged*.

Local Anesthetics

- Affect small myelinated fibers first.
- Unmyelinated C-fibers, then
  ↓
- Small myelinated nerve fibers (pain, temp), then
  ↓
- Larger A fibers (touch proprioception, Golgi tendon).

NEUROTRANSMITTERS

Excitatory

- Depolarize (more positive) the postsynaptic membrane potential.
  - Brings it closer to threshold.
  - ↑ probability of AP in postsynaptic neuron.
- Creates an excitatory postsynaptic potential (EPSP).

Note: EPSPs can combine, using summation (2 forms, see below) to reach threshold and initiate an AP.

Inhibitory

- Hyperpolarize (more negative) the postsynaptic membrane potential.
  - Moves it away from threshold.
  - ↓ probability of AP in postsynaptic neuron.
- Creates an inhibitory postsynaptic potential (IPSP).
- Result of ↑ membrane permeability to either Cl- or K+.
- Examples of inhibitory NTs:
  - Glycine.
  - GABA.
    - Both bind receptors and open Cl- channels (↑ Cl- permeability).

Note: The inhibitory or excitatory effects of NTs depend on their binding characteristics to receptors.

SUMMATION

Spatial Summation

- Two excitatory inputs arrive at a postsynaptic neuron simultaneously.
  - Converging circuit.
  - Arrival of impulses from *multiple* presynaptic fibers at same time.

Temporal Summation

- Two excitatory inputs arrive at a postsynaptic neuron in rapid succession.
  - ↑ frequency of nerve impulses from a *single* presynaptic fiber.

NERVE CONDUCTION

- Nerve impulse = Action potential spreads along plasma membrane.

Saltatory Conduction

- Occurs in myelinated fibers (remember: Schwann cells and oligodendrocytes).
- ↑ velocity of nerve transmission along myelinated fibers.
- Conserves energy because:

- Only the Ranvier node depolarizes.
  - Less energy for Na⁺/K⁺ ATPase to reestablish resting ion gradients.
  - Na⁺/K⁺ pumps reestablish concentration gradient only Ranvier nodes.
  - Allow repolarization to occur with less transfer of ions.
- Electrochemical basis behind saltatory conduction is ↓ **membrane capacitance.**

MYELIN

- Prevents movement of Na⁺ and K⁺ through the membrane.
  - Na⁺, K⁺ conductance only at Ranvier nodes.
- ↓ membrane capacitance.
- ↑ membrane resistance.

Saltatory conduction is a faster way to conduct an impulse down the axon (up to 100 m/sec).

> Conduction velocity depends on:
> - Diameter of nerve fiber.
>   - ↑ diameter ↑ → resistance to flow → ↑ velocity.
> - Presence of myelin sheath.

NODES OF RANVIER

- Exposed nerve membrane where depolarization occurs.
  - Continue fueling spread of AP during nerve transmission.
- Located every 0.2–2 mm along the myelin sheath.
- APs could not be produced if the myelin sheath were continuous.
- APs travel down axon and "jump" from node to node.

CONTINUOUS CONDUCTION

- Occurs in unmyelinated fibers.
- Nerve transmission (AP) travels along entire membrane surface.
- Relatively slow conduction (1.0 m/sec).

Problems with Nerve Conduction

WALLERIAN DEGENERATION

- Axon is cut.
- The axon remnant distal to the cut (away from the cell body) degenerates because axonal transport is interrupted.
- Regeneration of axons possible if endoneurial sheath is intact.
  - Occurs at a rate of 2–4 mm/day.
  - If cell body is irreversibly injured, the entire neuron degenerates.

NEUROPRAXIA

- Transient block (bruise).
- Incomplete paralysis or loss of sensation.
- Rapid recovery.

AXONOTMESIS

- Axon damaged, but connective sheath remains intact.
- Wallerian degeneration occurs distally but then regeneration can occur.

NEUROTMESIS

- Complete transaction of nerve trunk.
- Results in:
- Motor
  - Flaccid paralysis.
  - Atrophy of end-organ.
- Sensory
  - Total loss of cutaneous sensation.

▶ SYNAPSE

Functional connection, anatomical junction between

- Nerve axon (presynaptic axon) and
- Target cell
  - Nerve (postsynaptic neuron)
  - Muscle (NMJ)
  - Gland

PRESYNAPTIC NEURONS

- Transmit information toward a synapse.

SYNAPTIC CLEFT

- Space between presynaptic terminal and postsynaptic cell.

POSTSYNAPTIC NEURONS

- Transmit away from a synapse.

NERVE IMPULSES

- Travel in only one direction because synapses are polarized.

Note: Depolarization of the presynaptic cell initiates a response in the postsynaptic cell either by release of NTs (most common) or by direct passage of electrical current.

Note: Site of interneuronal communication can involve one axon to one dendrite, one axon to many dendrites, or many axons to one dendrite.

Neuronal Excitability

- Nerves are excited (APs generated) electrically or chemically.
  - Ligand-gated (NT binding) (most common).
  - Voltage gated channels.
  - Mechanically gated (stretching).

Types of Synapse

- Chemical synapse (most common).
  - Ligand-gated: Use NTs.
- Electrical synapse.

CHEMICAL SYNAPSE

- Most common type.
- Consists of:
  - Presynaptic membrane.
    - Synaptic vesicles within this terminal contain a NT.
  - Synaptic cleft.
    - Space between the presynaptic and postsynaptic membranes.
  - Postsynaptic membrane.
    - Membrane of postsynaptic neuron that contains specific receptors for the NT.

SYNAPTIC TRANSMISSION

- Release of NTs.
- NTs are stored in synaptic vesicles within the presynaptic axon terminal.
- AP depolarizes the presynaptic membrane, causing:
  - Voltage gated Ca^{2+} channels opened (on the presynaptic membrane).
    - ↑ Ca^{2+} influx.
  - Ca^{2+} causes the synaptic vesicles to fuse with membrane.
  - NTs are released by exocytosis into synaptic cleft.
  - NTs diffuse across cleft.
  - Bind to specific receptors on postsynaptic cell.
- The time required for this process to occur is called synaptic delay.

CHEMICAL NEUROTRANSMITTERS

- Mediate most connections.
- Small molecule NTs (contained within vesicles):
  - Glutamate, GABA, glycine, ACH, 5HT, NE, Epi, etc.
- Neuropeptides (large dense vesicles):
  - Somatostatin, endorphins, enkephalins, opioids, etc.

ELECTRICAL SYNAPSE

- Gap junctions; minority.
- Cytoplasm of adjacent cells is connected by gap junctions.
- Allows passage of local electrical currents (ions and small molecules) (from APs in presynaptic neuron) to pass directly to postsynaptic neuron.
  - Rare in the CNS.
  - Common in cardiac and smooth muscle.
  - Ensure a group of neurons act together; Synchronize groups of neurons.
  - Important in embryonic development (morphogenic gradients).

▶ NEUROMUSCULAR JUNCTION (NMJ)

Synapse between lower motor neuron (efferent nerve) and muscle.

- Presynaptic terminal (lower motor neuron axon)
  - Releases Ach.
- Postsynaptic membrane (skeletal muscle membrane).
  - Displays nicotinic receptor (N_M).

Sequence

Ach binds N_M.
↓
Na^+ channels open on the motor end-plate.
↓
Muscle fiber depolarized.
↓
Voltage gated Na^+ channels on the sarcolemma open.
↓
AP stimulated in skeletal muscle fiber.
↓
AP travels down the transverse tubules.
↓
Ca^{2+} release from the sarcoplasmic reticulum.
↓
Muscle contraction.

Acetylcholine Metabolism

- Synthesized in the presynaptic terminal of the motor neuron from which it is released.
    - Acetyl CoA + Choline – (choline acetyltransferase)→ ACh (acetylcholine).
- Stored in synaptic vesicles.
- Released into synaptic cleft (generates effect).
- Breakdown:
    - Ach – (acetylcholinesterase [AchE])→ acetate + choline.

Note: In the NMJ, AChE is located on the muscle end-plate.
Note: If AChEs are inhibited, get prolongation of end-plate potential (EPP).

> Two enzymes involved in ACh metabolism:
> - Choline acetyltransferase: ACh generation.
> - Acetylcholinesterase (AChE): ACh breakdown.

▶ SPECIAL SENSES

Vision

General eye anatomy. See also Chapter 2.

Eyeball

- Grossly divided into two segments:
- **Anterior segment**
    - Consists of two chambers (anterior and posterior).
    - Filled with aqueous humor (watery fluid).

- **Posterior segment**
  - Filled with vitreous humor (thick, gelatinous material).

STRUCTURAL COMPONENTS

- **Sclera**
  - Tough, white outer layer.
  - Maintains size and form of the eyeball.
- **Cornea**
  - Transparent dome on the anterior eye surface.
  - Protective function.
  - Helps focus light on retina at back of eye.
- **Choroid**
  Lining of the inner aspect of the eyeball beneath the retina; very vascular.

COMPONENTS THAT CONTROL LIGHT ENTERING THE EYE AND FOCUS LIGHT ON THE RETINA

- **Pupil**
  - Circular opening (black area) in the middle of the iris.
  - Light enters the eye to reach retina through this opening.
  - Lens is located behind this aperture.
  - Size of the pupil is controlled by muscles in the iris.
- **Iris**
  - Circular colored area of the eye (amount of pigment in the iris determines the color of the eye).
  - **Miosis**: Constriction of pupil:
    - Sphincter pupillae (iris sphincter) closes iris.
    - Response to:
      - Increased light.
      - Drugs (e.g., narcotics).
      - Pathologic conditions.
      - Parasympathetic stimulation.
  - **Mydriasis**: Dilation of the pupil (term often used for prolonged papillary dilation):
    - Dilator pupillae (iris dilator) opens iris.
    - Response to:
      - Decreased light.
      - Sympathetic stimulation (fight or flight).
      - Drug.
      - Disease.

- **Lens**
- Directly behind the iris and pupillary opening.
- Focuses light on the retina.
- Controlled by ciliary muscle (within the ciliary body).
- **Ciliary body**
- Functions:
  - Accommodation.
    - Ciliary muscle alters the lens refractory power (to focus light on the retina).
  - Produces aqueous humor.
  - Hold lens in place.

- **Retina**
  - Innermost layer of the eye on the posterior surface.
  - Receives visual stimuli.

- Communicates via CN II with the brain (visual cortex).
- Photoreceptors (visual receptors) of retina:
    - **Rods**
        - Contain rhodopsin (photopigment).
        - Perceive different degrees of brightness: Responsible for night vision (dark adaptation).
        - Relative lack of color discrimination.
        - Located mostly at the periphery of the retina.
    - **Cones**
        - Each contains one of three photopigments.
        - Each being sensitive to a particular wavelength of light.
    - Three types: Red, green, blue.
        - Primarily responsible for color vision.
    - Principal photoreceptors during daylight or in brightly lit areas.
        - Located in the center of the retina, especially in the fovea.

Note: Rods are more abundant, have higher sensitivity, and lower acuity compared with cones.

- **Photopigments**
    - Four photopigments:
        - Rhodopsin (rods).
        - Red, green, and blue (cones).
    - Each photopigment contains:
        - Opsin (protein) bound to
        - Retinal (a chromophore molecule).
    - The difference among the opsin molecules allows a photopigment to have specificity for a particular type or color of light.

Note: Retinal is constant among all photopigments and is produced from vitamin A.

VISUAL PATHWAY

See Figure 10–6.

Light
↓
(passes through cornea, lens, aqueous humor, vitreous humor and onto retina)
↓
Retina (rods & cones)
↓
Bipolar neurons
↓
Ganglion cells
↓
Optic disc
↓
Optic nerve (exits through optic foramen)
↓

Optic chiasm
↓
Lateral geniculate (of thalamus)
↓
Optic radiations
↓
Visual cortex (area 17) and visual association cortex (18, 19)

LESIONS ALONG THE VISUAL PATHWAY

- Left anopsia
- Bitemporal hemianopsia
- Right Homonomous hemianopsia
- Right hemianopsia with macular sparing

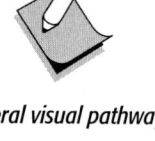

General visual pathway: Light enters eye → retina → optic nerve (CN II) → visual cortex (occipital lobe).

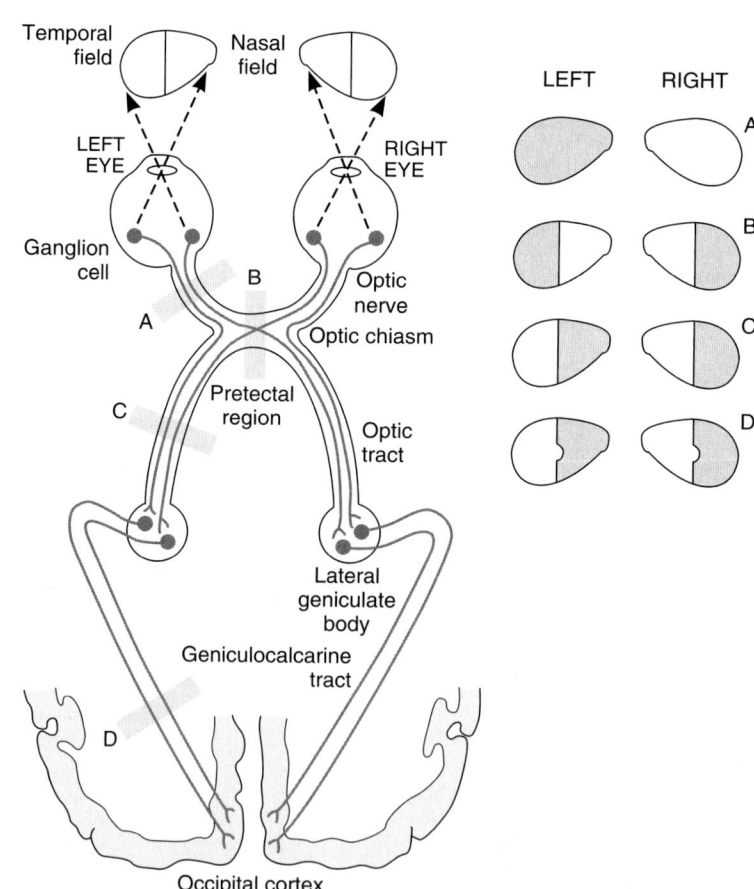

FIGURE 10–6. Visual pathway.

Reproduced, with permission, from Ganong. *Review of Medical Physiology*, 22nd ed. McGraw-Hill, 2005.

Disturbances of Vision

	Myopia (Nearsightedness)	Hyperopia (Farsightedness)	Astigmatism	Presbyopia
Problem	Eyeball too long.	Eyeball too short.	Curvature of lens is not uniform.	Loss of lens elasticity with advancing age.
	Focal point of far objects is focused in front of the retina. Near objects are focused correctly.	Focal point of near objects is focused behind the retina. Distant objects are focused correctly.		Eye cannot focus sharply on nearby objects.
Treatment	Concave lenses.	Convex lenses.	Cylindric lenses.	Often with bifocals.

▶ HEARING

Anatomy of the Ear

EXTERNAL EAR

- Auricle (Pinna)
  - Directs sound waves.
- External auditory canal (meatus)
  - Contains hair and cerumen (wax).
  - Serves as resonator and conduit.

MIDDLE EAR

- Tympanic cavity.
- Air-filled cavity in temporal bone.
  - Auditory tube: Equalizes pressure.
  - Ossicles (malleus, incus, stapes): Transmit sounds to oval window.

INNER EAR

See Figure 10–7.

- Formed by bony labyrinth and membranous labyrinth.
- Vestibule (saccule and utricle)
  - Associated with sense of balance.
- Semicircular canals
  - Concerned with equilibrium.
- Cochlea (two membranes: vestibular and basilar)
  - Responsible for hearing.
  - Spiral organ (organ of Corti).
    - Receptors (hair cells) for hearing.
    - Basic functional unit of hearing.
    - Transforms fluid vibrations from sound waves (mechanical energy) into a nerve impulse (electrical energy).

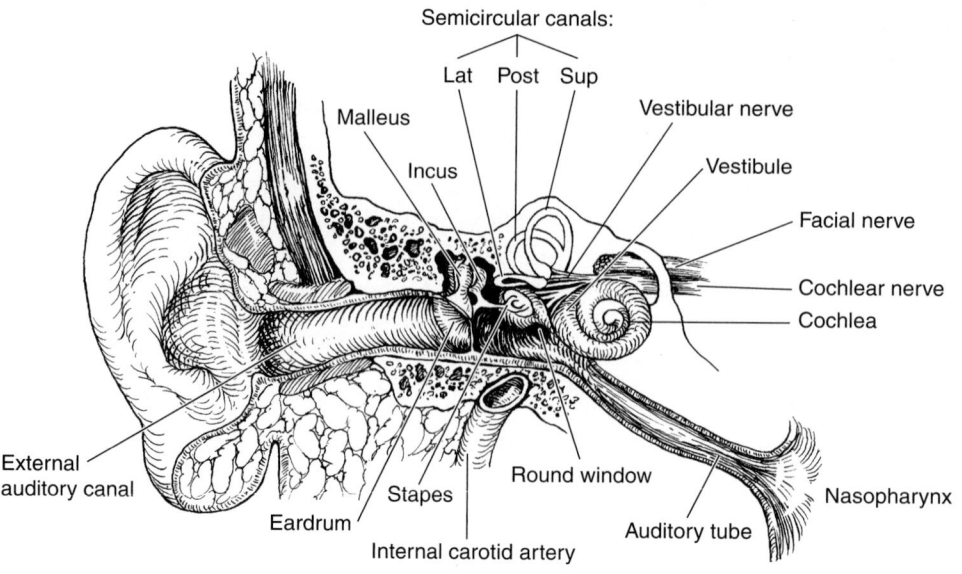

FIGURE 10-7. Inner ear.

Reproduced, with permission, from Ganong. *Review of Medical Physiology*, 22nd ed. McGraw-Hill, 2005.

Hearing

- Ability to detect sound.
- Human hearing range = 20–20,000 Hz.

CHARACTERISTICS OF A SOUND WAVE

- **Pitch**
    - Related to the frequency of the sound wave.
    - ↑ frequency = ↑ pitch.
        - Frequency is measures in hertz (Hz) or cycles per second.
- **Loudness** (amplitude)
    - Related to the intensity and the amplitude of the wave.
    - ↑ amplitude = ↑ intensity = ↑ loudness.
        - Intensity is measured in decibels (dB).
- **Timbre** (quality)
    - Related to the presence of additional sound-wave frequencies superimposed on the principal frequency.

Pitch = Frequency.
Loudness = Amplitude.

HEARING PATHWAY

Sound vibration
↓
Tympanic membrane
↓
Ossicles (malleus->incus->stapes)
↓
Oval window
↓

Waves in perilymph
↓
Bending of hairs (stereocilia)
↓
Hair cell depolarization within tectorial membrane or organ of Corti in cochlea
↓
Short axons to spiral ganglion (located within bony modiolus)
↓
Long axons form the cochlear nerve
↓
Synapse w/cochlear nuclei (dorsal and ventral)
↓
Superior olivary nucleus (ipsi- and contralaterally)
↓
Lateral lemniscus
↓
Inferior colliculus
↓
Medial geniculate of thalamus
↓
Transverse temporal gyrus (Heschl's gyrus)

Note: Superior olivary nuclei are important in sound localization.
Note: Presbycusis = hearing loss that gradually occurs because of changes in the inner or middle ear in individuals as they grow older.

Unlike other sensory systems, hearing has bilateral central representation (i.e., sound from one ear reaches auditory cortex in both hemispheres).

▶ TASTE

- Direct detection of chemical composition via contact with chemoreceptor cells.
- Food broken down; taste-producing molecules bind with protein from Ebners glands.
    - These bound molecules stimulate taste bud receptors.

▶ TASTE BUDS

- Made of gustatory receptor cells that synapse with sensory nerve fibers.
- Located:
    - Within the fungiform and vallate papillae of the tongue:
        - **Fungiform papillae**
            - Rounded.
            - Located mostly at the tongue tip of the tongue.
            - Contain ~5 taste buds.

- **Vallate papillae**
  - In "V" arrangement on the back of the tongue Contain ~100 taste buds.
- On the mucosa of the epiglottis, palate, and pharynx.

Note: **Filiform papillae** on dorsum of the tongue do **not** usually contain taste buds.

> *There are five basic tastes:*
> - Sweet
> - Sour
> - Bitter
> - Salt
> - Umami (MSG [monosodium glutamate])
>
> Each taste is sensed on all parts of the tongue, by each type of taste bud.

TASTE PATHWAY

Taste bud, receptor cell
↓
CN VII, IX, X
↓
Nucleus of the solitary tract (within medulla)
↓
Ipsilateral VPM of thalamus
↓
Insular cortex (to facial area of post-central gyrus).

TASTE DISTURBANCES

See Figure 10–8.

- **Ageusia:** Complete loss of taste.
- **Dysgeusia:** Disturbed sense of taste.

▶ SMELL

- Detection of inhaled odors.
- Chemoreceptor cells associated with the olfactory nerve (CN I).

Smell Pathway

See Figure 10–9.

Odorant particles (dissolve in mucous from Bowman's glands)
↓
Bipolar olfactory cells (within nasal mucosa)
↓
Olfactory nerve (pass through cribriform plate)
↓

Olfactory bulb (synapse with mitral and tufted cells)
  ↓
Olfactory tract
  ↓
Primary olfactory cortex and amygdala.

DISTURBANCES OF SMELL

- **Anosmia:** Absence of smell.
    - Disease of olfactory mucous membranes (common cold, allergic rhinitis).
    - Kallman syndrome.
- **Hyposmia:** Diminished smell.
- **Dysosmia:** Distorted smell.

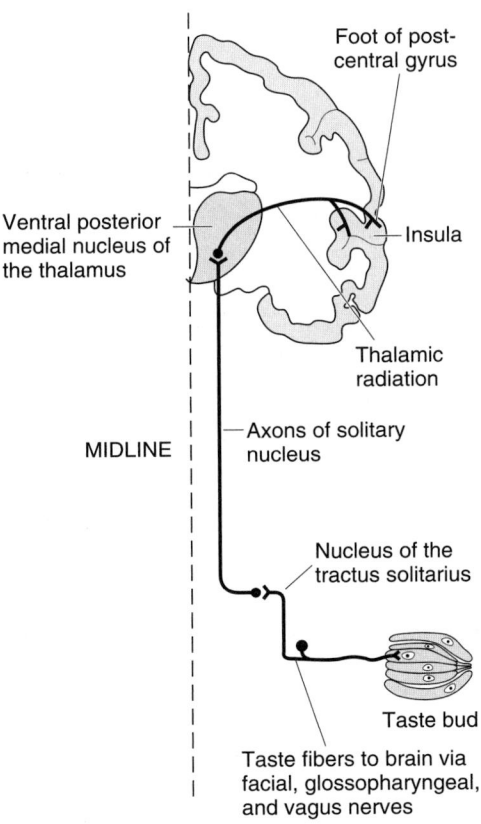

FIGURE 10-8. Taste disturbances.

Reproduced, with permission, from Ganong. *Review of Medical Physiology*, 22nd ed. McGraw-Hill, 2005.

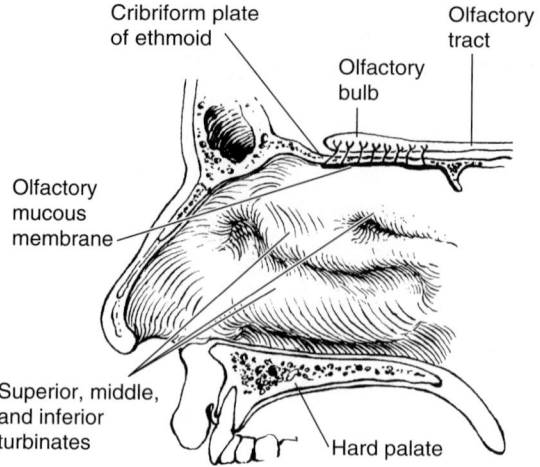

FIGURE 10-9. Smell pathway.

Reproduced, with permission, from Ganong. *Review of Medical Physiology*, 22nd ed. McGraw-Hill, 2005. (Reproduced from Waxman, St. TG. *Clinical Neuroanatomy*, 25th ed. McGraw-Hill, 2003).

CHAPTER 11
Muscle Physiology

Muscle	330
MAJOR CELLULAR COMPONENTS	330
INNERVATION	331
Skeletal Muscle	331
HISTOLOGY	331
CONNECTIVE TISSUE	332
MOTOR INNERVATION	332
CONTRACTION	332
CONTRACTION (TWITCH) SPEED	333
FIBER TYPES	333
MUSCLE RECEPTORS	334
SPINAL REFLEXES	334
Cardiac Muscle	334
HISTOLOGY	334
INNERVATION	334
MUSCLE CONTRACTION	334
Smooth Muscle	335
HISTOLOGY	335
INNERVATION	335
MUSCLE CONTRACTION	335

▶ MUSCLE

- The largest tissue type in the human body.
- Convert chemical energy to mechanical energy.
- Three types:
  - Skeletal
  - Cardiac
  - Smooth

Major Cellular Components

- **Sarcolemma:** The plasma membrane of muscle cells.
- **Sarcoplasm:** The cytoplasm of muscle cells.
- **Sarcoplasmic reticulum (SR):** A network of channels extending throughout the sarcoplasm that stores Ca^{2+}.
- **Myofilaments:** Mediate muscle contraction. Located in the sarcoplasm.
  - **Thin filaments:** ~6–8 nm in diameter.
    - Actin
    - **Troponin:** Attached to each tropomyosin molecule.
    - **Tropomyosin:** Blocks actin binding sites during rest.
  - **Thick filaments:** ~15 nm in diameter.
    - Myosin

Comparison of Skeletal, Cardiac, and Smooth Muscle

Characteristic	Skeletal	Cardiac	Smooth
Striations	Yes	Yes	No
Nucleation	Multinucleated	Single	Single
Nucleus location	Peripheral	Central	Central
Innervation	Motor	Autonomic	Autonomic
Movement	Voluntary	Involuntary	Involuntary
Contraction by	A.P.	Intrinsic	A.P./hormones
Syncytium	No	Yes	Yes
Ca^{2+} source	SR	SR/extracellular	SR/extracellular
T-tubules	Yes	Yes	No
Regulation	Actin	Actin	Myosin
Troponin	Yes	Yes	No

Innervation

- Afferent nerves: Sensory receptor → CNS.
- Efferent nerves: CNS → muscle cell.

▶ SKELETAL MUSCLE

Histology

See Figure 11–1.

- Cells are long and **multinucleated.**
- Nuclei are generally elongated and peripherally located.
- The major structural unit is the **myofibril:**
  - **Thick filaments** (contain myosin).
  - **Thin filaments** (contain actin, troponin, and tropomyosin).
  - Myosin cross-bridges link the two filaments.
- The **sarcomere** is the functional (contractile) unit of the myofibril.
- **Cross-striations** are apparent due to alternating light and dark banding of the myofibrils.
  - **A band:** Dark band containing myosin. Never changes length.
  - **H band:** Light band that bisects the A band.
  - **I band:** Light band that contains actin.
  - **Z line:** Dark band that bisects the I band.

Myasthenia gravis is an autoimmune disease in which the acetylcholine receptors on the sarcolemma are blocked, diminishing the number of muscle fibers responsive to the action potential.

Weight lifting causes muscle **hypertrophy,** increasing skeletal muscle cell size, not number. Contrarily, muscle disuse causes a decrease in muscle size.

The d**A**rk band is the **A** band.
The l**I**ght band is the **I** band.

HAZI (hazy):

The **H** band bisects the **A** band.
The **Z** line bisects the **I** band.

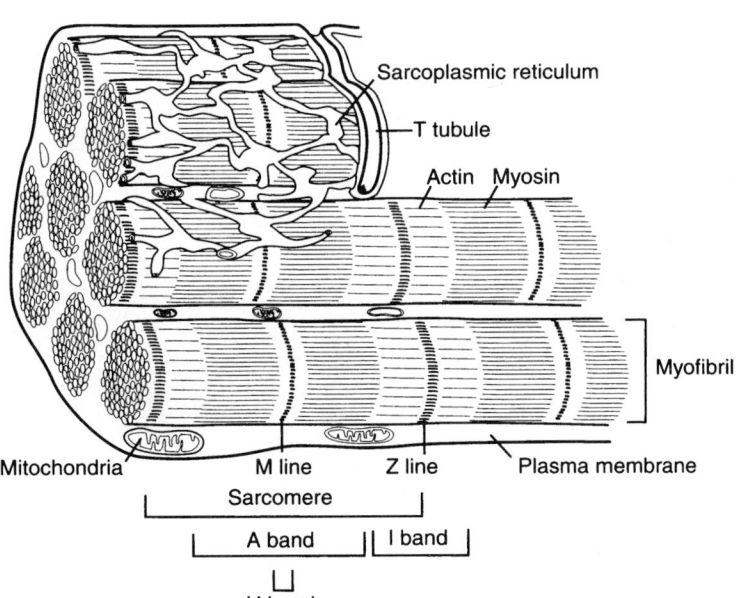

FIGURE 11–1. Skeletal muscle histology.

Reproduced, with permission, from Bhushan V. *First Aid for the USMLE Step 1.* McGraw Hill, 2006.

A sarcomere is defined as the area between two Z lines.

Each **motor unit** consists of the following:

- *Motor neuron*
- *Synaptic cleft*
- *Associated muscle fibers*

Connective Tissue

- Contains a rich supply of blood vessels and nerves required for nerve conduction.
- Divided into three layers:
    - **Epimysium:** Surrounds the entire muscle.
    - **Periomysium:** Surrounds muscle bundles (fascicles).
    - **Endomysium:** Surrounds each muscle fiber.

As thin and thick filaments overlap, the H and I bands are shortened, thereby contracting each sarcomere.

Motor Innervation

- One motor neuron innervates several skeletal muscle fibers.
- When an action potential reaches the neuromuscular junction, **acetylcholine** is released from vesicles within the axon terminus and binds to postsynaptic nicotinic receptors on the sarcolemma.
- This, in turn, increases the membrane permeability of Na$^+$ and K$^+$ and depolarizes the muscle cell.
- All motor neurons are arranged in various positions within the **ventral horn** of the spinal cord.

*Occurs via **actin-linked** regulation.*

Contraction

- The sliding filament model of muscle contraction.
- See Figure 11–2.
- The action potential travels along the sarcolemma and through a system of **t-tubules,** which extend from the outer surface of the muscle fiber to the SR of two adjacent sarcomeres.

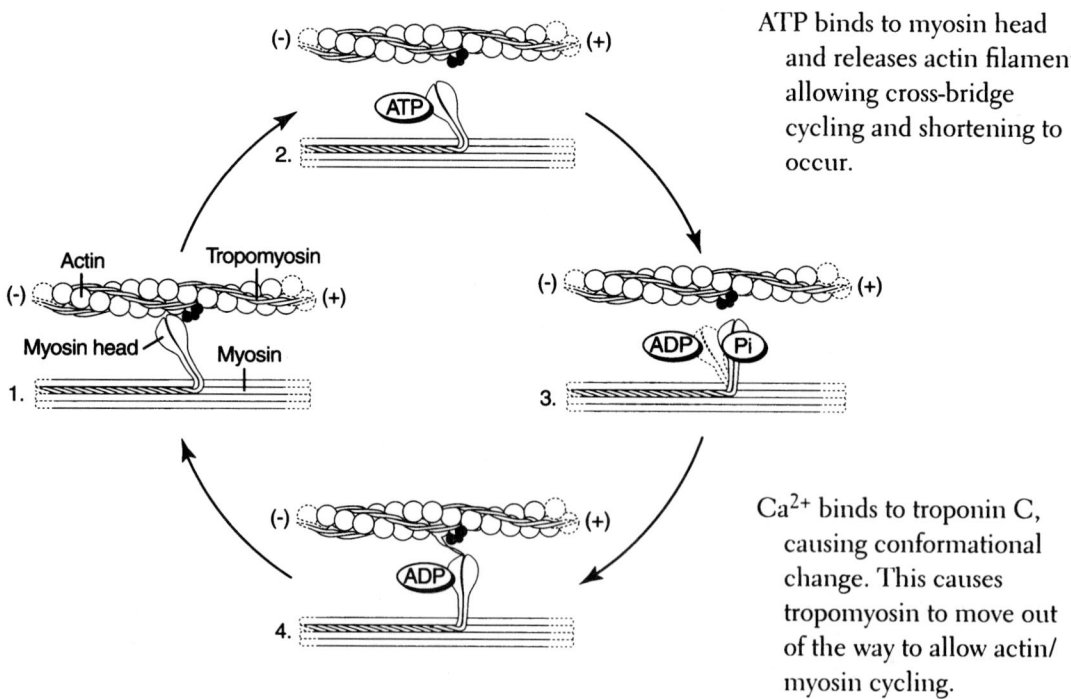

FIGURE 11-2. Skeletal muscle contraction.

Reproduced, with permission, from Bhushan V. *First Aid for the USMLE Step 1.* McGraw-Hill, 2006.

- Ca^{2+} released from the terminal cisternae of each SR bind to **troponin C**, which is attached to the **tropomyosin** molecule of thin filaments. This causes a conformational change in the shape of tropomyosin, allowing the actin filament to interact with the myosin cross-bridge.
- An **ATP** molecule bound to myosin is hydrolyzed to ADP + P_i. When the ADP + P_i is released from myosin, the actin filament is pulled closer toward the center of the sarcomere, shortening its length.
- As long as Ca^{2+} and ATP are available, this cycle continues, further contracting the muscle. If more muscle force is needed, more motor units are activated.
- During relaxation, Ca^{2+} is taken up by the SR, causing the release of actin from the myosin cross-bridges. Tropomyosin returns to its normal configuration, blocking this interaction.

> *The sources of ATP for muscle contraction arise from:*
> - *Glycogen stores → glycolysis.*
> - *TCA cycle → oxidative phosphorylation.*
> - ***Creatine phosphate***

Contraction (Twitch) Speed

Comparison of Skeletal Muscle by Twitch Speed

Characteristic	Slow (Type I)	Fast (Type II)
Color	Red	White
Function	Postural endurance	Rapid/powerful movement
Contraction speed	Slow	Fast
ATPase activity	Low	High
ATP source	Oxidative phosphorylation	Anaerobic glycolysis of stored glycogen
Percent mitochondria	High	Low
Percent myoglobin	High	Low
Percent SR	Low	High
Rate of fatigue	Low	High
Fiber diameter	Small	Large

> ***One Slow Fat Red Ox:***
>
> Type I
> Slow twitch
> Lipid accumulation
> Red fibers
> Oxidative phosphorylation

> ***Two Fast Skinny White Chickens:***
>
> Type II
> Fast twitch
> Low lipid accumulation
> White fibers
>   (like chicken breasts)

Fiber Types
- **Extrafusal fibers**
  - Make up the majority of skeletal muscle.
  - Innervated by **α-motor neurons.**
- **Intrafusal fibers**
  - Located in the bulk of the muscle.
  - Innervated by **γ-motor neurons.**
    - **Nuclear bag fibers:** Transmit information about *length* and *tension*. Innervated by fast *Type Ia* afferent nerve fibers.
    - **Nuclear chain fibers:** Transmit information about *length*. Innervated by slow *Type II* afferent nerve fibers.

*The two fiber types run **parallel** and attach to tendons at either end.*

Muscle Receptors

- **Muscle spindles:** Detect muscle fiber *length* and *tension*. Innervated by *Type Ia* and *Type II* afferent nerve fibers.
- **Golgi tendon organs:** Detect muscle fiber *tension*. Innervated by *Type Ib* afferent nerve fibers.

*Muscle spindles are composed of intrafusal fibers and run **parallel** to the main extrafusal fibers.*

Spinal Reflexes

STRETCH REFLEX

- Receptor: Muscle spindles.
- Sensitivity: Length and tension.
- Action: Muscle contraction.

*The stretch reflex maintains muscle **tone.***

TENDON (INVERSE MYOTATIC) REFLEX

- Receptor: Golgi tendon organs.
- Sensitivity: Tension.
- Action: Muscle relaxation.

▶ CARDIAC MUSCLE

Histology

- Cells have a similar contractile structure and **striated** appearance.
- Fibers are firmly linked by *desmosomes*.
- Nuclei are centrally located.
- Cells have many **branches**, which communicate to adjacent cardiac muscle cells via *gap junctions*.
- **Intercalated discs** coordinate the action of cardiac muscle cells.
- Cells do *not* undergo mitosis; injury results in fibrosis with loss of function at that site.

*Cardiac muscle behaves as a **functional syncytium.***

*An increase in cardiac demand causes a **compensatory hypertrophy**, increasing cardiac cell size, not number.*

The sinuatrial (SA) node is known as the pacemaker of the heart.

*Occurs via **actin-linked regulation**, but relies more on extracellular Ca^{2+} than skeletal muscle because its SR is less extensive.*

The plateau in the cardiac muscle action potential is due to the influx of Ca^{2+}.

Innervation

- Mediated by its own **intrinsic contractile activity.**
- There are **no motor units.**
- The **autonomic nervous system** (both sympathetic and parasympathetic fibers) controls the *rate* and *strength* of myocardial depolarization.

Muscle Contraction

- Ca^{2+} enters the myocytes via specific **calcium channels**, which are regulated by **cAMP protein kinases.**
- The influx of Ca^{2+} enables the release of more Ca^{2+} from the SR, initiating troponin-C binding and eventual muscle contraction.
- Relaxation occurs when Ca^{2+} exits the myocytes through a regulated Ca^{2+}-Na^{+} exchange system.

SMOOTH MUSCLE

Histology

- Commonly found in tubular organs such as blood vessels, the GI tract, and the respiratory tract, but also in ciliary bodies of the eye and hair follicles.
- Cells are small in diameter but very long.
- Nuclei are single and centrally located.
- Myofibrils are **not striated.**
- **No t-tubules** are present.
- SR system is poorly developed.

Innervation

- Mediated by the **autonomic nervous system** (both sympathetic and parasympathetic).
- However, there is a considerable synaptic distance from the nerve terminal to the sarcolemma because the autonomic axons terminate in the surrounding connective tissue.
- Because not all smooth muscle cells are directly innervated, they rely on cell–cell *gap junctions* to propagate the action potential.

Muscle Contraction

See Figure 11–3.

- Ca^{2+} (from the SR or extracellular sources) enters the smooth muscle cell cytoplasm and binds to **calmodulin**.
- Calmodulin activates **myosin light-chain kinase**, which transfers a Pi from an ATP molecule to the myosin light-chain.
- The phosphorylation of myosin enables it to interact with actin in the same manner as skeletal and cardiac muscle.
- Relaxation occurs when Ca^{2+} is taken up by the SR or plasma membrane and the myosin light-chain kinase becomes inactivated.
- Each contraction cycle requires one ATP.

Smooth muscle behaves as a **functional syncytium.**

Smooth muscle contraction can also be stimulated by **hormones** such as epinephrine and oxytocin.

Occurs via **myosin-linked regulation**; thin filaments **lack troponin**, so they are always ready to interact with myosin.

Maintains contraction for extended periods of time because the cross-bridges detach very slowly, allowing them to stay attached longer.

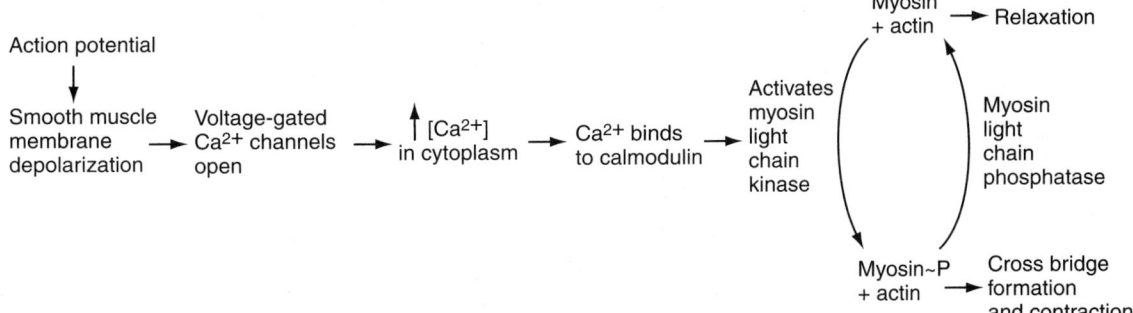

FIGURE 11–3. Smooth muscle contraction.

Reproduced, with permission, from Bhushan V. *First Aid for the USMLE Step 1.* McGraw-Hill, 2006.

CHAPTER 12

Circulatory and Cardiac Physiology

Blood Flow and Cardiodynamics	339
BLOOD FLOW	339
RESISTANCE	339
PROPERTIES OF FLOW	340
VELOCITY OF BLOOD FLOW	340
OXYGEN EXCHANGE	342
Blood Volume	342
Capacitance	342
Total Peripheral Resistance	343
Blood Pressure	344
Determinants of Cardiac Function	345
CARDIAC OUTPUT	345
HEART RATE AND CONTRACTILITY	346
VENOUS RETURN	347
PRESSURE–VOLUME LOOP	348
Electrophysiology	350
ELECTRICAL CONDUCTION OF THE HEART	350
Electrocardiogram (EKG)	352
Regulatory Mechanisms	354
BAINBRIDGE REFLEX	354
BARORECEPTORS	354
CHEMORECEPTORS	355
HORMONAL REGULATION SYSTEMS	356
EXERCISE	356
Hematocrit (HCT)	356
Hemoglobin Concentration	356
Anemia	357
CONSEQUENCES OF ANEMIA	357
CYANOSIS	358

Erythropoietin	358
NEGATIVE FEEDBACK	**358**
Coagulation and Hemostasis	358
VIRCHOW'S TRIAD	**358**
HEMOSTASIS	**358**
COAGULATION	**358**

► BLOOD FLOW AND CARDIODYNAMICS

Blood Flow

- F = P/R (flow = pressure/resistance).
- Flow is proportional to pressure difference at two ends of vessel.
- Flows from high pressure to low pressure.
- Inversely proportional to resistance along the vessel.
- Greatest in
    - Large straight vessels.
    - Low turbulence.
    - Low viscosity.
    - Low resistance.

PERFUSION PRESSURE

- Pressure at the arterial end minus pressure at venous end.

Resistance

- Poiseuille's law ($F = P\pi R^4/8\eta L$) describes the flow rate of liquid through a tube.
- The resistance to flow ($R = 8\pi L/\pi r^4$) is determined by
    - η = viscosity.
        - Hematocrit (HCT)
            - Affect is greater in larger vessels than smaller.
            - Overall vascular resistance is not affected unless severe (e.g., polycythemia).
        - Decrease in deformation of cells.
        - Plasma concentration (e.g., increase in protein, multiple myeloma).
    - L = length of tube.
    - r = radius.
        - Type and size of vessel.
        - Regulation of tone (sympathetic nervous system, medications, local factors).
        - Pathologic narrowing of vessel.
- $R \pi l/r^4$.
- If radius (r) increases by 2, the resistance (R) drops 16 x. ** most powerful relationship with resistance.

The RADIUS has the most powerful relationship with resistance.

SERIES RESISTANCE

- $R_{total} = R_1 + R_2 + R_3 + R_4 \ldots$

PARALLEL RESISTANCE

- Recruitment of capillaries serves to lower the resistance and therefore increase the flow.
  $1/R_{total} = 1/R_1 + 1/R_2 + 1/R_3 + 1/R_4 \ldots$

Resistance and conductance are inversely related.

Properties of Flow

See Figure 12–1.

*Resistance to flow of blood offered by the entire systemic circulation is called **total peripheral resistance (TPR)**.*

- **Laminar flow** (streamline)
  - In straight vessels.
  - Layer closest to vessel surface does not move.
  - Layer in center moves at maximum velocity.
  - Laminar flow occurs up to a certain critical velocity.
    - Turbulent flow occurs above critical velocity.
- **Turbulent flow**
  - Occurs above critical velocity.
  - Reynolds number.
  - Represents probability for turbulent flow.
  - Related to:
    - Velocity.
    - Diameter of vessel.
    - Blood viscosity.
    - Examples of turbulence:
  - Constricted, atherosclerotic vessel.
  - Ascending aorta.
  - Anemia.

Velocity of Blood Flow

When the vena cava is somewhat collapsed, as it often is, it has a lower cross-sectional area and a higher velocity of blood flow when compared to the aorta.

- Fastest to slowest:
  - Aorta.
  - Vena cavae.
  - Large veins.
  - Small arteries.
  - Arterioles.
  - Capillaries.

See Figure 12–2 for systemic blood flow and changes in pressure and velocity.

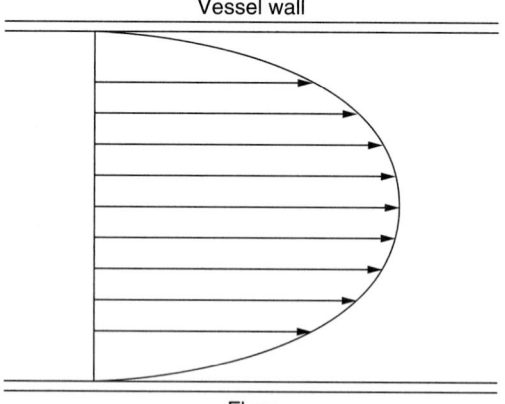

FIGURE 12–1. Properties of flow.

Reproduced, with permission, from Ganong WF. *Review of Medical Physiology*, 22nd ed. McGraw-Hill, 2005.

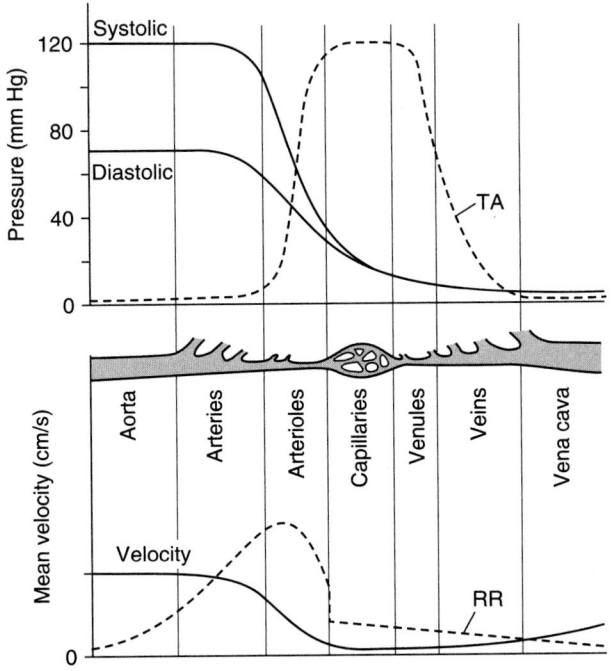

FIGURE 12-2. Systemic blood flow—changes in pressure and velocity.

Reproduced, with permission, from Ganong WF. *Review of Medical Physiology*, 22nd ed. McGraw-Hill, 2005.

LAPLACE'S LAW

- Wall stress = Pr/t.
  - P = pressure.
  - r = radius.
  - t = wall thickness.
- **In vessels:** A thin-walled, distended vessel, under large amounts of pressure has more wall tension/stress and is at greater risk for rupture.
- **In the heart:** A dilated, thin-walled myocardium, under increasing pressure and volume has higher wall tension (and the myocardial oxygen demand is elevated).
  - P within the ventricle depends on afterload (e.g., TPR, aortic stenosis).
  - r within the ventricle depends on preload (amount of venous return).
  - (t) thickness of the ventricle: Increased thickness decreases wall stress to a point, then
  - Oxygen demand increases because of greater muscle mass.
  - Oxygen supply decreases by narrowing coronary vessels.

Blood Vessel Types and Characteristics

Arteries*	Arterioles	Capillaries	Veins
Oxygenated blood carried under high-pressure from heart to body. Muscular walls. High pressure. Low compliance.	Regulate blood flow into capillaries. *Primary resistance vessels* Tissue metabolites, humoral factors affect vasoconstriction and vasodilation.	Nutrient, oxygen, and waste exchange. Thin walls.	Carry deoxygenated blood back to heart. Large lumens. High compliance (volume reservoirs). May have valves.

*Pulmonary and umbilical arteries carry deoxygenated blood. Pulmonary vein carries oxygenated blood.

Oxygen Exchange

CAPILLARIES

- Greatest total area.
- Large surface area.
- Slowest velocity of an individual blood cell.
  - Allows time for oxygen, nutrient exchange/diffusion.

ARTERIOLES

- Account for:
  - Largest drop in BP (~50% drop from arteries to arterioles).
  - Highest proportion of peripheral vascular resistance.
- Pressure decreases as blood moves through systemic circulation.
  - This pressure gradient is required for blood flow.

At rest most capillaries are closed. In active tissue they dilate and perfuse. In inflammation capillary leakiness is mediated by substance P, bradykinin, etc.

▶ BLOOD VOLUME

Most is held within the **systemic venous circulation**:

- >60% in systemic veins.
- >10% in systemic arteries.
- <10% in arterioles and capillaries.
- 9% in pulmonary vessels.
- 7% in heart.

Venules are small veins that collect blood from capillaries (coalesce into larger veins).

▶ CAPACITANCE

- Ability to hold blood volume.
- Act as a reservoir.

- Veins.
  - Capacitance vessels.
  - Dilate to accommodate blood volume.
  - Hold 50–60% of blood volume.

In hypovolemia, veins/venules constrict.

- Sympathetic mediated.
- Compensatory.
  - No clinical manifestations with 15–20% blood loss.
  - Helps maintain mean systemic filling pressure in the face of blood loss.
  - Preload is maintained with venous constriction.

Arterial constriction system has much less effect on mean systemic filling pressure.

- Arterial system contains relatively small amount of blood.
- Arterial constriction increases afterload.

Capillaries do not constrict because they lack smooth muscle in their walls.

Comparison of Pulmonary and Systemic Circulations

	Pulmonary Circulation[a]	Systemic Circulation[b]
BP	↓	↑
Resistance	↓	↑
Compliance	↑ (store blood without changing BP).	↓
Circuit[c]	Right heart → pulmonary artery → lungs → pulmonary vein → left heart (oxygenated).	Left heart → aorta → systemic arteries/arterioles/capillaries → venules/veins → SVC, IVC → right heart (deoxygenated).

[a]Pulmonary arteries supply only the lung gas exchange areas (alveoli).
[b]Systemic circulation supplies the body with oxygenated blood. Note that the bronchial arteries are part of the systemic circulation that supplies the lung tissue and bronchi for cellular metabolism (*not* gas exchange).
[c]Volume of blood flow is 5L/min in both circuits (systemic and pulmonary).

▶ TOTAL PERIPHERAL RESISTANCE

- TPR (Peripheral vascular resistance).
- Vascular resistance of the systemic circulation.
- Mean arterial pressure minus central venous pressure divided by the cardiac output (MAP – CVP)/CO.
- Increases with sympathetic activation; arteriolar constriction.

> Because MAP = CO × TPR, the sympathetic/adrenergic system ↑ MAP by both:
> - ↑ CO (via ↑ HR and SV).
> - ↑ TPR (by vasoconstriction, $\alpha 1$).

	↑TPR	↓TPR
Example	Cold	Exercise

	Vasoconstriction α_1 (sympathetic nervous system).	Vasodilation
		• Especially in skeletal muscle
		  • β_2 (sympathetic nervous system).
		• Local metabolites
		  • Lactate.
		  • K^+.
		  • Adenosine.

Sympathetic activation ↓ venous compliance and ↑ venous return (returns more blood to heart). This ↑ CO, via the Starling mechanism, and more blood is pumped back into arterial circulation.

Factor	Regulates
TPR	Blood flow from systemic circulation into venous circulation.
CO	Blood flow from veins back into arterial system.
Compliance	Amount of blood in systemic veins.

▶ BLOOD PRESSURE

- Systolic pressure/diastolic pressure (120/80).
- **Pulse pressure** = SBP − DBP.
  - Normal is (120 − 80) = 40.
  - Increases with age because of stiffened arteries (atherosclerosis, arteriosclerosis).
- **Mean arterial pressure (MAP)** = ~DBP + pulse pressure/3.
  - MAP = CO × TPR.
  - Vascular compliance − increase in volume/increase in pressure.
  - Average pressure throughout the course of the cycle.
  - MAP is slightly less than halfway between SBP and DBP because diastole is longer than systole.

Hypertension: Wall:lumen ratio ↑, arteriolar and capillary density ↓. See pathology for further discussion of pathogenesis.

Pulse Pressure

Narrow	Wide
Decreased arterial compliance (stiff, less distensible wall) • HTN/Atherosclerosis • Aortic stenosis • Cardiac tamponade • Heart failure Decreased SV (less blood ejected with each beat)	AV malformations Aortic regurgitation

DETERMINANTS OF CARDIAC FUNCTION

Cardiac Output

- Cardiac output (CO) = Amount of blood pumped per minute.
- CO = HR × SV.
- Stroke volume (SV).
    - Amount of blood ejected with each beat.
    - SV = ~EDV − ESV.
    - Average SV is 70–80 ml.
- HR
    - Bradycardia = <60 bpm.
    - Tachycardia = >100 bpm.
- Average resting CO is ~5.6 L/min for men (10–20% less for women).
- Varies depending on body activity, age, body size, and condition of heart.
- CO = O_2 consumption/ ([O_2] pulmonary vein − [O_2] pulmonary artery).

EJECTION FRACTION

- Proportion of end diastolic blood pumped out during diastole.

EF = EDV-ESV/EDV (or SV/EDV).

FRANK–STARLING MECHANISM

- Most important determinant of CO is venous return. (See Figure 12–3.)
- ↑ venous return (EDV): ↑ ventricular filling in diastole: ↑ preload.

↓

- ↑ cross bridges between actin and myosin.

↓

- ↑ contraction force of cardiac muscle.

↓

- ↑ CO.

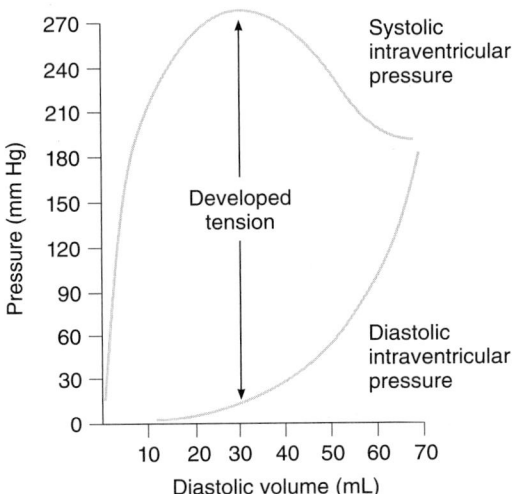

FIGURE 12–3. Frank–Starling mechanism.

Reproduced, with permission, from Ganong WF. *Review of Medical Physiology*, 22nd ed. McGraw-Hill, 2005.

- The fibrous pericardium prevents the heart from overdistending during diastole, keeping it working at an effective point on Starling's curve. With compensatory cardiac enlargement (occurring slowly) the pericardium also expands, becoming more lax. In this case the ventricle can overfill (fall off Starling's curve).
- Conversely, a pericardium that is too stiff, (or a pericardial space filled with fluid) results in underfilling or incomplete filling of the ventricle, leading to diastolic dysfunction and reduced stroke volumes.

Determinants of Cardiac Function

Myocardial Oxygen Supply	Myocardial Oxygen Demand
Arterial O_2 content Coronary blood flow ■ Coronary perfusion pressure ■ Patency	HR Contractility Wall stress (LaPlace's law)

Imbalance between myocardial oxygen supply and demand causes ischemia (angina) and myocardial infarction (MI).

Heart Rate and Contractility

- Increase with sympathetic activation and certain drugs.
- However, remember that sympathetic activation also ↑TPR.
- Remember, CO = HR × SV.

	Heart Rate	Contractility
Effect	Chronotrope	Inotrope
	A chronotrope ↑ HR by increasing rate of SA node depolarization. ↑HR will ↑CO until very high rate – when filling time is ↓.	Sympathetic or drug-mediated stimulation causes ↑ intracellular Ca^{2+}, which ↑ contraction force. ↑ force of contraction ↑ SV (and therefore CO).

- LaPlace's Law = Wall stress = Pr/t
  - P = pressure → **afterload**.
  - r = radius → **preload**.

	Preload	Afterload
	Filling of the ventricles (EDV)	Force against which the heart contracts
Determinants	Venous return* Radius of the ventricle (chamber size and expansion)	TPR (sympathetic activation, atherosclerosis) BP Aortic outflow tract (e.g., narrowed in aortic stenosis—fixed increase in afterload)

*Frank–Starling mechanism says that venous return (preload) has a greater effect on CO than does TPR (afterload). The best way to ↑ CO is to ↑ preload (↑venous return).

Venous Return

See Figure 12–4.

- **Skeletal muscle contraction**
  - Contraction pushes blood in veins back to heart.
  - Rhythmic contraction of leg muscles + presence of valves increase/allow venous return.
  - Counteracts force of gravity (that tends to pool blood in feet).
- **Compliance**
  - Intrathoracic pressure
    - ↑ intrathoracic pressure: ↑ venous compliance : ↓ venous return.
    - ↓ intrathoracic pressure : ↓ venous compliance : ↑ venous return.
  - Sympathetic nervous system
    - ↑ sympathetic tone : ↓ venous compliance (some constriction): ↑ venous return.

At very high heart rates (e.g., >150–200) CO actually falls. ↑↑↑HR → ↓diastolic filling → ↓SV → ↓CO. So even though ↑HR (which ordinarily ↑CO), the ↓SV is to such a great extent that CO actually ↓ (so will BP↓).

Coarctation of the aorta increases afterload. There is a difference when measuring BP between arms and legs (or left and right arms, pre-versus post-ductus). This type of differential BP may also be present in older patients with atherosclerosis or dissection.

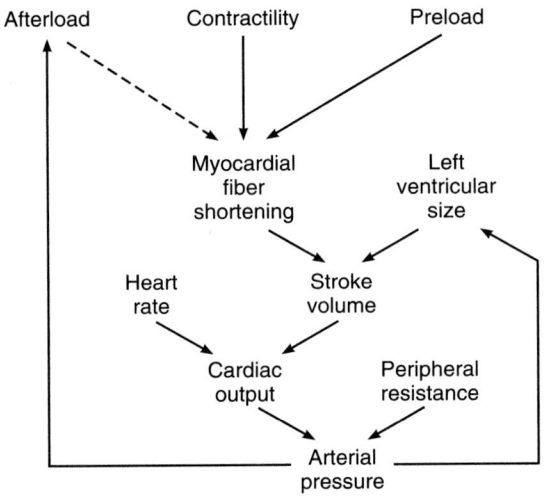

FIGURE 12–4. Venous return.

Reproduced, with permission, from Ganong WF. *Review of Medical Physiology*, 22nd ed. McGraw-Hill, 2005.

Cardiac Cycle

	Diastole (Filling Phase)[a]	Isovolumetric Contraction	Systole (Ejection Phase)	Isovolumetric Relaxation
AV valves	Open	Closed	Closed	Closed
Pulmonic, aortic valves [b]	Closed	Closed	Open	Closed
Heart sound		S1 ("lub")[c] Sound of the AV valves (mitral and tricuspid) closing. This sound begins systole (ventricular contraction).		S2 ("dub") Sound of the semilunar valves (aortic and pulmonic) closing. This sound begins diastole (ventricle filling).[d]
	Blood enters ventricles through the open AV valves: ■ 70–80% passive. ■ 20–30% b/c atrial "kick" (contraction). Diastole is the long phase of the cycle.		Blood is ejected out the open aortic and pulmonic valves.	

[a] The coronary arteries are perfused during diastole.
[b] The aortic valve closes before the pulmonic, causing a splitting of S2 (this is accentuated on inspiration).
[c] S1 is louder and longer than S2.
[d] The pericardium helps regulate ventricular filling. (See the earlier section on the "Frank–Starling Mechanism.")

Pressure–Volume Loop

See Figure 12–5.
See Figure 12–6 for the cardiac cycle.

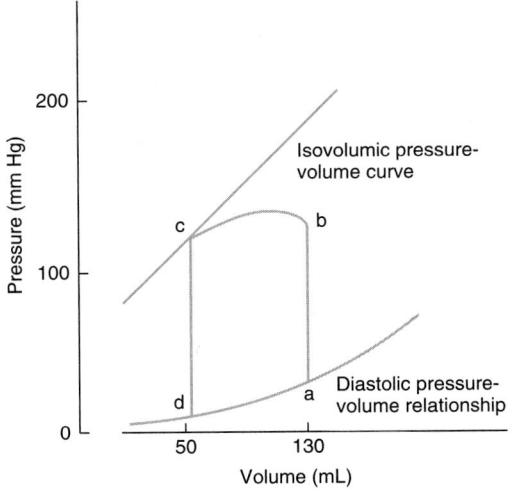

FIGURE 12-5. Pressure-loop volume.

Reproduced, with permission, from Ganong WF. *Review of Medical Physiology*, 22nd ed. McGraw-Hill, 2005.

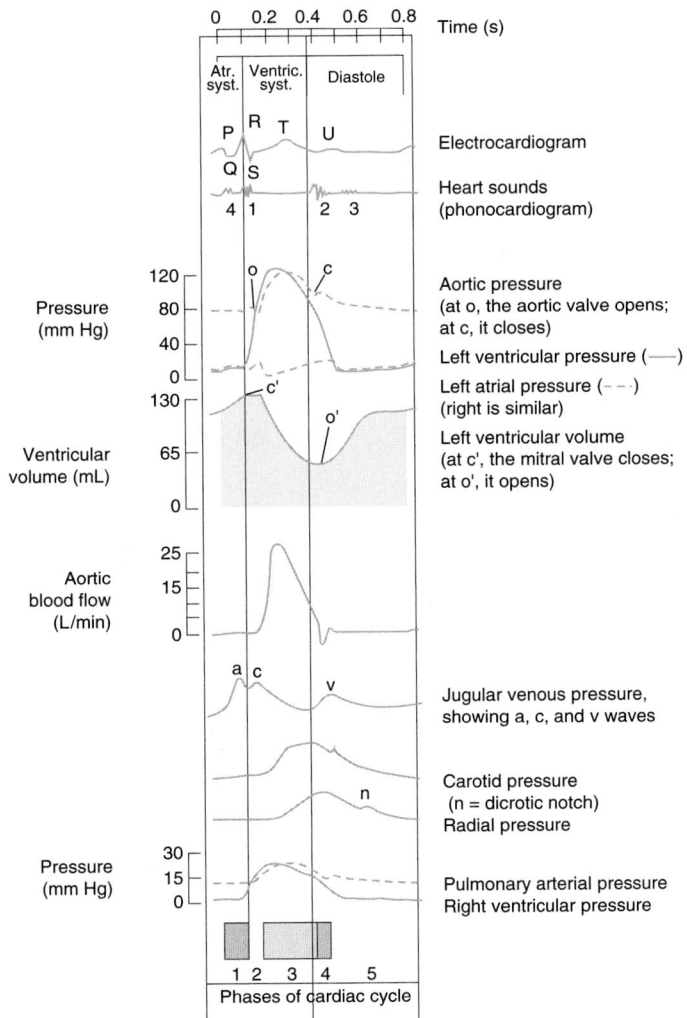

FIGURE 12-6. Cardiac cycle.

Reproduced, with permission, from Ganong WF. *Review of Medical Physiology*, 22nd ed. McGraw-Hill, 2005.

Heart Murmurs with Valvular Disease

Diastolic	Systolic
Aortic insufficiency	Aortic stenosis
Mitral stenosis	Mitral regurgitation

▶ ELECTROPHYSIOLOGY

Electrical Conduction of the Heart

See Figure 12–7.
- **Automaticity**
    - The spontaneous phase 4 depolarization that generates Aps.
    - This electrical signals conduct to atrial tissue, causing it to contract.
    - SA node → AV node → ventricular bundles (His/Purkinje) → ventricular myocytes → *ventricular contraction*.
- **Refractory period**
    - Long refractory period of heart allows relaxation (diastolic filling) and prevents the heart from going into reentry (arrhythmia).
    - Takes 0.22 seconds for AP to spread through the heart.
    - Ventricular muscle's refractory period is 0.25–0.30 second.
    - Atrial muscle's refractory period is 0.15 second.

> *As opposed to cardiac muscle, skeletal muscle has short a refractory period.*
> - This allows successive stimulation, a short time after initial contraction.
> - Tetany serves to increase strength of contraction.

Absolute Refractory Period	Relative Refractory Period
During this, another AP cannot be elicited, regardless of magnitude of stimulus. Determined by Na^+ channel inactivation/gate closure.	Immediately follows the absolute refractory period. Continues until the membrane potential returns to resting level. During this, it is possible to generate another AP but need larger stimulus.

Cardiac Conductive Tissues

Nodal/Pacemaker Tissue	Cardiac Myocytes
	Gap junctions relay electrical signals, causing contraction.
Phases 0–4.	Phases 0–4.
Phase 0 dependent on Ca^{2+}.	Phase 0 dependent on Na^+.

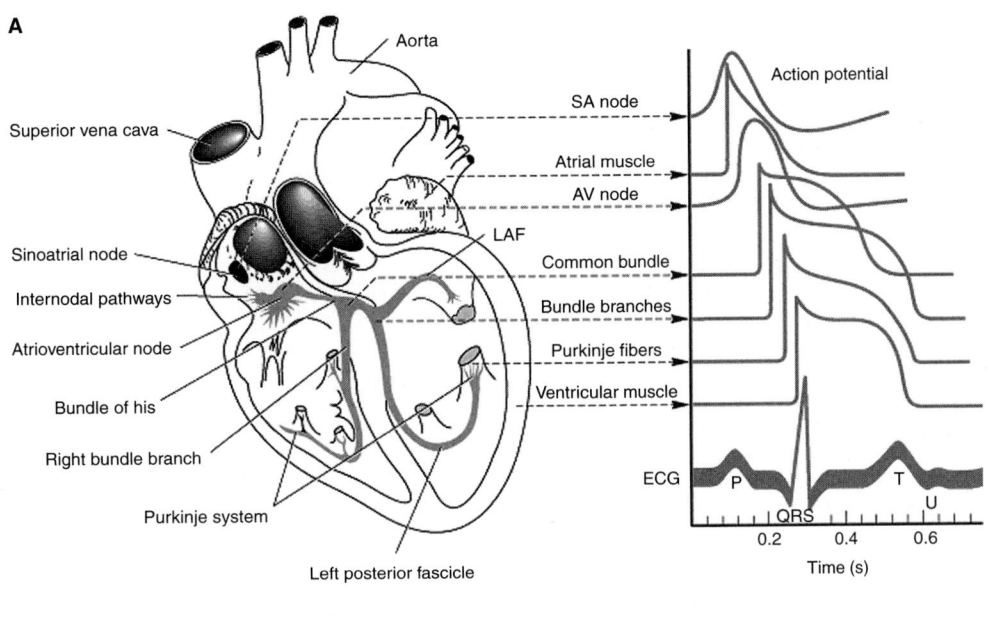
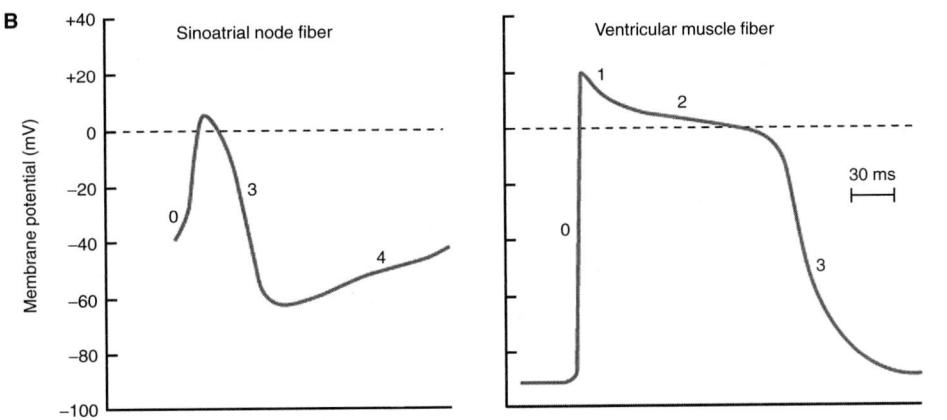

FIGURE 12-7. Electrical conduction of the heart.

Reproduced, with permission, from Ganong WF. *Review of Medical Physiology*, 22nd ed. McGraw-Hill, 2005.

Nodal/Pacemaker Conduction System

SA Node	Internodal Pathways	Av Node	His-Purkinje System
Located in post wall of RA near opening of SVC. Pacemaker of the heart (starts the depolarization). Depolarizes at intrinsic rate that drives depolarization of rest of heart. Transmits signals faster than AV. Atria contract before ventricles, preventing fast, arrythmogenic beats from reaching the ventricle.	Transmits depolarization wave from the SA node to the LA and AV node.[a]	Located in the lower right interatrial septum. The impulse is delayed in AV node (~0.13s) (slow conduction rate). Atria to contract before ventricles.	Fiber network arising in AV node. Purkinje fibers originate from R and L bundle branches.[b] Extend to papillary muscles and lateral walls of ventricles. Depolarization wave travels extremely fast through bundle branches and Purkinje fibers. Total elapsed time is 0.03 sec.

[a] Aside from AV node, the atria and ventricles are electrically isolated.
[b] HIS-Purkinje fibers fan across subendocardial surface of ventricles from endocardium outward through the myocardium. As cardiac impulse spreads, these fibers cause ventricles to depolarize and contract.

▶ ELECTROCARDIOGRAM (EKG)

- Records the flow of electrical impulses through the heart.

See Figure 12–8 for EKG waves.

- To read EKG:
    - Remember that a single lead corresponds to an anatomic territory.
    - Look at multiple leads together for voltage abnormalities and axis deviations.
    - Look at a single lead for arrhythmias.

EKG Leads

Standard Bipolar	Standard Unipolar	Chest leads
I—right arm (−), left arm (+) II—right arm (−) and left leg (+) III—left arm (−) and left leg (+)	AVR—right arm (+) AVL—left arm (+) AVF—left leg (+)	V1, V2, V3, V4, V5, V6 represent 6 places along chest wall.

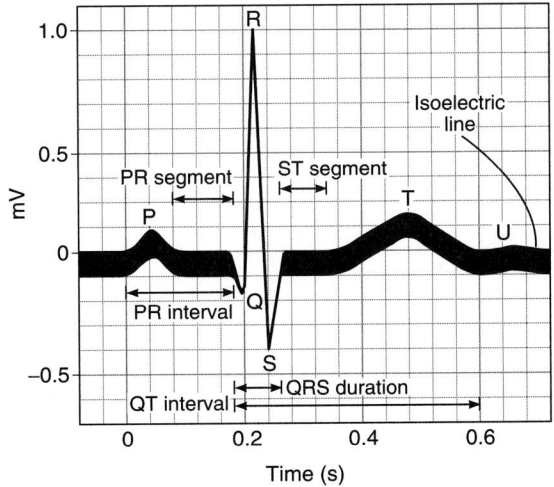

FIGURE 12-8. Waves of the EKG.

Reproduced, with permission, from Ganong WF. *Review of Medical Physiology*, 22nd ed. McGraw-Hill, 2005.

EKG Waves

P	PR Interval	QRS	ST Segment	T[a,b,c]
Atrial depolarization.	Length between depolarization of atria and depolarization of ventricles (~0.16s).	Ventricular depolarization During phase 0, atrial repolarization occurs within QRS. Highest Na^+ influx; maximum ventricular Na^+ channel conductance. Shape of QRS complex is dictated by spread of the AP throughout the ventricular muscle.	Length corresponds to AP duration in ventricular muscle. Entire ventricle is depolarized. During phase 2, prolonged calcium conductance through slow channels.	Ventricular repolarization.
Prior to atrial contraction	Varies w/ HR (↑HR : ↓ PR).	Prior to contraction.	Isoelectric.	

[a] U wave is occasionally found in EKGs. This is caused by repolarization of papillary muscle, or it can be seen with hypokalemia.
[b] QT interval is the period between ventricular depolarization and repolarization (~0.35s).
[c] The isoelectric point between T and P waves (ventricle is at resting membrane potential) occurs during ventricular diastole (when ventricle is filling with blood) and is shortened at high HRs.

REGULATORY MECHANISMS

Autonomic Control of the Heart

	Sympathetic	Parasympathetic
Control center	Medulla	Medulla
Nerve	T1–4	Vagus nerve (CN X)
NT	NE	Ach
HR	↑	↓
	↑ SA nodal discharge. ↑ Rate of depolarization through heart. ↑ Intracellular Ca^{2+}. ↑ Ventricular contraction force.	↓ SA nodal discharge. ↓ Rate of depolarization through heart.

The right vagus nerve supplies the SA node; the left vagus nerve innervates the AV node.

Bainbridge Reflex

- Stretch of atria (with ↑ blood volume) causes ↑ HR and, therefore, ↑ CO.
- Mediated by stretch receptors in atria.
- Receptor cells are sensitive to pressure and stretch.
    - Mediated by vagal (CN X) afferents to the medulla.
        - Efferent loop is slowing of vagal output.
- Pumps more blood out of pulmonary system to the systemic system.
    - This helps prevent pulmonary edema.

Receptors

Receptor type	Baroreceptor	Chemoreceptor
Effect exerted	HR, BP	Respiration > vasomotor

Baroreceptors

- Modulate intravascular pressure and HR over a short time period.
- Activated by ↑ BP.
- Causes ↓ HR, vasodilation, ↓ BP.

BARORECEPTOR REFLEX

- ↑ BP → ↑ parasympathetic afferent output (CN IX, X) → medulla → ↑ vagal efferent tone (CN X) (↓ sympathetic tone) → ↓ HR, ↓ BP (vasodilation, venodilation) → ↓ CO.

Carotid Sinus[a]	Aortic Arch Baroreceptor[a]
Spindle-shaped dilation of receptors at the common carotid artery bifurcation (superior border of thyroid cartilage).	Receptors in the aortic arch.
Afferent = CN IX.	Afferent = CN X.

[a]These receptors are located in the adventitia of the vessels. They are extensively branched, knobby, coiled, and intertwined ends of myelinated nerve fibers (resemble Golgi tendon organs).

Stretch receptors in the atria and pulmonary circulations are stimulated by expansion of blood volume; they do not directly respond to changes in systemic arterial BP.

Carotid Sinus Syndrome

- Excessive stimulation of both carotid sinuses (e.g., convulsive seizures) can lead to momentary loss of consciousness.

Response to Sudden Standing

- ↓ BP in brain, upper body sensed by baroreceptors →
- ↓ parasympathetic firing (CN IX, X); (sympathetic discharge → ↑HR, ↑ conduction velocity, ↑ cardiac contractility, ↑peripheral resistance ↑vasoconstriction), ↓ renal blood flow ↑α-1 vasocontriction of afferent artery; β-1 on JGA → ↑renin → ↑ angiotensin-II → aldosterone) → ↑ blood back to heart (↑preload because venoconstriction of large veins) → ↑ CO → return/maintain BP.

Hemorrhage or Hypovolemia

Compensations:

- Baroreceptor reflex (↑ sympathetic, ↓ parasympathetic tone).
    - ↑ epinephrine from adrenal medulla.
    - ↓ vagal output from medulla (↓ carotid sinus, ↓ aortic baroreceptor firing).
- RAAS (Renin-Angiotensin-Aldosterone system). See renal also.
    - AT-II, aldosterone.
- ADH
    - Capillary fluid shift.

Chemoreceptors

- Detect changes in blood oxygen, carbon dioxide, and hydrogen ion concentrations.
- Modulate respiratory center in brain (regulate respiratory activity).

Carotid Body	Aortic Body
Afferent CN IX	Afferent CN X

CHEMORECEPTOR PATHWAY

- See also Chapter 13, "Respiratory Physiology."
- ↑CO_2, ↑H^+, and/or ↓O_2 → stimulates chemoreceptors (carotid, aortic bodies) → ↑ parasympathetic afferent output (CN IX, X) → medulla (respiratory center) → ↑ ventilation → (↑BP, ↑HR secondary to simultaneous secretion of catecholamines from the adrenal medulla).

Hormonal Regulation Systems

See Chapter 14, "Renal, Fluid, Acid–Base Physiology."

Exercise

- Mechanisms to meet ↑ demand to muscles during exercise (↑supply)
- ↑CO because ↑ HR and ↑SV.
- Sympathetic nervous system
  - β_2 adrenergic receptors in muscle
    - Vasodilate
    - ↑ Blood flow to muscles
  - β_1 receptors in heart
    - ↑ HR
    - ↑ Contraction force (inotropic)
    - ↑ CO
  - α_1 in other parts of body
    - Vasoconstriction
    - ↑Arterial pressure
- Enhanced venous return (↑ preload)
  - ↓ venous compliance
  - Pumping effect of the skeletal muscle
  - Vasoconstriction
- Local metabolites (released as O_2↓0)
  - Adenosine, CO_2, lactic acid
    - Vasodilate: ↓vascular resistance, ↑ blood flow

Note: During exercise ↑ CO is slightly > ↓ TPR, so MAP ↑.

During exercise initially ↑ SV, then later ↑ HR (which is important, >50% of maximal work capacity is reached).

SVR ↓ during exercise (vasodilation, β_2, local metabolites). Blood flow to skeletal muscle can increase 20-fold during strenuous exercise.

AUTOREGULATION OF BLOOD FLOW

- As blood flow ↑ to muscles during exercise, the adenosine is washed out.
- ↓ adenosine → arterioles and small arteries vasoconstrict → keeping blood flow at a normal rate (in face of ↑arterial pressure).

▶ HEMATOCRIT (HCT)

- Percentage of RBCs in blood sample
- Normal:
  - Male: 44–46.
  - Female: 40–42.
- Venous HCT is typically higher than arterial HCT because of "chloride shift."

▶ HEMOGLOBIN CONCENTRATION

- See also Chapter 6, "Biological Compounds" and Chapter 13, "Respiratory Physiology," for discussion of hemoglobin (Hb).

- Normal
    - Male: 15–16 g/dl.
    - Female: 13–14 g/dl.
- Severe anemia
    - <7.5 g/dl.

▶ ANEMIA

- ↓ HCT.
- ↓ RBC and/or ↓ Hb concentration.

Consequences of Anemia

- ↓ oxygen transport in blood.
- Fatigue, respiratory compensation, cardiac compensation.
- Hypoxia in the tissues.
    - Causes small arteries and arterioles to dilate (so ↑ blood return to the heart (preload).
- Hypoxia in the pulmonary circulation results in vasoconstriction of those vessels.

Compensations with Anemia

Cardiac Compensation	Respiratory Compensation
↑ CO Chemoreceptors sense ↑O_2. • ↑SV (↑ pulse pressure). • ↑HR (try to deliver more O_2 to tissues). ↓HCT → ↓blood viscosity. • ↓ resistance to flow → ↓ PVR. • ↑ blood returns to the heart (↑ preload).	Bohr effect O_2–Hb curve shifts to the right (→). Unloads more O_2 to the tissues. • ↑2, 3-DPG. • ↑CO. • ↑RBC H^+.

Types of Anemia

↓ Production	↑ Destruction
Fe deficiency	Blood loss
Folate deficiency	Hemolysis
B_{12} deficiency	Hemoglobinopathies

Note: Carbon monoxide poisoning

- CO competes with oxygen for Hb binding sites; CO has greater affinity.
- Normal Hb level.
- O_2 content ↓.

Cyanosis

- Deoxygenated hemoglobin in tissues gives the skin/mucous membranes a blue tint.
- Does **not** occur in severe anemia because you need >5 gm of deoxygenated Hb per 100 ml of blood to appreciate.

▶ ERYTHROPOIETIN

- Glycoprotein hormone produced in kidneys.
- ↑ RBC production by bone marrow.
- Acts at the hemocytoblast (pluripotent stem cell).
- ↓ Erythropoiesis → **anemia**.
- ↑ Erythropoiesis → **polycythemia**.
  - ↑ blood viscosity, sluggish blood flow.

Negative Feedback

- ↓ O_2 tension (anoxia/hypoxia) → ↑ erythropoietin.
- ↑ O_2 → ↓ erythropoietin.

▶ COAGULATION AND HEMOSTASIS

Virchow's Triad

- Endothelial injury
- Stasis
- Hypercoaguability

Tissue factor (tissue thromboplastin) is part of the extrinsic pathway (it is not present in blood).

Hemostasis

- Three parts:
  - Vasoconstriction
  - Platelet aggregation/plug
  - Coagulation

Both intrinsic and extrinsic pathways are activated when blood vessels are damaged.

Coagulation

See Figure 12–9.

- Intrinsic and extrinsic pathways
  - Prothrombin is cleaved to thrombin.
    - Converted by prothrombin activator (Factor V_a).
  - Fibrinogen cleaved to fibrin.
    - Converted by thrombin.
  - Fibrin forms the clot and cross-links with the platelets.

In cirrhosis, proteins, including prothrombin and fibrinogen, are deficient.

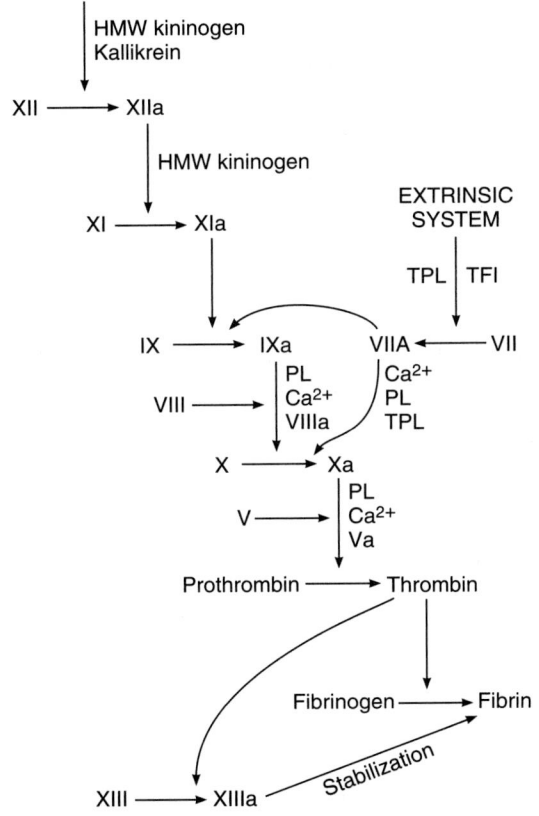

FIGURE 12-9. Intrinsic and extrinsic pathways of coagulation.

Reproduced, with permission, from Ganong WF. *Review of Medical Physiology*, 22nd ed. McGraw-Hill, 2005.

CHAPTER 13
Respiratory Physiology

Lung Volumes	362
Lung Mechanics	363
INSPIRATION	363
EXPIRATION	363
Gas Exchange in the Lungs	365
Hemoglobin	365
O_2-HB DISSOCIATION CURVE	365
BOHR EFFECT	366
HALDANE EFFECT	366
AMOUNT OF O_2 IN BLOOD	366
CARBON DIOXIDE	368
HYPOXEMIA	368
HYPERCARBIA	369
HYPERVENTILATION	370
Respiratory Regulation	370
RESPIRATORY DRIVE	370
ACID–BASE BALANCE AND RESPIRATORY CHANGES	372
HEHRING–BREUER REFLEX	373
PULMONARY CHEMOREFLEX	373
HIGH ALTITUDE	374

▶ LUNG VOLUMES

See Figure 13–1.

Lung volumes

Inspiratory reserve volume (IRV)	Air inspired with maximal inspiratory effort (after inspiring at TV).	Inspiratory capacity (IC)	Maximum air inspired up to TLC (limited by elastic recoil of lung).
Tidal volume (TV)	Air inspired or expired with a normal breath.	(TV + IRV)	
Expiratory reserve volume (ERV)	Air pushed out after passive expiration (FRC – RV).	Functional residual capacity (FRC)	Air left in lungs after a normal passive expiration.
Residual volume (RV)	Air remaining in lungs after maximal exhalation; cannot be measured by spirometry.	(ERV + RV)	

RV is increased in older individuals and in chronic obstructive pulmonary disease (COPD) or asthma because of air trapping.

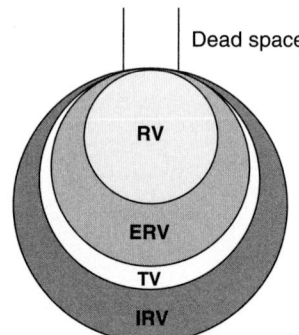
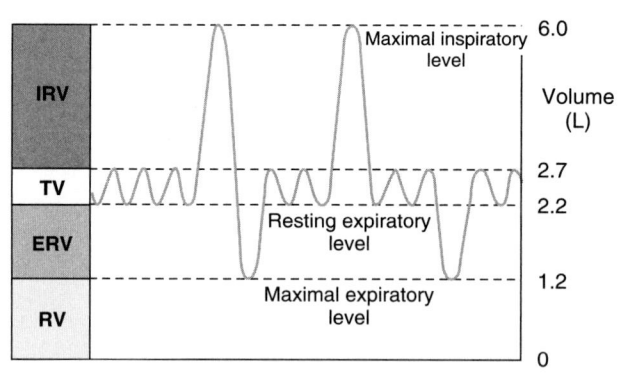

FIGURE 13–1. Lung volumes.

Reproduced, with permission, from Ganong WF. *Review of Medical Physiology*, 22nd ed. McGraw-Hill, 2005.

- Total lung volume (TLV) = IRV + TV + ERV + RV.
- Vital capacity (VC) = TLV − RV.

▶ LUNG MECHANICS

Inspiration

- Active process
  - Requires muscular effort.
    - Mostly diaphragm at rest.
    - Intercostals used on exertion.
- Inspiratory effort causes:
  - ↓ intrapleural pressure.
  - ↓ alveolar pressure.
  - Pressure gradient from mouth to alveoli.
  - Gas flow down pressure gradient.

Expiration

- Passive process (usually).
  - Due to lung recoil.
- Relaxation of inspiratory muscles causes:
  - ↑ Intrapleural pressure (intrapleural pressure becomes less negative).
  - ↑ Alveolar pressure.
  - Pressure gradient from alveoli to mouth.
  - Gas flow down pressure gradient.

VC = greatest amount of air that one can exchange in a forced respiration (inhalation + expiration).

FUNCTIONAL RESIDUAL CAPACITY

- FRC = At rest.
- Balance between inspiratory and expiratory forces.
  - Collapsing forces = Expanding forces.
- Muscle contraction is needed to ↑ or ↓ lung volume from FRC.

Collapsing Forces	Expanding Forces
Favors ↓ lung volume. ■ Elastic connective tissue of the lungs	Favors ↑ lung volume. ■ Elastic connective tissue of chest wall
↑ Surface tension helps *counteract* collapse. ■ Surfactant coating the alveoli	

ALVEOLAR PRESSURE

- Atmospheric pressure in resting position.
- 760 mm Hg (at FRC).

INTRAPLEURAL PRESSURE

- Pressure within pleural cavity between outer surface lung and inner surface chest cavity.
- 756 mm Hg (at FRC).

Alveolar Ventilation

- (V_A) = RR × (TV − dead space air volume).
- Amount of gas that reaches the functional respiratory units (i.e., alveoli) per minute.
- Amount of atmospheric air that can undergo gas exchange.
- Good gauge for breathing effectiveness.

Respiratory Rate

- Breaths per minute.

Tidal Volume

- TV = amount of air brought into/out of lungs with a normal breath.
- 500 mL
  - 350 mL used for alveolar ventilation.
  - 150 mL dead space.

Dead Space

- V_D = Volume of air not participating in gas exchange.
- Anatomic dead space
  - Typically 150 mL.
  - Volume of nonventilated gas in airways.
  - No gas exchange occurs within the nasal passages, pharynx, trachea, bronchi.
- Physiologic dead space
  - Due to alveoli that are ventilated but not perfused.
  - Usually insignificant, unless there is disease.

Minute Ventilation

- TV × RR.

Zones of the Lung

Conducting zone (no gas exchange)	Trachea Main bronchi Bronchioles Terminal bronchioles
Respiratory zone (gas exchange occurs)	Respiratory bronchioles Alveoli

- Conducting zone airways contain mucous-secreting cells:
  - Goblet cells
  - Mucous cells

- Respiratory zone, alveolar wall has:
  - Type I epithelial cells
  - Type II epithelial cells ↓ pneumocytes)
    - Produce surfactant
  - See also Chapter 2.

GAS EXCHANGE IN THE LUNGS

- O_2 uptake, CO_2 elimination by the blood
    - O_2 diffusion (alveolus → blood)
    - CO_2 diffusion (alveolus ← blood)
- Depends on:
    - **Partial pressure gradient**
        - Pressure difference between two sides of the membrane.
        - Diffusion occurs from high to low pressure (down the gradient).
            - $PAO_2 > PaO_2$ (alveolar > pulmonary arterial); O_2 diffuses from alveoli → blood.
            - PCO_2 blood > PCO_2 in alveolus; CO_2 diffuses from blood → alveoli.
    - **Gas solubility**
        - Number of molecules dissolved in the liquid ↑ partial pressure of gas ↑.
        - Solubility is an intrinsic property of the gas.
        - Solubility ↑ as partial pressure ↑ (Henry's law).
    - **Thickness of membrane** (alveolus)
        - Rate of diffusion is inversely proportional to the diffusion distance.
            - ↑ diffusion as ↓ alveolar thickness.
    - **Alveolar surface area**
        - Rate of diffusion is directly proportional to surface area.
            - ↓ surface area (e.g., emphysema), ↓ diffusion, ↓ gas exchange.

HEMOGLOBIN

- See also Biological Compounds, Chapter 6.
- Carries O_2 from lungs to tissues.
- Carries CO_2 from tissues to lungs.
- Normally:
    - 98% saturated with O_2 in lungs (arterial).
    - 75% saturated in tissues (venous).
    - 300 million Hb molecules in each erythrocyte.
        - Synthesis begins in erythroblasts.

O_2-Hb Dissociation Curve

See Figure 13–2.

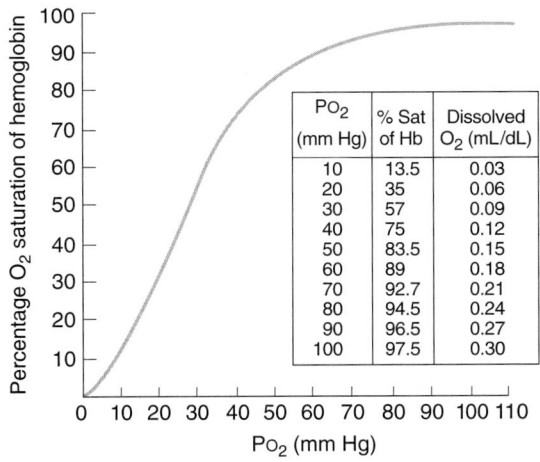

FIGURE 13-2. O_2–Hb dissociation curve.

Reproduced, with permission, from Ganong WF. *Review of Medical Physiology*, 22nd ed. McGraw-Hill, 2005.

The PO_2 determines the affinity of Hb for O_2 binding by causing a conformational change of Hb.

CO has 240 times the affinity for Hb as O_2 does. It therefore interferes with unloading of O_2 from Hb.

Shift	Left Shift	Right Shift
Effect	Favors O_2 uptake (e.g., at lungs).	Favors O_2 release (to tissues).
Causes	↑ Ph. ↓ 2, 3-DPG. ↓ temperature. CO.	↓ pH. ↑ PCO_2. ↑ 2, 3-DPG. ↑ temperature.
	When PO_2 is low, Hb has a greater affinity for O_2 binding at the lungs.	When PO_2 is high, Hb does not bind O_2 as readily. O_2 is released to the tissues.
		Exercising muscle: Temperature ↑, pH goes ↓ (lactic acid ↑), 2, 3-DPG ↑.

2, 3-DPG is a product of glycolysis via the Ebden–Myerhoff pathway (see biochemistry section).

Example: O_2-Hb curve shifts to the right (→) in anemia. This helps unload O_2 to the tissues. It occurs because there is ↑ 2, 3-DPG, ↑ CO_2, and ↑RBC H+'s (↓pH).

Venous blood carries more CO_2 than arterial blood, and CO_2 uptake is facilitated in the tissues and CO_2 release is facilitated in the lungs.

AV fistula: Venous PCO_2 is lower than normal (because it bypassed the tissues); likewise venous PO_2 is higher (some O_2 is not dropped off at the tissues).

Bohr Effect

Curve shifts right (→) in an acidic environment (↓pH) to help unload O_2 to the tissues.

- Hb has decreased affinity for O_2 when pH ↓.
- H^+'s ↑ as pH ↓.
- The H^+'s bond more actively to deoxygenated Hb than to oxyhemoglobin.
- As CO_2 ↑, pH ↓, curve shifts to the right (→).

Haldane Effect

- Oxygen tension affects the affinity of Hb for CO_2.
- High oxygen tension—lungs:
  - Hb ↑ O_2 binding; ↓ affinity for CO_2.
    - CO_2 released in the lungs (as ↓ O_2–Hb).
- Low oxygen tension—tissues:
  - Hb ↓ O_2 binding; ↑ affinity for CO_2 (binds H^+, forms carbamino compounds).
  - CO_2 uptake in the tissues (as ↓ O_2–Hb).

Amount of O_2 in Blood

Dissolved O_2	O_2–Hb
Partial pressure of O_2 in blood (PO_2)	$Hb + O_2 \leftrightarrow HbO_2$ $Hb4(O_2)4$
Small fraction of the total O_2 carried in the blood. - 0.003 mL/dL blood/mm Hg PO_2.	Hb-O_2 depends on: - PO_2. O_2 content (pulmonary function, anemia). Hb concentration. - Hb affinity for O_2. %Hb bound with O_2 = O_2 saturation.

OXYGEN CONTENT

- Total amount of oxygen carried in blood ($PO_2 + O_2$–Hb).
- Determined mostly by the amount of hemoglobin and its saturation.
- Amount of hemoglobin is affected by anemia (production, loss, or destruction).
- The more hemoglobin in blood, the more O_2 that can be carried.

OXYGEN SATURATION

- The amount of Hb saturated with O_2.
- Corresponds to O_2–Hb curve.
- Determined by:
  - PO_2 (important; see table corresponding $SaO_2 : PO_2$).
  - O_2 affinity of Hb altered by:
    - Changes in Hb molecule.
      - Intrinsic (hemoglobinopathies).
      - Extrinsic (e.g., changes in pH, PCO_2, temperature, etc.)
      - Competition for Hb binding (e.g. CO poisoning).

NORMAL VALUES

- Oxygen content (per 1 gm Hb) = 1.34 mL of O_2.
- Hemoglobin concentration = ~15 gm/dL.
  - Women: 12–16 gm/dL.
  - Men: 14–18 gm/dL.
  - Infants: 14–20 gm/dL.
- Oxygen concentration = ~20 gm-mL/dL (or 15 gm/dL × 1.34 mL)—just 20.1 mL.

Remember: Blood Hb concentration does not affect O_2 saturation of Hb or PaO_2 (both PaO_2 and SaO_2 are independent of the Hb concentration).

Remember: With anemia, ↑ CO as compensation to maintain adequate oxygenation to the tissues.

OXYGEN-CARRYING CAPACITY OF BLOOD

Depends on:

- Oxygenation (from lungs).
  - FiO_2.
  - PaO_2 (gradient).
  - Effective gas exchange (no dead space or shunt).
- Hb concentration.
- Hb avidity for oxygen.
  - CO.
  - Left shift of curve.
- Perfusion.
  - Cardiac function.
  - Patency of vessels.
  - Adequacy of forward flow.

> **Key Points:**
> - Most O_2 in blood is carried by Hb.
> - Only a small amount of oxygen is dissolved in blood under normal conditions.
> - PO_2 (difference/gradient between alveolus and capillary) is what drives oxygen transfer to the blood.

Carbon Dioxide

See Figure 13–3.

- Carbon dioxide (CO_2) is carried in blood as:
  - **Bicarbonate in serum** (most).
  - Bicarbonate in RBC.
  - Carbaminohemoglobin
    - CO_2^+ NH_2 group of Heme (**not** Fe_2^+ of Heme like O_2 or CO).
  - Dissolved in blood (PCO_2).

Carbonic anhydrase is not present in the serum. Bicarbonate can be produced in serum by nonenzymatic means, but the process is slow.

CHLORIDE SHIFT

- Bicarbonate carried in serum is generated within the RBC.
- It is transported to the serum in exchange for Cl^-.
- Cycle:
  - CO_2 in blood diffuses passively into RBC.
  - Carbonic anhydrase (within RBC) combines intracellular CO_2 with H_2O to form bicarbonate and H^+.
  - Bicarbonate passes across the RBC membrane into serum in exchange for Cl^-.

Hypoxemia in COPD is secondary to both hypoventilation (↑ PCO) and V/Q mismatch (A-a gradient).

Hypoxemia

- Low oxygen level in blood (PO_2 <80).
- Causes of hypoxemia:
  - ↓ FiO_2
  - Hypoventilation
  - V/Q mismatch
  - Shunt
  - Diffusion limitation

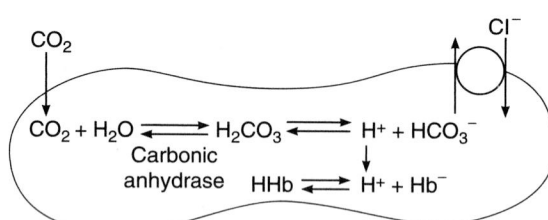

FIGURE 13–3. Carbon dioxide (CO_2) as carried in the blood.

Reproduced, with permission, from Ganong WF. *Review of Medical Physiology*, 22nd ed. McGraw-Hill, 2005.

Causes of Hypoxemia

↓ Fio$_2$	Hypoventilation	V/Q Mismatch	Shunt	Diffusion Limitation (↓ DLCO)
↓ fraction of inspired O$_2$ (usually 21%). ■ High altitude ■ Incorrect ventilator settings	↓ respiratory drive (central). ■ Narcotics ■ Medullary injury ↓ ability for chest excursion (peripheral) ■ Polio ■ Chest trauma (rib fracture) ■ Diaphragmatic injury ■ Phrenic nerve paralysis	Unequal ventilation and perfusion. Segment of lung is ventilated but not perfused (= dead space). ■ Asthma ■ COPD ■ Interstitial lung disease ■ Alveolar disease ■ Pulmonary vascular disease	Segment of lung is perfused but not aerated. Intraalveolar filling ■ Atelectasis ■ Pneumonia ■ Pulmonary edema ■ Intracardiac shunt ■ Vascular shunt	↓ surface area of blood gas barrier. ■ Pneumonectomy ■ Emphysema Thick blood–gas barrier ■ Diffuse interstitial fibrosis ■ Sarcoidosis ■ Asbestosis ■ ARDS ↓ Hb to carry oxygen ■ Anemia ■ PE

HYPOXIC VASOCONSTRICTION

- Mechanism to minimize V/Q mismatch.
- Example:
  - Shunt (air cannot get into alveolus).
    - Peanut occluding bronchiole (child).
    - Atelectasis.
- Blood perfuses past that alveolus.
- No/minimal gas exchange occurs.
- Response is vasoconstriction of the pulmonary vasculature in that region.
  - ↓ amount of blood going to nonventilated segment of lung.
- If this vasoconstriction secondary to hypoxia exists for long enough,
  - Get permanent secondary changes to the pulmonary vasculature.
  - Pulmonary hypertension.

Hypercarbia

- ↑ CO$_2$ in blood.
- Occurs because of either or both of the following:
  - ↑ CO$_2$ production.
  - ↓ V$_A$ (alveolar ventilation)—hypoventilation.
- Compensation: Hyperventilation.

Note: Extreme hypercarbia (CO$_2$ ↑↑) depresses the CNS (including respiratory center) whereby respiratory compensation does not occur. Result is CO$_2$ **narcosis:**

- Headache.
- Confusion.
- Coma.

Hyperventilation

- ↑ Rate and depth of breathing exceeding requirement for O_2 delivery and CO_2 removal
- Stimulated by:
  - **↓ PO_2 in normal circumstances** (non-COPD).
  - Chemoreceptor stimulation (↑CO_2, ↑H^+, ↓PO_2).
  - Effect on brain—emotional situations, anxiety.
- Results in:
  - ↓ CO_2: hypocapnia (hypocarbia).
  - Respiratory alkalosis (pH ↑).
  - ↑cerebrovascular resistance.
  - ↓ cerebral blood flow.
  - ↑PO_2 (and arterial oxygen concentration).

Effect of CO_2 on Cerebral Circulation

↑ PCO_2	↓ PCO_2
Vasodilation → ↑ cerebral blood flow.	Vasoconstriction → ↓ cerebral blood flow.

SYMPTOMS OF HYPERVENTILATION

- Related to ↓ cerebral blood flow.
- Example: Anxiety → ↑ventilation → ↓ CO_2 → ↓ cerebral blood flow → neurologic symptoms:
  - Faintness/dizziness.
  - Blurred vision.
  - Also experience sensation of:
    - Suffocation.
    - Chest tightness.
- Terminate hyperventilation attack must:
  - ↑ PCO_2.
    - Breathing in and out of a plastic bag.
    - Inhale 5% CO_2 mixture.

Note: In shock, hyperventilation is caused by chemoreceptor stimulation (secondary to ↓ PO_2 (hypoxia) and ↑ H^+ (acidosis) because of local stagnation of blood flow.

▶ RESPIRATORY REGULATION

Respiratory Drive

- Based on arterial PCO_2, specifically H^+.
- The H^+ (derived from CO_2) that acts at central chemoeceptors (Medulla).

PATHWAY

- As ↑ PCO_2 → CO_2 diffuses from cerebral blood vessels into CSF → carbonic acid (H_2CO_3) is formed → dissociates into bicarbonate (HCO_3^-) and protons ($H+$s) → these protons ($H+$s) stimulate the central chemoreceptors → ↑ventilation.

↑Respiratory Drive

- Central chemoreceptors (medulla)
  - ↑ PCO_2 (as its byproduct, H^+, in CSF or brain interstitial fluid sensed in medulla).
- Peripheral chemoreceptors (carotid or aortic bodies)
  - ↑ H^+ (in blood or brain interstitial fluid).
  - ↓ PO_2 (in blood).

Function of Respiratory Regulation

- Keep alveolar PCO_2 stable (prevent hypercarbia or hypocarbia).
- Buffer acid–base changes.
- Prevent hypoxemia (↑ PO_2 when it falls).

↑ PCO_2 (↑ $H+$ sensed in medulla) → ↑ respiration (blow off more CO_2) → ↓ PCO_2 → ↓ respiration.

↓ inspired O_2 has no effect on respiratory drive unless O_2 is <60 mm Hg; then it stimulates carotid and aortic chemoreceptors, resulting in ↑ respiration.

Distinguish carotid and aortic bodies from carotid sinus and aortic baroreceptors (the latter two control changes in blood pressure and HR). CN IX (glossopharyngeal) provides afferent innervation for both carotid body and carotid sinus; CN X (vagus) is afferent for both aortic body and aortic baroreceptors.

Respiratory Chemoreceptors

Receptors	Central Medullary chemoreceptors	Peripheral Carotid and aortic bodies (See Figure 13–4).
Affected by	↑ H^+ CSF, brain interstitial fluid.	↑ PCO_2. ↑ H^+. ↓ PO_2 (<60 mm Hg).
	Major regulators of ventilation. **Not** respond to PO_2. **Not** respond to arterial PCO_2; it is PCO_2 that diffuses across into CSF then is converted to H^+.	Less important than central chemoreceptors (medulla). However, they respond more quickly and regulate abrupt changes in PCO_2

	Carotid Body	**Aortic Body**
Afferent	CN IX	CN X
Efferent	Phrenic, intercostals nerves	Phrenic, intercostals nerves

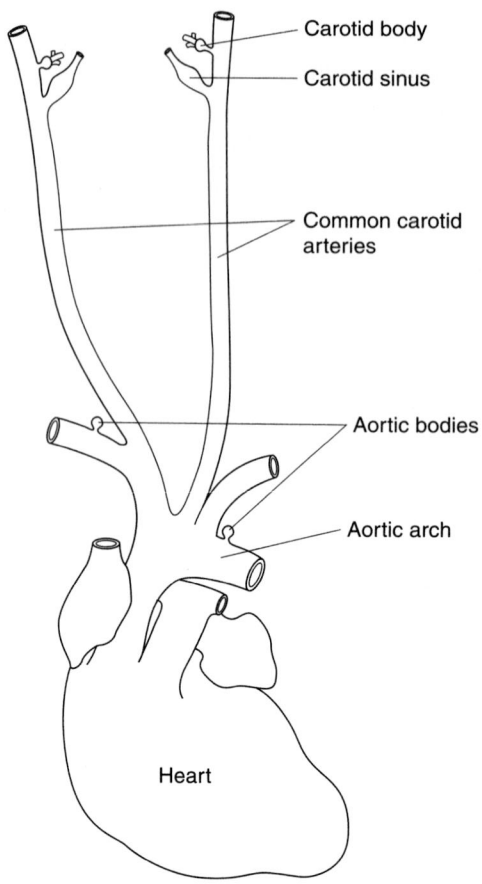

FIGURE 13-4. Carotid and aortic bodies.

Reproduced, with permission, from Ganong WF. *Review of Medical Physiology*, 22nd ed. McGraw-Hill, 2005.

Acid–Base Balance and Respiratory Changes

- See chart in Chapter 14.
- Primary respiratory processes: Respiratory acidosis and alkalosis → metabolic compensation.
- Primary metabolic processes: metabolic acidosis and alkalosis → respiratory compensation.

Primary Metabolic Process	Respiratory Compensation	Mechanism
Metabolic acidosis. ■ Diabetic ketoacidosis. 　■ Kussmaul breathing.	↑ respiration (hyperventilate). ■ Blow off CO_2. ■ ↓ alveolar CO_2. *Respiratory alkalosis*	↑ H^+ stimulates central and peripheral chemoreceptors.
Metabolic alkalosis. ■ ↓ HCL. 　■ Vomiting. 　　NG suctioning	↓ respiration (hypoventilate) ■ ↑ alveolar CO_2. ■ ↑ H^+. *Respiratory acidosis*	↓ H^+ ↓ stimulation to the central and peripheral chemoreceptors.

Hering–Breuer Reflex

- Inflate lungs → expiration.
- Deflate lungs → inspiration.
- Mediated by myelinated slow responding receptors.
- Vagus nerve.

Pulmonary Chemoreflex

- Lung hyperinflation causes:
    - First apnea.
    - Then:
        - Rapid breathing (tachypnea).
        - Bradycardia.
        - Hypotension.
    - Mediated by:
        - J (juxtacapillary) receptors.
            - C fiber endings (unmyelinated) close to pulmonary vessels.

The pulmonary chemoreflex is analogous to the Bezold–Jarisch reflex in the heart.

Pulmonary capillaries (endothelial cells and alveolar capillary bed) contain ACE (angiotensin converting enzyme). ACE converts angiontensin-I to angiotensin-II (RAAS system).

	Stretch Receptors	**J Receptors**	**Irritant Receptors**
Located	Airway smooth muscle.	Alveolar walls.	Between airway epithelial cells
Stimulated by	Lung distention.	Engorgement of capillary or alveolar walls with fluid (e.g., CHF).	Noxious substances (e.g., dust, pollen) Histamine
Causes	Expiration (prevents overinflation; Hering–Breuer reflex).	Rapid shallow breathing.	Coughing, bronchoconstriction.

Kussmaul breathing is rapid deep labored breathing in people with acidosis, in particular diabetic ketoacidosis.

Respiratory Conditions

Condition	Description
Dyspnea	Difficulty breathing; unpleasant sensation.
Apnea	Cessation of breathing, usually transient (central versus peripheral).
Hyperapnea	Abnormally deep and rapid breathing.
Hypercapnea	↑ CO_2 in arterial blood, secondary to underbreathing (↓ ventilation).
Hypocapnea	↓ CO_2 in arterial blood, secondary to overbreathing (↑ ventilation).
Respiratory arrest	Cessation of breathing.
Hyperventilation	↑ alveolar ventilation (greater than metabolic requirements); leads to ↓ PCO_2 (with ↓ cerebral perfusion, fainting/syncope).
Hypoventilation	↓ alveolar ventilation (less than needed for metabolic requirements); leads to ↑ PCO_2.

High Altitude

- ↓ FiO_2
- Results in:
    - Alveolar hypoxia (↓ PAO_2).
    - Arterial hypoxemia (↓ PaO_2).
    - Secondary to ↓ barometric pressure.
- Compensation:
    - Pulmonary vasoconstriction (because of alveolar hypoxia).
    - ↑ erythropoietin (↑ HCT, ↑ O_2 carrying capacity).
    - ↑ mitochondrial density.
    - ↑ 2, 3-DPG (shifting O_2–Hb curve to the right, release O_2 to tissues).
    - ↑ respiratory rate (because of arterial hypoxia, secondary to ↓ barometric pressure; sensed by *peripheral chemoreceptors*; feeding back to medulla to ↑ respiratory rate).
    - Respiratory alkalosis (secondary to ↑ RR).
    - ↑ renal bicarbonate excretion, ↓ in H^+ excretion (compensation for respiratory alkalosis).

CHAPTER 14

Renal, Fluid, Acid–Base Physiology

Body Fluid Distribution	376
TOTAL BODY WATER	376
Fluid Movement	377
STARLING FORCES	377
BALANCE OF FLUIDS	377
OSMOSIS	378
EDEMA	378
VOLUME EXPANSION AND CONTRACTION	378
Acid-Base Physiology	379
HENDERSON–HASSELBACH EQUATION	380
ISOELECTRIC POINT	380
ZWITTERIONS (DIPOLAR IONS)	380
BUFFER	380
CONTROL OF ACID–BASE BALANCE	380
Urinary System	381
AMMONIA	381
NEPHRON	381
RENAL BLOOD SUPPLY	382
FILTRATION	382
Countercurrent Mechanism	384
COUNTERCURRENT EXCHANGE	384
Effective Renal Plasma Flow (ERPF)	385
Renal Blood Flow	385
Glomerular Filtration Rate	385
Renal Clearance	386
Hormonal Response to Volume Changes	386

▶ BODY FLUID DISTRIBUTION

Total Body Water

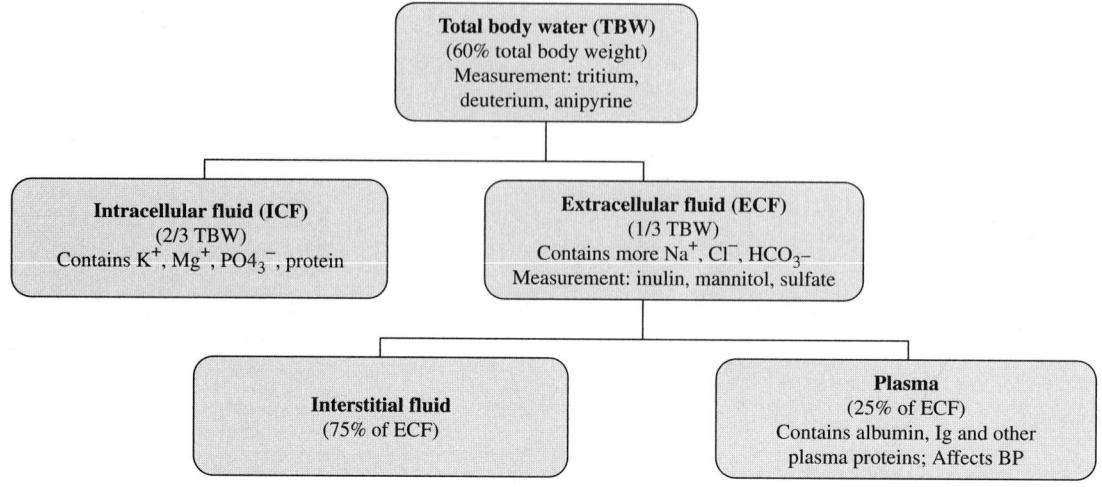

Intra- and Extracellular Fluids

	Extracellular Fluid	Intracellular Fluid
[Na]	142	10
[K]	4	140
%Body weight	15–20	35–40
Components (%BW)	Blood plasma (4–5) Interstitial fluid (11–15) Transcellular fluid ■ CSF ■ Intraocular ■ Synovial ■ Pericardial ■ Pleural ■ Peritoneal	NA

Skin epidermis is nourished by way of diffusion of interstitial fluid (tissue fluid) from capillary beds in the dermis; this fluid bathes the cells.

► FLUID MOVEMENT

Starling Forces

- Forces that move fluid
  - Hydrostatic pressure
  - Oncotic pressure
- Fluid equilibrates between the intravascular and interstitial spaces.
- Fluid in the interstitial space
  - Is taken up by cells (becomes intracellular fluid)
  - Returns to the capillaries or
  - Returns to circulation via lymphatics.

Balance of Fluids

Hydrostatic Pressure	Oncotic Pressure (Colloid Osmotic Pressure)
"push"	"pull"
Force created by the column of fluid (water force promoting movement from one space to the other) "water pushes toward the other space"	Force exerted by proteins, large molecules (that do not themselves readily diffuse) "Pulls water toward the protein"

- These forces force water from the intravascular space to interstitium or vice versa. Both hydrostatic and oncotic pressure exist for the intravascular space and the interstitium.
  - A combination of these forces dictates the movement of fluid.
  - **Fluid movement** = $k[(P_c + \Pi_i) - (P_i + \Pi_c)]$.
    - k = capillary perfusion coefficient.
    - P_c = capillary hydrostatic pressure.
    - Π_i = interstitial oncotic pressure.
    - Π_c = capillary oncotic pressure.
    - P_i = interstitial hydrostatic pressure.
- Promote fluid from capillaries to interstitium: $P_c + \Pi_i$.
- Promote fluid from interstitium to capillaries: $P_i + \Pi_c$.
- See Figure 14–1 for fluid capillary exchange.

See discussion of plasma proteins in Chapter 6, Biological Compounds.

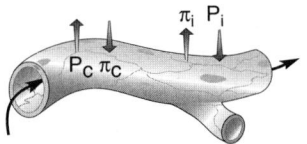

FIGURE 14-1. Fluid capillary exchange.

Reproduced, with permission, from Bhushan V. *First Aid for the USMLE Step 1*. McGraw-Hill, 2006.

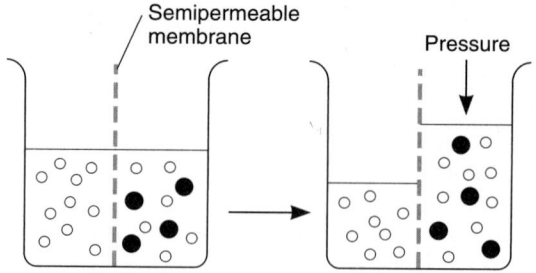

FIGURE 14-2. Osmosis.

Reproduced, with permission, from Ganong WF. *Review of Medical Physiology*, 22nd ed. McGraw-Hill, 2005.

Osmosis

See Figure 14–2.

- **Osmosis:** *Simple diffusion* of **water** caused by a concentration gradient.
- **Osmotic pressure:** The pressure developed as a result of net osmosis into a solution; depends on the *number* of solute particles present.
- **Osmolarity:** Osmotic pressure expressed in osmols/kg of *solution*.
- **Osmolality:** Osmotic pressure expressed in osmols/kg of *water*.

▶ EDEMA

- Excess fluid in the interstitial space

Cause	↑ P_c	↓ Π_c	↑ Π_i	↓ P_i
Examples	CHF Cirrhosis	Nephrotic syndrome Protein-losing enteropathy Cirrhosis Malnutrition	Lymphatic blockage • Elephantiasis • Lymph node resection	

OTHER CAUSES OF EDEMA

- Increased capillary permeability (burns, sepsis, anaphylaxis/angioedema, ARDS).
- Inappropriate renal sodium and water retention.

Volume Expansion and Contraction

EXTRACELLULAR FLUID (ECF) EXPANSION

- Excess fluid in the intervascular or interstitial spaces.
- Evidence in physical examination.
  - Rales
  - Edema
  - Hypertension
  - Bulging fontanelle

INTRACELLULAR FLUID (ICF) EXPANSION

- Excess fluid intracellularly.
- Gauged by serum Na+
  - Low serum Na+ = intracellular expansion.
  - If chronic, formation of intracellular osmolytes prevents drastic influx of H₂O and cell burst.

Expansion	Examples	ECF Volume	ICF Volume	ECF Osmolarity	HCT	[Na+]	[Albumin]	UNa+
(Hypo-) H₂O > Na+	SIADH	↑	↑	↓	↓	↓	↓	↑
(Iso-) H₂O = Na+	Isotonic NS	↑	–	–	↓	–	↓	↑
(Hyper-) H₂O < Na+	Hypertonic NS	↑	↓	↑	↓	↑	↓	↑

Expansion	Examples	ECF Volume	ICF Volume	ECF Osmolarity	HCT	[Na+]	[Albumin]	UNa+
(Hyper-) H₂O > Na+	Sweating, fever, DI	↓	↓	↑	↑	↑	↑	↓
(Iso-) H₂O = Na+	Diarrhea	↓	–	–	↑	–	↑	↓
(Hypo-) H₂O < Na+	Adrenal insufficiency	↓	↑	↓	↑	↓	↑	↓

Solutions

Solution	Characteristics	Effect on Cells	Example
Hypertonic	Solute > solvent	Shrink	>0.9% NaCl
Isotonic	Solute = solvent	No change	0.9% NaCl
Hypotonic	Solute < solvent	Swell	<0.9% NaCl

Isotonic solutions separated by a semipermeable membrane do not cause net movement of water or solutes. The osmotic potential is the same on either side of the membrane.

▶ ACID-BASE PHYSIOLOGY

Process	pH	HCO₃/PaCO₂	Compensation	pH	HCO₃/PaCO₂
Metabolic acidosis	↓	HCO₃⁻ ↓	Respiratory (*hyperventilate*)	↑	PaCO₂ ↓
Metabolic alkalosis	↑	HCO₃⁻ ↑	Respiratory (*hypoventilate*)	↓	PaCO₂ ↑
Respiratory acidosis	↓	PaCO₂ ↑	Metabolic (*conserve HCO₃*)	↑	HCO₃ ↑
Respiratory alkalosis	↑	PaCO₂ ↓	Metabolic (*excrete HCO₃*)	↓	HCO₃ ↓

Henderson–Hasselbach Equation

- pH = pKa + log [A-]/[HA].
- pH = pK when an acid is half neutralized.

Isoelectric Point

Glycine has a net negative charge at any pH above its isoelectric point, so it moves toward the positive electrode (anode). At any pH below its isoelectric point (pI), glycine exhibits a net positive charge and moves toward the negative electrode (cathode).

- pH where the number of positive charges equals the number of negative charges.
- Solute has no electric charge at this pH.
  - Does not move an electric field (pI for that solute).
- Allows separation of proteins or amino acids based on charge.

Zwitterions (Dipolar Ions)

- Physiologic pH: Amino acids have both
  - negatively charged carboxyl group ($-COO^-$) and
  - positively charged amino group ($-NH_3^+$).

Buffer

- System to minimize pH changes
- Consists of
  - weak acid (proton donor)
  - conjugate base (a salt)(proton acceptor)
- Releases H^+ ions when the pH rises.
- Accepts H^+ when the pH drops.

BUFFER SYSTEMS

In the oral cavity, the carbonic acid system helps neutralize dietary and bacteria-generated acids.

- Sodium bicarbonate: carbonic acid buffer.
  - The major buffer in extracellular fluid, blood.
  - Breaks down to CO_2 and H_2O with respiratory elimination.
- Blood pH is ~ 7.4.
  - Range 7.35–7.45.
  - Usually >7.4: slightly alkaline/basic.
- Primary determinant is the bicarbonate and CO_2 ratio.
  - pH = pKa + log $[HCO_3^-]/0.03 \times pCO_2$.
  - pH = 6.1 + log$[HCO_3^-]/(0.03 \times pCO_2)$.
    - 6.1 is the pKa of the bicarb-CO_2 buffer system.

Control of Acid–Base Balance

- **Renal**
  - In tubules: H_2CO_3 (carbonic anhydrase) → $H_2O + CO_2$ → $H^+ + HCO_3^-$.
    - H^+ secreted, then excreted.
    - HCO_3^- reabsorbed.
    - NH_4, (ammonium), phosphates are excreted to compensate for acidity.
- **Buffers**
  - Bicarbonate
  - Hemoglobin
  - Albumin

- **Respiratory**
  - Blow off CO_2 (elevated CO_2 stimulates respiration).

▶ URINARY SYSTEM

- Regulates water and solute balance.
- Removes nitrogenous wastes (as urea) from blood.
  - Urea is a byproduct of protein breakdown.
    - Urea cycle in liver.

Kidney Function

Filtration	Hormonal
Water and solute balance Excretion of wastes	Erythropoietin (stimulates RBCs) Renin (stimulates angiotensin, aldosterone system)

Urine

Characteristics	Contents
Clear, yellow Slightly acidic pH Specific gravity 1.005–1.030	Na Cl K Ca Mg Sulfates Phosphates HCO_3 Uric acid Ammonia Creatinine Urobilinogen

Kidneys ordinarily excrete 1–2 L per day in urine.

180 L of glomerular filtrate are produced each day (99% reabsorbed).

Ammonia

- Waste product
- Sources:
  - Amino acids
    - Liver
    - Kidneys
    - Amines
    - Purines and pyrimidines

The urea cycle in the liver is important for disposal of ammonia.

Nephron

See Chapter 2, Histology.

- Functional and structural unit of the kidney
  - Glomerulus
  - Bowman's capsule/space

- Tubules
  - Proximal convoluted
  - Loop of Henle
  - Distal convoluted
- Collecting duct
- Renal pelvis
- Ureter

Glomerulus is a tuft of capillaries (endothelial cells) that interface with Bowman's capsule (epithelial cells). Filtration occurs at this interface.

Renal Blood Supply

See Figure 14–3.

- Renal arteries branch from the aorta.
- Left renal artery is longer than the right.
  - Renal artery
  - Interlobar arteries
  - Arcuate arteries
  - Interlobular arteries
  - Afferent arteriole
  - Glomerulus
  - Efferent arteriole

Majority of glomerular filtrate occurs at the proximal convoluted tubule (just distal to Bowman's space).

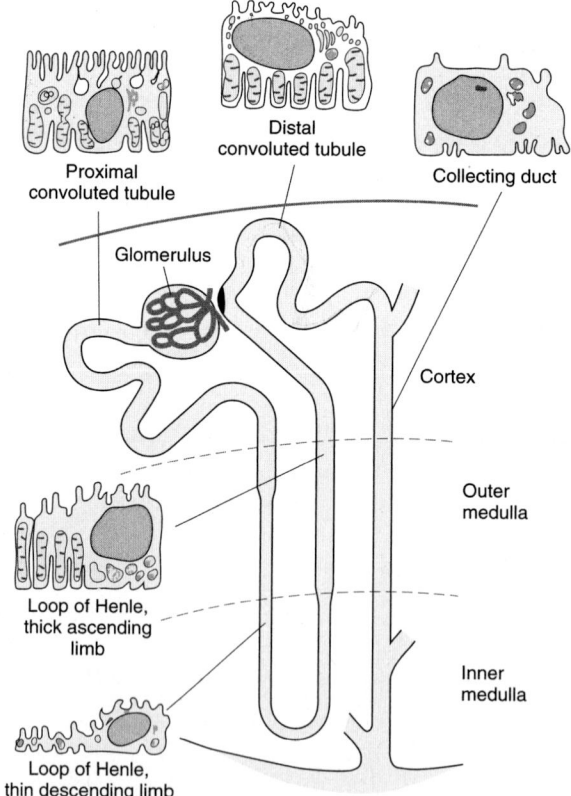

FIGURE 14–3. Renal blood supply.

Reproduced, with permission, from Ganong WF. *Review of Medical Physiology*, 22nd ed. McGraw-Hill, 2005.

Filtration

- Renal blood flow delivered to glomerulus.
- Filtrate passes:
  - Epithelial cell barrier (glomerulus). *endothelial cell*
  - Epithelial cell barrier (Bowman's capsule).
- Filtrate enters Bowman's space, the first part of the tubule.

Reabsorption	Secretion	Excretion
Tubule back to circulation.	From tubular cell or circulation into tubular fluid.	Tubular fluid (and solute) that ends up as urine.

Substance	Reabsorption	Comments
H_2O	Proximal tubule Loop of Henle (descending) Distal tubule, collecting duct	Ascending loop is impermeable to H_2O. ADH
Na	Proximal tubule (70%) Loop of Henle Distal tubule Collecting duct	Cl and H_2O follow passively Na/K/2Cl, impermeable to H_2O Na/K/2Cl cotransport Aldosterone Na^+ channel
Glucose	Proximal tubule	

Function of Nephron Segments

Segment	Reabsorption	Secretion
Proximal convoluted tubule.	H_2O, Na^+, K^+, Cl^-, HCO_3^-, amino acids, glucose, proteins.	H^+, ammonia
Descending loop of Henle.	H_2O (Impermeable to Na^+)	
Ascending loop of Henle.	Na^+, K^+, Cl^- (Impermeable to H_2O)	
Distal convoluted tubule.	Na^+, Cl^- Ca^{2+} (Regulated by **PTH**)	
Collecting duct.	H_2O (Regulated by **ADH**) Na^+ (Regulated by **aldosterone**)	K^+, H^+, ammonia, drugs

Reabsorption occurs by active transport, facilitated diffusion, and solvent drag. It can be paracellular or transcellular.

At plasma concentrations <250 mg/dL all filtered glucose is reabsorbed in the proximal tubule and excretion is zero. With glucose concentration >350 mg/dL the additional filtered glucose cannot be reabsorbed and is spilled into the urine (excreted). Glucosuria (as in diabetes) occurs when the Tm has been exceeded (plasma glucose concentration > 350 mg/dL).

Reabsorption of NaCl (and impermeability to water) by the thick ascending loop is the basis of the countercurrent multiplier system.

See Figure below.

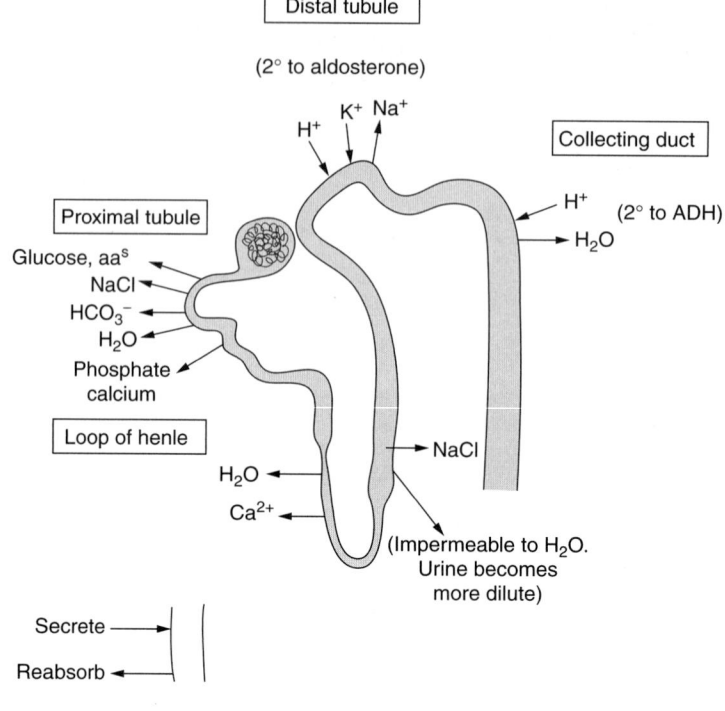

Filtration.

In the absence of ADH aquaporins are not expressed on the collecting duct membrane, therefore water reabsorption at the medullary collecting duct is much less pronounced and dilute urine is excreted.

If the vasa recta coursed straight through medulla, then water would move from the blood in the capillary into the interstitium (and interstitial solute would move into the capillary). This would dissipate the countercurrent gradient and decrease the concentrating ability.

▶ COUNTERCURRENT MECHANISM

- Countercurrent multiplier.
- Creation of a gradient to allow for concentrated urine.
- Occurs in:
  - Loop of Henle.
  - Collecting tubules (cortical and medullary).
  - Because these are anatomically located in both the medulla and cortex.
  - Mechanism:
  - Ascending loop:
    - **Active Na reabsorption (pumping)**
    - **Impermeability to water**
- This preferential egress of Na but not water creates:
- Dilute tubular fluid.
- Hyperosmotic interstitium.
- Urine is dilute at cortical collecting duct (water > Na).
- Urine concentrates as it descends medullary collecting duct.
- Because of the gradient created by hyperosmotic medulla.
- Gradient ("pulls" water from the tubule).
- In presence of ADH
  - Aquaporins promote egress of water along this gradient.

Countercurrent Exchange

- Allows the hyperosmotic medullary gradient to be maintained.
- Hairpin (or loop) configuration of vasa recta capillaries.
- Minimizes removal of excess medullary interstitial solute.
- Maintains gradient so that urine can be concentrated.

EFFECTIVE RENAL PLASMA FLOW (ERPF)

- Volume of plasma flowing through the peritubular capillaries.
- Determined by calculation of paraaminohippuric acid (PAH).
  - PAH is completely secreted into the proximal tubule and excreted into the urine.
  - Therefore the volume of plasma cleared of PAH is ~ = ERPF.
- PAH is both filtered and secreted and used to estimate renal plasma flow.

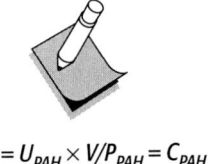

$ERPF = U_{PAH} \times V/P_{PAH} = C_{PAH}$

RENAL BLOOD FLOW

Response to decreased renal blood flow.
- Decreased renal blood flow (e.g., renal artery stenosis).
- Decrease in glomerular hydrostatic pressure (initially).
- Decrease in GFR.
  - Decreases NaCl delivery to the macula densa (Cl- more important).
  - Causes JG cells to secrete renin.
  - AT-II is formed (aldosterone released).
  - AT-II constricts efferent arteriole.
  - Increases glomerular hydrostatic pressure.
  - GFR back to normal.

GLOMERULAR FILTRATION RATE

- GFR = rate of filtrate formation at the glomerulus.
- Surrogate of renal function
- Determined by:
  - Hydrostatic pressures (Bowman's space and glomerulus).
  - Oncotic (colloid) pressures (Bowman's space and glomerulus).
  - Capillary filtration coefficient.
- Calculate using Cr or inulin clearance.
  - Freely filtered.
  - Not reabsorbed.
  - Minimally secreted into the urine.

GFR Increased ↑	GFR Decreased ↓

Increased renal perfusion (blood flow)
 ■ E.g., dopamine, fenoldopam
 ■ Afferent arteriole vasodilation
   ■ Increases glomerular capillary hydrostatic pressure.
 	
 Efferent arteriole vasoconstriction
   ■ Increases glomerular capillary hydrostatic pressure.
   ■ However excessive constriction here will decrease RBF and GFR.
 Decreased plasma oncotic pressure
   ■ E.g., decrease plasma proteins
	Decreased renal perfusion
	 ■ E.g., renal artery stenosis, low BP
	 Afferent arteriole vasoconstriction
	 Efferent arteriole vasodilation
	   ■ E.g., ACE-I
	 Increased hydrostatic pressure in Bowman's space
	   ■ E.g., blocked ureter, outflow obstruction

$GFR = U_{Inulin} \times V/P_{Inulin} = C_{Pinulin}$

▶ RENAL CLEARANCE

- Rate of substance is cleared from plasma.
- Clearance = (urine concentration × urine flow rate)/plasma concentration.
  - Use Cr or inulin clearance to estimate GFR.
  - Cr and inulin are freely filtered by the glomerulus.
  - Not secreted or reabsorbed.
  - Filtration rate and excretion rate are equal in steady state.

Excretion rate = GFR − reabsorption + secretion.

Inulin clearance = rate insulin cleared from plasma/unit time = $U_{Inulin} \times V/P_{Inulin} = C_{PInulin}$ = GFR.
Note: inulin is a starch.

Net reabsorption:
Solute clearance is less than that of inulin.
Net secretion:
Solute clearance is greater than that of inulin.

When GFR decreases by 50%, Cr clearance is decreased by about 50%. Cr excretion is decreased and plasma Cr level is increased.

Cr clearance is used to assess renal function in the clinical setting.

Hormones and the Kidney

	Released from	Release Stimulated by	Site of Action	Effect
ADH	Posterior pituitary	Thirst ↑ Na^+ (↑ osmolarity) ↓ extracellular fluid.	Distal Tubule Collecting Duct Aquaporins	↑ H_2O resorption ↓ serum Na ↑ blood volume
Renin	Juxtaglomerular apparatus	↓ Renal BP (or pO_2) ↓ GFR ↓ Cl- delivery to macula densa Sympathetic stimulation. B1 receptors	Cleaves AT (made in liver) into AT-I ACE (in pulmonary capillaries). AT-I* → AT-II	AT-II Vasoconstrictor ↑ PVR efferent arteriole vasoconstrictor ↑ GFR Na^+, H_2O retention stimulates release of aldosterone.
Aldosterone	Adrenal cortex (zona glomerulosa).	Renin via AT-II ↑ K^+	Collecting duct	NaCl, H_2O reabsorption. K^+ excretion HCO_3 reabsorption.

*AT-I and AT-II = angiotensin I and II

▶ HORMONAL RESPONSE TO VOLUME CHANGES

See Figure 14–4.

- See the following chart for hormonal response to volume changes under normal circumstances.

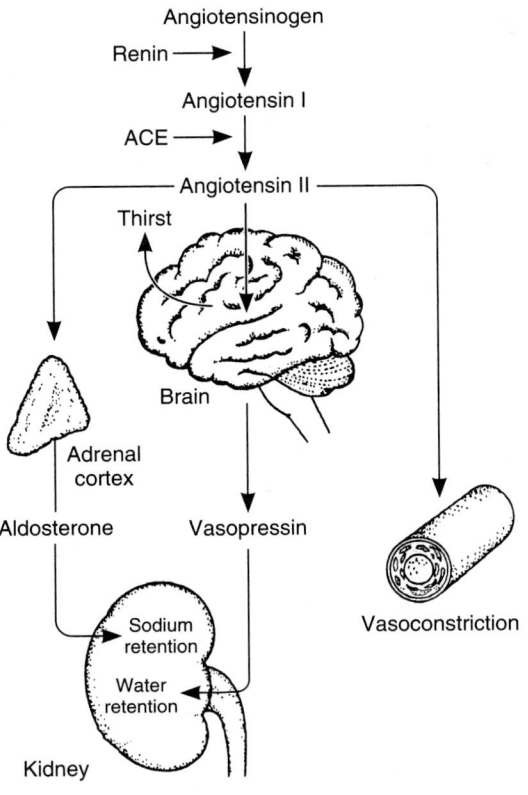

FIGURE 14-4. Hormonal response to volume changes.

Reproduced, with permission, from Ganong WF. *Review of Medical Physiology*, 22nd ed. McGraw-Hill, 2005.

Volume Expansion	Volume Contraction
↓ ADH	↑ ADH
↓ renin-aldosterone	↑ renin-aldosterone
↑ ANP, BNP (natriuretic peptides) ↑renal Na⁺ excretion	↓ ANP, BNP (natriuretic peptides) – ↓ renal Na⁺ excretion
↑ baroreceptor response (↓ HR, ↓ BP)	↓ baroreceptor response (↑ HR, ↑ BP)

CHAPTER 15

Gastrointestinal Physiology

Gastrointestinal System	390
NERVOUS CONTROL	390
Gastric Secretions	391
STAGES OF GASTRIC SECRETION	392
CHYME	392
GI Contractions	392
PERISTALSIS	392
SEGMENTATION (MIXING)	392
TONIC CONTRACTIONS	393
DIGESTION AND ABSORPTION	393
EXOCRINE PANCREAS	394
BILE	395
Liver	395
LIVER FUNCTIONS	395
CHOLESTEROL SYNTHESIS	396
UREA CYCLE	396
GLUCOSE METABOLISM	396
GLUCOSE	396
PROTEIN METABOLISM	397
JAUNDICE	397

GASTROINTESTINAL SYSTEM

- Functions to digest and absorb nutritive substances, vitamins, nutrient, and fluids.

Nervous Control

- Extrinsic
  - Mostly vagus (CN X, parasympathetic).
- Intrinsic
  - Enteric nervous system
    - **Myenteric plexus** (Auerbach's plexus): Between outer longitudinal and middle circular muscle layers.
    - **Submucous plexus** (Meissner's plexus): Between the middle circular layer and the mucosa.

Hormonal Control

Hormone	Stimulus	Action
Gastrin[a]	Peptides, amino acids in gastric lumen; stomach distention.	Stimulates HCl secretion and gastric motility.
Cholecystokinin[b]	Fats, fatty acids, amino acids in duodenum.	↑ pancreatic digestive enzyme secretion. ↑ gallbladder contraction.
Secretin[b]	↓ pH in duodenum. HCL into duodenum.	↑ HCO_3^- from pancreas (neutralizes H^+ in duodenum). ↓ gastric motility. ↓ gastric acid secretion. ↑ bile secretion from gallbladder.
GIP[b,c]	Fats and glucose in duodenum.	↓ gastric motility. ↓ gastric acid secretion. ↑ insulin release (β cells) in setting of ↑ BGL.

[a]Gastrin is produced/secreted from G cells (enteroendocrine) in the stomach in response to a meal.
[b]Cholecystokinin, secretin, and GIP are all produced/secreted from duodenum.
[c]GIP = gastric inhibitory peptide.

ENTERO GASTRONE

- Includes:
  - Secretin
  - Cholecystokinin
  - Gastric inhibitory peptide (GIP)

- All are released by small intestine in response to chime entering the duodenum:
  - Acidity (HCL)
  - Fats (FFAs)
  - Amino acids
- These hormones then enter the bloodstream.
  - Target organ is stomach.
    - ↓ gastric motility (↓ pyloric pump).
    - ↓ gastric emptying.

> **Enterogastric reflex**
> - Duodenum distends with chyme.
> - Pyloric pump inhibited.
> - ↓ gastric motility and emptying.

▶ GASTRIC SECRETIONS

- Gastric glands make 2–3 L secretions per day.
- pH of gastric secretion is 1.0–3.5.
- Secretions include:
  - **Mucous**
    - Adheres to stomach wall.
    - Lubricates the walls.
    - Protects the gastric mucosa from acidic secretions.
      - Mucous is alkaline.
  - **HCL**
    - Assists in digestion.
    - ↑ by Ach, gastrin, and histamine.
  - **Pepsinogen**
    - Converted to pepsin (when in contact with HCl).
    - Pepsin is a proteolytic enzyme.
  - **Intrinsic factor**
    - Binds vitamin B_{12} to allow for its absorption.
  - **Gastrin**
    - Hormone, bloodstream to parietal (oxyntic) cells in gastric glands.
    - Stimulates HCl secretion.

> **Peptic ulcers can result from:**
> - ↑ HCl (acid oversecretion).
> - ↓ mucous (↓ ability of mucosal barrier to protect against acid).
> - Also contribution by *H. pylori*.

Gastric Secretions by Region

Stomach Region	Gland(s)	Secretion(s)
Cardiac	Cardiac glands	Mucous
Fundus (and body)*	Gastric or fundic glands ■ Mucous neck cells ■ Parietal (oxyntic) cells ■ Chief cells ■ Enteroendocrine cells	Mucous HCl and IF Pepsinogen Gastrin
Pylorus	Pyloric glands	Mucous

*In the fundus there are 3 to 7 glands in the base of each gastric pit.

Stages of Gastric Secretion

- **Cephalic phase**
    - Smell, sight, taste, thought of food triggers reflexes to stimulate gastric secretion (parasympathetic activation).
- **Gastric phase**
    - Begins when food enters the stomach.
    - Stomach wall distends and ↑ pH triggers gastrin release.
    - Accounts for ~70% of gastric secretion.
- **Intestinal phase**
    - Begins when acidic, high-osmolarity food enters the intestine.
    - Gastric secretion is inhibited via
        - Enterogastric reflex.
        - Hormonal mechanisms (e.g., secretin).

Chyme

- Semiliquid contents of the stomach.
    - Consist of partially digested foods and gastric secretions.
    - Passes through pyloric valve into duodenum.
- Volume and composition of chyme affects gastric motility, gastric emptying.
- Chyme is broken down by digestive enzymes in the small intestine.

Gastric Emptying

Increased by	Decreased by
Eating	CCK
Gastric distention	Secretin
Gastrin	GIP
Vagal input (parasympathetic)	Duodenal distention (enterogastric reflex)

▶ GI CONTRACTIONS

Three major types.

Peristalsis

- Coordinated contractions with relaxation ahead.
- Propels chyme forward (from proximal to distal).
- Controlled by the enteric nervous system.
    - Local reflexes (stimulated by distention).

Segmentation (Mixing)

- Most common in the small intestine.
- Rhythmic contractions in a piece of gut.
- Chops chyme and mixes it with digestive enzyme juices.

- Ensures chyme comes into maximum contact with the gut wall.
  - ↑ surface area for digestion and absorption.
- Stimulated by distention.
- Occurs at rate of 11–12 cycles per minute in duodenum.
- Progressively slower rate as you progress further down distally in the gut.
  - About 6–7 cycles per minute in terminal ileum.

Tonic Contractions

- Long duration—minutes to hours.
- Examples are sphincters located along GI tract.

Contractions in the GI tract are influenced by mechanical, neural, and hormonal inputs. Myenteric (intrinsic) and parasympathetic (extrinsic) stimulation both increase contractile force.

Digestion and Absorption

Component	Digestion Enzyme[a]	Location	Absorption
Carbohydrates	Amylase (saliva)[b] Amylase (pancreas) Disaccharidases • Sucrase • Lactase • Maltase	Upper GI (mouth, stomach) Duodenum, small intestine Small intestine • Brush border	Na$^+$ cotransport* • Glucose • Galactose Facilitated diffusion • Fructose
Proteins	Pepsin Trypsin Chymotrypsin Carboxypeptidase Peptidases	Stomach Pancreas Small intestine • Brush border	Na$^+$ cotransport* or Facilitated diffusion
Fats	Lingual lipase Pancreatic lipase	Upper GI (mouth, stomach) Small intestine	Diffusion into enterocyte Exocytosis into lymph

[a]No human enzymes can hydrolyze cellulose.
[b]Ptyalin (a-amylase) is secreted by parotid glands. It hydrolyzes starch (into the disaccharide maltose).

Disaccharide Absorption

- Disaccharides and small glucose polymers are hydrolyzed at brush border by disaccharidases:
  - Lactase
  - Sucrase
  - Maltase
  - α-dextrinase
- Hydrolization forms:
  - Monosaccharides
  - Glucose
  - Galactose
- Disaccharides are absorbed by Na cotransport (secondary active transporters are driven by the sodium gradient).
- Fructose absorption is mediated by facilitated diffusion.

Protein Absorption

- Proteins are broken down by peptidases on brush border.
- Protein breakdown gives rise to
  - Dipeptides
  - Amino acids
- Absorption immediately follows breakdown
  - Via secondary active transporters using sodium or hydrogen gradients.

Triglycerides Digestion and Absorption

- Triglycerides make up majority of dietary lipid.
- Digestion starts with lingual lipase.
- Bile salts (amphipathic)
  ↓
- Emulsify triglycerides (in duodenum)
  ↓
- Pancreatic lipase, which breaks down emulsified triglycerides into:
  ↓
- Monoglyceride + free fatty acids (FFAs)
  ↓
- Monoglycerides + FFAs stay associated with bile salts as:
  ↓
- *Micelles* (smaller fat droplets)
  ↓
- Contact brush border and are absorbed into enterocyte by simple diffusion
  ↓
- Endoplasmic reticulum where reconstituted as triglycerides
  ↓
- Packaged as chylomicrons (triglycerides + cholesterol, lipoproteins, and other lipids)
  ↓
- *Chylomicrons* into lymphatics by exocytosis.

Triglycerides need to be broken into monoglyceride and free fatty acids.

Exocrine Pancreas

- Pancreatic secretion stimulated by:
  - Ach
  - Cholecystokinin
  - Secretin

- Enzymatic secretions from pancreatic acinar cells.
  - Protein breakdown:
    - Trypsin
    - Chymotrypsin
    - Carboxypepsidase
  - Carbohydrate breakdown:
    - Amylase
  - Fat breakdown:
    - Lipase
    - Cholesterol esterase
    - Phospholipase
- Enzymes are secreted in inactive form.
  - Activated in small intestine (contact acidic chyme).
- Pancreatic ductal cells secrete fluid high in bicarbonate.
  - pH of pancreatic secretions is 8.0 to 8.3.

Bile

- Produced by the liver.
- Stored in the gallbladder.
- pH ~7.8.
- Helps with lipid digestion and absorption.
  - Emulsification
  - Release (gallbladder contraction) stimulated by:
  - Cholecystokinin (hormone produced by wall of upper intestine).

pHs of secretions

Secretion*	pH
Gastric	1.0–3.5
Pancreatic	8.0–8.3
Bile	7.8
Intestinal	7.5–8.0

*Intestinal secretions are mainly mucous. They are secreted by goblet cells and enterocytes.

▶ LIVER

Liver Functions

- Stores minerals and vitamins.
- Stores iron (Fe) as ferritin.
- Synthesizes cholesterol.
- Conjugates steroids.
- Metabolizes carbohydrates:
  - Regulates blood glucose level:
    - Glucose metabolism.
    - Glucose/carbohydrate storage.
    - Gluconeogenesis.
- Metabolizes lipids:
  - Synthesizes lipoproteins.
  - Regulates lipid metabolism.

- Metabolizes protein:
  - Deaminates AAs → urea (urea cycle).
  - Synthesizes AAs.
  - Synthesizes plasma proteins (e.g., fibrinogen, prothrombin, clotting proteins).
- Detoxifies; reduces or eliminates toxic elements (e.g., alcohol detoxification).
- Destroys damaged red blood cells.
- Phagocytosis of foreign antigens.
- Serves as bile reservoir.
  - Secretes bile.

Cholesterol Synthesis

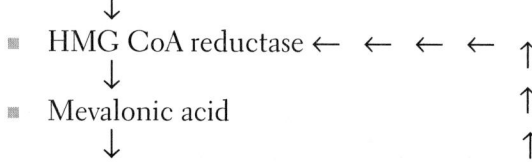

Cholesterol synthesis in the liver is regulated by negative feedback. Cholesterol allosterically inhibits HMG CoA reductase (↓ cholesterol formation from acetyl CoA).

- See also Chapter 7.
- Cholesterol is important for:
  - Bile salts (formed from cholesterol in liver)
  - Steroid hormones
  - Vitamin D
- Made from acetyl CoA
  ↓
- HMG CoA reductase ← ← ← ← ↑
  ↓   ↑
- Mevalonic acid   ↑
  ↓   ↑
- Cholesterol (negative feedback to HMG CoA reductase).

Urea Cycle

Nonprotein nitrogen in the blood is made up primarily of urea.

- See also Chapter 7.
- Urea is the fate of most of the ammonia channeled to the liver.
- Deamination of amino acids results in ammonia (NH_3).
- Ammonia is toxic, fatal if it accumulates.
- Urea cycle converts NH_3 into urea:
  - $2\ NH_3 + CO_2 \rightarrow$ urea.
  - Hydrolysis of arginine gives rise to urea.
- Ornithine regulates turn of the cycle (see biochemistry).
- Urea then passes to bloodstream to kidneys and is excreted in urine.

Glucose Metabolism

- See also Chapter 7.
- Glucose is required by all tissues, especially brain and RBCs.
- Liver maintains blood glucose level:
  - Liver releases glucose during exercise and between meals.
  - Released glucose is from one of two sources:
    - Glycogenolysis (breakdown of stored glycogen).
    - Gluconeogenesis (formation of new glucose).

Glucose

- Glucose is the major fuel source derived from carbohydrate ingestion.
- The presence of glucose in urine occurs only when a person has exceeded the renal threshold (K_M) for glucose (e.g., uncontrolled DM).

- During fasting liver glycogen ↓ because glycogenolysis occurs (to deliver glucose to the bloodstream).
- Skeletal muscle lacks glucose-6-phosphatase, so cannot deliver glucose to the bloodstream.
- The brain has no significant stores of glycogen and is completely dependent on blood glucose. The brain oxidizes nearly 140 g per day of glucose to CO_2 and H_2O, making ATP.

GLUCONEOGENESIS

- Synthesis of glucose from noncarbohydrate compounds.
- Mostly occurs in liver.
- ~10% occurs in kidneys.
- During prolonged starvation, the kidneys become major glucose-producing organs.

GLYCOGENESIS

- Glucose uptake to liver (via GLUT proteins).
- Glucokinase
    - Enzyme present only in the liver (expressed significantly only after a meal).
    - Converts glucose to glucose-6-phosphate, using ATP to catalyze the phosphorylation.

Protein Metabolism

- Deamination of amino acids.
    - Convert to carbohydrates or fats for energy source.
- Amino acid synthesis.
    - Nonessential amino acids can be synthesized in the liver.

Jaundice

- Yellowish discoloration of skin, sclera, and tissues.
- Secondary to hyperbilirubinemia (high levels of bile pigment bilirubin in the blood).
- Jaundice is common manifestation of liver disease.
- Occurs at any age and in either sex.

Other tissues use hexokinase to do the same thing as glucokinase.

See the section on plasma constituents. Liver plasma protein synthesis accounts for 90% of plasma proteins.

Under the tongue is the first location to spot jaundice.

Causes of Jaundice

Prehepatic (Hemolytic)	Hepatic (Hepatocyte Damage)	Posthepatic (Obstructive)
Hemolytic anemia Malaria	Hepatitis Alcoholic liver disease Primary biliary cirrhosis	Choledocholithiasis Pancreatic head cancer

BILIRUBIN

- Derived from broken-down hemoglobin.
- Carried to liver and is conjugated (converted into diglucuronide derivative).
- Excreted into the intestine as a component of bile.
- Normal plasma bilirubin concentration = 0.5 mg/100 mL.
- In jaundice, can rise to 40 mg/100 mL.

CHAPTER 16
Nutrition

Vitamins	400
FAT SOLUBLE VITAMINS	**400**
WATER SOLUBLE VITAMINS	**401**
VITAMIN DEFICIENCIES	**402**
Minerals	403
MAJOR MINERALS	**403**
MINOR MINERALS	**404**

▶ VITAMINS

- Essential organic compounds required for growth and metabolism.
- Most act as **coenzymes**.

Fat Soluble Vitamins

See Table 16–1.
See Figure below for synthesis of biologically active vitamin D.

Excess fat-soluble vitamins accumulate in body fat. Excess water-soluble vitamins are eliminated in urine.

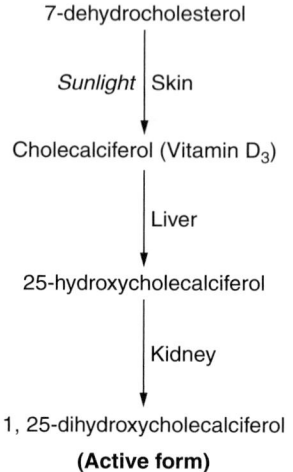

Synthesis of biologically active vitamin D.

TABLE 16–1. The Fat-Soluble Vitamins.

Vitamin	Function	Deficiency	Other Facts
Vitamin A (Retinol)	Epithelial development and maintenance. Growth and remodeling of bone.	Night blindness. Xerophthalmia (ocular tissue keratinization). Dry skin. *Enamel* irregularities.	Constituent of the visual pigments **rhodopsin** (rods) and **iodopsin** (cones).
Vitamin D (Calciferol)	Growth and mineralization of bone and teeth. Ca^{2+} and $(PO_4)^{3-}$ metabolism.	**Rickets** (children). **Osteomalacia** (adults).	*Most toxic* of fat-soluble vitamins.
Vitamin E (Tocopherol)	**Antioxidant** (prevents free radical formation).	Neurologic dysfunction (premature infants).	*Least toxic* of fat-soluble vitamins.
Vitamin K (Phylloquinone) (Menaquinones) (Menadione)	Activation of **prothrombin** and vit. K dependent clotting factors **(II, VII, IX, X)**. Synthesis of γ-carboxyglutamate (chelates Ca^{2+}).	Diminished blood clotting. ↑ PT and INR (extrinsic clotting pathway).	Warfarin (Coumadin) blocks hepatic synthesis of vit. K dependent clotting factors. Synthesized by intestinal bacteria.

Water Soluble Vitamins

See Table 16–2.

TABLE 16–2. The Water-Soluble Vitamins

VITAMIN	FUNCTION	DEFICIENCY	OTHER FACTS
Vitamin B_1 (thiamine)	Metabolism of carbohydrates and amino acids. Decarboxylation of α-ketoacids.	**Beriberi:** Peripheral nerve damage. **Wernicke–Korsakoff syndrome:** CNS damage.	Deficiency associated with alcoholism and malnutrition.
Vitamin B_2 (riboflavin)	Component of **FAD** and **FMN.**	**Cheilosis.** Dermatitis. Photosensitivity. Glossitis.	Synthesized by intestinal bacteria.
Vitamin B_3 (niacin)	Component of **NAD** and **NADP.**	**Pellagra.**	Formed from **tryptophan.**
Vitamin B_5 (pantothenic acid)	Component of **Coenzyme A.** Fatty acid synthesis.	Dermatitis. Fatigue. Sleep impairment. Diarrhea.	
Vitamin B_6 (pyridoxine)	Precursor of **pyridoxal phosphate** (a coenzyme in transamination reactions).	Fatigue. Depression. Impaired growth. Convulsions.	Formed from **pyridine.** Deficiency associated with oral contraceptive use.
Vitamin B_6 (pyridoxine)	Precursor of **pyridoxal phosphate** (a coenzyme in transamination reactions).	Fatigue. Depression. Impaired growth. Convulsions.	Formed from **pyridine.** Deficiency associated with oral contraceptive use.
Vitamin B_{12} (cobalamin)	Formation of **methionine.** Converts **methylmalonyl CoA** → **succinyl CoA.** *Intrinsic factor* required for GI absorption.	**Pernicious anemia.** Glossitis.	Not found in plant foods (only animal sources). Synthesized by intestinal bacteria.
Folic acid	Synthesis of **purines** (adenosine and guanine) and **thymidine** (required for DNA formation).	**Megaloblastic anemia.** Glossitis.	*Most common vitamin deficiency in U.S.* Inhibited by antimetabolites (e.g., methotrexate).

TABLE 16-2. The Water-Soluble Vitamins (Continued)

Vitamin	Function	Deficiency	Other Facts
Biotin (vitamin H)	Protein and amino acid synthesis. Converts **acetyl CoA → malonyl CoA** in fatty acid synthesis.	Fatigue. Depression. Muscle pain. Hair loss. Dermatitis.	Inactivated by **avidin** (a protein in egg whites). Synthesized by intestinal bacteria.
Vitamin C (ascorbic acid)	Coenzyme for the hydroxylation of **proline** and **lysine** (in collagen synthesis).	**Scurvy:** Delayed wound healing, poor bone matrix formation, ↑ permeability of oral mucosa, capillary fragility.	Deficiency associated with gingival disease.

Vitamin Deficiencies

Pellagra

- Deficiency: Vitamin B_3 (niacin).
- Clinical effects: Three Ds.
    - Dementia
    - Dermatitis
    - Diarrhea

Folic acid is essential for neural tube formation.

Megaloblastic Anemia

- Deficiency: Folic acid.
- Megaloblasts: Large-nucleated cells.

Vitamin B_{12} malabsorption also occurs with Crohn's disease.

Pernicious Anemia

- Deficiency: Vitamin B_{12} (cobalmin).
- Form of megaloblastic anemia plus:
    - **Neurologic dysfunction.**
    - ↓ intrinsic factor (destruction of gastric parietal cells).

▶ MINERALS

- Essential elements required for structural and metabolic function.

Major minerals

See Table 16–3 for the major minerals.

- Greater than 0.005% of body weight.

TABLE 16-3. The Major Minerals

ELEMENT	FUNCTION
Calcium	**Bone** and **tooth** formation Muscle contraction Nerve function Blood clotting
Chlorine	Membrane function (major *negative* ion in *extracellular fluid*) Water balance Digestion
Magnesium	Protein synthesis
Phosphorous	**Bone** and **tooth** formation Component of ATP Acid–base balance
Potassium	Membrane function (major *positive* ion in *intracellular fluid*) Acid–base balance Nerve function Water balance
Sodium	Membrane function (major *positive* ion in *extracellular fluid*) Acid–base balance Nerve function Water balance
Sulfur	**Cartilage** and **tendon** formation

*A deficiency in **calcium** results in osteopenia and osteoporosis. Their diagnosis is based on bone density scans.*

Minor minerals

See Table 16–4 for the minor minerals.

- Less than 0.005% of body weight.

Transferrin *transports copper and iron in blood plasma.*

TABLE 16–4. The Minor Minerals

Element	Function	Deficiency
Chromium	Glucose metabolism.	
Cobalt	Constituent of **Vitamin B$_{12}$** (cobalmin).	Pernicious anemia
Copper	**Iron** metabolism. Maturation of collagen and elastin (cofactor for **lysyl oxidase**).	Microcytic anemia
Fluoride	Converts hydroxyapatite → fluorapatite (reduces solubility of enamel). Excreted by the kidney. Passes the placental barrier. Deposited in other calcified tissues.	↑ caries risk
Iodine	Constituent of **thyroid hormones.** Energy metabolism.	**Cretinism** (children) **Myxedema** (adults)
Iron	Constituent of **hemoglobin** and **myoglobin.** Constituent of **cytochromes.** Stored as **ferritin** and **hemosiderin.**	Microcytic anemia
Manganese	Cofactor of several enzymes.	
Molybdenum	Constituent of some enzymes.	
Selenium	Fat metabolism. Skeletal muscle function.	Cardiomyopathy
Zinc	**Collagen** metabolism (constituent of MMPs). Taste acuity. Stabilizes cell membranes. Cell-mediated immunity.	Delayed wound healing Hypogonadism

CHAPTER 17

Endocrine Physiology

Hormone Types and Classification	407
STEROID HORMONES	407
AMINE HORMONES	407
PEPTIDE HORMONES	407
Hormone Mechanisms	408
SECOND MESSENGER	408
Pituitary and Hypothalamus	409
HYPOTHALAMUS	409
PITUITARY GLAND	410
HYPOTHALAMIC–PITUITARY ENDOCRINE ORGAN AXIS	410
DIABETES INSIPIDUS	412
SYNDROME OF INAPPROPRIATE ADH SECRETION (SIADH)	413
SOMATOSTATIN	414
SEX HORMONES	414
PUBERTY	414
Reproduction	416
MENSTRUATION	416
OOGONIA	417
CORPUS LUTEUM	418
Pancreas	418
DIABETES MELLITUS	419
DIABETES INSIPIDUS	419
Adrenal Gland	419
ADRENAL CORTEX	419
ADRENAL MEDULLA	422
Thyroid Gland	424
HYPOTHALAMIC–PITUITARY–THYROID AXIS	424
NEGATIVE FEEDBACK LOOP	424
THYROID GLAND	424
HYPO- AND HYPERTHYROIDISM	426

Calcium and Phosphorus Metabolism 427
    HORMONES AND CALCIUM REGULATION **429**

Hormones and the Kidney 429
    ERYTHROPOIETIN **429**
    ALDOSTERONE **430**

▶ HORMONE TYPES AND CLASSIFICATION

Steroid Hormones

- Derivatives of cholesterol
    - *Cyclopentanoperhydrophenanthrene* core
- Sex hormones
    - Estradiol
    - Progesterone
    - Testosterone
- Adrenal hormones
    - Cortisol
    - Aldosterone
- **Not** water soluble
- Action:
    - Bind to intracellular receptors.
    - Form hormone response elements (HREs), complexes that activate or inactivate genes.

Amine Hormones

- Derived from amino acids
- Tyrosine
    - Thyroid hormones
        - Thyroxine (T_4)
        - Triiodothyronine (T_3)
    - Catecholamines
        - Norepinephrine
        - Epinephrine
        - Dopamine
- Tryptophan
    - Melatonin

Peptide Hormones

- Made in precursor form (pre-hormone).
- Transported in blood unbound.
- Secreted in secretory vesicles.
- Action:
    - Bind to plasma membrane receptor.
    - Generate second messenger.
- Peptide hormones include:
    - Anterior pituitary hormones: growth hormone (GH), thyroid-stimulating hormone (TSH), follicle-stimulating hormone (FSH), luteinizing hormone (LH), prolactin
    - Posterior pituitary hormones: Antidiuretic Hormone (ADH), oxytocin
    - Pancreatic hormones: insulin and glucagons
    - Parathyroid hormone (PTH).

Small Peptides	Larger Peptides	Glycoproteins
TRH	Insulin*	LH
GnRH	GH	FSH
Somatostatin	PTH	TSH
	hCG	

*Insulin works by ↑ tyrosine kinase activity of cytoplasmic portions of transmembrane receptors.

▶ HORMONE MECHANISMS

- A certain hormone affects its target cells (not necessarily all body cells).
- **Target cells** have hormone-specific receptors:
  - Intracellular receptor (steroid hormones)
  - Plasma membrane receptor (amine and peptide hormones)

Second Messenger

Protein kinases are involved in cAMP, cGMP, and IP3 pathways.

- Signals received at cell surface (extracellular receptor) are relayed to targets in the cytoplasm or nucleus by second messengers.
- Three major classes:
  - Cyclic nucleotides (cAMP, cGMP).
  - IP3 and DAG.
  - Ca^{2+} ions.

Second Messengers Used by Common Hormones

cAMP	cGMP	IP3, DAG
Epinephrine*	ANP	ADH
Glucagon	NO	TSH
ACTH		Angiotensin
PTH		
TSH		
FSH		
LH		

*When glucagon, epinephrine, and PTH activate cAMP → ↑ glycolysis, ↑ gluconeogenesis.

AC is a protein enzyme located on the inner surface of the plasma membrane.

cAMP is metabolized by phosphodiesterase. So, phosphodiesterase shuts off the response of the second messenger.

cAMP Mechanism

See Figure 17–1.

- Hormone/factor binds extracellular receptor (G protein coupled receptor).
- G protein activated.
- Adenylate cyclase (AC) activated.
- ATP –(AC)→ Camp.
- ↑ Camp.
  - Activates Protein Kinase A.
  - Stimulates gene transcription.
    - CREB (cAMP response element binding protein).

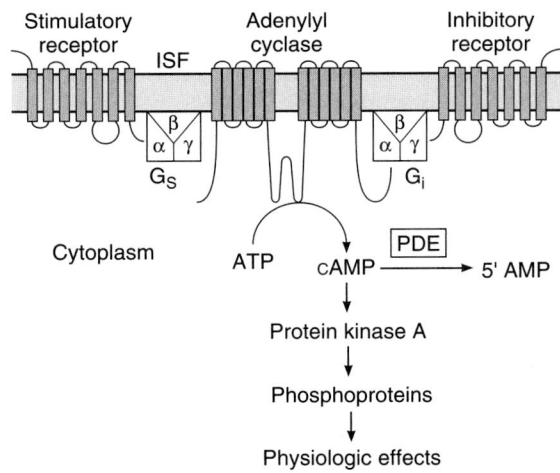

FIGURE 17-1. **cAMP mechanism.**

Reproduced, with permission, from Ganong WF. *Review of Medical Physiology*, 22nd ed. McGraw-Hill, 2005.

▶ PITUITARY AND HYPOTHALAMUS

Hypothalamus

- Part of forebrain involved in homeostasis control.
- Controls anterior and posterior pituitary.

HYPOTHALAMIC CONTROL OF THE ANTERIOR PITUITARY

- Hypothalamic releasing and inhibitory factors control secretion of anterior pituitary hormones.
- These factors are:
  - Secreted within the hypothalamus then,
  - Transported to anterior pituitary via small blood vessels (portal system).
    - Hypothalamic–hypophyseal portal system.

	Hypothalamic Hormone	Anterior Pituitary Hormone
Releasing	Gonadotropin-releasing hormone (GnRH)	↑ FSH, ↑ LH
	Thyrotropin-releasing hormone (TRH)	↑ TSH
	Corticotropin-releasing hormone (CRH)	↑ ACTH
	Growth hormone–releasing hormone	↑ GH
Inhibitory	Dopamine (DA)	↓ prolactin
	Somatostatin	↓ GH

Hypothalamic Control of the Posterior Pituitary

- Posterior pituitary hormones are synthesized in cell bodies of neurosecretory cells (located in hypothalamus).
- Axons project to and deliver hormones to pars nervosa of posterior pituitary.
- Brain neural inputs influence their release.

Hypothalamic Neurosecretory Cells	Hormones Produced
Supraoptic and Paraventricular nuclei	ADH Oxytocin

Pituitary Gland

See Figure 17–2.

- Formed from:
    - Diencephalon (posterior pituitary).
    - Rathke's pouch (anterior pituitary).
        - In week 5 of development, Rathke's pouch and diencephalon come in contact.

GH is the only anterior pituitary hormone that does not act directly on a target gland.

Hypothalamic–Pituitary Endocrine Organ Axis

See Figures 17–3 and 17–4.

- **Hypothalamus:** Releasing factors
- **Pituitary:** Trophic hormones
- **Endocrine organ:** Hormones
    - Hormones exert metabolic affect.
    - Hormones give feedback on the system.

Neither ADH nor oxytocin is produced in the posterior pituitary (made in hypothalamus).

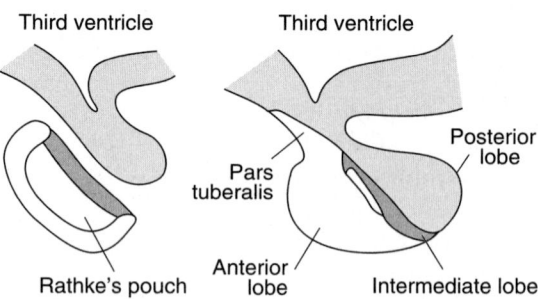

FIGURE 17-2. Pituitary gland.

Reproduced, with permission, from Ganong WF. *Review of Medical Physiology*, 22nd ed. McGraw-Hill, 2005.

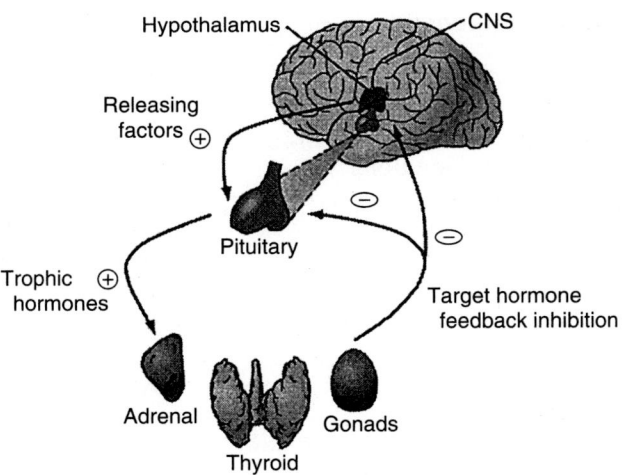

FIGURE 17–3. Hypothalamic-pituitary endocrine organ axis.

Reproduced, with permission, from DLK, Braunwald E, Fauci AS, Hauser SL, Longo DL, Jameson JL, Isselbacher KJ, eds. *Harrison's Principles of Internal Medicine,* 16th ed. McGraw-Hill, 2004.

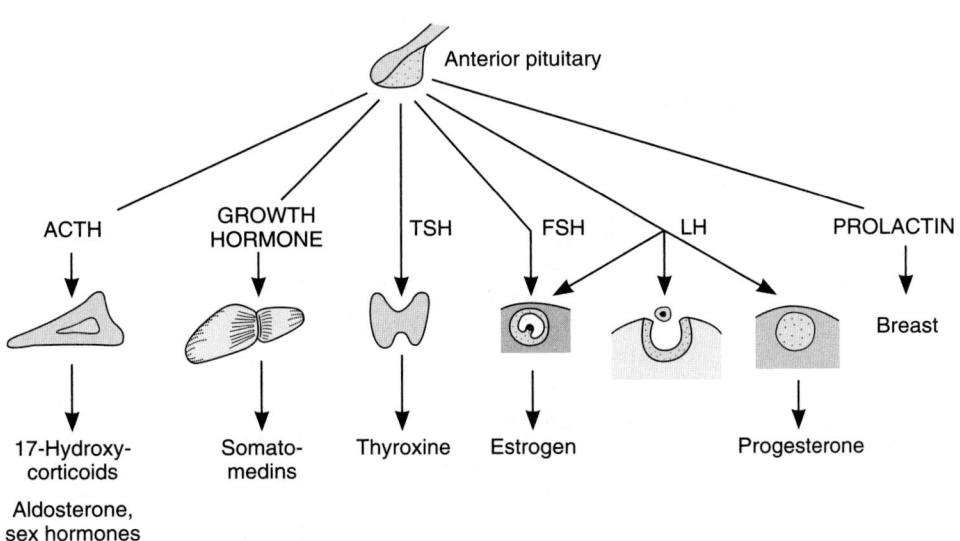

FIGURE 17–4. Hypothalamic-pituitary endocrine organ axis.

Reproduced, with permission, from Ganong WF. *Review of Medical Physiology,* 22nd ed. McGraw-Hill, 2005.

Posterior Pituitary Hormones

Hormone	ADH	Oxytocin
Produced	Hypothalamus (mainly, supraoptic nuclei)	Hypothalamus (supraoptic and paraventricular nuclei)
Stored	Posterior pituitary	Posterior pituitary
↑ release	↑ plasma Na^+ ↑ plasma osmolarity ↓ blood volume ↓ BP Nicotine Sweating SIADH	Suckling Cervical dilation Estrogen (↑ uterine oxytocin receptors)
↓ release	Ethanol Caffeine Drinking (↑ H_2O) Diabetes insipidus (DI)	Stress—catecholamines
Action	H_2O reabsorption of water from collecting duct: ↑ aquaporin expression Produce small volume of concentrated urine Conserve intravascular H_2O Helps control BP	Milk letdown* (ejection of milk with breast feeding) Uterine contraction with birthing Maternal behavior

Body fluid volume stays close to normal in DI provided the patient drinks enough water (↑ thirst) to make up for the ↑ passage of water in the urine.

*Oxytocin causes contraction myoepithelial cells surrounding sac-like alveoli of the mammary glands to induce milk let-down.

Diabetes Insipidus

- Distinguish from diabetes mellitus.
- Shares in common with diabetes mellitus:
  - Polydipsia.
  - Polyuria (very dilute).
- Different mechanism
  - ↓ ADH (or ADH doesn't work).
  - ↓ tubular reabsorption of H_2O in the kidney.
    - Pass large amount of dilute urine.
    - Hypertonic serum.
      - ↑ thirst.

Causes of Diabetes Insipidus

Central Diabetes Insipidus (↓ ADH)	Nephrogenic Diabetes Insipidus (ADH Normal OR ↑)
↓ ADH to stimulate renal tubule ■ ↓ activity of posterior pituitary gland ■ Destruction of supraoptic nuclei (hypothalamus)	Renal tubule does not respond to ADH ■ Congenital and familial ■ Drug induced (e.g., lithium)

↓ ADH (or ADH doesn't work) = DI (polydipsia, polyuria).

Syndrome of Inappropriate ADH Secretion (SIADH)

- Non-osmotically driven (ADH secretion)
- Hyponatremia (↑ Na⁺)
- Hypotonicity
- Concentrated Urine
- Elevated Urine Na⁺

Anterior Pituitary Hormones

Hormone	Prolactin (Lactogenic or Luteotropic Hormone)	Growth Hormone
Produced	Acidophils of pars distalis/anterior pituitary	Acidophils of pars distalis/anterior pituitary
↑ release	TRH ↓ dopamine, with pregnancy or lactation	GHRH ↓ plasma glucose concentration ↑ plasma level of amino acids (especially arginine) Gigantism Acromegaly
↓ Release	↑ dopamine (prolactin inhibitory factor)	Somatostatin Somatomedins Obesity Hyperglycemia Pregnancy Dwarfism
Action	Stimulates milk production by mammary glands (during pregnancy for breast development and after delivery of the child for lactation)	Exerts effect on almost all tissues ↑ all aspects of bone growth ↑ rate protein synthesis in all cells ↑ mobilization of fats; use fat for energy ↓ rate of carbohydrate utilization - Cells shift from using carbohydrates to fat in presence of GH
		Works by way of IGF-1
Dwarfism	↓ GH (undersecretion) in children.	
Gigantism	↑ GH (oversecretion) in children.	
Acromegaly	↑ GH (oversecretion) in adults (after growth plate fuses).	

GH is released in a pulsatile fashion (rate of GH increases and decreases within minutes).

GH (e.g., GH supplements) causes positive nitrogen balance; nitrogen intake exceeds output.

Lactogenesis is production of milk by mammary glands. Prolactin and oxytocin work together to facilitate breast-feeding: milk production then milk letdown.

Prolactin is under predominant inhibitory control. Normally high level of baseline dopamine is transmitted to the anterior pituitary, allowing for minimal prolactin secretion. Then, with pregnancy or lactation, dopamine formation is suppressed, allowing anterior pituitary to secrete prolactin.

Somatostatin

- Peptide hormone
- Secreted by:
  - Median eminence of hypothalamus.
  - Delta cells of pancreatic islets.
- Functions to **inhibit** release/secretion of:
  - GH (somatotropin) and thyrotropin (TSH) by anterior pituitary.
  - Insulin (from beta cells of pancreas).
  - Glucagon (from alpha cells of pancreas).
  - Gastrin (by gastric mucosa).

Sex Hormones

- FSH and LH.
- GnRH from hypothalamus stimulates release of both FSH and LH.

Progesterone is made by the ovaries.

All estrogens have an aromatic A ring (unlike other steroid hormones).

Comparison of major sex hormones

	FSH	LH
Males	Sertoli (sustentacular) cells - Sperm production, maturation	Leydig (interstitial) cells - Produce testosterone

Females	Ovary
	- Graafian follicle development
	- Steroid production
	  - Estradiol (during follicular phase)
	  - Progesterone (during luteal phase)
		Ovary
		- Steroid production
		- Estrogen-induced LH surge stimulates ovulation
		  - Forms corpus luteum

Puberty

See Figures 17–5 and 17–6.

- Age 10–15.
- ↑ GnRH (from the hypothalamus)
  - Stimulates anterior pituitary:
    - ↑ FSH
    - ↑ LH
  - Stimulates gonadal tissue (growth and function)
    - Ovaries
    - Testes
- Secondary sex characteristics appear (see following chart).
- During early childhood, a boy does not secrete gonadotropins and so has little circulating testosterone.
- On completion of puberty a male has full adult sexual capabilities and is capable of reproduction.
- Females reach puberty 1 to 2 years earlier than males. Puberty in females is heralded by menarche (first menses).

Secondary Sex Characteristics

Males (↑ Testosterone)	Females (↑ Estrogens)*
Enlargement of penis, scrotum, testis, hair growth, voice changes	Enlargement of vagina, uterus, uterine tubes; deposition of fat in breasts and hips

*Estrogen is effective at very low concentrations and generates a slowly developing long-term response in target tissues by binding to an intracellular receptor.

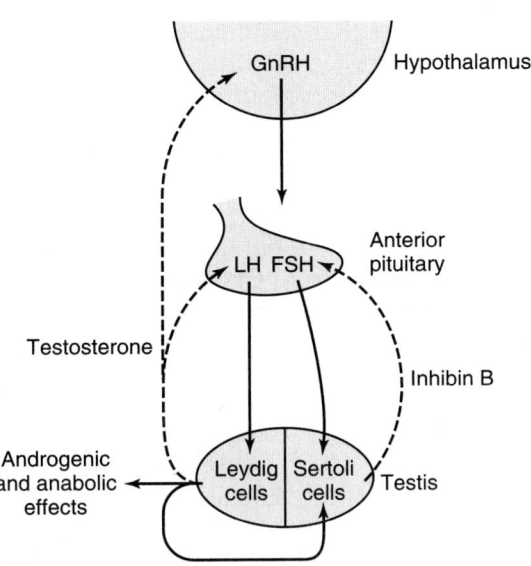

FIGURE 17-5. Puberty in the male.

Reproduced, with permission, from Ganong WF. *Review of Medical Physiology*, 22nd ed. McGraw-Hill, 2005.

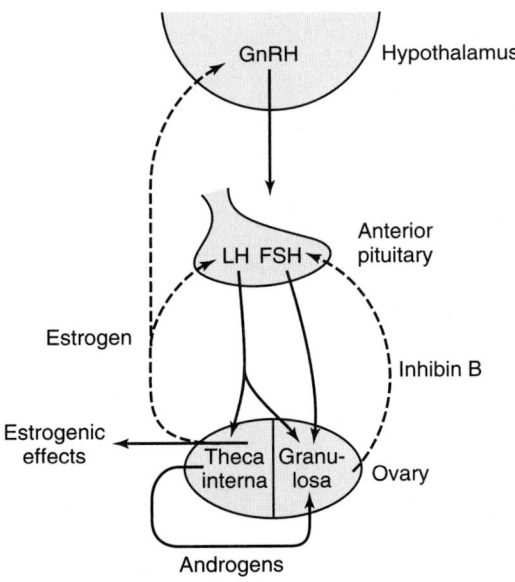

FIGURE 17-6. Puberty in the female.

Reproduced, with permission, from Ganong WF. *Review of Medical Physiology*, 22nd ed. McGraw-Hill, 2005.

Precocious Puberty

- Puberty occurs at an abnormally early age.
- Adrenal cortex: ↑ hormones similar to male and female sex hormones.

▶ REPRODUCTION

Menstruation

See Figure 17–7.

- Average menstrual cycle is 28 days (range 22–34).
- Without estrogen and progesterone, the endometrial lining is shed as menstrual fluid during menstruation/menses.
- Usually lasts about 3–5 days and involves loss of about 50 mL of blood.

	Follicular Phase	**Ovulation***	**Luteal Phase**
Days	1–14	15	16–28
Events	FSH, LH: Stimulate ovarian follicle. ↑ estrogen secretion.	LH surge: Caused by estrogen ~day 14 or 15. Stimulates ovulation.	↓ FSH, LH levels.
	Estrogen: Endometrium proliferation.	Ovulation occurs 14 days before menses (regardless of cycle length).	Corpus luteum forms. ↑ estrogen and progesterone.
	Late in this phase: Estrogen levels ↑ *peak*. FSH secretion ↓. LH secretion ↑.		If no fertilization: Corpus luteum degenerates. ↓ estrogen and progesterone levels. Feedback to hypothalamus: ↑ GnRH (cycle begins again).

*Oral contraceptive pills (OCPs) contain synthetic estrogen-like and progesterone-like substances that inhibit ovulation. OCPs suppress LHRH (GnRH) (by hypothalamus) → prevent the LH surge (by pituitary) → prevent ovulation.

Ovulation

- Stimulated by estrogen-induced LH surge.
- Ovulation is the discharge of an ovum (oocyte) from the mature follicle (graafian follicle) of the ovary.

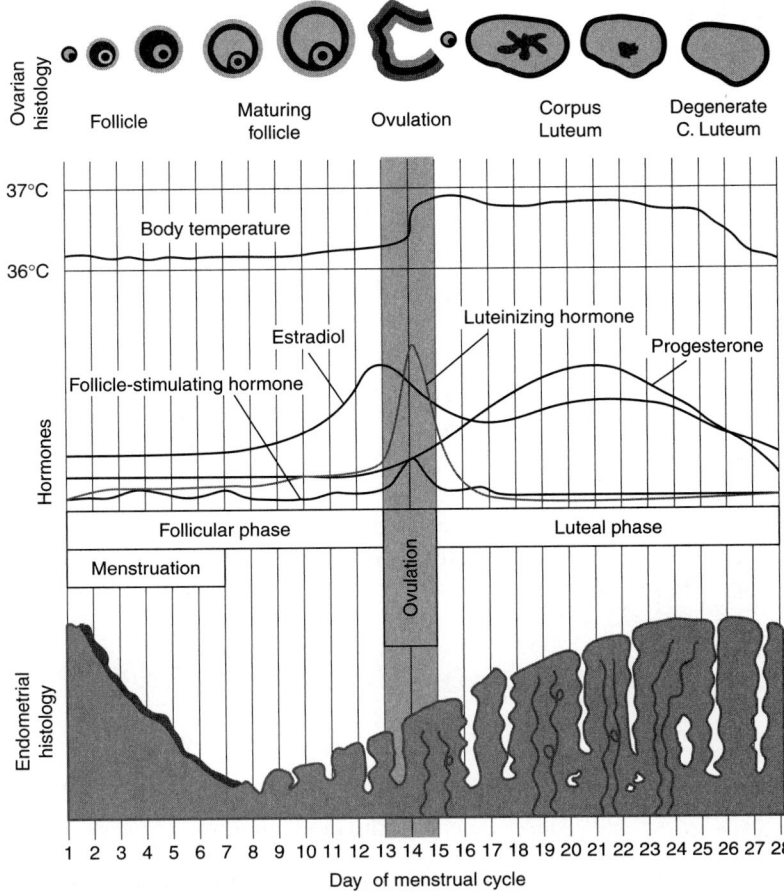

FIGURE 17-7. Female reproductive cycle.

Permission is granted to copy, distribute, and/or modify this document under the terms of the GNU free Documentation License, Version 1.2 or any later version published by the Free Software Foundation; with no Invariant Sections, no Front-Cover Texts, and no Back-Cover Texts. A copy of the license is included in the section entitled "GNU Free Documentation License." (http://en.wikipedia.org/wiki/Menstrual_cycle)

The LH surge leads to final maturation of the follicle, rupture of follicle, and ovulation. In the absence of LH, even in the presence off large amounts of FSH, the follicle will not progress to ovulation.

Key points of the female sexual cycle:

- Only a single mature ovum is released (normally) from the ovaries each month.
- So only a single fetus can begin to grow at a time.
- Uterine endometrium is prepared for implantation of the fertilized ovum at the time of ovulation.

Oogonia

- See the embryology section, Chapter 4.
- Source of oocytes
- Primordial follicles
    - Stimulated by FSH (from ant pituitary) to form:
    - *Primary oocytes* (in first meiotic division) and become:
    ↓
- Primary follicles
    - With Primary oocytes
    - Form the antrum (cavity) to become:
    ↓
- Secondary follicles
    - Primary oocytes complete first meiotic division.
    ↓
- Mature graafian follicles
    - With *secondary oocytes* (in second meiotic division).
    - LH surge causes release of secondary oocyte (egg) into abdominal cavity (ovulation).

*Human Choriogonadotropin (**hCG**), produced by the placenta, stimulates corpus luteum to persist and to secrete/produce progesterone and estradiol.*

- Egg swept by fimbraie into infundibulum/ostium of Fallopian tube (uterine tube, oviduct) to be fertilized.

Fertilization	OR	No fertilization
↓		↓
Zygote implants on uterus		Egg discarded

Corpus Luteum

- Ruptured mature ovarian follicle forms a yellow mass of cells after ovulation (egg release).
- **No** fertilization:
  - Corpus luteum retrogresses into corpus albicans.
    - Becomes a mass of scar tissue.
    - Disappears.
- **Yes** fertilization and pregnancy:
  - Corpus luteum persists (for several months).
    - Granulosa cells secrete hormones.
      - Progesterone > estrogen.

▶ PANCREAS

FSH and LH work together to cause ovulation and formation of corpus luteum.

Insulin conserves proteins, carbohydrates, and fats in the body: ↑ protein synthesis (inhibits protein breakdown), ↑ glycogenesis (inhibits glucose breakdown), and ↑ triglyceride synthesis (inhibits lipolysis).

Removal of anterior lobe of pituitary gland results in ↑ sensitivity to insulin.

Hormone	Insulin	Glucagon
Secreted	Pancreas Beta cells of islets of Langerhans	Pancreas Alpha cells in islets of Langerhans
↑ release	↑ **BGL (hyperglycemia) major stimuli.** ↑ amino acids, especially arginine, lysine, leucine. Glucagon. GH. Cortisol. Parasympathetic stimulation.	↓ BGL (hypoglycemia). ↓ amino acids (especially arginine). Cholecystokinin secretion. Sympathetic stimulation. ■ Epinephrine, NE secretion.
↓ release	↓ BGL (hypoglycemia). Sympathetic stimulation.	↑ BGL. Insulin. Somatostatin. Free fatty acids. Ketoacids.
Action	↓ BGL. ■ ↑ glucose uptake and utilization. ■ ↑↑ GLUT transporters. ↑ glycogenesis in liver. ■ ↑ glucose → glycogen. ↑ synthesis of triglycerides, proteins.	↑ BGL. ↑ glycogenolysis in liver. ■ Glycogen → glucose. ↑ free fatty acids. ↑ amino acids. ↑ urea production. It does not stimulate glycogen breakdown in the muscle.

Diabetes Mellitus

- Metabolic syndrome characterized by hyperglycemia.
- Secondary to either or both
  - Insulin deficiency.
  - Reduced effectiveness of insulin.
- Most common endocrine disorder involving the pancreas.
  - Pancreas itself may be entirely normal in cases of insulin resistance.

Diabetes Insipidus

- Distinguish from diabetes mellitus.
- Not a problem with the pancreas and insulin, but rather with ADH secretion or action.

Polyuria in diabetes mellitus (DM) is a result of osmotic diuresis, secondary to sustained hyperglycemia. (Distinguish from polyuria in DI).

Normal blood glucose level (BGL) = 80–100 mg/dl.

ADRENAL GLAND

Adrenal Cortex

- Steroid hormones
- Cholesterol core

Histologic layers of the adrenal cortex, from outermost to innermost:

- *Salt (aldosterone) = Glomerulosa.*
- *Sugar (cortisol) = Fasciculata.*
- *Sex (androgens) = Reticularis.*

CRH–ACTH–Cortisol Axis

- Hypothalamus
- CRH acts on (travels via portal system)
  ↓
- Anterior pituitary (basophils of pars distalis)
- ACTH acts on
  ↓
- Adrenal cortex (zona fasciculata)
- Cortisol (travels via bloodstream → systemic effects)

Negative Feedback Loop

- CRH → ACTH → cortisol.
- Cortisol feeds back and inhibits both the hypothalamus and anterior pituitary.
- ACTH
  - Controls production and secretion of cortisol.
  - Secretion is controlled by hypothalamus.
  - Secreted in bursts, causing cortisol levels to rise and fall.
  - Bursts are most frequent in the early morning; ~ 75% of the daily production of cortisol occurs between 4 am and 10 am.

Corticosteroids = aldosterone (mineralocorticoid) + cortisol (glucocorticoid).

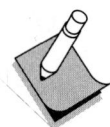

Action of cortisol is to help deal with stressors and provide the brain with adequate energy sources.

Cortisol is produced in the body (endogenous). Hydrocortisone is a synthetic corticosteroid (exogenous). Other synthetic forms: decadron, methylprednisolone.

Patients taking exogenous cortisol for a long time suppress the adrenal–ACTH (pituitary) axis. Lack of stimulation from ACTH causes atrophy of adrenal cortex. Adrenal insufficiency occurs when exogenous therapy is ceased.

Cortisol

Secreted	Adrenal cortex (zona fasiculata)	
↑ release	■ Stress. ■ Illness. ■ Trauma. ■ Surgery. ■ Temperature extremes. ■ Psychological. ■ Cushing's syndrome or disease. (See Figure 17–8.)	
↓ release	Adrenal axis suppression (e.g., pharmacologically induced). Addison's disease. Waterhouse–Frederickson.	

Action	■ ↑ BGL.
	■ ↑ glucagon and epinephrine action; ↓ insulin action.
	■ ↑ gluconeogenesis.
	    ■ ↓ glucose uptake.
	    ■ ↑ lipolysis.
	■ ↑ fatty acids.
	■ ↑ proteolysis (protein breakdown).
	■ ↑ amino acids.
	Anti-inflammatory action.
	Effects on immune system, bone, calcium absorption from GI, CNS.	

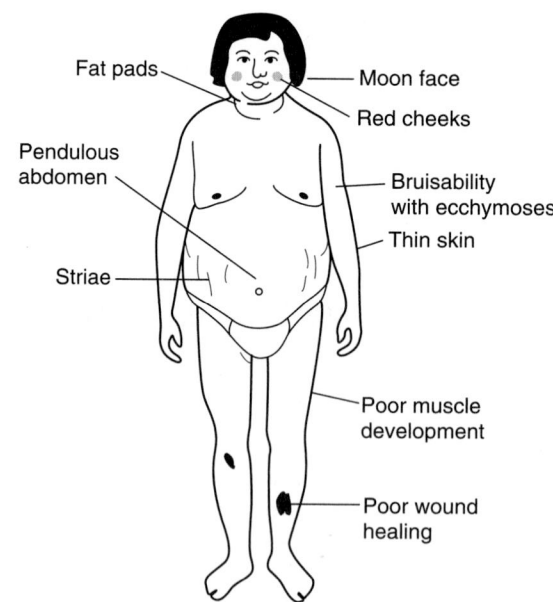

FIGURE 17-8. Cushing's syndrome.

Reproduced, with permission, from Ganong WF. *Review of Medical Physiology*, 22nd ed. McGraw-Hill, 2005.

Cushing's Syndrome vs. Cushing's Disease

	Cushing's Syndrome	**Cushing's Disease**
Cause	↑ cortisol. Exogenously administered glucocorticoids (cortisol-like medications). Endogenous ↑ cortisol (cortisol-secreting adrenalcortical tumor). Ectopic ACTH production (e.g., oat cell carcinoma).	↑ cortisol Secondary to ACTH (ACTH-secreting pituitary tumor)
Symptoms	Usually no ↑ pigmentation. Central obesity. Moon facies. Buffalo hump. Exophthalmos (retroorbital fat). Skin atrophy. Striae. (Hyperpigmentation if ↑ ACTH). Proximal muscle wasting/weakness. Bone loss. Glucose intolerance/DM-2 picture. HTN ■ ↑ sensitivity to cathecholamines, ↑ angiotensinogen, ↑ aldosterone receptors. Thromboembolism. Irritability, anxiety, panic attacks. Depression, Insomnia. ↑ Infection.	Hyperpigmentation

ADDISON'S DISEASE

- Adrenocortical insufficiency.
- ↓ corticosteroids (glucocorticoids and mineralocorticoids).
- Can occur with any age and M = F.
- In primary Addison's, cutaneous pigmentation tends to disappear following therapy, but oral pigmentation usually persists.

	Primary Addison's Disease	**Secondary Addison's Disease**
Cause	↓ cortisol Destruction of adrenal cortex<ul><li>>90% cortex must be destroyed before symptoms</li><li>70% unknown Likely autoimmune</li><li>30% identifiable cause</li><li>Infection (e.g., Tb) Cancer/neoplasm Amyloidosis Hemorrhage in the gland</li></ul>	↓ cortisol ↓ or lack of ACTH<ul><li>Abruptly stopping chronic exogenous corticoids (e.g., prednisone); usually temporary</li><li>↓ pituitary function: surgical removal, apoplexy, tumor, infection</li></ul>
Symptoms	↑ skin pigmentation (bronzing of skin) ↓ BP (hypotension) ↓ Na^+, Cl^-, HCO_3^- ↑ K^+ ↓ BGL Malaise Weight loss Depression	No ↑ skin pigmentation
Oral signs	Diffuse intraoral pigmentation<ul><li>Gingiva</li><li>Tongue</li><li>Hard palate</li><li>Buccal mucosa</li></ul>	No oral pigmentation
Treatment	Cortisol (exogenous, as hydrocortisone or prednisone)	

The adrenal medulla is a neural crest derivative.

> **NE can be released in two ways:**
> - By adrenal medulla into bloodstream.
> - Directly within an organ:
>   - Via sympathetic innervation.
>   - Postganglionic sympathetic (adrenergic) neuron that stores NE.
>
> **Note:** Effects are more widespread when NE is released into bloodstream by adrenal medulla than within an organ from a postganglionic sympathetic nerve ending.

Adrenal Medulla

See Figures 17–9.

- Specialized ganglion of sympathetic nervous system
- Preganglionic sympathetic fibers (cholinergic)
- Synapse directly on chromaffin cells in the adrenal medulla
- Chromaffin cells then secrete into the circulation:
  - Epinephrine (80%)
  - Norepinephrine (NE) (20%)

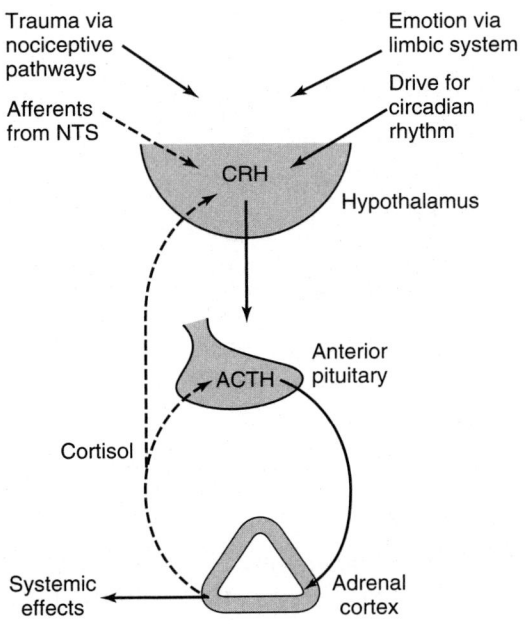

FIGURE 17-9. Adrenal medulla.

Reproduced, with permission, from Ganong WF. *Review of Medical Physiology*, 22nd ed. McGraw-Hill, 2005.

EPINEPHRINE AND NOREPINEPHRINE

- Direct acting adrenergic agonists
- Biosynthesized from tyrosine (amino acid)
- Released from adrenal medulla from storage vesicles in response to:
    - Sympathetic stimulation (fright, startle)
    - Exercise
    - Cold
    - ↓ BGL
- Function: (regulators of carbohydrate and lipid metabolism, cardiovascular effects)
    - ↑ Fatty acids
        - ↑ Triacylglycerol breakdown (lipolysis).
    - ↑ BGL.
        - ↑ Glycogen breakdown (glycogenolysis).
            - Activates muscle glycogen phosphorylase.
        - ↑ Gluconeogenesis.
    - ↑ CO (especially epinephrine).
        - ↑↑ rate, force, and amplitude of heart beat.
    - ↑ BP.
        - ↑ Vasoconstriction in skin, mucous membranes, kidneys.
    - Bronchodilation.
        - ↑ Relaxes bronchiolar smooth muscle.

Catecholamines (epinephrine, norepinephrine, and dopamine) are products of tyrosine metabolism.
Pathway:
Tyrosine → DOPA → dopamine → norepinephrine → epinephrine.

THYROID GLAND

See Figure 17–10.

Hypothalamic–Pituitary–Thyroid Axis

- TRH-TSH-Thyroid hormone axis
- Hypothalamus: TRH released (travels via portal system).
  ↓
- Anterior pituitary (basophils of pars distalis): TSH acts on
  ↓
- Thyroid gland (TSH receptor): Thyroid hormones (T_3, T_4) (travel via bloodstream → systemic effects).

Negative Feedback Loop

Stress can inhibit TSH secretion secondary to neural influences that inhibit secretion of TRH from hypothalamus.

See Figure 17–10.

- TRH → TSH → thyroid hormones.
- Thyroid hormones feedback and inhibit both the hypothalamus and anterior pituitary.
  - ↑ thyroid hormones: ↓ both TRH and TSH secretion.
  - ↑ TSH: ↓ TRH secretion.

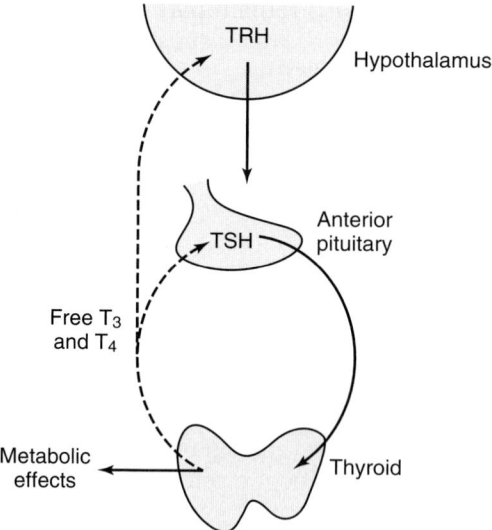

FIGURE 17-10. Thyroid gland.

Reproduced, with permission, from Ganong WF. *Review of Medical Physiology*, 22nd ed. McGraw-Hill, 2005.

Thyroid Gland

- Well vascularized gland.
  - One of highest rates of blood flow per gram of tissue of any organ.
- Composed of follicles, filled with colloid.
  - Colloid contains thyroglobulin (tyrosine containing glycoprotein).
    - Thyroglobulin contains thyroid hormones within its molecule.

THYROID CELLS (FOLLICULAR CELLS)

Three functions:

- Collect and transport iodine.
- Synthesize and secrete (into colloid) thyroglobulin.
- Remove thyroid hormones from thyroglobulin and secrete them into the circulation.

THYROGLOBULIN

- Glycoprotein hormone (10% carbohydrate).
- Contains many tyrosine residues (incorporated into thyroid hormones).
- Synthesized by thyroid follicular cell.
- Secreted/stored in colloid region of follicles.

THYROID HORMONE PRODUCTION

- Thyroglobulin is iodinated (within the colloid).
  - Iodine attaches to tyrosine molecules.
  - Thyroid hormones (T_3, T_4) remain part of the thyroglobulin molecules until secreted.

THYROID HORMONE SECRETION

- Colloid is taken up into the cytoplasm of the thyroid follicular cells.
  ↓
- Peptide bonds between iodinated residues and thyroglobulin are hydrolyzed.
  ↓
- Thyroglobulin releases thyroid hormones as free T_4 and T_3.
  ↓
- T_4 (mostly) and T_3 are discharged into the bloodstream/capillaries (systemic effects).

Thyroid hormones are lipophillic hormones. They exert effect via gene transcription.

T_4 acts as pro-hormone to T_3 (enzymatic removal of one iodine atom) in the peripheral tissues. T_3 is a more potent hormone.

THYROID HORMONES

- Necessary for normal growth and development.
  - ↑ cellular metabolism, growth.
  - ↑ differentiation of tissues, especially brain, neural tissues.
- Affect many metabolic processes and metabolic rate ↑ HR, ↑ cardiac contractility.
- ↑ O_2 consumption and heat production.
- ↑ glycogenolysis.
- ↑ gluconeogenesis.
- ↑ GI carbohydrate absorption.
- ↑ lipolysis.
- ↑ protein breakdown.

Hypo- and Hyperthyroidism

	HYPOTHYROID	**HYPERTHYROIDISM**
Diseases	Cretinism (children) Myxedema (adults)	Grave's disease* Plummer's disease Solitary toxic adenoma Toxic multinodular goiter Hashimoto's thyroiditis TSH-secreting pituitary tumor
Symptoms	Weight gain Cold intolerance Low-pitched voice Mental and physical slowness Constipation Dry skin Coarse hair Puffiness of face, eyelids, hands.	Restlessness, irritability Fatigue Heat intolerance (sweating) ↑ temperature Tachycardia Fine hair Diarrhea Tremor (shakiness) ↑ Basal metabolic rate Weight loss Generalized osteoporosis Oral manifestations: If hyperthyroid in childhood, can get: ■ Premature eruption of teeth ■ Loss of deciduous dentition

*Grave's disease is the most common form of hyperthyroidism; 50% get exophthalmos (secondary to TSH-receptor antibodies in circulation).

GRAVE'S DISEASE

- Most common form of hyperthyroidism.
- Caused by binding of immunoglobulin antibodies to TSH receptors in the thyroid.
    - Stimulates production of thyroxin.
- Typical signs
    - Goiter (enlarged thyroid)
    - Exophthalmos (bulging eyes)

PLUMMER'S DISEASE

- Toxic multinodular goiter.
- Multiple secreting thyroid nodules (adenomas) within gland.
- Uncommon in adolescents and young adults (↑ with age).
- Exophthalmos is rare.

▶ CALCIUM AND PHOSPHORUS METABOLISM

Regulation	Normal Serum Value	
	Calcium	**Phosphorus**
	8.5–10.5 mg/dl	3.0–4.5 mg/dl
PTH	↑ Ca^{2+} ↑ bone resorption ↑ renal tubular reabsorption	↓ P ↓ renal tubular reabsorption ↑ renal P excretion
Vitamin D	↑ Ca^{2+} ↑ GI absorption of Ca^{2+}	

↓ calcium in diet = ↑ PTH secretion, ↑ bone resorption (to compensate).

	Hypocalcemia	**Hypercalcemia**
Effect	Irritability/excitability nerves and muscles Tetany	Cardiac and CNS depression

Hormones and Calcium Regulation

Hormone	Parathyroid Hormone	Calcitonin
Secreted	Parathyroid gland (chief cells).	Thyroid gland (parafollicular [C-cells]).
↑ release	▪ ↓ plasma Ca^{2+}.	▪ ↑ plasma Ca^{2+}.
↓ release	▪ ↑ plasma Ca^{2+}.	▪ ↓ plasma Ca^{2+}.
Action	↑ plasma Ca^{2+}. ▪ ↑ Bone resorption ▪ Directly. ▪ By osteoclasts. ↑ Ca^{2+} reabsorption in kidney. ↑ GI absorption of Ca^{2+} (via vitamin D). ↓ Plasma phosphate. ▪ ↑ phosphate excretion in urine (via vitamin D).	↓ plasma Ca^{2+}. ▪ ↑ Ca^{2+} deposition in bone. ▪ ↓ bone resorption. ↓ GI absorption of Ca^{2+}. ↑ Ca^{2+} renal excretion. ↓ plasma phosphate. ▪ ↑ phosphate renal excretion.

- PTH is the most important hormone in Ca^{2+} metabolism (principal controller of Ca^{2+} and phosphate metabolism) and is involved in remodeling of bone. Plasma Ca^{2+} is major controller of PTH secretion.
- PTH Stimulates 1-alpha hydroxylase in the kidneys.
- Compared to PTH, calcitonin has only a minor role in regulating blood calcium (in fact, calcitonin is not required in adult humans). Calcitonin is important during bone development.

	Hypoparathyroidism	**Hyperparathyroidism**
Example(s)	Congenital (DiGeorge syndrome). Iatrogenic (surgery) Infiltration/destruction (sarcoidosis) Idiopathic <ul><li>↓ bone resorption</li><li>↓ renal Ca^{2+} reabsorption</li><li>↑ renal phosphate reabsorption</li><li>↓ 1, 25-dihydroxycholecalciferol*</li></ul>	Parathyroid adenoma Parathyroid carcinoma (rare) Multiple endocrine neoplasm (MEN) von Recklinghausen's disease <ul><li>↑ bone resorption</li><li>↑ renal Ca^{2+} reabsorption</li><li>↓ renal phosphate reabsorption</li><li>↓/↓ 1, 25-dihydroxycholecalciferol</li></ul>
Calcium	↓ plasma Ca^{2+} (↑ Ca^{2+} in bone)	↑ plasma Ca^{2+} (↓ Ca^{2+} in bone)
Phosphate	↑ plasma phosphate	↓ plasma phosphate
Symptom(s)	Tetany Mental status changes (MS Δ's) seizures ↓ Cardiac contractility Vomiting	Bone pain Pathologic fractures Osteitis fibrosa cystica Brown tumors of bone Nephrolithiasis Muscular weakness

*1, 25-dihydroxycholecalciferol = active form of vitamin D.

Hormones and Calcium Regulation

See Chapter 15, "Gastrointestinal Physiology."

▶ HORMONES AND THE KIDNEY

See Chapter 14.

Erythropoietin

- Released by kidneys.
- Stimulates RBC production.

Hormone	Erythropoietin
Secreted	Kidney (peritubular capillary interstitial cells)
↑ release	↓ PO_2 (hypoxemia) - Anemia - Lung disease - Cardiac disease - High altitudes
↑ release	Normal PO_2 ↑ RBC volume
Action	↑ RBCs - EPO receptors on erythroid progenitors ↑ replication - ↑ maturation

Aldosterone

See Figure 17–11.

- Released by adrenal cortex zona glomerulosa.

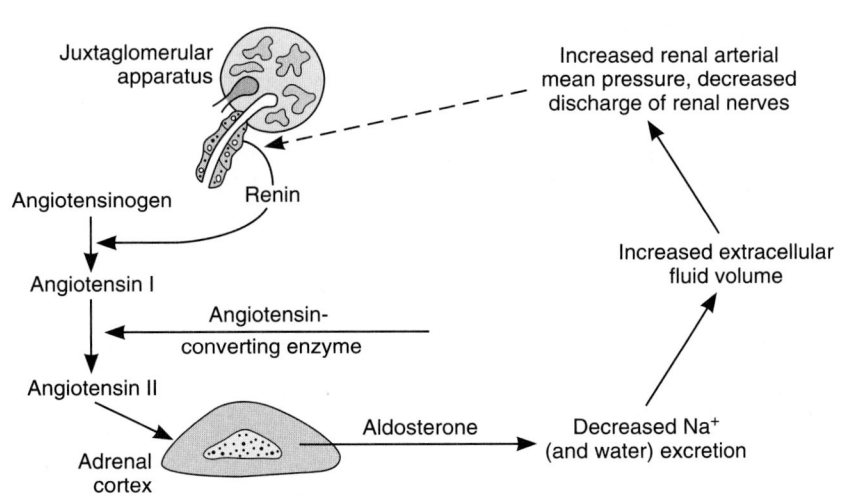

FIGURE 17–11. Adrenal Cortex.

Reproduced, with permission, from Ganong WF. *Review of Medical Physiology*, 22nd ed. McGraw-Hill, 2005.

↓ Na⁺ → Juxtaglomerular (JG) cells secrete renin → rennin cleaves angiotensinogen into AT-I → AT-I (converted by ACE) → AT-II. AT-II then stimulates adrenal cortex to release aldosterone.

In Addison's disease there is hyposecretion of both aldosterone and cortisol.

Hormone	Aldosterone (Mineralocorticoid)
Secreted	Adrenal cortex (zona glomerulosa).
↑ release	↑ K⁺. ↑ AT-II (via ↑ renin).
↓ release	↓ K⁺. ↓ AT-II (via ↓ renin).
Action	Site of action is distal nephron—DCT, collecting ducts. ■ ↑ plasma volume (↑ H_2O reabsorption). ■ ↑ plasma Na⁺ (↑ Na⁺ reabsorption). ■ ↓ plasma K⁺ (↓ K⁺ reabsorption; ↑ K⁺ excretion).

SECTION 3
Microbiology-Pathology

- Microbiology
- Oral Microbiology and Pathology
- Reactions to Tissue Injury
- Immunology and Immunopathology
- Systemic Pathology
- Neoplasia

CHAPTER 18
Microbiology

General Microbiology	435
CELL TYPES	435
MICROORGANISMS	435
INFECTIONS	436
Sterilization and Disinfection	437
STERILIZATION	437
DISINFECTION	438
PASTEURIZATION	438
SANITIZATION	439
INFECTION CONTROL	439
Bacteriology	441
BACTERIA	441
PATHOGENESIS	441
BACTERIAL VIRULENCE FACTORS	442
CLASSIFICATION	444
MEDICALLY RELEVANT BACTERIA	446
BACTERIAL VACCINES	454
ANTIBIOTIC DRUGS	454
Virology	458
VIRUSES	458
PATHOGENESIS	460
CLASSIFICATION	461
HEPATITIS VIRUSES	467
VIRAL VACCINES	469
ANTIVIRAL DRUGS	469
BACTERIOPHAGES (PHAGES)	469
PRIONS	470
Mycology	470
FUNGI	470
PATHOGENESIS	471

CLASSIFICATION	471
ANTIFUNGAL DRUGS	472

Parasitology 474
PARASITES 474

▶ GENERAL MICROBIOLOGY

Cell Types

See Table 18–1.

- Prokaryotes
- Eukaryotes

Microorganisms

See Table 18–2.

- Bacteria
- Viruses
- Fungi
- Parasites

TABLE 18–1. Comparison of Prokaryotic and Eukaryotic Cells

Cell Type	Membrane-Enveloped Nucleus	Membrane-Bound Organelles	Ribosome Size	Nucleic Acid Location	DNA Type	Replication
Prokaryote	No	No	70S	Nucleoid (cytoplasm)	Circular	Binary Fission
Eukaryote	Yes	Yes	80S	Nucleus	Linear	Mitosis

TABLE 18–2. Comparison of Major Microorganisms Implicated in Infectious Diseases

Micro-Organism	Cell Type	Outer Surface	Nucleic Acid	Ribosomes	Mitochondria	Replication
Bacteria	Prokaryotic	Cell wall of peptidoglycan.	RNA and DNA	70S	No	Binary fission
Viruses	Noncellular	Protein capsid and lipoprotein envelope.	RNA or DNA	None	No	Assembly within host cells.
Fungi	Eukaryotic	Cell wall of chitin.	RNA and DNA	80S	Yes	Budding (yeasts) Mitosis (molds)
Parasites	Eukaryotic	Cell membrane	RNA and DNA	80S	Yes	Mitosis

Infections

EPIDEMIOLOGY

- An **endemic** infection occurs at minimal levels within a population.
- An **epidemic** infection occurs more frequently than normal within a population.
- A **pandemic** infection occurs worldwide.

BACTERIAL AND VIRAL INFECTIONS

- **Bacteremia**: The presence of bacteria in the bloodstream. If the bacteria cannot be cleared by host immune cells, **sepsis** results.
- **Viremia**: The presence of viruses in the bloodstream.

INFECTIOUS STATES

- **Acute**: Short-term active infection with symptoms.
- **Chronic**: Long-term active infection with symptoms.
- **Subclinical**: Infection is detectable only by serological tests.
- **Latent**: No active growth of microorganisms but potential for reactivation.
- **Carrier**: Active growth of microorganisms with or without symptoms.

Pus is a creamy substance that contains dead neutrophils, necrotic cells, and exudates.

INTERACTIVE ASSOCIATIONS

- **Commensalism**: The association of two organisms living close together in which one benefits from the other.
- **Symbiosis**: The essential association of two organisms that live close to each other with or without mutual benefit.
- **Mutualism**: A form of symbiosis in which two organisms live together with mutual benefit.

INFECTIOUS SWELLINGS

- **Abscess**: An *acute inflammatory lesion* consisting of a localized collection of pus surrounded by a fibrous wall.
- **Granuloma**: A *chronic inflammatory lesion* consisting of granulation tissue: fibrosis (fibroblasts), angiogenesis (new capillaries), and inflammatory cells (macrophages, lymphocytes, plasma cells, epithelioid cells, and multinucleated giant cells).
- **Cyst**: A fluid-filled sac lined with epithelium.
- **Cellulitis**: An acute, diffuse swelling along fascial planes that separate muscle bundles.

Ludwig's angina is a rapidly occurring cellulitis involving the submandibular, sublingual, and submental fascial spaces, bilaterally. Because it can cause airway obstruction, emergency treatment is critical.

SEPSIS

Common signs and symptoms of sepsis:

- Fever
- Fatigue
- Nausea/vomiting
- Chills
- Diarrhea

Sepsis is most commonly caused by Staphylococcus aureus and Escherichia coli.

STERILIZATION AND DISINFECTION

Sterilization

See Table 18–3.

TABLE 18–3. Common Sterilization Techniques

Sterilization Technique	Mechanism of Action	Common Use	Characteristics
Moist heat (**autoclaving**)	Denatures proteins.	Normal cycle heats to **121°C (250°F) for 15–20 minutes**, yielding 15 lb/in^2 of vapor pressure. Fast cycle heats to 134°C (270°F) for 3 minutes, yielding 30 lb/in^2 of vapor pressure.	Most common form of sterilization. Can corrode or dull carbon-steel instruments.
Dry heat	Denatures proteins.	Heats to 160°C (320°F) for 2 hours, or 170°C (340°F) for 1 hour.	Does *not* corrode or dull instruments.
Chemical vapor (chemiclave)	Denatures and alkylates nucleic acids and proteins.	Heats to 132°C (270°F) for 20–30 minutes, yielding 25 lb/in^2 of vapor pressure.	Uses a combination of alcohol and formaldehyde. Does *not* corrode or dull instruments.
Ethylene oxide gas	Alkylates nucleic acids and proteins.	Sterilization is slow, taking 8–10 hours.	Requires an appropriate chamber and ventilation system. Used mostly in hospitals for heat-sensitive materials.
Formaldehyde	Alkylates nucleic acids and proteins.	Commonly used as a 37% solution in water (Formalin).	Less efficacious compared to other methods of sterilization.
Glutaraldehyde (2%)	Alkylates nucleic acids and proteins.	Sterilization is slow, taking 10 hours.	Associated with hypersensitivity. Used mostly for heat-sensitive materials.
Filtration	Physically and electrostatically traps microorganisms larger than the pore size.	Commonly uses a nitrocellulose filter with a 0.22 μm pore size.	The preferred method of sterilizing **liquid solutions.**

- The killing of *all* microorganisms, including bacterial spores.
- Heat sterilization (moist heat and dry heat) is the most reliable mode of sterilization because it can be easily biologically tested.
- Cleaning instruments before sterilization helps to minimize microbial concentrations and maximize sterilization efficacy.

Spore tests (with Bacillus stearothermophilus) are recommended on a weekly basis.

Disinfection

- The killing of many, but not all, microorganisms.

DISINFECTANTS

See Table 18–4.

Disinfectant effectiveness is determined by killing activity against Mycobacterium tuberculosis.

- Disinfectants are used only on *inanimate objects* such as countertops and chairs.

ANTISEPTICS

See Table 18–5.

- Chemicals that kill microorganisms on the surface of *skin and mucous membranes*.
- Many antiseptics can also be used as disinfectants.

Human immunodeficiency virus (HIV) is relatively easy to kill on most environmental surfaces.

Pasteurization

- A method of heat-killing milk-borne pathogens such as *Mycobacterium tuberculosis, Salmonella, Streptococcus, Listeria,* and *Brucella*.
- Heats milk to 62°C for 30 minutes, then cools rapidly.

TABLE 18-4. Common Disinfectants

DISINFECTANT	FAMILY	MECHANISM OF ACTION	CHARACTERISTICS
Phenols	Phenol	Disrupts cell membranes and denatures proteins.	Rarely used today because they are extremely caustic.
Quarternary ammonium compounds	Cationic detergent	Disrupts cell membranes.	Also used as antiseptics.
Chlorine	Chlorine	Oxidatively inactivates sulfhydryl-containing enzymes.	It is the active component of hypochlorite (bleach).

TABLE 18-5. Common Antiseptics

ANTISEPTIC	FAMILY	MECHANISM OF ACTION	CHARACTERISTICS
Iodine and iodophors	Iodine	Oxidatively inactivates sulfhydryl-containing enzymes.	Most effective skin antiseptics. Associated with hypersensitivity.
Ethanol and isopropyl alcohol (70–90%)	Alcohol	Disrupts cell membranes and denatures proteins.	Most widely used skin antiseptic. Used on skin prior to venipuncture or immunizations. Isopropyl alcohol can be used as a waterless handwash.
Hydrogen peroxide	Peroxide	Oxidatively inactivates sulfhydryl-containing enzymes.	Effective only against *catalase-negative* organisms.
Chlorhexidine gluconate (0.12%)	Bis-biguanide	Disrupts cell membranes (due to its cationic properties).	Highly substantive. Used as a handwash and a mouthrinse.
Triclosan	Bis-phenol	Disrupts cell membranes.	Used as a handwash and as an ingredient in some dentifrices.

Sanitization

- A method of treating public water supplies to reduce microbial loads.

Infection Control

REGULATIONS VS. RECOMMENDATIONS

- The **Centers for Disease Control and Prevention (CDC)** is the major agency responsible for infectious disease epidemiology, surveillance, and prevention. It provides *recommendations* and *guidelines* for infection control procedures used by healthcare workers.
- The **Occupational Safety and Health Administration (OSHA)**, a division of the U.S. Department of Labor, is responsible for composing and enforcing infection control *laws* and *regulations* that must be followed by healthcare workers. OSHA may use CDC recommendations and guidelines in drafting its mandates.

Universal Precautions

- All human blood (and other body fluids that contain visible blood) are treated as infectious for HIV, hepatitis B virus (HBV), and other bloodborne pathogens.
- The greatest risk for bloodborne infection among healthcare workers is **HBV**.
- **Engineering controls** (sharps disposal containers, etc.) and **work practice controls** (prohibiting food storage near potentially contaminated material, etc.) must be used to eliminate or minimize exposure.
- All reusable equipment and instruments that contact a patient's blood, saliva, or mucous membranes must be sterilized.
- All environmental and working surfaces must be cleaned and disinfected after contact with a patient's blood or other potentially infectious materials.
- All disposable sharps (needles, blades, etc.) must be discarded in closable, puncture-resistant containers.
- All other regulated wastes (disposable equipment, gauze, etc.) must be discarded in closable containers.
- All containers of sharps, regulated wastes, and potentially infectious material must be labeled "biohazard."
- Appropriate **personal protective equipment (PPE)**, including gloves, face shields or masks, eye protection, long-sleeve gowns/coats, surgical caps, and shoe covers must be worn (depending on the degree of exposure risk).
- Gloves are required during the handling and cleaning of blood-soiled equipment.
- Latex-free gloves *(vinyl* or *nitrile)* must be provided for patients or employees with rubber latex hypersensitivity.

Handwashing *is the most important infection control practice for reducing nosocomial infections and must be performed after removal of personal protective equipment.*

Preexposure Protocol

- Dentists *must* offer the HBV vaccine to their employees at no cost.
- If the employee declines, a declination form must be signed.
- The employee must be given the free vaccine if he or she changes his or her mind.

Postexposure Protocol

- If someone is exposed to or comes into contact with infectious material, *immediate* aggressive washing and first aid of the site is required.
- The dentist *must* provide **confidential** medical evaluation and follow-up at no cost to the employee.
- The medical evaluation includes blood collection and testing from the source individual and the employee.
- The follow-up includes postexposure prophylaxis, counseling, and evaluation.
- The employee has the right to decline blood collection and testing.
- The dentist does *not* have the right to know the test results of the employee or the source individual.

► BACTERIOLOGY

Bacteria

- Prokaryotic cells of various shapes and sizes.
- All bacteria (except *Mycoplasma* sp.) contain a selectively permeable **plasma membrane** surrounded by a **peptidoglycan cell wall** of differing thicknesses.
- A gelatinous **polysaccharide capsule** surrounds the cell wall, which functions in virulence (prevents opsonization and phagocytosis), antigenicity, and bacterial adhesion.

Peptidoglycan is a cross-linked polysaccharide consisting of alternating N-acetylmuramic acid and N-acetylglucosamine residues.

Pathogenesis

BACTERIAL GROWTH CURVE

See Figure 18–1.

- **Lag phase:** Increased metabolic activity as the bacteria prepare to divide.
- **Log phase:** Exponential growth and division.
- **Stationary phase:** Cell growth plateaus as the number of new cells balances the number of dying cells due to the depletion of required nutrients.
- **Death phase:** Exponential increase in bacterial cell death.

*Salivary **lysozyme** cleaves the glycosidic bonds of the peptidoglycan molecule.*

BACTERIAL GENETIC EXCHANGE

- Genetic information is exchanged *between* bacteria in three ways (conjugation, transduction, and transformation), creating genetic variability and antibiotic resistance.
- Transfer of DNA *within* a bacterial cell occurs via **transposons**, which are portions of DNA that move from one site on the chromosome to another (or to a plasmid).
- Regardless of the mode of exchange, the DNA becomes integrated in the host cell chromosome by **recombination**.
  - **Conjugation:** DNA transfer from a donor cell (F^+ cell) *directly* to a recipient cell (F^- cell) through a conjugation tube (**sex pilus**). Usually, the F^+ DNA is transferred as a separate **F plasmid** (F factor); however, the F factor is sometimes incorporated into the F^+ chromosome, allowing partial or complete chromosomal transfer. These F^+ cells are called **Hfr** (high-frequency recombination) cells.

*Bacteria reproduce by **binary fission**, in which one parent cell divides into two progeny cells. Bacterial growth is thus exponential.*

There are only a few natural transformers: Streptococcus sp., Haemophilus sp., Neisseria gonorrhoeae, and Helicobacter pylori.

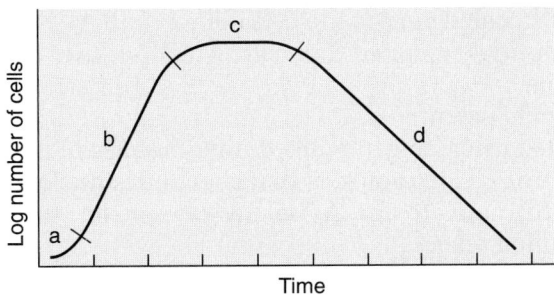

FIGURE 18–1. Bacterial growth curve.

Reproduced, with permission, from Levinson W. *Medical Microbiology and Immunology*, 8th ed. McGraw-Hill, 2004.

- **Transduction:** DNA transfer via a virus (**bacteriophage**).
- **Transformation:** DNA itself (from either donor cell lysis or laboratory extraction) is taken up by a recipient cell, transforming its phenotype.

Bacterial Virulence Factors

MEDIATORS OF BACTERIAL ADHESION/ATTACHMENT

- Capsule
- Glycocalyx
- Surface proteins (adhesins)
- Fimbriae

MEDIATORS OF EVASION OF HOST DEFENSES

- Capsule
  - Prevents opsonization and phagocytosis.
- Surface proteins
  - **M protein:** Antiphagocytic (from group A streptococci).
  - **Protein A:** Inhibits complement (from *Staphylococcus aureus*).
- Enzymes
  - **Coagulase:** Promotes fibrin clot formation.
  - **IgA protease:** Degrades IgA.
  - **Leukocidins:** Destroy polymorphonuclear neutrophils (PMNs) and macrophages.

MEDIATORS OF HOST TISSUE DESTRUCTION

- Enzymes
  - **Collagenases (metalloproteinases):** Degrade collagens.
  - **Hyaluronidase:** Degrades hyaluronic acid.
  - **Lecithinase:** Hydrolyzes lecithin to destroy plasma membranes.
  - **Streptodornase (DNase):** Depolymerizes DNA.
  - **Streptolysin O:** Causes β-hemolysis (oxygen-labile).
  - **Streptolysin S:** Causes β-hemolysis (oxygen-stable).
  - **Pneumolysin:** Causes β-hemolysis.
  - **Streptokinase:** Activates plasminogen to dissolve clots.
  - **Staphylokinase:** Activates plasminogen to dissolve clots.
  - **Exfoliatin:** Epidermolytic protease causing scalded skin syndrome.
- Toxins
  - **Exotoxin:** Located *outside* the cell wall.
    - **Polypeptides** secreted by *both* gram-positive and gram-negative bacteria.
    - Extremely potent toxins.
    - Detected using enzyme-linked immunosorbent assay (ELISA).
    - **Enterotoxins** are exotoxins that affect intestinal endothelial cells.
      - **Botulinum toxin:** A potent neurotoxin that inhibits acetylcholine release.

- **Tetanus toxin:** A neurotoxin that inhibits glycine release.
- **Diphtheria toxin:** Inhibits protein synthesis.
- **Anthrax toxin:** Edema factor, lethal factor, protective antigen.
- **Toxic shock syndrome toxin (TSST):** A superantigen that promotes cytokine release from T-cells and macrophages.
- **Exotoxin A:** An enterotoxin.
- **Exotoxin B:** A cytotoxin that destroys tissue rapidly.
- **Alpha toxin:** Lecithinase.
- **Erythrogenic toxin:** A superantigen that causes scarlet fever.
- **Endotoxin:** Located *within* the cell wall. (See Figures 18–2 and 18–3.)
  - Endotoxin is a **lipopolysaccharide (LPS).**
  - **Lipid A** is the toxic component of LPS.
  - Found *only* in gram-negative bacteria.

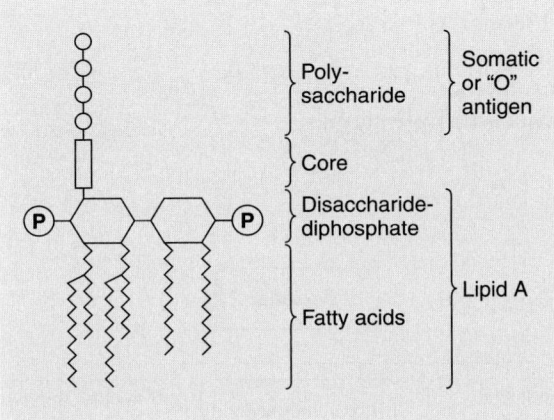

FIGURE 18-2. Endotoxin (LPS) structure.

Reproduced, with permission, from Levinson W. *Medical Microbiology, and Immunology*, 8th ed. McGraw-Hill, 2004.

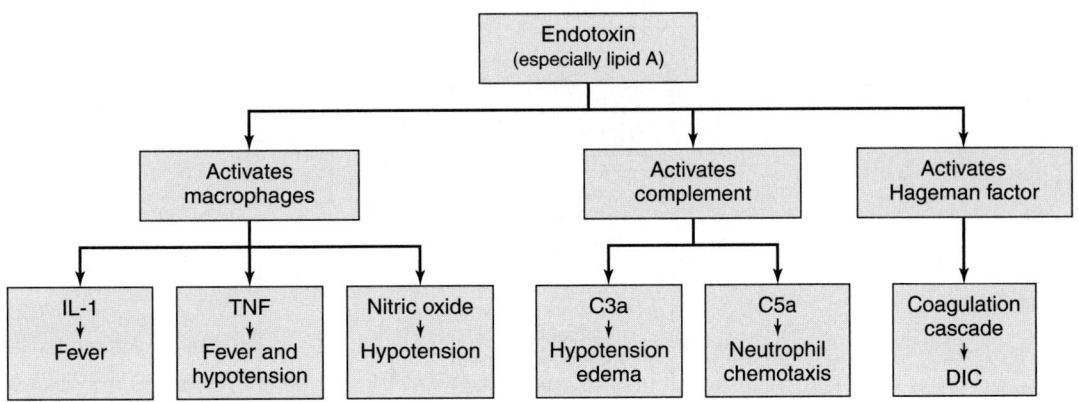

FIGURE 18-3. Mode of action of endotoxin.

Reproduced, with permission, from Levinson W. *Medical Microbiology and Immunology*, 8th ed. McGraw-Hill, 2004.

SPECIALIZED BACTERIAL STRUCTURES

- **Flagella:** Long appendages that provide bacterial motility.
- **Pili (fimbriae):** Shorter appendages that mediate bacterial attachment to cells.
- **Glycocalyx:** A sticky polysaccharide coating that enables bacterial adherence to surfaces (e.g., teeth, heart valves, catheters).

Classification

See Figure 18–4.

- By shape:
    - **Cocci:** Round
        - **Diplococci:** Pairs
        - **Streptococci:** Chains
        - **Staphylococci:** Clusters
    - **Bacilli:** Rods
    - **Spirochetes:** Spiral
    - **Pleomorphic:** Multiple shapes

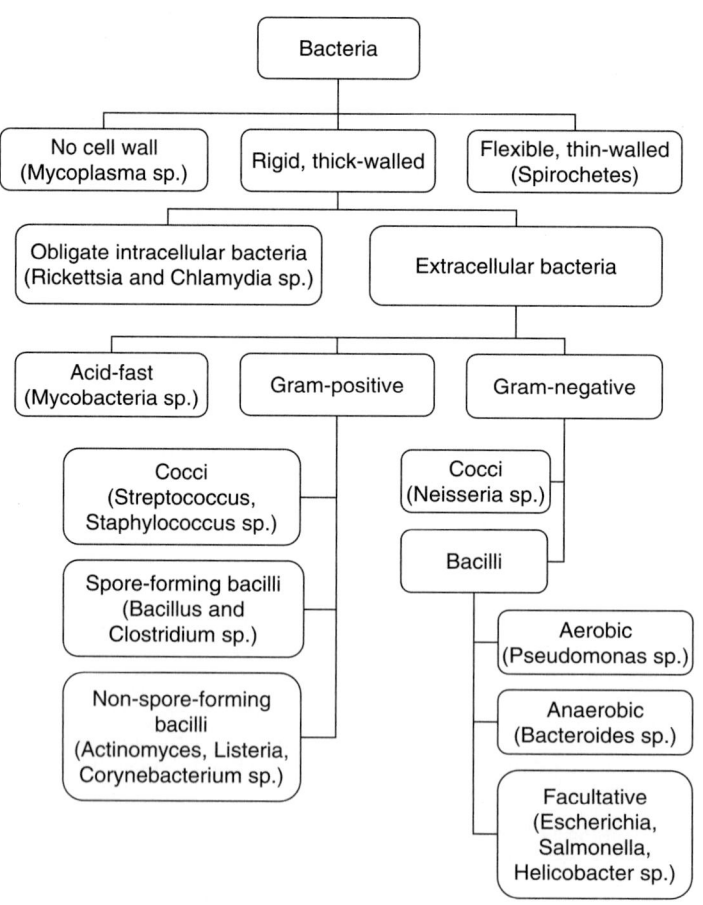

FIGURE 18-4. **Classification of bacteria.**

- By diagnostic stain (based on cell wall type) (see Table 18-6).
  - **Gram stain:** Separates almost all bacteria into two categories:
    - Gram-positive.
    - Gram-negative.
  - **Acid-fast stain:** Stains *Mycobacteria* sp.
- By oxygen requirements:
  - **Obligate aerobic:** Require oxygen for growth.
  - **Obligate anaerobic:** Cannot grow in oxygenated environments because they lack *superoxide dismutase* (rids O_2 radicals) and/or *catalase* (rids H_2O_2).
  - **Facultative anaerobic:** Grow aerobically when oxygen is present, but use fermentation pathways in its absence.
- By spore production:
  - **Spores** are thick-walled cells produced only by certain **gram-positive rods:** *Bacillus* (aerobic) and *Clostridium* (anaerobic) species.
  - They are formed in low-nutrient states (during the **stationary phase** of bacterial cell growth) and remain dormant, often in soil.
  - When nutrients are restored, they germinate to form new bacteria.
  - Spores are extremely **heat resistant.**

*Mycobacteria cell walls contain **mycolic acid**, not peptidoglycan.*

Only sterilization procedures (autoclaving, ethylene oxide gas, etc.) are sporicidal.

TABLE 18-6. Comparison of Gram-Positive and Gram-Negative Bacteria

Gram Stain	Stain Color	Peptidoglycan Wall	Major Wall Constituent	Periplasmic Space	Endotoxin
Gram-positive	Purple	Thick	Lipoteichoic acid (LTA)	No	No
Gram-negative	Pink	Thin	Lipopolysaccharide (LPS)	Yes	Yes (LPS)

Medically Relevant Bacteria

GRAM-POSITIVE COCCI

- *Streptococci*
    - Grow in pairs or chains.
    - Many are part of the normal human flora.
    - Do *not* produce catalase.
    - Classified by lysis of erythrocytes (hemolysis) when plated on blood agar. (See Tables 18–7 and 18–8.)
    - Beta-hemolytic *Strep* are further classified by **Lancefield groups** (Group A, B, C, D, etc.).
    - **Sherman classification** (rarely used) is based on phenotypic tests:
        - Pyogenic
        - Viridans
        - *Lactococci*
        - *Enterococci*
- *Staphylococci*
    - Grow in grapelike clusters.
    - Produce pyogenic (suppurative) infections.
    - Produce **catalase** (rids H_2O_2).

See Table 18–9.

Streptococci hemolysis:

Alpha: **A**lmost (incomplete)
Beta: **B**est (complete)
Gamma: **G**arbage (none)

TABLE 18-7. Classification of *Streptococci* by Hemolysis

CLASSIFICATION	HEMOLYSIS	CHARACTERISTICS	ASSOCIATED DISEASE
Alpha	Incomplete		Caries Endocarditis Upper respiratory tract infections
Beta	Complete	Lancefield group is determined by the **C carbohydrate** composition of the cell wall.	
Group A		Type of group A is determined by the **M protein** located on outer surface of cell.	Pyogenic infections Pharyngitis Glomerulonephritis Meningitis Scarlet fever Rheumatic fever
Group B			Neonatal meningitis Neonatal sepsis
Group C			Rare in humans
Group D			Urinary tract infections Endocarditis
Gamma	None		

TABLE 18-8. Comparison of Major *Streptococci*

Species	Hemolysis	Major Virulence Factors	Disease
S. pyogenes	Beta (Group A)	**Hyaluronidase** **Streptokinase** **Erythrogenic toxin** **Streptolysin O and S** Exotoxin A and B	Pyogenic infections Pharyngitis Glomerulonephritis Meningitis Scarlet fever Rheumatic fever
S. agalactiae	Beta (Group B)	Capsular polysaccharide	Neonatal meningitis Neonatal sepsis
S. bovis	Beta (Group D)	None	Endocarditis
Enterococci	Beta (Group D)	None	Urinary tract infections
S. pneumoniae ▪ Lancet-shaped diplococcus	Alpha	Capsular polysaccharide Pneumolysin IgA protease	Pneumonia (elderly) Meningitis (elderly) Upper respiratory tract infections
Viridans group	Alpha	None	Caries Endocarditis

TABLE 18-9. Comparison of Major *Staphylococci*

Species	Coagulase	Hemolysis	Major Virulence Factors	Disease
S. aureus	+	Beta	**Protein A** **β-lactamase** **Enterotoxin** Hyaluronidase Staphylokinase TSST Exfoliatin	Abscess Gastroenteritis Endocarditis Toxic shock syndrome. Scalded skin syndrome.
S. epidermidis	−	Gamma	Glycocalyx	Infection of IV catheters and prosthetic implants. Endocarditis
S. saprophyticus	−	Gamma	None	Urinary tract infections.

MICROBIOLOGY—PATHOLOGY

MICROBIOLOGY

GRAM-POSITIVE BACILLI

See Table 18–10.

- Spore-forming.
- Non-spore-forming.

TABLE 18–10. Comparison of Major Gram-Positive Bacilli

Bacterium	Oxygen Requirement	Major Virulence Factors	Disease
Spore-forming			
Bacillus anthracis	Aerobic	D-glutamate capsule Anthrax toxin	Anthrax - Malignant pustule - Transmitted cutaneously or by inhalation
Bacillus cereus	Facultative	Enterotoxins	Food poisoning - Ingestion of reheated grains and rice (fried rice)
Clostridium botulinum	Anaerobic	Botulinum toxin - Botox derives from exotoxin A	Botulism - CN paralysis - Muscle paralysis - Respiratory failure - Ingestion of undercooked canned foods, fish, ham, pork
Clostridium tetani	Anaerobic	Tetanus toxin	Tetanus - Associated with puncture wounds - Spastic paralysis - Trismus
Clostridium perfringens	Anaerobic	Alpha toxin	Gas gangrene - Necrotizing faciitis - Myonecrosis Food poisoning - Ingestion of reheated meats
Clostridium difficile	Anaerobic	Exotoxin A and B	Antibiotic-associated pseudomembranous colitis (especially clindamycin)
Non-spore-forming			
Cornybacterium diphtheriae - Club-shaped	Aerobic	Diphtheria toxin	Diphtheria - Firm, gray tonsilar pseudomembranes

TABLE 18-10. Comparison of Major Gram-Positive Bacilli (Continued)

Bacterium	Oxygen Requirement	Major Virulence Factors	Disease
Listeria monocytogenes ▪ Motile via actin rockets	Aerobic	Listeriolysin O	Neonatal meningitis Neonatal sepsis Gastroenteritis
Actinomyces israelii	Anaerobic	None	Actinomycosis ▪ Slow-growing, lumpy abscesses. ▪ Characteristic **sulfur granules** are bacterial colonies.

Gram-Negative Cocci

See Table 18–11.

TABLE 18-11. Comparison of Major Gram-Negative Cocci

Bacterium	Oxygen Requirement	Major Virulence Factors	Disease
Neisseria meningitidis	Aerobic	Polysaccharide capsule Endotoxin (LPS) IgA protease	Meningitis (children and young adults) Waterhouse–Friderichsen syndrome
Neisseria gonorrhoeae	Aerobic	Endotoxin (LOS) Fimbriae IgA protease	Gonorrhea Septic arthritis

GRAM-NEGATIVE BACILLI

See Table 18–12.
- Enteric
- Respiratory
- Zoonotic

*Haemophilus aegyptius (Koch–Weeks bacillus) causes acute contagious conjunctivitis (**pink eye**). Transmitted by hand-to-hand contact.*

TABLE 18–12. Comparison of Major Gram-Negative Bacilli

BACTERIUM	OXYGEN REQUIREMENT	MAJOR VIRULENCE FACTORS	DISEASE
Enteric bacilli (associated with the enteric tract)			
Escherichia coli	Facultative	Enterotoxin Endotoxin	Urinary tract infection. Traveler's diarrhea Neonatal meningitis
Salmonella sp. - Animal sources include eggs, poultry, pets.	Facultative	Endotoxin	Enterocolitis Typhoid fever Septicemia → osteomyelitis - Often in patients with sickle cell anemia.
Shigella sp.	Facultative	Enterotoxin Endotoxin	Enterocolitis Dysentery - Bloody diarrhea
Vibrio cholerae - Comma-shaped.	Facultative	Enterotoxin Endotoxin	Cholera - Watery diarrhea
Campylobacter jejuni - Comma-shaped.	Facultative (5% O_2)	Enterotoxin Endotoxin	Enterocolitis (children)
Helicobacter pylori	Facultative	Endotoxin	Gastritis Peptic ulcers Gastric carcinoma (associated)
Klebsiella pneumoniae	Facultative	Endotoxin	Pneumonia Urinary tract infection. - Patients often have chronic respiratory disease, alcoholism, or diabetes.

TABLE 18-12. Comparison of Major Gram-Negative Bacilli (Continued)

Bacterium	Oxygen Requirement	Major Virulence Factors	Disease
Pseudomonas aeruginosa ■ Produces a blue-green pigment in culture.	Aerobic	Exotoxin Endotoxin	Sepsis Pneumonia Urinary tract infection. Otitis externa Often occurs in hospitalized patients with burns or cystic fibrosis.
Bacteroides sp.	Anaerobic	Endotoxin Fimbriae	Abscess Periodontitis (associated)
Respiratory bacilli (associated with respiratory tract)			
Haemophilus influenzae	Facultative	Endotoxin	Meningitis (children) Epiglottitis Upper respiratory tract infection. Otitis media
Legionella pneumophila	Facultative	Endotoxin	Pneumonia (legionnaires' disease) Patients tend to be older, smokers, and alcoholics.
Bordetella pertussis	Aerobic	Pertussis toxin Tracheal cytotoxin Adenylate cyclase Endotoxin Fimbriae	Pertussis (whooping cough)
Zoonotic bacilli (transmitted by animals)			
Brucella sp.	Facultative	Endotoxin	Brucellosis (undulant fever) ■ Transmitted by contaminated dairy products, or direct contact with goats, sheep, pigs, cattle
Francisella tularensis	Facultative	Endotoxin	Tularemia ■ Transmitted by infected ticks (especially from rabbits), or direct contact from wild animals
Yersinia pestis	Facultative	Exotoxin Endotoxin F-1, V, and W antigens	Plague ■ Transmitted by infected fleas (especially from rats and prairie dogs)
Pasteurella multocida	Facultative	Endotoxin	Cellulitis ■ Transmitted by animal bites

MYCOBACTERIA

- Aerobic bacilli.
- Cell wall has high lipid (mycolic acid) content.
- Stains with **acid-fast** stain (carbolfuchsin).

See Table 18–13.

OTHER BACTERIAL TYPES

(See Table 18–14.)

- *Mycoplasma* sp.
- *Chlamydia* sp.
- *Rickettsia* sp.
- Spirochetes.

TABLE 18-13. Comparison of Major *Mycobacteria* Species

	MAJOR VIRULENCE FACTORS	CHARACTERISTICS	DISEASE
Mycobacterium tuberculosis	Cord factor Tuberculoproteins	Inhalation of airborne droplets **Primary TB:** Causes granulomatous lesions and hilar lymphadenopathy **(Ghon complex)** in lungs **Secondary TB:** Causes *caseous granulomas,* which may lead to miliary or disseminated infection Treated with rifampin, isoniazid, and pyrazinamide **PPD skin test** elicits type IV (delayed) hypersensitivity reaction	Tuberculosis
Mycobacterium leprae	Lepromin proteins	**Tuberculoid type:** Cell-mediated immune response and granulomas in nerves **Lepromatous type:** Foam cells containing bacteria in skin	Leprosy

TABLE 18-14. Comparison of Wall-less, Obligate Intracellular, and Spirochete Bacteria

Bacterium	Characteristics	Disease
Wall-less bacteria		
Mycoplasma pneumoniae	**Smallest bacterium** Cell membrane contains **cholesterol**	Atypical pneumonia
Obligate intracellular bacteria		
Chlamydia trachomatis	Forms cytoplasmic inclusions. Most common cause of **STDs** Trachoma is most common cause of preventable **blindness** IC can be contracted in a swimming pool	Trachoma Inclusion conjunctivitis (IC)
Rickettsia rickettsii	Causes vasculitis. Transmitted by infected ticks	Rocky Mountain spotted fever
Rickettsia prowazekii	Causes vasculitis. Transmitted by infected lice	Epidemic typhus
Spirochetes		
Treponema pallidum	**Primary:** Painless chancre (ulcer) at site of local contact **Secondary:** Highly infectious maculopapular rash and condyloma lata on skin and mucosa **Tertiary:** Gumma (granuloma) formation often on tongue or palate Treated with penicillin	Syphilis
Borelia burgdorferi	Transmitted by infected ticks **Stage 1:** Erythema migrans **Stage 2:** Neuropathies (Bell's palsy) **Stage 3:** Arthritis and CNS disease Most often occurs in CT, NY, PA, NJ Treated with doxycycline or amoxicillin	Lyme disease

Bacterial Vaccines

Vaccinations can confer two types of acquired immunity. (See also Chapter 21, "Immunology and Immunopathology.")

- **Active immunity:** Whole bacteria, capsular polysaccharides, or toxoids elicit immunity.
    - **Live attenuated vaccine**
        - Tuberculosis
        - Tularemia
    - **Killed vaccine**
        - Cholera
        - Typhoid fever
        - Pertussis
    - **Toxoid vaccine:** Contains inactivated exotoxin.
        - Tetanus
        - Diphtheria
    - **Capsular polysaccharide vaccine**
        - Pneumonia (*Strep. pneumoniae*)
        - Meningitis (*N. meningitidis* and *H. influenzae*)
- **Passive immunity:** Preformed antibody preparations elicit immunity.
    - **Antitoxin vaccine:** Contains antibodies to bacterial exotoxins.
        - Tetanus
        - Diphtheria
        - Botulism

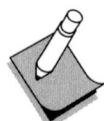

A **toxoid** is an inactivated bacterial exotoxin.

An **antitoxin** is an antibody to a bacterial exotoxin.

Antibiotic Drugs

See Table 8-15.

CLASSIFICATION

- By spectrum:
    - Broad: Effective against several types of bacteria.
    - Narrow: Effective against only one or a few types of bacteria.
- By activity:
    - Bacteriocidal: Kills bacteria.
    - Bacteriostatic: Inhibits bacterial growth (host immune cells kill bacteria).

Concomitant administration of bacteriocidal and bacteriostatic antibiotics has an antagonistic effect because each interferes with the other's mechanism of action.

PENICILLINS

- Inhibit peptidoglycan cross-linking by blocking transpepdidase during last stage of cell wall synthesis
- Bacteriocidal
- Contain β-lactam rings, which are cleaved by bacterial β-lactamase (penicillinase), inactivating the drug
- 10% risk of hypersensitivity
    - First generation
        - Narrow spectrum: G(+) cocci/bacilli and some G(−) aerobic cocci
            - Penicillin G
            - Penicillin V
    - Second generation (β-lactamase resistant)
        - Narrow spectrum: Target G(−) β-lactamase-producing staphylococci (especially *S. aureus*)
            - Methicillin
            - Nafcillin

Most antibacterial activity occurs during the log phase of bacterial growth.

TABLE 18-15. Comparison of Common Antibiotics Used in Dentistry

Drug Class	Mechanism of Action	Activity	Spectrum
Penicillins	Inhibit peptidoglycan cross-linking by blocking transpepdidase during last stage of cell wall synthesis.	Cidal	Narrow ↓ Broader
Cephalosporins	Inhibit peptidoglycan cross-linking by blocking transpepdidase during last stage of cell wall synthesis.	Cidal	Narrow ↓ Broader
Metronidazole	Inhibits DNA synthesis.	Cidal	Narrow
Fluoroquinolones	Inhibit DNA gyrase (topoisomerase).	Cidal	Broader
Aminoglycosides	Inhibit protein synthesis by binding to 30S ribosomal subunits (block the formation of the initiation complex).	Cidal	Broader
Macrolides	Inhibit protein synthesis by binding to 50S ribosomal subunits (block the release of tRNA).	Static	Narrow
Clindamycin	Inhibit protein synthesis by binding to 50S ribosomal subunits (blocks the release of tRNA).	Static	Narrow
Tetracyclines	Inhibit protein synthesis by binding to 30S ribosomal subunits (block aminoacyl-tRNA binding).	Static	Broad
Sulfonamides	Inhibit folic acid synthesis by competing with p-aminobenzoic acid (PABA).	Static	Broad

- Oxacillin
- Cloxacillin
- Dicloxacillin
- Third generation (extended spectrum)
    - Broader spectrum: Also include some G(–) bacilli.
        - Ampicillin
        - Amoxicillin
- Combinations
    - An extended spectrum penicillin with a β-lactamase inhibitor.
    - Broader spectrum: Target more G(–) bacilli including β-lactamase staphylococci (especially S. aureus)
        - Amoxicillin and clavulanic acid
        - Ampicillin and sublactam

Cephalosporins

- Inhibit peptidoglycan cross-linking by blocking transpepdidase during last stage of cell wall synthesis
- Bacteriocidal
- Contain β-lactam rings
- 10% cross-hypersensitivity with penicillins
  - First generation
    - Narrow spectrum: G(+) cocci (but not enterococci) and some G(−) bacilli
      - Cefazolin
      - Cephalexin
      - Cefadroxil
  - Second generation
    - Broader spectrum: Fewer G(+) cocci, but more G(−) bacilli.
      - Cefaclor
      - Cefprozil
      - Cefoxitin
  - Third generation
    - Broader spectrum: Fewer G(+) cocci (except some enterococci), but more G(−) bacilli, and anaerobes
      - Cefpodoxime
      - Cefixime
  - Fourth generation
    - Broader spectrum: Fewer G(+) cocci (except more enterococci), but more G(−) bacilli, and anaerobes
      - Cefepime

Vancomycin

- Inhibits peptidoglycan cross-linking by binding to D-alanyl-D-alanine during cell wall synthesis
- Bacteriocidal
- Narrow spectrum: Mostly G(+) cocci and bacilli (especially penicillinase-resistant *S. aureus*)

Macrolides

- Inhibit protein synthesis by binding to 50S ribosomal subunits (block the release of tRNA)
- Bacteriostatic
- Associated with GI upset
  - Erythromycin
    - Narrow spectrum: G(+) cocci/bacilli, some G(−) anaerobes, and *Mycoplasma* sp.
    - Inhibits cytochrome P450
  - Clarithromycin
    - Broader spectrum: Targets more anaerobes
  - Azithromycin
    - Broader spectrum: Targets more anaerobes

CLINDAMYCIN

- Inhibit protein synthesis by binding to 50S ribosomal subunits (blocks the release of tRNA)
- Bacteriostatic (in low doses)
- Narrow spectrum: G(+) and some G(–) anaerobes (*Bacteroides* sp.)
- Associated with diarrhea and **pseudomembranous colitis** (caused by an overgrowth of *Clostridium difficile*)

TETRACYCLINES

- Inhibit protein synthesis by binding to 30S ribosomal subunits (block aminoacyl-tRNA binding)
- Bacteriostatic
- Broad spectrum: G(+) and G(-) aerobes/anaerobes, spirochetes, *Mycoplasma* sp., *Chlamydia*, and *Rickettsia*
- Divalent and trivalent cations inhibit absorption
- Associated with staining of teeth during their calcification
    - Tetracycline
    - Doxycycline
    - Minocycline

METRONIDAZOLE

- Inhibits DNA synthesis
- Bacteriocidal
- Narrow spectrum: Targets anaerobes and some protozoa
- Often used to treat pseudomembranous colitis

FLUOROQUINOLONES

- Inhibit DNA gyrase (topoisomerase)
- Bacteriocidal
- Broader spectrum: G(+) and G(–) aerobes/facultatives and mycobacteria, but not anaerobes
- Divalent and trivalent cations inhibit absorption
    - Ciprofloxacin
    - Ofloxacin

AMINOGLYCOSIDES

- Inhibit protein synthesis by binding to 30S ribosomal subunits (block the formation of the initiation complex)
- Bacteriocidal (in clinical doses)
- Broader spectrum: G(+) and G(–) aerobes
- Associated with ototoxicity and nephrotoxicity
    - Streptomycin
    - Gentamycin

SULFONAMIDES

- Inhibit folic acid synthesis by competing with *p*-aminobenzoic acid (PABA).
- Bacteriostatic
- Broad spectrum: Targets G(+), many G(−), *Actinomyces* sp., and *Chlamydia* sp.
- Associated with hypersensitivity, renal toxicity, and hematopoietic toxicity
  - Sulfadiazine
  - Sulfamethoxazole
  - Trimethoprim

CHLORAMPHENICOL

- Inhibits protein synthesis by binding to 50S ribosomal subunits (blocks peptidyl transferase)
- Bacteriostatic
- Broad spectrum: Some G(+) cocci, G(−) aerobes/anaerobes, spirochetes, *Rickettsia* sp., *Chlamydia* sp., *Mycoplasma* sp., and *Salmonella* sp.
- Associated with bone marrow toxicity

TOPICAL ANTIBIOTICS

- Neomycin: An aminoglycoside
- Polymyxin B: Alters cell membrane permeability
- Bacitracin: Inhibits cell wall synthesis

ANTIBIOTIC PROPHYLAXIS PRIOR TO DENTAL TREATMENT

See Table 18–16.

- It is sometimes necessary to premedicate patients for the prevention of bacterial endocarditis or infection of prosthetic implants prior to certain dental procedures.
- The American Dental Association standardizes the current guidelines.

TABLE 18–16. Guidelines for Antibiotic Prophylaxis

SITUATION	DRUG	DOSAGE
Standard prophylaxis	Amoxicillin	Adults: 2 g PO 1 hr before procedure. Children: 50 mg/kg PO 1 hr before procedure.
Unable to take oral medications.	Ampicillin	Adults: 2 g IM or IV within 30 min before procedure. Children: 50 mg/kg IM or IV within 30 min before procedure.
Allergic to penicillins	Clindamycin	Adults: 600 mg PO 1 hr before procedure. Children: 20 mg/kg PO 1 hr before procedure.
	Cephalexin or cefadroxil	Adults: 2 g PO 1 hr before procedure. Children: 50 mg/kg PO 1 hr before procedure.

TABLE 18-16. Guidelines for Antibiotic Prophylaxis (Continued)

Situation	Drug	Dosage
	Azithromycin or clarithromycin	Adults: 500 mg PO 1 hr before procedure. Children: 15 mg/kg PO 1 hr before procedure.
Allergic to penicillins and unable to take oral medications.	Clindamycin	Adults: 600 mg IV within 30 min before procedure. Children: 20 mg/kg IV within 30 min before procedure.
	Cefazolin	Adults: 1 g IM or IV within 30 min before procedure. Children: 25 mg/kg IM or IV within 30 min before procedure.

▶ VIROLOGY

Viruses

See Figure 18–5.

- Characterized by single- or double-stranded DNA or RNA (never both) surrounded by a protein **capsid.**
- The combination of the nucleic acid and the protein capsid is known as the **nucleocapsid.**
- Some viruses have an outer membrane called an **envelope**, which is composed of plasma membrane **lipoproteins** and glycoproteins obtained as the virus leaves its host cell (**budding**).
- Viral proteins mediate viral attachment, protect the nucleic acid, and serve as antigens. Other proteins include DNA or RNA polymerases.
- Do *not* contain mitochondria or ribosomes; must replicate within living host cells.
- Not visible by light microscopy.

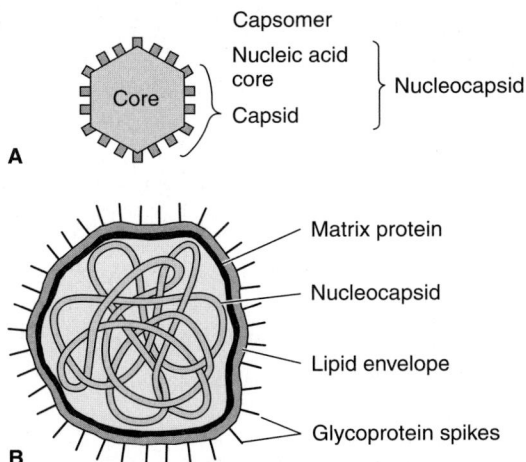

FIGURE 18-5. Comparison of non-enveloped and enveloped viruses.

Reproduced, with permission, from Levinson W. *Medical Microbiology and Immunology*, 8th ed. McGraw-Hill, 2004.

Pathogenesis

VIRAL GROWTH CURVE

See Figure 18–6.

One virion can replicate to form hundreds of progeny viruses.

- **Latent phase:** Viral penetration to viral release.
- **Eclipse phase:** Viral penetration to viral assembly within host cell.
  - No infectious virus can be detected during this phase.
- **Rise phase:** Viral assembly to viral release.

VIRAL REPLICATION

See Figure 18–7.

*The host cellular morphologic and functional changes associated with viral replication and release are known as the **cytopathic effect (CPE)**. The CPE is often specific for a particular virus. Not all viruses cause CPE.*

- **Attachment:** Determined by the specificity of viral proteins to host cells.
- **Penetration:** Via receptor-mediated endocytosis (e.g., pinocytosis).
- **Uncoating:** Viral nucleic acid is spilled into the cytoplasm.
- **Transcription and Translation:**
  - All **DNA viruses** (except poxviruses) replicate in the *nucleus* using host cell RNA polymerase.
  - All **RNA viruses** (except retroviruses and orthomyxoviruses) replicate in the *cytoplasm* using their own RNA polymerase. Transcription is only necessary for viruses whose RNA has *negative polarity* (a virus's RNA that has positive polarity serves as the mRNA itself).
  - All **retroviruses** use their own **reverse transcriptase** for transcription.
- **Assembly:** The new viral nucleic acid and capsid proteins are packaged.
- **Release:** Either by *budding* through the host plasma membrane (creating a viral envelope) or by host plasma membrane *rupture*.

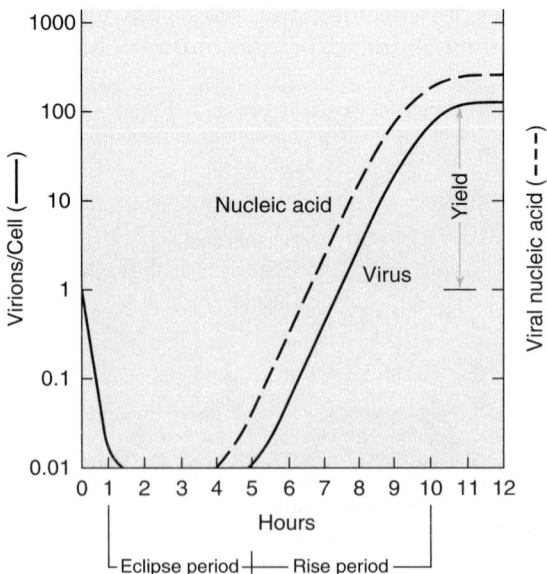

FIGURE 18-6. Viral growth curve.

Reproduced, with permission, from Levinson W. *Medical Microbiology and Immunology*, 8th ed. McGraw-Hill, 2004.

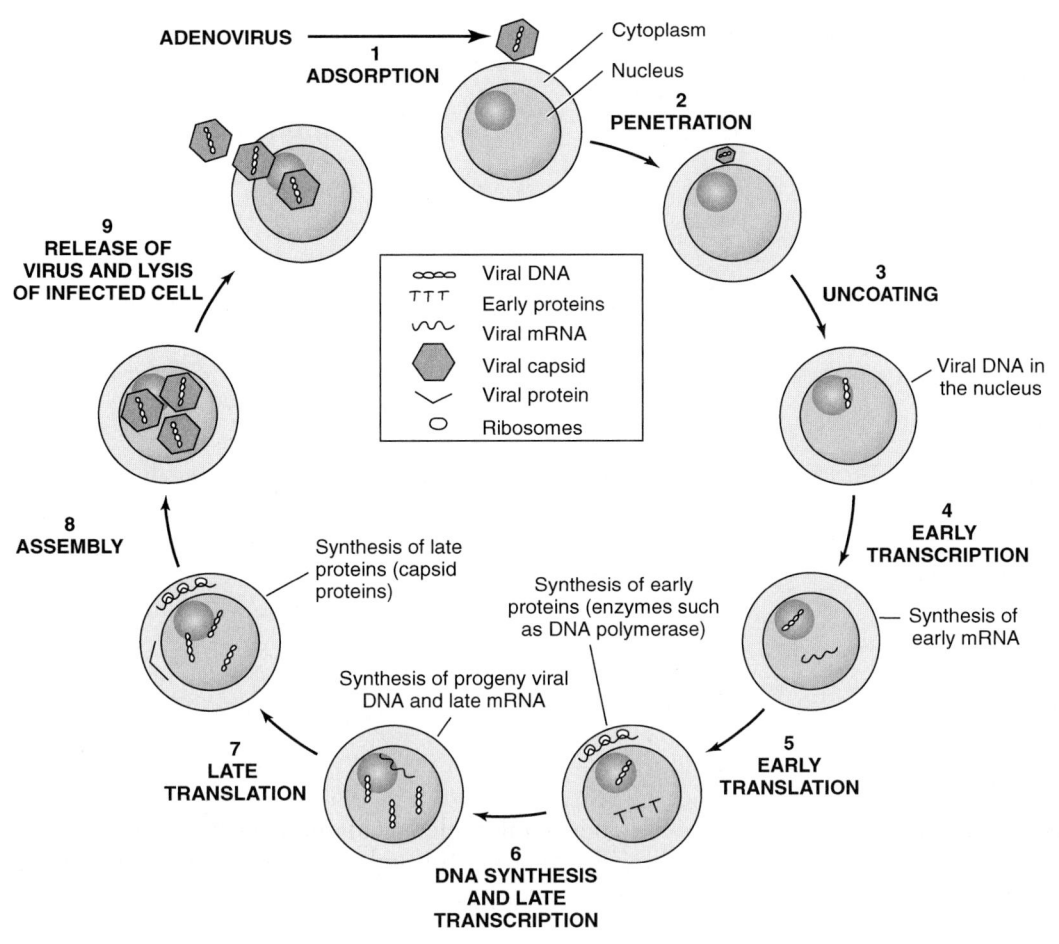

FIGURE 18-7. **Viral growth cycle.**

Reproduced, with permission, from Levinson W. *Medical Microbiology and Immunology*, 8th ed. McGraw-Hill, 2004.

VIRAL ANTIGENIC CHANGES

- Antigenic changes contribute to the cause of epidemics and pandemics.
- Commonly associated with **influenza viruses** (orthomyxoviruses).
- There are two modes of antigenic change:
    - **Antigenic drifts:** Minor changes caused by genomic mutations.
    - **Antigenic shifts:** Major changes caused by genomic re-assortment.

Classification

RNA NON-ENVELOPED VIRUSES

See Table 18–17
- Picornavirus
- Calicivirus
- Reovirus

*Influenza viruses have two envelope glycoprotein spikes, **hemagglutinin** and **neuraminidase**, which exhibit the majority of antigenic changes.*

TABLE 18–17. RNA Non-enveloped Viruses in Order of Increasing Size

Family	Nucleic Acid	Virus	Disease	Antiviral Treatment	Vaccine
Picornavirus ■ Smallest RNA virus	Single, linear	Poliovirus	Polio	None	Yes
		Coxsackie A virus	Herpangina ■ Palate, tongue Hand-foot-and-mouth disease ■ Gingiva, buccal mucosa Acute lymphonodular pharyngitis Aseptic meningitis	None	No
		Coxsackie B virus	Pleurodynia Myocarditis Pericarditis Aseptic meningitis	None	No
		Rhinovirus	Common cold	None	No
		HAV	Hepatitis A	None	Yes
Calicivirus	Single, linear	Norwalk virus	Gastroenteritis (adults)	None	No
		HEV	Hepatitis E	None	No
Reovirus	Double, linear	Rotavirus	Gastroenteritis (infants)	None	No
		Orbivirus ■ Only virus transmitted by ticks	Colorado tick fever	None	No

*Poliovirus, coxsackieviruses, and hepatitis A virus are **enteroviruses**.*

Roboviruses *are rodent-borne viruses. Examples include hantavirus (Sin nombre virus).*

Arboviruses *are arthropod-borne viruses. Examples include West Nile virus, yellow fever virus, Colorado tick fever virus, and eastern/western encephalitis virus.*

RNA-Enveloped Viruses

See Table 18–18.

- Deltavirus
- Flavivirus
- Togavirus
- Orthomyxovirus
- Retrovirus
- Paramyxovirus
- Rhabdovirus
- Filovirus
- Coronavirus
- Bunyavirus

TABLE 18-18. RNA Enveloped Viruses in Order of Increasing Size

Family	Nucleic Acid	Virus	Disease	Antiviral Treatment	Vaccine
Deltavirus	Single, circular	HDV	Hepatitis D	α-interferon	Yes
Flavivirus	Single, linear	Japanese Encephalitis virus	Encephalitis	None	Yes
		Yellow fever virus	Yellow fever	None	Yes
		West Nile virus	Encephalitis	None	No
		HCV	Hepatitis C Hepatocellular carcinoma (associated)	α-interferon Ribavirin	No
Togavirus	Single, linear	Rubella virus	Rubella German measles "3-day measles" Erythematous rash	None	Yes
		Eastern/western encephalitis virus	Encephalitis	None	Yes (equine)
Orthomyxovirus ■ Exhibit various **antigenic changes** ■ Replicate in nucleus	Single, linear	Influenza viruses	Influenza Reye's syndrome (association)	Amantidine Rimantidine Zanamivir Oseltamivir	Yes
Retrovirus ■ Uses reverse transcriptase ■ Replicate in nucleus	Single, linear	HTLV	Adult T-cell leukemia/ lymphoma Chronic progressive myelopathy	None	No
		HIV ■ Infects CD4 T-helper cells. ■ Diagnosis confirmed by Western blot.	AIDS	Zidovudine Lamivudine Stavudine Indinavir Ritonavir	No

TABLE 18-18. RNA Enveloped Viruses in Order of Increasing Size (Continued)

Family	Nucleic Acid	Virus	Disease	Antiviral Treatment	Vaccine
Paramyxovirus	Single, linear	Measles virus	Measles (rubeola) ■ Nonpruritic maculopapular brick-red rash. ■ Multiple white lesions (Koplik's spots) are often seen on the buccal mucosa.	None	Yes
		Mumps virus	Mumps ■ Parotitis, orchitis, deafness	None	Yes
		RSV ■ Infants only	Bronchiolitis Pneumonia	Ribavirin	No
		Parainfluenza viruses	Croup Bronchiolitis Common cold	None	No
Rhabdovirus	Single, linear	Rabies virus	Rabies	None	Yes
Filovirus	Single, linear	Ebola virus	Ebola hemorrhagic fever	None	No
Coronavirus	Single, linear	Coronavirus	Common cold SARS	None	No
Bunyavirus	Single, circular	Hantavirus (Sin Nombre virus)	Hantavirus pulmonary syndrome.	None	No

HIV contains two strands of RNA (diploid) and reverse transcriptase. The two important envelope proteins are gp120 (mediates attachment to CD4) and gp41 (mediates fusion to the host cell). The nucleocapsid is composed of p24 and p7. (See Figure 18–8.)

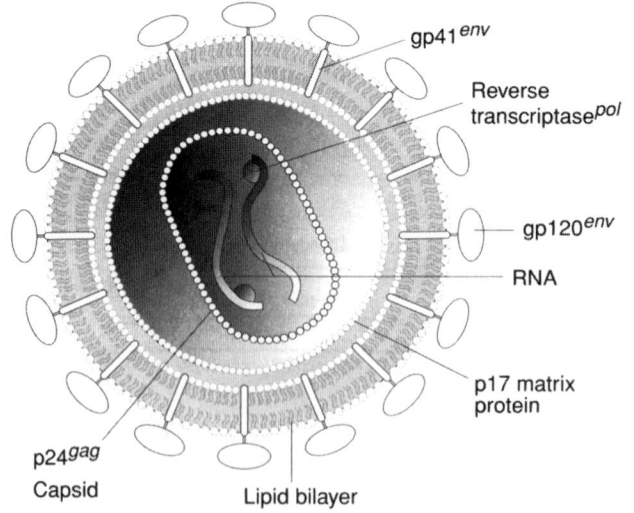

FIGURE 18-8. HIV.

Reproduced, with permission, from Bhushan V. *First Aid for the USMLE Step 1.* McGraw-Hill, 2006.

DNA NON-ENVELOPED VIRUSES

See Table 18–19.

- Parvovirus
- Papovavirus
- Adenovirus

TABLE 18-19. Major DNA Non-enveloped Viruses in Order of Increasing Size

Family	Nucleic Acid	Virus	Disease	Antiviral Treatment	Vaccine
Parvovirus - Smallest DNA virus	Single, linear	B19 virus	Aplastic anemia - Especially in patients with sickle cell anemia. - Erythema infectiosum (Fifth disease) Fetal infections	None	No
Papovavirus	Double, circular	HPV	Papillomas; warts Condyloma acuminatum; genital warts Verruca vulgaris Cervical cancer	Podophyllin α-interferon Cidofovir	No
Adenovirus	Double, linear	Adenovirus	Pharyngitis Conjunctivitis Pneumonia Common cold	None	Yes

*Reye's syndrome is a potentially deadly disease that typically occurs in children aged 4–12 years. It is associated with the use of **aspirin** to treat influenza or varicella (chickenpox).*

DNA ENVELOPED VIRUSES

See Table 18–20.

- Hepadnavirus
- Herpesvirus
- Poxvirus

TABLE 18-20. Major DNA Enveloped Viruses in Order of Increasing Size

Family	Nucleic Acid	Virus	Disease	Antiviral Treatment	Vaccine
Hepadnavirus	Double, circular	HBV	Hepatitis B	α-interferon	Yes
			Hepatocellular carcinoma (associated)	Lamivudine	
Herpesvirus - Lies dormant in **sensory nerve ganglia**, especially trigeminal ganglion.	Double, linear	HSV-1	Gingivostomatitis Herpes labialis Keratoconjunctivitis Encephalitis	Acyclovir Penciclovir Valacyclovir Famciclovir	No
		HSV-2	Herpes genitalis Neonatal encephalitis Aseptic meningitis		
		VZV	Varicella—primary - Chickenpox - Pruritic, macular lesions that become pustular and crusted. - Reye's syndrome (associated) Zoster—recurrent - Shingles - Usually localized to a single dermatome.	Acyclovir Famciclovir Valacyclovir	Yes
		CMV	Congenital abnormalities Cytomegalic inclusion disease	Ganciclovir Valganciclovir Foscarnet	No
		EBV	Infectious mononucleosis - Transmission via saliva - **Heterophile test** used for screening Burkitt's lymphoma (association) Nasopharyngeal carcinoma (association)	None (self-limiting in 2–3 weeks)	No

TABLE 18-20. Major DNA Enveloped Viruses in Order of Increasing Size (Continued)

Family	Nucleic Acid	Virus	Disease	Antiviral Treatment	Vaccine
		HHV-8	B-cell lymphoma (association) Hairy leukoplakia (association) Kaposi's sarcoma	None	No
Poxvirus ■ Largest DNA virus Replicates in cytoplasm	Double, linear	Variola virus	Smallpox ■ Eradicated	None	Yes
		MCV	Molluscum contagiosum	None	No

Hepatitis Viruses

Classification

See Table 18–21.

Signs and Symptoms of Viral Hepatitis

- Fatigue
- Myalgia
- Loss of appetite
- Nausea
- Diarrhea
- Constipation
- Fever
- Jaundice

TABLE 18-21. Comparison of Major Hepatitis Viruses

Virus	Nucleic Acid	Viral Class	Envelope	Transmission	Characteristics
HAV	ss RNA	Picornavirus	No	Fecal-oral	Usually self-limiting; recovery within four months.
HBV	ds DNA	Hepadnavirus	Yes	Bloodborne	Increased incidence of HCC if chronic.
HCV	ss RNA	Flavivirus	Yes	Bloodborne	Increased incidence of chronic liver disease, cirrhosis, HCC.
HDV	ss RNA	Deltavirus	Yes	Bloodborne	Requires presence of HBsAg for replication.
HEV	ss RNA	Calicivirus	No	Fecal-oral	Causes occasional epidemics in underdeveloped countries.

HCV is the most common reason for liver transplantation in the United States.

Hepatitis viruses are extremely heat resistant (moreso than HIV). Proper autoclaving kills all hepatitis viruses.

An individual vaccinated for HBV will show serology positive only for anti-HBs.

TESTS OF LIVER FUNCTION

- Bilirubin
- ALT (alanine aminotransferase)
- AST (aspartate aminotransferase)

SEROLOGY

See Figure 18–9 and Table 18–22.

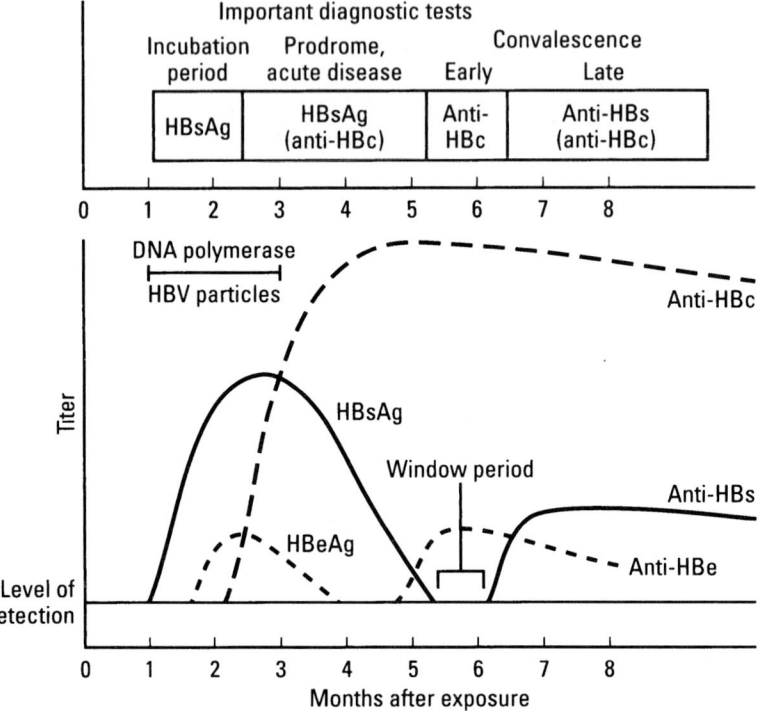

FIGURE 18-9. Serologic findings associated with acute HBV.

Reproduced, with permission, from Bhushan V. *First Aid for the USMLE Step 1*. McGraw-Hill, 2006.

TABLE 18-22. Serological Profiles of Hepatitis Infections

VIRUS	ACUTE INFECTION	CHRONICITY	PERCENT CHRONICITY	IMMUNITY
HAV	IgM Anti-HAV	None	None	Anti-HAV
HBV	**IgM Anti-HBc** HBsAg HBeAg	HBsAg HBeAg Anti-HBc	10% (adults) 30–90% (infants)	**Anti-HBs** Anti-HBc Anti-HBe
HCV	Anti-HCV	Anti-HCV	80%	Anti-HCV
HDV	IgM Anti-HDV	Anti-HDV	6%	Anti-HBs Anti-HDV
HEV	IgM Anti-HEV	None	None	Anti-HEV

Viral Vaccines

Vaccinations can confer two types of acquired immunity. (See also Chapter 21, "Immunology and Immunopathology.")

- **Active immunity:** Live attenuated viruses, killed viruses, or purified viral protein subunits elicit immunity. Slow onset. Long-lasting (memory).
  - **Live attenuated vaccine:** Stimulates IgA, IgG, and T-cell responses.
    - Measles
    - Mumps
    - Rubella
    - Polio (Sabin), oral
    - Varicella-zoster
    - Smallpox
  - **Killed vaccine:** Stimulates mostly IgG responses.
    - Influenza
    - Polio (Salk), injection
    - Rabies
    - Hepatitis A
  - **Subunit vaccine:** Contains purified viral protein subunits.
    - Hepatitis B—HBsAg
- **Passive immunity:** Preformed antibody preparations elicit immunity. Fast onset. Short life span.
  - **Immune globulin vaccine**
    - Hepatitis B
    - Rabies
    - Varicella-zoster

Live attenuated vaccines provide longer and greater immunity than killed vaccines, but they have the potential to revert to virulence or can be excreted and transmitted to non-immune individuals.

Adjuvants *are often added to vaccines to slow their absorption and increase their effectiveness.*

Antiviral Drugs

INTERFERONS

- Glycoproteins that originate from infected host cells to protect other non-infected host cells.
- Do not directly affect viruses, but instead **nonspecifically prevent their replication** within host cells by inducing resistance.

Bacteriophages (Phages)

- Viruses that infect bacterial cells.
- Replication can occur by two pathways (see Figure 18–10).
  - **Lytic cycle:** The process by which some phages replicate within the host cell, producing hundreds of new progeny phage. The host cell is ultimately destroyed.
  - **Lysogenic cycle:** The process by which some phages incorporate their DNA in the host cell chromosome. The integrated viral DNA is called a **prophage**. Replication occurs only when the host DNA is damaged, excising the viral DNA. The host cell is usually not destroyed.

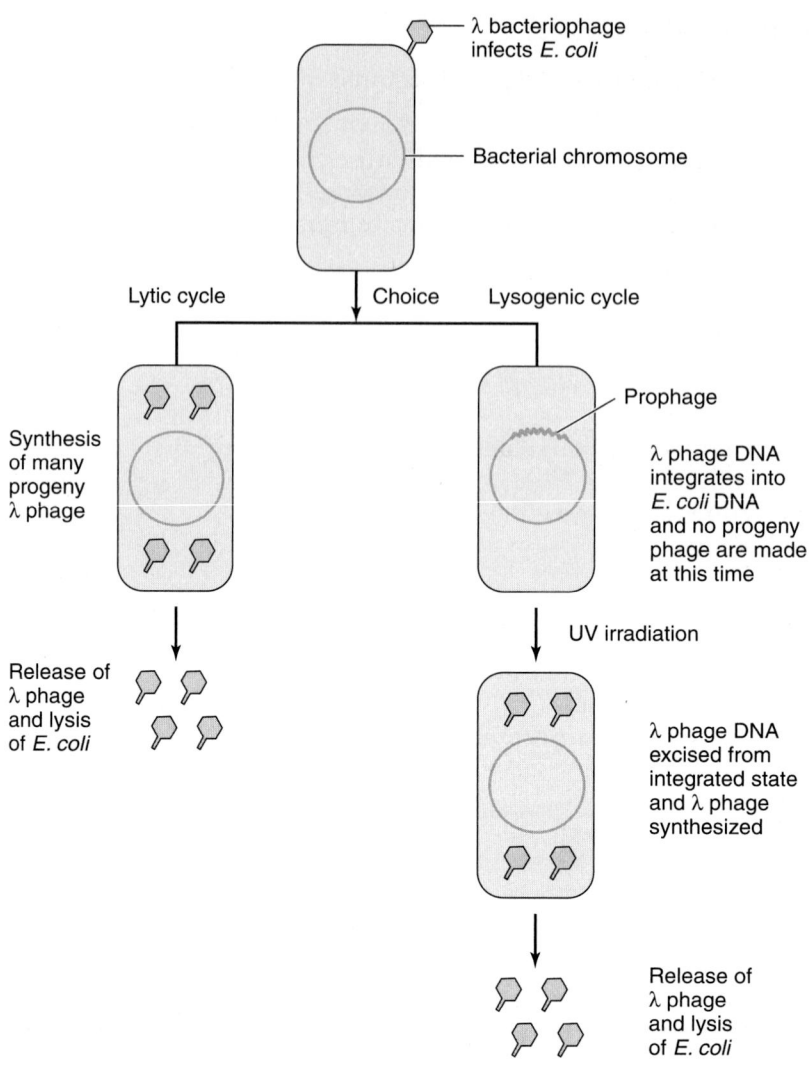

FIGURE 18-10. Bacteriophage replication.

Reproduced, with permission, from Levinson W. *Medical Microbiology and Immunology*, 8th ed. McGraw-Hill, 2004.

Prions

- Infectious agents composed entirely of protein (no nucleic acid).
- Do *not* elicit inflammatory or antibody responses.
- Cause **transmissible spongiform encephalopathies**:
    - Creutzfeldt–Jacob disease (in humans).
    - Mad cow disease (in cows).

▶ MYCOLOGY

Fungi

- Gram-positive, eukaryotic microorganisms.
- All are either obligate (the majority) or facultative aerobes.
- None are obligate anaerobes.
- Cell walls predominantly composed of **chitin**.
- Cell membranes contain **ergosterol**.

FUNGAL REPRODUCTION

- **Sexual:** Mating and formation of **spores**.
    - Zygospores
    - Ascospores
    - Basidiospores
- **Asexual:** Budding and formation of **conidia**.
    - Arthrospores
    - Chlamydospores
    - Blastospores
    - Sporangiospores

Pathogenesis

- **Fungal infection:** Leads to a largely **cell-mediated immune response** and granuloma formation.
- **Mycotoxicosis:** Induced by ingestion of fungal toxins.
- **Allergic response:** Type I hypersensitivity reactions to inhalation of fungal spores.

Classification

See Table 18–23.

- Yeasts
- Molds

Most fungal spores and conidia are killed at temperatures greater than 80°C for 30 minutes.

Aflatoxins *are hepatocarcinogenic toxins produced by Aspergillus flavus, generally found in contaminated grains and peanuts.*

*Some fungi exhibit **dimorphism**—they exist as molds at ambient temperatures but as yeasts at warmer (body) temperatures.*

TABLE 18–23. Comparison of Yeasts and Molds

FUNGUS	MORPHOLOGY	REPRODUCTION
Yeasts	Single cells.	Asexual budding
Molds	Long filaments (**hyphae**), which form a mat-like structure (**mycelium**).	Mitosis

Medically Relevant Fungi

- Systemic and cutaneous fungal infections. (See Table 18–24.)
- Opportunistic fungal infections. (See Table 18–25.)

Opportunistic infections induce disease in immunocompromised patients, such as those with AIDS or who take immunosuppressive medications.

Antifungal Drugs

See Table 18–26.

- The vast majority of the antifungal drugs prescribed by dentists are used to treat *candidiasis*, the major fungal infection that affects the oral cavity.

TABLE 18–24. Major Systemic and Cutaneous Fungal Infections

Fungus	Disease	Type	Characteristics	Treatment
Blastomyces dermatitidis	Blastomycosis	Dimorphic	Endemic in North America. Inhalation of microconidia produces respiratory infection.	Itraconazole Amphotericin B
Coccidioides immitis	Coccidioidomycosis	Dimorphic	Endemic in southwest US and Latin America. Inhalation of **arthrospores** produces respiratory infection.	Amphotericin B Itraconazole Ketoconazole Fluconazole
Histoplasma capsulatum	Histoplasmosis	Dimorphic	Endemic in Ohio and Mississippi River valleys. Found in soil often contaminated by **bird/bat droppings**. Inhalation of microconidia produces respiratory infection. **Yeast cells located within host macrophages.**	Itraconazole Amphotericin B Fluconazole
Trichophyton sp. *Epidermophyton* sp. *Microsporum* sp.	Dermatophytosis	Molds	Tinea corporus (**ringworm**). Tinea capitis (scalp itch). Tinea cruris (jock itch). Tinea pedis (athlete's foot). Tinea unguium (nail fungus).	Miconazole Clotrimazole Tolnaftate **Griseofulvin**

TABLE 18-25. Major Opportunistic Fungal Infections

Fungus	Disease	Type	Characteristics	Susceptibility
Aspergillus fumigatus	Aspergillosis	Mold	Inhalation of conidia causes respiratory infection and aspergilloma (**fungus ball**) formation in lungs.	AIDS Organ transplantation.
Candida albicans	**Candidiasis** Vaginitis Angular cheilitis Median rhomboid glossitis	Yeast	Part of normal human flora of mouth, vagina, GI tract, and skin. Appears as budding yeasts or **pseudohyphae.**	AIDS Prolonged use of antibiotics.
Cryptococcus neoformans	Cryptococcosis	Yeast	Inhalation of spores causes respiratory infection, meningitis, and pneumonia.	AIDS
Mucor sp. Rhizopus sp. Absidia sp.	Mucormycosis	Molds	Inhalation of conidia causes respiratory, skin, **paranasal sinus, and brain infections.**	**Diabetes (ketoacidosis)** Leukemia Burns

TABLE 18-26. Common Antifungal Drugs to Treat Candidiasis

Drug	Mechanism of Action	Common Forms
Nystatin	Binds to ergosterol.	Topical Oral suspension
Amphotericin B	Binds to ergosterol.	Topical Oral suspension Intravenous
Clotrimazole	Inhibits ergosterol synthesis.	Troche
Ketoconazole	Inhibits ergosterol synthesis. Blocks fungal cytochrome P450.	Tablet
Fluconazole	Inhibits ergosterol synthesis. Blocks fungal cytochrome P450.	Tablet

*Most antifungal drugs target the **ergosterol** component of fungal cell membranes, altering their permeability.*

▶ PARASITOLOGY

Parasites

CLASSIFICATION

- **Protozoa**
  - *Unicellular*, eukaryotic microorganisms that lack a cell wall and largely infect blood cells, intestinal and urogenital tissue, and meninges.
- **Metazoa (helminths)**
  - *Multicellular* worms that often infect the intestines, brain, liver, and other tissues.

PHYLOGENY

See Figure 18–11.

*Parasitic infections generally elicit an **IgE-mediated** host immune response accompanied by marked **eosinophilia**.*

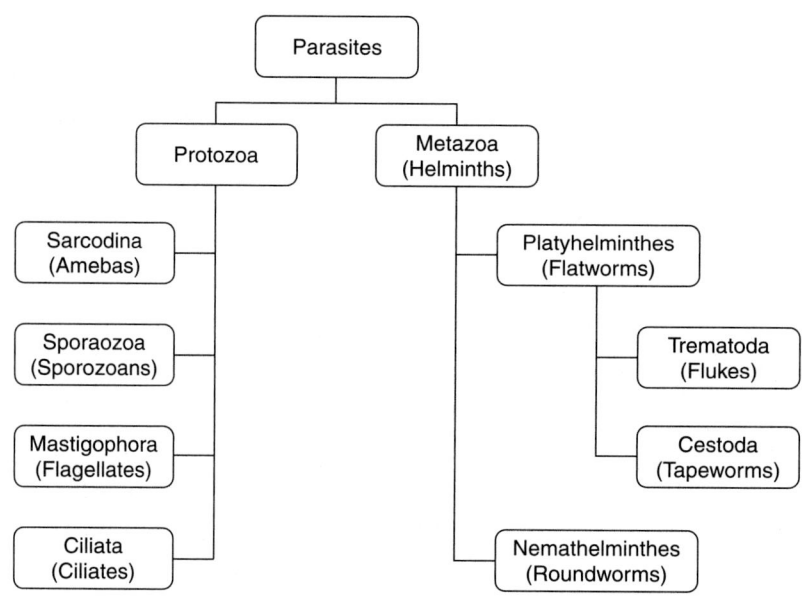

FIGURE 18-11. Phylogeny of parasites.

Reproduced, with permission, from Levinson W. *Medical Microbiology and Immunology*, 8th ed. McGraw-Hill, 2004.

Medically Relevant Parasites

- Protozoa. (See Table 18–27.)
- Metazoa (helminths). (See Table 18–28.)

TABLE 18-27. **Common Protozoa Associated with Human Infection**

Protozoan	Disease	Transmission	Characteristics	Treatment
Entamoeba histolytica	Amebiasis Dysentery Liver abscess	Fecal-oral	Exists as a **trophozoite** (motile ameba in host intestines) and a nonmotile cyst (in contaminated food/water).	Metronidazole
Giardia lamblia	Giardiasis Diarrhea	Fecal-oral	Exists as a trophozoite (intestinal) and a nonmotile cyst (contaminated food/water).	Metronidazole
Cryptosporidium parvum	Cryptosporidiosis Diarrhea	Fecal-oral	Associated with immuno-compromised patients (AIDS).	None
Trichomonas vaginalis	Trichomoniasis Vaginitis Urethritis (males)	Sexually	Exists only as a trophozoite.	Metronidazole
Plasmodium vivax *Plasmodium ovale* *Plasmodium malariae* *Plasmodium falciparum* (most fatal)	Malaria Influenza-like onset	Female *Anopheles* **mosquitoes** Infected blood products	Sporozoites differentiate into **merozoites** in the liver. **Hypnozoites** are latent forms that cause relapses. Causes lysis of **erythrocytes.**	Chloroquine Primaquine Mefloquine
Toxoplasma gondii	Toxoplasmosis ■ CNS infection Seizures Associated with AIDS	Fecal-oral **Transplacental**	Exists as a trophozoite (intestinal) and a nonmotile cyst (uncooked meat and **cat feces**).	Sulfadiazine Pyrimethamine
Pneumocystis carinii (*Pneumocystis jiroveci*)	Pneumonia	Inhalation	Fungus by DNA analysis. Associated with immuno-compromised patients (AIDS).	Trimethoprim Sulfamethoxazole Pentamidine

TABLE 18-28. Common Metazoa (Helminths) Associated with Human Infection

Metazoan	Disease	Transmission	Characteristics	Treatment
Taenia solium	Taeniasis (tapeworm)	Ingestion of undercooked **pork.**	**Cysticercosis** (larvae accumulation)	Praziquantel Albendazole
Taenia saginata	Taeniasis (tapeworm)	Ingestion of undercooked **beef.**	Does not cause cysticercosis.	Praziquantel
Enterobius vermicularis	Enterobiasis (pinworm)	Ingestion of worm eggs.	**Most common worm** in US. Associated with **perianal pruritis.**	Mebendazole
Trichinella spiralis	Trichinosis	Ingestion of undercooked meat (pig, bear).	Larvae only grow in **striated muscle.** Associated with muscle pain, **periorbital edema,** fever, eosinophilia.	None

CHAPTER 19

Oral Microbiology and Pathology

Oral Microbiology	478
PLAQUE	478
CALCULUS	479
MATERIA ALBA	479
Oral Pathology	479
CARIES	479
PLAQUE-INDUCED GINGIVITIS	480
CHRONIC PERIODONTITIS	480
AGGRESSIVE PERIODONTITIS	481
NECROTIZING PERIODONTAL DISEASES	481
CANDIDIASIS	482
Chemical Plaque Control	482

ORAL MICROBIOLOGY

- Even though the oral cavity harbors more than 300 species of bacteria, most are part of the normal oral flora. A few, however, are heavily associated with both dental and periodontal diseases.

Plaque

- An organized **biofilm** of microorganisms, organic components (polysaccharides, proteins, glycoproteins), inorganic components (calcium, phosphorus), desquamated cells (epithelial cells, leukocytes), and food debris.
- It adheres to teeth, dental prostheses, and oral mucosal surfaces and is also found in the gingival sulcus and periodontal pockets.
- Dental plaque is classified as *supragingival* and *subgingival* based on its position along the tooth surface. (See Table 19–1.)
- As plaque matures, there is a transition from the early aerobic environment characterized by Gram-positive facultative species to an exceedingly oxygen-deprived milieu in which Gram-negative anaerobes predominate.

PLAQUE FORMATION

- **Pellicle formation:** Salivary and GCF **glycoproteins** bind to oral mucosal, tooth, and dental prosthesis surfaces *almost immediately* via electrostatic and van der Waals forces. It prevents tissue desiccation and provides surface lubrication, but also promotes bacterial adherence.
- **Bacterial colonization:** Occurs within a few hours of pellicle formation. Gram-positive facultative species (*Streptococcus* sp., *Actinomyces* sp., *Lactobacillus* sp.) are the first to colonize through the binding of their adhesins and fimbriae to the pellicle.
- **Maturation:** Coaggregation of bacterial species that do not initially colonize tooth and gingival epithelial surfaces.

Periodontal health is characterized by the predominant inhabitants of the oral cavity, mostly gram-positive facultative species such as Streptococcus sanguis, Streptococcus mitis, Actinomyces viscosus, Actinomyces naeslundii, and a few beneficial gram-negative species such as Veillonella parvula and Capnocytophaga ochracea.

Chlorhexidine gluconate is the most effective antiplaque mouthrinse due to its substantivity.

As a plaque biofilm extends from a supragingival to a subgingival environment, there is a shift in the microbial flora from mostly gram-positive, facultative cocci to predominantly gram-negative, anaerobic bacilli and spirochetes.

TABLE 19–1. Comparison of Supragingival and Subgingival Plaque

PLAQUE	LOCATION	FORM	DOMINANT BACTERIAL SPECIES	AFFECTED BY DIET AND SALIVA
Supragingival	At or coronal to the gingival margin.	Attached to gingival epithelial and tooth surfaces.	Gram-positive facultative cocci.	Yes
Subgingival	Apical to the gingival margin.	Attached to gingival epithelial and tooth surfaces, and also loosely adherent.	Gram-negative anaerobic bacilli and spirochetes.	No

Calculus

- Calcified bacterial plaque that forms on teeth and dental prostheses.
- 70–90% of calculus is composed of inorganic components (calcium, phosphorus), the majority of which are crystalline (**hydroxyapatite**).
- The remaining 10–30% of calculus is organic, consisting of protein—**carbohydrate** complexes, desquamated cells (epithelial cells, leukocytes), and microorganisms.
- **Saliva** is the main mineral source for *supragingival calculus*, but **GCF** provides most of the mineral for *subgingival calculus*.
- Plaque becomes 50% mineralized in about 2 days and close to 90% mineralized in about 12 days.

Calculus does not directly irritate the gingiva, but provides a fixed nidus for the continued accumulation of perio-pathogenic plaque bacteria.

Calculus Formation

- **Epitactic concept:** The predominant theory of calculus formation, which suggests that seeding agents (protein–carbohydrate complexes or bacteria) induce small foci of mineralization, which ultimately enlarge and coalesce to form a calcified mass.

Materia alba

- Loosely adherent matter largely composed of desquamated cells, food debris, and other components of dental plaque that is easily washed away.

▶ ORAL PATHOLOGY

Caries

Characteristics

- Cariogenic bacteria synthesize glucans (dextrans) and fructans (levans) from their metabolism of dietary sucrose, which contribute to plaque formation and their adherence to tooth surfaces.
- As a consequence, **lactic acid** is formed, reducing salivary pH and creating sites of enamel demineralization and cavitation.
- The *frequency* of carbohydrate intake is more detrimental than the *quantity* because it maintains a prolonged decrease in pH.

Stephan Curve

See Figure 19–1.

- Rapid drop in salivary pH within a few minutes after fermentable carbohydrate (e.g., sucrose) intake.
- Enamel demineralization occurs once the pH falls below 5.5.
- Recovery to a normal salivary pH can take 15–40 minutes.

Classification

- Pit and fissure
- Smooth-surface
- Root
- Recurrent

Recurrent caries occurs around an existing restoration. It may occur on the crown or the root.

- **Streptococcus sp.** (S. mutans, S. sanguis, S. salivarius) generally cause pit and fissure, smooth-surface, and root caries.
- **Lactobacillus sp.** (L. casei, L. acidophilus) generally cause pit and fissure caries.
- **Actinomyces sp.** (A. viscosus, A. naeslundii) generally cause root caries.

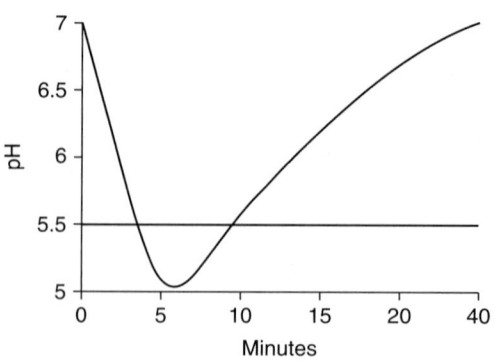

FIGURE 19-1. The Stephan curve.

PREDOMINANT MICROBIAL FLORA

- Generally **gram-positive, facultative cocci and bacilli.**
- *Streptococcus mutans* is the primary etiologic agent of caries.

Plaque-Induced Gingivitis

CHARACTERISTICS

- Presence of plaque.
- Absence of attachment loss.
- Gingival inflammation, starting at the gingival margin.
- Can be modified by systemic factors, medications, or malnutrition.
- Reversible with removal of plaque (and modifying factor).

*Gingivitis associated with sex steroid fluctuations (pregnancy, puberty, menstrual cycle, oral contraceptive use) is associated with elevated proportions of **Prevotella intermedia**, which uses these steroids as growth factors.*

PREDOMINANT MICROBIAL FLORA

- Variable microbial pattern containing predominantly **gram-positive and gram-negative facultative and anaerobic cocci, bacilli, and spirochetes** such as *Streptococcus sanguis, Streptococcus mitis, Actinomyces viscosus, Actinomyces naeslundii, Peptostreptococcus micros, Fusobacterium nucleatum, Prevotella intermedia,* and *Campylobacter rectus.*

Chronic Periodontitis

- Formerly known as **adult periodontitis.**

Recurrent periodontitis describes a return of periodontitis after successful treatment.

Refractory periodontitis describes periodontitis that does not respond well to treatment.

CHARACTERISTICS

- Presence of plaque.
- Presence of attachment loss.
- Amount of periodontal destruction is *consistent* with presence of microbial deposits (subgingival plaque and calculus).
- Most prevalent in adults but can occur in children and adolescents.
- Generally progresses at a slow to moderate rate but may have periods of rapid progression.
- Can be modified by other local factors, systemic factors, medications, smoking, or emotional stress.

PREDOMINANT MICROBIAL FLORA

- Variable microbial pattern containing predominantly **gram-negative, anaerobic bacilli and spirochetes** such as *Porphyromonas gingivalis*, *Tanerella forsythensus* (formerly *Bacteroides forsythus*), *Treponema denticola*, *Prevotella intermedia*, *Fusobacterium nucleatum*, *Eikenella corrodens*, and *Campylobacter rectus*.

Aggressive Periodontitis

- Formerly known as **juvenile periodontitis** or **early-onset periodontitis**.

CHARACTERISTICS

- Presence of plaque.
- Presence of attachment loss.
- Amount of periodontal destruction is generally *inconsistent* with presence of microbial deposits.
- Familial aggregation.
- Usually affects individuals younger than 30 years but can occur in older patients.
- Generally progresses rapidly but may be self-arresting.
- Phagocyte abnormalities are common.
- Hyper-responsive monocyte/macrophage phenotype is common.
- Can be modified by other local factors, systemic factors, medications, smoking, or emotional stress.

PREDOMINANT MICROBIAL FLORA

- Similar to chronic periodontitis with often elevated proportions of *Actinobacillus actinomycetemcomitans* and/or *Porphyromonas gingivalis*.

Necrotizing Periodontal Diseases

- Formerly known as **trench mouth** or **Vincent's disease**.

CHARACTERISTICS

- Presence of plaque.
- Interproximal gingival necrosis ("punched-out" papillae).
- Marginal gingival pseudomembrane formation.
- Attachment loss may or may not be present.
- Gingiva bleeds easily.
- Pain.
- Fetor oris.
- Commonly associated with emotional stress, malnutrition, smoking, or immunosuppression (HIV).

CLASSIFICATION

- **Necrotizing ulcerative gingivitis (NUG):** No attachment loss.
- **Necrotizing ulcerative periodontitis (NUP):** Attachment loss present.

PREDOMINANT MICROBIAL FLORA

- Variable microbial flora with elevated proportions of **spirochetes** (*Treponema* sp.), *Prevotella intermedia*, and *Fusobacterium* sp.

Candidiasis

CHARACTERISTICS

- An opportunistic fungal infection.
- Commonly associated with immunosuppression (HIV), ill-fitting dentures, chronic xerostomia (Sjögren's syndrome), or prolonged use of antibiotics.

CLASSIFICATION

- **Pseudomembranous candidiasis (thrush):** Whitish patches of desquamative epithelium, which can be easily wiped off, leaving a slightly bleeding surface.
- **Atrophic (erythemaous) candidiasis:** Painful bright-red, smooth, "beefy" lesions on the tongue, palate, or other mucosal surfaces, usually associated with ill-fitting dentures.
- **Chronic hyperplastic candidiasis:** Asymptomatic whitish plaques commonly found on the buccal mucosa near the commissures that cannot be removed, resembling oral leukoplakia.

PREDOMINANT MICROBIAL FLORA

- *Candida albicans*.

CHEMICAL PLAQUE CONTROL

- In general, chemical plaque control is not meant to replace mechanical plaque control.
- See Table 19–2 for commercial products for chemical plaque control.

Only two mouthrinses have been ADA approved for the treatment of gingivitis: prescription-only 0.12% chlorhexidine gluconate (Peridex) and an OTC phenolic/essential oil compound (Listerine).

Only one dentifrice has been ADA approved for the treatment of gingivitis: an OTC preparation containing 0.3% triclosan (Total).

TABLE 19–2. Commercially Available Products for Chemical Plaque Control

Chemical	Product	Inhibits	Characteristic
Chlorhexidine gluconate (0.12%)	Peridex PerioGuard	Plaque Gingivitis **(Most potent inhibitor)**	Side effects include extrinsic staining, altered taste perception, and supragingival calculus formation.
Phenolic/essential oil compound	Listerine	Plaque Gingivitis	Contains highest alcohol content (26.9%).
Triclosan	Total	Plaque Gingivitis	
Stannous fluoride	Gel-Kam Gum Care	Plaque Gingivitis	Side effects include extrinsic staining. ADA approved *only* for anti-caries properties.
Cetylpyridinium chloride	Scope Cepacol Viadent	Plaque	Only Viadent has been shown to inhibit *both* plaque and gingivitis.

CHAPTER 20
Reactions to Tissue Injury

Inflammation and Repair	486
CELL INJURY	486
CELL DEATH	490
INFLAMMATION	491
INFLAMMATORY MEDIATORS	493
WOUND REPAIR	495

> **INFLAMMATION AND REPAIR**

Cell Injury

MODES OF CELL INJURY

- Hypoxia
- Physical trauma
- Microorganisms
- Immunologic reactions
- Chemical/pharmacologic insult
- Nutritional imbalances
- Genetic defects
- Aging

> *Heart, brain, and lungs are very vulnerable to hypoxia. Results from:*
> - *Vascular ischemia.*
> - *↓ blood oxygen (e.g., anemia, pulmonary disease).*
> - *↓ tissue perfusion (e.g., shock, cardiac failure).*
> - *CO poisoning.*

CHEMICAL INJURY

Chemical-Induced Cell Injury

Chemical	Findings
Carbon monoxide (CO)	Systemic hypoxia
Carbon tetrachloride (CCl_4)	Hepatocellular damage ("fatty liver")
Mercury	Renal tubular necrosis Pneumonitis GI ulceration Gingival lesions
Cyanide	Prevents cellular oxidation Odor of bitter almonds
Methanol	Blindness
Lead	Basophilic stippling of RBCs

FREE RADICAL INJURY

- Induced by activated oxygen species.
- Initiate autocatalytic reactions.
- Cellular damage:
  - Membrane lipid peroxidation
  - Nucleic acid denaturation
  - Cross-linking of proteins
- Generated from:
  - Redox reactions
  - Radiation (UV light)
  - Drugs and chemicals
  - Reperfusion injury

- Antioxidants:
  - Superoxide dismutase ($2O_2 + 2H^+ \rightarrow H_2O_2 + O_2$)
  - Catalase ($2H_2O_2 \rightarrow O_2 + 2H_2O$)
  - Vitamin E
  - Ceruloplasmin

TYPES OF CELL INJURY

- Reversible cell injury
  - Cellular and organelle swelling (due to Ca^{2+} influx).
  - Bleb formation.
  - Ribosomal detachment from ER.
  - Clumping of chromatin (due to ↓ pH).
  - Increased lipid deposition (due to ↓ protein synthesis).
- Irreversible cell injury
  - Extensive plasma membrane damage.
  - Massive Ca^{2+} influx.
  - Diminished oxidative phosphorylation within mitochondria (due to accumulation of Ca^{2+}-rich densities).
  - Release of lysosomal enzymes into the cytoplasm (due to lysosomal rupture).
  - Nuclear fragmentation (**karyorrhexis**).
  - Cell death.

The outcome of cell injury depends largely on the severity and duration of the insult, but also on the cell type and its adaptive mechanisms.

CELLULAR REACTIONS TO INJURY

See Table 20–1.

TABLE 20–1. Cellular Reactions to Injury

CELLULAR REACTION	DEFINITION	RESULTS
Atrophy	Decrease in cell mass	Decrease in tissue or organ size (usually secondary to decreased neurovascular supply, nutrition, endocrine stimulation)
Hypertrophy	Increase in cell mass	Increase in tissue or organ size (usually secondary to increased tissue workload)
Aplasia	Complete lack of cells	**Agenesis** (tissue or organ absence)
Hypoplasia	Decrease in cell numbers	Decrease in tissue or organ size
Hyperplasia	Increase in cell numbers	Increase in tissue or organ size (e.g., glandular breast proliferation associated with pregnancy)
Metaplasia	Morphological change from one cell type to another	Usually occurs in response to stress (e.g., conversion of columnar epithelium to stratified squamous)

Hypertrophy and hyperplasia can occur simultaneously (e.g., uterine enlargement during pregnancy).

> **Gingival overgrowth** is often drug related:
> - Phenytoin (Dilantin)
> - Ca^{2+} channel blockers (e.g. nifedipine)
> - Cyclosporin

ENZYMATIC CELLULAR DEGRADATION

- **Autolysis:** Cellular degradation caused by *intracellular* enzymes indigenous to the cell itself.
- **Heterolysis:** Cellular degradation caused by enzymes *extrinsic* to the cell.

ENDOGENOUS PIGMENTATION

See Table 20–2.

TABLE 20–2. Comparison of Endogenous Pigments

PIGMENT	CHARACTERISTICS	ASSOCIATED PATHOLOGY
Lipofuscin	Yellow-brown "Wear-and-tear" pigment Derived from lipid peroxidation Has no effect on cell function Accumulates in heart, liver, brain	Brown atrophy Age
Bilirubin	Yellowish Major bile pigment Derived from heme **Jaundice:** Bilirubin accumulation	Biliary tree obstruction Hepatocellular injury Hemolytic anemias
Hemosiderin (see Table below)	Golden brown Derived from heme Aggregates of ferritin micelles (iron storage sites) Identified with Prussian blue stain Accumulates in phagocytes of: • Bone marrow • Liver • Spleen	Hemosiderosis Hemochromatosis
Melanin	Brown-black Derived from *tyrosine* Synthesized in melanocytes Accumulates in skin, eyes, hair	**Increased melanin:** Physiologic pigmentation Suntan Addison's disease **Decreased melanin:** Albinism Vitiligo
Ceroid	Derived from lipofuscin (via auto-oxidation) Accumulates in hepatic Kupffer cells	Hepatocellular injury

Hemosiderin Accumulation

Process	Definition	Associations	Tissue Injury
Hemosiderosis	Increased hemosiderin accumulation (in tissue macrophages).	Hemorrhage Thalassemia	No
Hemochromatosis (Bronzed disease)	More extensive hemosiderin accumulation (throughout body).	↑ Iron absorption ↓ Iron utilization Hemolytic anemias Blood transfusions	Yes

PATHOLOGIC CALCIFICATIONS

See Table 20–3.

- Abnormal deposition of calcium salts in normally noncalcified tissues.
- Types of calcifications:
  - Dystrophic
  - Metastatic

TABLE 20-3. Types of Pathologic Calcification

Calcification Type	Definition	Serum Ca^{2+}	Pathogenesis	Common Locations
Dystrophic	Calcification of degenerate or necrotic tissue	Normal	Enhanced by *collagen* and *acidic phosphoproteins* (e.g., osteopontin)	Hyalinized scars Degenerated leiomyoma foci Caseous nodules (Tb) Damaged heart valves Atherosclerotic plaques
Metastatic	Calcification of normal tissue	Abnormal	Precipitation caused by tissue *acidity* and increased Ca^{2+} concentration *Associated with:* Hyperparathyroidism Vitamin D intoxication Bone destruction (e.g., metastatic cancer) Sarcoidosis	Stomach Lungs Kidneys

Eggshell calcification:
- Thin layer of calcification around intrathoracic lymph nodes.
- Seen on chest X-ray.
- Associated with silicosis.

Calcinosis:
- Calcification in or under the skin.
- Associated with *scleroderma* and *dermatomyositis.*

Cell Death

NECROSIS

See Table 20–4.

- Most common form of cell death resulting from irreversible injury.
- Characterized histologically by a vacuolated cytoplasm, calcification, and nuclear changes.
- Cellular degradation:
  - **Autolysis:** Caused by intracellular enzymes of necrotic cell.
  - **Heterolysis:** Caused by enzymes outside the necrotic cell.
- Three major forms of necrosis:
  - Coagulative
  - Liquefactive
  - Caseous

Nuclear Changes Associated with Cell Death

Nuclear Change	Description
Pyknosis	Nuclear shrinkage and chromatin condensation.
Karyolysis	Nuclear dissolution and chromatin fading (basophilia).
Karyorrhexis	Nuclear fragmentation.

TABLE 20–4. Major Types of Necrosis

NECROSIS	CHARACTERISTICS	EXAMPLE
Coagulative	Ischemia Protein denaturation Tissue architecture preserved Infarct area is triangular shaped	Myocardial infarction
▪ Gangrenous	Ischemic coagulation Putrefaction	Gangrene
Liquefactive	Enzymatic digestion Suppuration Loss of tissue architecture	Focal bacterial infections
▪ Fat	Adipose liquefaction Fatty acids released	Acute pancreatitis
Caseous	Granulomatous inflammation Clumped cheesy material	Tuberculosis

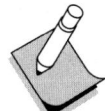

Coagulative necrosis is the most common form of necrosis.

Infarction: *Tissue death secondary to ↓ O_2 supply (↓ blood supply).*

Apoptosis

- Programmed cell death that occurs in both physiologic and pathologic states.
- Does *not* result in an inflammatory response.
- Induced by several cytosolic proteases.
- Leads to nuclear pyknosis and karyorrhexis, cell shrinkage, and ultimately phagocytosis by macrophages or neighboring parenchymal cells.

Inflammation

- A *vascular* and *cellular* response to tissue injury, resulting in the isolation of the causative agent, elimination of necrotic cells and tissues, and host tissue repair.
- There are two basic types of inflammatory response:
  - Acute
  - Chronic

Acute Inflammation

See Table 20–5 for two stages of acute inflammation.

- The initial response to tissue injury, largely consisting of leukocyte infiltration, which rids the affected area of infectious agents (mostly bacteria) and degrades necrotic tissues resulting from the damage.
- **PMNs** are the first leukocytes to respond.
- The presence of *monocytes* and *macrophages* marks the transition from acute to chronic inflammation.
- Its outcome may include the following (see also the section "Wound Repair" later in this chapter):
  - **Regeneration:** Complete resolution of affected tissues.
  - **Repair:** Fibrosis (scarring) of affected tissues.
  - **Abscess:** Formation of pus (neutrophils, necrotic cells, and exudate).
  - **Chronic inflammation:** See the section "Chronic Inflammation."

Acute inflammation generally precedes chronic inflammation, although some types of injury can directly induce a chronic inflammatory response.

> The five classic signs of acute inflammation:
>
> - **Redness (rubor):** From vasodilation and ↑ vascular permeability.
> - **Heat (calor):** From vasodilation and ↑ vascular permeability.
> - **Swelling (tumor):** From edema.
> - **Pain (dolor):** From inflammatory mediators and pressure due to edema.
> - **Loss of function (functio laesa):** From swelling and pain.

TABLE 20–5. The Two Stages of Acute Inflammation

Stage	Events	Characteristics
Vascular	Vasodilation and increased vascular permeability, predominantly mediated by **histamine-producing cells** (mast cells, basophils, and platelets)	Formation of an exudative **edema** (a straw-colored *protein-rich exudate* of extravascular fluid)
Cellular	Margination, adhesion, diapedesis, and chemotaxis of leukocytes (predominantly polymorphonuclear neutrophils [**PMNs**]) toward the site of injury	Phagocytosis and leukocyte degranulation leads to *microbial cell lysis,* but also host tissue damage

*An **exudate** (exudative edema) is caused by an inflammatory increase in vascular permeability. A **transudate** (transudative edema) is caused by a noninflammatory alteration of either vascular hydrostatic or osmotic pressures.*

CHRONIC INFLAMMATION

- A prolonged inflammatory response consisting of *continuous* inflammatory cell infiltrates, tissue injury, and wound healing.
- Can be caused by *persistent* infections, foreign bodies, immune reactions, or unknown reasons.

The Three Stages of Chronic Inflammation

Stage	Events
Mononuclear cell infiltration	Migration of macrophages, lymphocytes, plasma cells, and eosinophils
Granulation tissue formation	Healing tissue consisting largely of fibrosis (fibroblasts), angiogenesis (new capillaries), and inflammatory cells
Host tissue destruction	Mediated by cytokines of host leukocytes

Comparison of Acute and Chronic Inflammation

Inflammation	Duration	Predominant Cells	Response	Maximum Healing Potential	Example
Acute	Days	Neutrophils Mast cells	Exudative	Regeneration	Pulpal abscess
Chronic	Weeks to years	Macrophages Lymphocytes Plasma cells	Proliferative	Repair (fibrosis)	Chronic Periodontitis

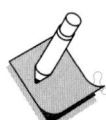

Neurons (CNS), alveolar (lung), cardiac (heart), and skeletal and smooth (muscle) cells do not have potential to regenerate.

*A **granuloma** consists of granulation tissue (fibrosis, angiogenesis, and inflammatory cells) frequently containing epithelioid cells and multinucleated giant cells.*

GRANULOMATOUS INFLAMMATION

- A specific type of *chronic inflammation* characterized by macrophages that have been transformed into **epithelioid cells** and are surrounded by lymphocytes, fibroblasts, and local parenchymal cells.
- Associated with tuberculosis, leprosy, sarcoidosis, syphilis, blastomycosis, histoplasmosis, coccidioidomycosis, Crohn's disease, and foreign body containment (e.g., sutures).

SYSTEMIC EFFECTS OF INFLAMMATION

- Fever
- Leukocytosis
  - Neutrophilia: Largely associated with *bacterial* infections.
  - Eosinophilia: Largely associated with *parasitic* infections.
  - Lymphocytosis: Associated with some *viral* infections (mumps, rubella).

Inflammatory Mediators

CYTOKINES

See Table 20-6 for inflammatory cytokines.

- Small peptides secreted by many cell types.
- Most are involved in host defense and immunity.
- There are four major categories of cytokines:
  - **Interleukins (IL):** Largest group of cytokines. Regulate leukocyte activity.
  - **Interferons (INF):** Interfere with virus replication.
  - **Tumor necrosis factors (TNF):** Regulate tumor suppression.
  - **Colony stimulating factors (CSF):** Regulate differentiation and growth of bone marrow elements.

TABLE 20-6. Important Inflammatory Cytokines

CYTOKINE	SECRETED BY	FUNCTION
IL-1	Monocytes Macrophages PMNs Fibroblasts Epithelial cells Endothelial cells	Produces fever Stimulates T_H cells Stimulates osteoclasts
IL-2	T_H-1 cells	Stimulates other T_H cells and T_C cells
IL-3*	T_H cells NK cells	Stimulates hematopoietic cells
IL-4	T_H-2 cells	Stimulates B cells and IgE
IL-5	T_H-2 cells	Stimulates B cells and IgA Stimulates eosinophils
IL-6	Monocytes Macrophages Fibroblasts T_H cells	Produces fever Stimulates B cells Stimulates T_H cells
IL-8	Monocytes Macrophages	Chemotaxis of PMNs
IL-10	T_H-2 cells	Inhibits T_H-1 cells
IL-12	Monocytes Macrophages	Stimulates T_H-1 cells
INF-γ	T_H-1 cells	Stimulates monocytes, macrophages, NK cells, and PMNs

TABLE 20-6. Important Inflammatory Cytokines (Continued)

Cytokine	Secreted By	Function
TNF-α TNF-β	Monocytes (α) Macrophages (α) T cells (β)	Stimulates adhesion molecules Stimulates T$_H$ cells Stimulates osteoclasts Cachexia
TGF-β	Monocytes Macrophages T cells B cells	The "anti-cytokine" Inhibits T cells, B cells, PMNs, monocytes, macrophages, NK cells Stimulates collagen formation and wound healing

* IL-3 is also known as colony stimulating factor (CSF)

INFLAMMATORY MEDIATORS

See Table 20–7.

TABLE 20-7. Major Inflammatory Mediators

Mediator	Secreted By	Vascular Response	Bronchial Response	Derive From	Major Function
Histamine	Mast cells Basophils	Dilation	Constriction	Histidine	Vasodilation Vascular permeability Primary mediator of **anaphylaxis**
Prostaglandins	Many tissues	Dilation	Variable	Arachidonic acid	Vasodilation Pain Fever
Leukotrienes (SRS-A)	Leukocytes Lung Endothelium Mast cells	Dilation	Constriction	Arachidonic acid	Vascular permeability Chemotaxis (LT-B$_4$) Primary mediator of **asthma**
Cytokines	Leukocytes Endothelium	None directly	None directly	Various	Fever (IL-1, IL-6, TNF-α) Chemotaxis (IL-8)

TABLE 20-7. Major Inflammatory Mediators (Continued)

Mediator	Secreted By	Vascular Response	Bronchial Response	Derive From	Major Function
Seratonin	Platelets Gastric mucosa	Constriction	No effect	Tryptophan	Vascular permeability
Bradykinin	In plasma	Dilation	Dilation	Kininogen	**Pain** Vascular permeability
Nitric oxide	Endothelium Macrophages	Dilation	Variable	Arginine	Vasodilation Tissue damage
Complement proteins	In plasma	Dilation	Constriction	Hepatocytes	Vascular permeability (C3a, C5a) Chemotaxis (C5a)
Lysosomal enzymes	Neutrophils Macrophages	No effect	No effect	Various	Bacterial killing Tissue damage
f-met-leu-phe (FMLP)	Bacterial cells	No effect	No effect	Various amino acids	Chemotaxis

Wound Repair

Stages of Wound Repair

- Inflammatory stage
    - Starts immediately after tissue injury and lasts 3–5 days.
    - The vascular and cellular phases of acute inflammation are activated. (See the section "Inflammation" earlier in this chapter.)
    - Fibrin clot formation.
    - Epithelial migration starts from opposing wound margins.
    - Local mesenchymal cells differentiate into fibroblasts.
- Fibroplastic stage
    - Starts 3–4 days after tissue injury and lasts 2–3 weeks.
    - Epithelial migration is completed and its thickness increases.
    - Collagen formation occurs as fibroblasts migrate across the fibrin network.
    - Angiogenesis and new capillary formation starts from the wound margins.
    - Fibrinolysis occurs as more connective tissue is formed.

Although there are three sequential stages, they are not mutually exclusive; their events commonly overlap.

- Remodeling stage
  - Starts 2–3 weeks after tissue injury and continues indefinitely.
  - Epithelial stratification is restored.
  - Collagen remodeling, re-orienting the fibers to provide better tensile strength.
  - Wound contraction and scar formation.

Methods of Wound Healing

See Table below.

- Primary intention
- Secondary intention

*During epithelialization, the free edges of the wound epithelium migrate toward each other until they meet, signaling a stop in lateral growth. This is known as **contact inhibition**.*

Comparison of Primary and Secondary Intention Wound Healing

Method	Definition	Characteristics	Examples
Primary	Occurs when wound margins are closely re-approximated	Faster healing with minimal scarring and risk of infection	Well-approximated surgical incisions or lacerations Well-reduced bone fractures Replaced periodontal flaps
Secondary	Occurs when there is a gap between the wound margins because close re-approximation cannot occur	Slower healing with granulation tissue formation and scarring	Extraction sockets Large burns and ulcers Poorly reduced bone fractures External-bevel gingivectomies

Regeneration

- Adaptive mechanism for restoring a tissue or organ.
- Occurs in several tissue types:
  - Liver
  - Bone
  - Cartilage
  - Intestinal mucosa
  - Surface epithelium
- Does *not* occur in several tissue types:
  - Skeletal muscle
  - Cardiac muscle
  - Neurons

Liver is a very uncommon site for infarction because of its regenerative capacity; can remove as much as 70% of hepatic tissue. Hepatocyte mitosis peaks at 33 hours.

CHAPTER 21

Immunology and Immunopathology

Immunology	498
THE IMMUNE SYSTEM	498
CELL-MEDIATED IMMUNITY	499
ANTIBODY-MEDIATED (HUMORAL) IMMUNITY	499
CELLULAR COMPONENTS OF THE IMMUNE SYSTEM	499
OPSONIZATION AND PHAGOCYTOSIS	502
IMMUNOGLOBULINS (ANTIBODIES)	503
COMPLEMENT	504
TRANSPLANTATION	506
HYPERSENSITIVITY	506
LABORATORY TESTS	509
IMMUNOPATHOLOGY	510

▶ IMMUNOLOGY

The Immune System

- Its primary purpose is to prevent microbial infection.
- Once infection occurs, the combined effects of the immune system elicit an inflammatory response, targeting the microbial antigens.

LINES OF DEFENSE

- Skin and mucous membranes
- Innate (natural) immunity
    - Functions *immediately* after microbial infiltration.
    - **Nonspecific** targeting of antigens.
    - Does *not* arise from previous infection or vaccination (**no memory**).
        - Natural killer (NK) cells
        - Polymorphonuclear neutrophils (PMNs)
        - Complement system
        - Nonspecific enzymes (lysozyme)
- Acquired (adaptive) immunity
    - Functions *days* after microbial infiltration.
    - **Specific** targeting of antigens.
    - Responds to millions of unique antigens (**exhibits diversity**).
    - Improves on multiple exposure to microorganisms (**has memory**).
    - Two types of acquired immunity (see Table below):
        - Cell-mediated
        - Antibody-mediated (humoral)

Comparison of the Two Types of Acquired Immunity

Acquired Immunity	Predominant Cells
Cell-mediated	T-lymphocytes
Antibody-mediated (humoral)	B-lymphocytes Immunoglobulins

CLASSIFICATION OF ACQUIRED IMMUNITY

- Active immunity
    - Occurs after exposure to foreign antigens.
    - Can be from a previous microbial infection or immunization (vaccination) with live attenuated or killed antigens.
    - Produces *both* antibodies and activated T-lymphocytes.
    - Produces long-term resistance (years) but has a *slow onset* (days).
- Passive immunity
    - Occurs after exposure to preformed antibodies from another host.
    - Can be passed from mother to fetus (IgG) during pregnancy or from mother to newborn (IgA) during breastfeeding.

- Can also be from immunization (vaccination) with immune globulins.
- Provides *only* antibodies.
- Has a short life-span (months), but provides *immediate* availability of antibodies.

ANTIGENS

- Molecules that react with antibodies to induce an immune response.
- Most are **proteins,** but many are also polysaccharides, lipoproteins, and nucleoproteins.
- The antibody-binding site on an antigen is called an **epitope.**
- A **hapten** is an antigen that cannot elicit an immune response on its own; it must be bound to a carrier protein.
- An **adjuvant** is a molecule that enhances the immune response to an antigen.

Many drugs, such as penicillin, are haptens.

***Freund's adjuvant,** commonly used for research, consists of killed M. tuberculosis suspended in lanolin and mineral oil.*

Cell-Mediated Immunity

- Host defense against many viruses, bacteria (especially intracellular infections), fungi, and parasites.
- Also important in granulomatous infections, tumor suppression, organ transplant rejection, and graft-versus-host reactions.
- Responsible for type IV (delayed) hypersensitivity.
- Mediated by T-lymphocytes (T_H cells, T_C cells), NK cells, and macrophages.

Antibody-Mediated (Humoral) Immunity

- Host defense against many bacteria (especially capsular- and toxin-induced infections) and some viruses.
- Mediated by B-lymphocytes (plasma cells, memory cells) and antibodies (immunoglobulins).

Cellular Components of the Immune System

T-CELLS

See Table 21–1.

- Differentiate in the **thymus.**
- Long life span, ranging from months to years.
- Have a **CD3-associated T-cell receptor (TCR),** which recognizes a unique antigen *only* in conjunction with MHC proteins.

*All nucleated cells exhibit **class I MHC** surface proteins, which are important in the recognition of self versus non-self.*
*Only antigen-presenting cells (APCs) exhibit **class II MHC** surface proteins, which bind and present antigen to T_H cells.*

> **CD8 lymphocytes function in two ways:**
> - Release perforins (disrupt cell membranes).
> - Induce apoptosis (programmed cell death).

*The process by which an antigen binds to a specific TCR (T-cell) or Ig (B-cell), activating that immune cell to clonally expand into cells of the same specificity is called **clonal selection**.*

TABLE 21–1. T-cells

T-Cell	Function	Characteristics
CD4 lymphocytes – Helper T-cells (T_H cells)		Respond to antigen associated with **class II MHC** proteins
T_H-1 cells	Signal CD8 cells to differentiate into cytotoxic T-cells; Signal macrophages in type IV (delayed) hypersensitivity reactions	Secrete IL-2 and INF-γ
T_H-2 cells	Signal B-cells to differentiate into plasma cells, producing antibodies	Secrete IL-4 and IL-5
CD8 lymphocytes, cytotoxic T-cells (T_C cells)	Kill virus-infected, tumor, and allograft cells	Respond to antigen associated with **class I MHC** proteins
Memory T-cells	Activated in response to re-exposure to antigen	Exist for years after initial exposure

B-Cells

See Table 21–2.

- Differentiate in the **bone marrow.**
- Short life span, ranging from days to weeks.

TABLE 21–2. B-cells

B-Cell	Function	Characteristics
Plasma cells	Synthesize immunoglobulins (antibodies)	*Only* **monomeric IgM** and **IgD** are expressed on their surfaces as antigen receptors
Mature B-cells	Antigen presentation	Express class II MHC proteins
Memory B-cells	Activated in response to re-exposure to antigen	Exist for years after initial exposure

Natural Killer (NK) Cells

- Lack a CD3-associated TCR and surface IgM or IgD.
- Are *not* specific to any antigen and do not need to recognize MHC proteins.
- Do *not* require previous exposure to antigen to function (have **no memory**).
  - Function: Kill virus-infected cells and tumor cells.

IgG antibodies enhance NK cell effectiveness via antibody-dependent cellular toxicity (ADCC).

Monocytes and Macrophages

- *Agranular* leukocytes.
- Derived from bone marrow histiocytes.
- Exist in plasma (monocytes) and in tissues (macrophages).
- Activated by bacterial LPS, peptidoglycan, and DNA, as well as T_H-1 cell-mediated INF-γ.
- Functions:
  - Phagocytosis: Via Fc and C3b receptors.
  - Antigen presentation: Express class II MHC proteins.
  - Cytokine production: IL-1, IL-6, IL-8, INF, and TNF.

*Monocytes and macrophages are major components of the **reticuloendothelial system**, which includes all phagocytic cells except for granulocytes (PMNs).*

Dendritic Cells

- *Agranular* leukocytes.
- Located primarily in the skin and mucous membranes.
- Function:
  - Antigen presentation: Express class II MHC proteins.

*Other phagocytes include **histiocytes** (fixed macrophages in various connective tissues), **microglia** (CNS), **dust cells** (lung), and **Kupffer cells** (liver).*

Polymorphonuclear Neutrophils

See Table 21–3.

- *Granular* leukocytes. Cytoplasmic granules (lysosomes) contain several bacteriocidal enzymes.
- Functions:
  - Phagocytosis
  - Cytokine production

***Langerhans' cells** are the major dendritic cells of the gingival epithelium.*

TABLE 21-3. Major Contents of PMN Cytoplasmic Granules

Granule Type	Enzymes
Primary (azurophilic)	Hydrolase
	Myeloperoxidase
	Neuraminidase
Secondary	Collagenase
	Lysozyme
	Lactoferrin

Antigen-presenting cells (APCs) express class II MHC proteins and present antigen to CD4 T-cells. The predominant APCs of the immune system are monocytes and macrophages, dendritic cells (Langerhans' cells), and B-cells.

Chemokines (IL-8, C5a, LT-B$_4$, FMLP) are chemotactic cytokines for PMNs and macrophages.

The two major opsonins are IgG and C3b.

EOSINOPHILS

- *Granular* leukocytes.
- Bind antigen-bound IgG or IgE, subsequently releasing cytoplasmic granules.
- Do *not* present antigen to T-cells.
- Functions:
  - Defense against **parasitic infections** (especially nematodes).
  - Mediate hypersensitivity diseases: Release histaminase, leukotrienes, and peroxidase.
  - Phagocytosis.

BASOPHILS AND MAST CELLS

- *Granular* leukocytes.
- Exist in plasma (basophils) and in tissues (mast cells).
- Bind antigen-bound **IgE**, subsequently releasing cytoplasmic granules (histamine, heparin, peroxidase, and hydrolase) and inflammatory cytokines.
- Function:
  - Mediate immediate hypersensitivity reactions such as **anaphylaxis**.

Opsonization and Phagocytosis

OPSONIZATION

- Enhances phagocytosis of microorganisms.
- Antibody (**IgG**) or complement protein (**C3b**) coat the outer surface of microorganisms, allowing phagocytes to bind and engulf them more efficiently.

PHAGOCYTOSIS

See Table 21–4.

- The process by which microorganisms, cell debris, dead or damaged host cells, and other insoluble particles are taken up and broken down by phagocytes.

TABLE 21–4. Stages of Phagocytosis

STAGE	EVENTS	CHARACTERISTICS
Adhesion	Plasma phagocytes (PMNs, monocytes) bind to vascular endothelium	Mediated by *selectins* and *cellular adhesion molecules (CAMs)*
Migration	Phagocytes migrate toward the microorganisms	**Diapedesis** is the movement of the phagocyte through the vascular endothelium. Mediated by *chemokines* (IL-8, C5a, LT-B$_4$, FMLP)
Ingestion	The phagocyte cell membrane forms *pseudopods*, which surround and engulf the microorganism	**Phagosome** formation occurs when the internalized endosome fuses with lysosomes. Mediated by *opsonization* (C3b, IgG)
Lysosomal degranulation	The lysosome empties its hydrolytic enzymes into the phagosome, killing the microorganism	Mediated by *lysosomal enzymes*

LYSOSOMAL CONTENTS

- Superoxide radicals (O_2^-)
  - $O_2 + e^- \rightarrow O_2^-$.
- Superoxide dismutase
  - Produces **hydrogen peroxide** (H_2O_2).
  - $2O_2^- + 2H^+ \rightarrow H_2O_2 + O_2$.
- Myeloperoxidase
  - Produces **hypochlorite ions** (ClO^-), which damage cell walls.
  - $Cl^- + H_2O_2 \rightarrow ClO^- + H_2O$.
- Lactoferrin
  - Chelates iron from bacteria.
- Lysozyme
  - Degrades bacterial cell wall peptidoglycan.
- Proteases
- Nucleases
- Lipases

Lysosomes are membrane-bound vesicles that contain hydrolytic enzymes necessary for intracellular digestion.

Immunoglobulins (Antibodies)

See Table 21–5.
- Y-shaped glycoproteins secreted by plasma cells. (See Figure 21–1.)
- Contain two identical **light polypeptide chains** (κ or λ), and two identical **heavy polypeptide chains** (α, γ, δ, ε, or μ) linked by **disulfide bonds**.

Catalase and other peroxidases (enzymes that break down H_2O_2) are located in membrane-bound organelles called **peroxisomes (microbodies)**. Bacteria that contain **catalase** *(Staphylococci sp.)* are able to resist the cidal effects of H_2O_2.

TABLE 21–5. Immunoglobulin Isotypes

ISOTYPE	SUBUNITS	LOCATION OF ACTION	FUNCTION	CHARACTERISTICS
IgA	1 or 2	Exocrine secretions	Prevents microbial attachment to mucous membranes	*2nd most abundant* antibody
IgD	1	B-cells	Uncertain	*Least abundant* antibody
IgE	1	Mast cells Basophils Eosinophils	Mediates type I hypersensitivity reactions **(anaphylaxis)**	Main host defense against **parasites** (especially helminths)
IgM	1 or 5	B-cells (monomer) Plasma (pentamer)	Main antimicrobial defense of **primary response** Activates complement Opsonizes B-cells	*Largest* antibody Most potent activator of complement Has highest avidity of all antibodies
IgG	1	Plasma	Main antimicrobial defense of **secondary response** Opsonizes bacteria Activates complement Neutralizes bacterial toxins and viruses	*Most abundant* antibody Crosses the **placenta** Has four subclasses ($IgG_{1, 2, 3, 4}$)

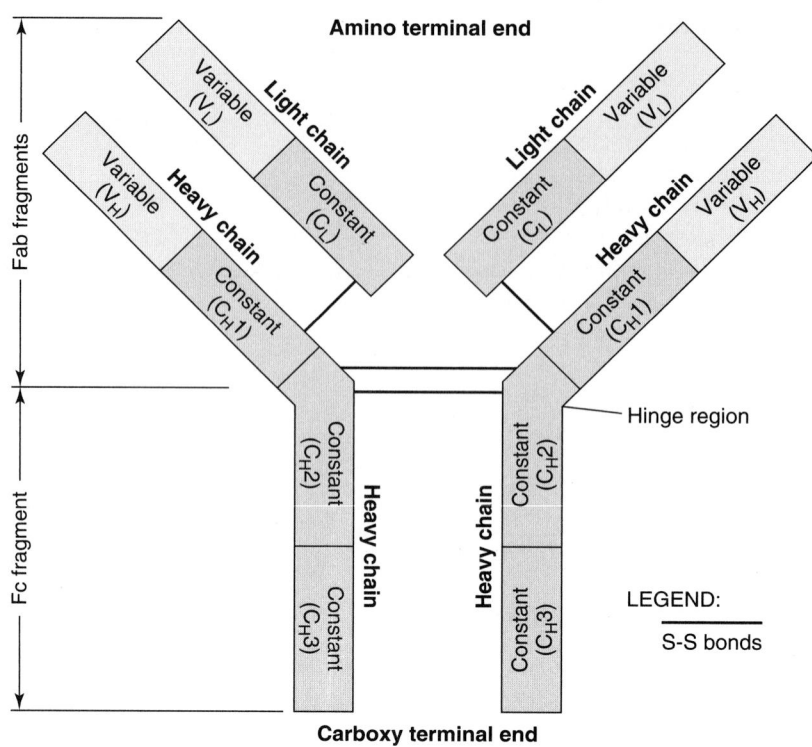

FIGURE 21-1. Immunoglubulin structure.

Reproduced, with permission, from Levinson W. *Medical Microbiology and Immunology*, 8th ed. McGraw-Hill, 2004.

IgA and IgM are the only antibodies that can exist as polymers, as a dimer and a pentamer, respectively. Only the polymeric forms contain a J chain, which initiates the polymerization process.

Secretory IgA (sIgA) differs from serum IgA in that it is more resistant to proteolytic degradation. It always exists as a dimer.

Only IgM and IgG can activate complement.

- The *constant regions* of the two heavy chains form the **F$_c$ site**, which binds to APCs or C3b. They define the immunoglobulin class **(isotype)**.
- The two *variable regions* of the heavy and light chains form the **F$_{ab}$ sites**, which are specific for binding antigen and determine the **idiotype**.
- Functions:
  - Neutralize bacterial toxins and viruses.
  - Opsonization (enhances phagocytosis).
  - Activate complement via the *classical pathway*.
  - Inhibit microbial attachment to mucosal surfaces.

Complement

See Tables 21–6 and 21–7 and Figure 21–2.

- Consists of about 20 plasma proteins.
- Synthesized in the **liver.**
- Augments other components of the immune system.
- All modes of activation lead to the production of C3.

TABLE 21-6. Pathways of Complement Activation

Pathway	Characteristics
Classic	Primarily activated by **antigen–antibody complexes** with **IgG$_{1,2,3}$** or **IgM**
Alternative	Primarily activated by bacterial **LPS (endotoxin)**
Lectin	Primarily activated by microorganisms containing cell-surface **mannan** (a polymer of mannose)

TABLE 21-7. Major Functions of Complement

Function	Events
Opsonization	Mediated by **C3b**
Chemotaxis	Mediated by **C5a**
Cell lysis (cytolysis)	**Membrane attack complex (MAC)** disrupts cell membrane permeability (composed of **C5b** and **C6-9**)

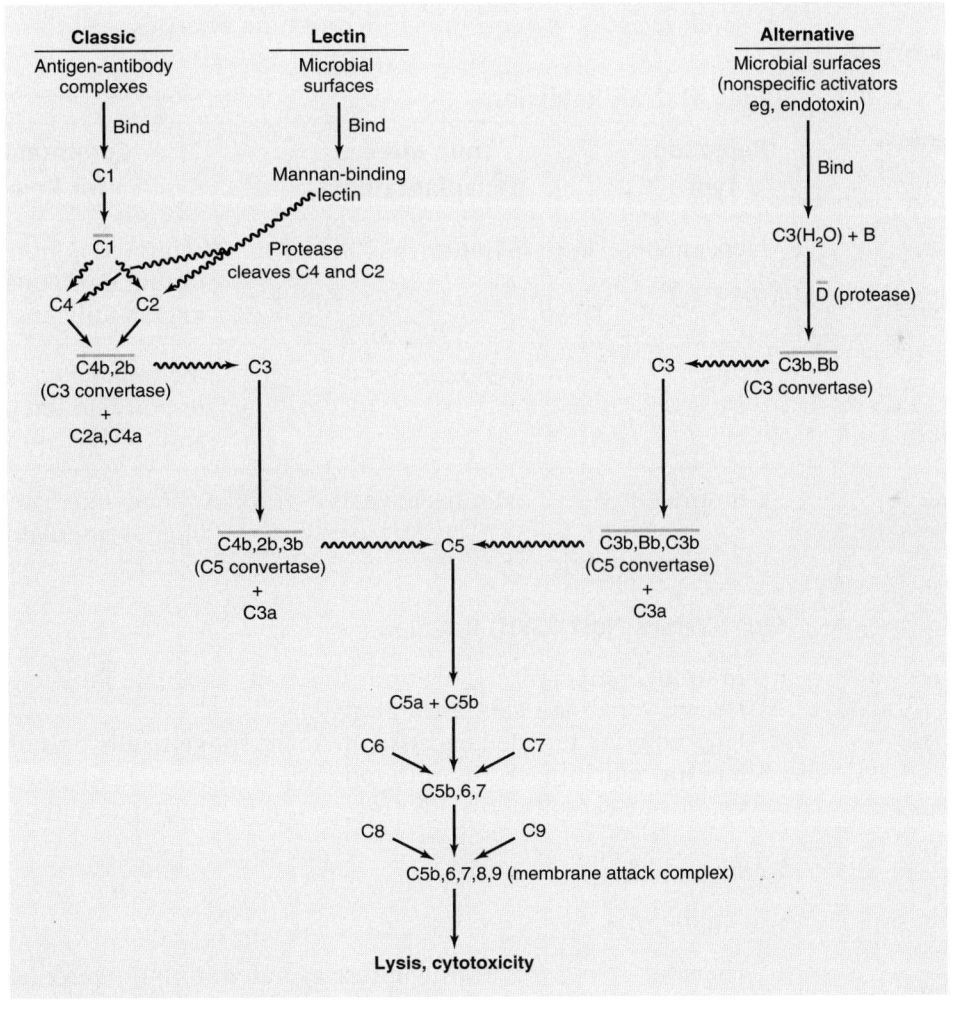

FIGURE 21-2. The complement system.

Reproduced, with permission, from Levinson W. *Medical Microbiology and Immunology*, 8th ed. McGraw-Hill, 2004.

Transplantation

TYPES OF GRAFT

- **Autograft:** Transplantation of tissue from one site to another within the same individual.
- **Isograft:** Transplantation of tissue between two genetically *identical* individuals in the same species.
- **Allograft:** Transplantation of tissue between two genetically *different* individuals in the same species.
- **Xenograft:** Transplantation of tissue between two different species.

GRAFT REJECTION

CD8 T_C cells elicit most of the destruction in graft rejection.

See Table below.

- **T-cell-mediated** immune response against donor alloantigens.
- The severity and rapidity of graft rejection is determined by the degree of differences between donor and recipient class I and II MHC proteins.
- If a *second* graft from the same donor is given to a sensitized recipient, an accelerated rejection response occurs due to the presence of presensitized T_C cells.
- Allografts are the most common grafts used for organ transplantation, blood transfusions, and other tissue grafts.
- Graft rejection can occur at different time intervals.

The most common types of hyperacute rejection are ABO blood mismatches.

Types of Graft Rejection

Rejection Type	Time after Transplantation	Common Reason for Rejection
Hyperacute	Minutes	Preformed antibody-mediated immune response to graft antigens
Acute	Weeks	T-cell-mediated immune response to foreign class I and II MHC proteins
Chronic	Months to years	Antibody-mediated necrosis of graft vasculature

GRAFT-VERSUS-HOST (GVH) REACTION

- Immunocompetent T-cells from the graft recognize the recipient's cells as foreign, eliciting their destruction.
- Host cells are targeted because the recipient generally undergoes radiation therapy, inducing severe immunocompromise.
- Occurs most commonly after *bone marrow transplants* and can be fatal.

Hypersensitivity

See Table 21–8.

- Hypersensitivity reactions elicit exaggerated immune responses, which are damaging and destructive to the host.
- See Chapter 20 for a list of the major inflammatory mediators.

TABLE 21-8. Hypersensitivity Reactions

Hypersensitivity Type	Major Mediator	Reaction	Associated Disease
Type I: Immediate (anaphylactic)	IgE	Antigen-bound IgE activates the release of inflammatory mediators from mast cells and basophils	Atopic allergy Angioedema Anaphylaxis
Type II: Cytotoxic	IgM IgG	IgM or IgG bind to host cell surface antigens, activating complement and producing MAC-mediated cell destruction	Hemolytic anemia ADCC Goodpasture's syndrome Erythroblastosis fetalis
Type III: Immune-complex	Antigen–antibody complexes	Antigen–antibody complexes (IgG, IgM, and IgA) are deposited in various tissues, activating complement and eliciting PMN/macrophage-mediated tissue destruction	Arthus reaction Serum sickness Glomerulonephritis RA SLE
Type IV: Delayed (cell-mediated)	T-cell	Macrophages present antigen, activating T-cells and producing lymphokine-mediated tissue destruction	Contact dermatitis Tuberculin (PPD) test Tuberculosis Sarcoidosis Leprosy

Hypersensitivity Reactions

See Figures 21–3 to 21–6.

- Type I: Immediate (anaphylactic).
- Type II: Cytotoxic.
- Type III: Immune-complex.
- Type IV: Delayed (cell-mediated).
    - The response generally starts hours or days after contact with antigen.

Atopic allergies *are common type I hypersensitivity reactions that have a strong genetic predisposition for excessive IgE production. Clinical manifestations include asthma, edema and erythema ("wheal and flare"), and urticaria (hives). Common allergens include pollens, animal danders, foods (shellfish and peanuts), drugs (penicillin), bee venom, and latex.*

Angioedema *is a more generalized version of type I hypersensitivity. It involves larger areas and deeper tissues beneath the skin and underlying tissues, causing a more diffuse swelling. May involve all or part of hands, feet, lips, eyelids, genitals, oral mucosa, and airway. Rapid (immediate) onset.*

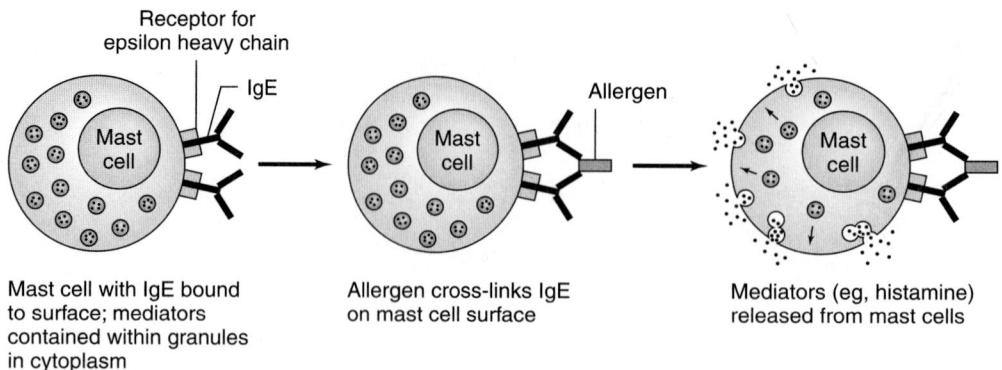

FIGURE 21-3. Type I: Immediate (anaphylactic) hypersensitivity.

Reproduced, with permission, from Levinson W. *Medical Microbiology and Immunology*, 8th ed. McGraw-Hill, 2004.

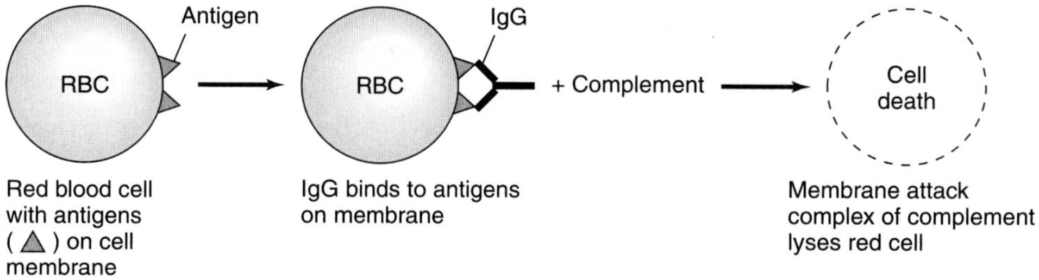

FIGURE 21-4. Type II: Cytotoxic hypersensitivity.

Reproduced, with permission, from Levinson W. *Medical Microbiology and Immunology*, 8th ed. McGraw-Hill, 2004.

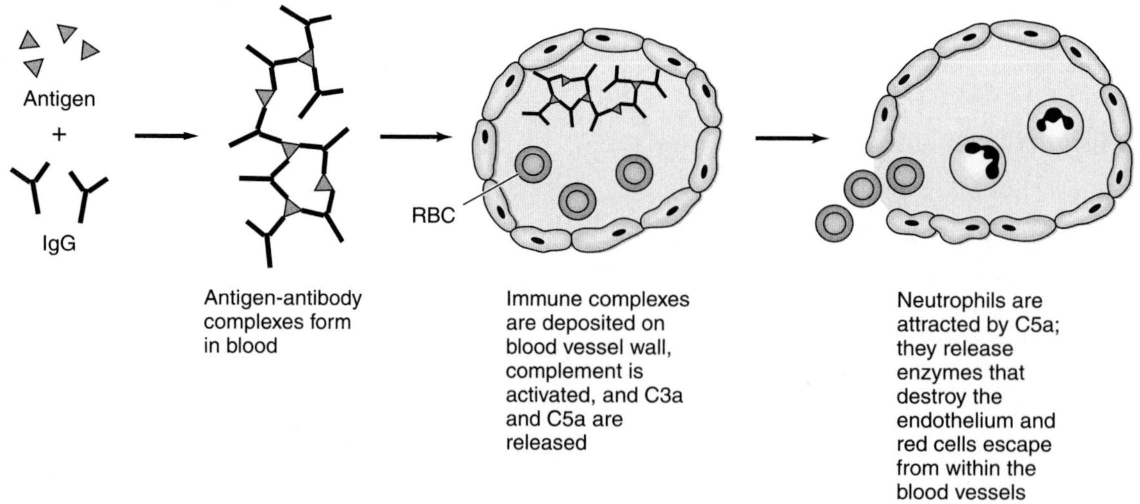

FIGURE 21-5. Type III: Immune-complex hypersensitivity.

Reproduced, with permission, from Levinson W. *Medical Microbiology and Immunology*, 8th ed. McGraw-Hill, 2004.

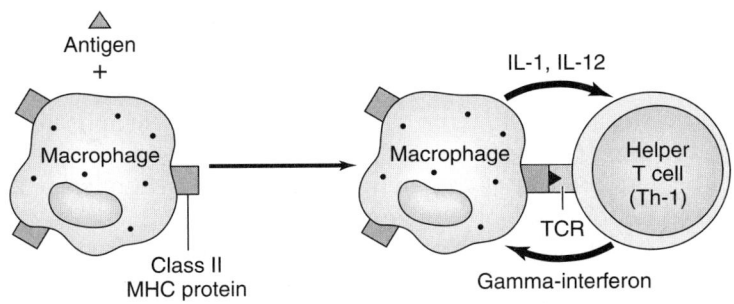

FIGURE 21-6. Type IV: Delayed (cell-mediated) hypersensitivity.

Reproduced, with permission, from Levinson W. *Medical Microbiology and Immunology*, 8th ed. McGraw-Hill, 2004.

Laboratory Tests

See Table 21–9.

- There are several methods for the detection and diagnosis of infectious diseases, autoimmune diseases, and blood typing.

*Anaphylaxis is the most severe form of type I hypersensitivity, leading to bronchoconstriction and hypotension (shock); can be life-threatening without treatment. Its treatment is **epinephrine** 0.3 mg (1:1,000) IM or 0.1mg (1:10,000) IV. Once vital signs are stabilized, antihistamines or corticosteroids can be administered.*

TABLE 21-9. Common Antigen–Antibody Laboratory Tests

Test	Function	Common Use
Agglutination	Antibody cross-links with a **particulate** antigen, creating visible clumping if positive.	ABO blood typing.
Precipitation	Antibody cross-links with a **soluble** antigen, creating visible precipitates if positive.	Detection of serum antigen or antibody.
Radioimmunoassay (RIA)	Radio-labeled antibodies cross-link with unlabeled (unknown) antigen, creating measurable radioactive complexes if positive.	Detection of serum antigen or hapten.
Enzyme-linked immunosorbent assay (ELISA)	Enzyme-labeled antibody binds to serum antibody–antigen complexes. A substrate is then added, activating the enzyme, and eliciting a color reaction (determined by spectrophotometry) if positive.	Detection of antigen or antibody in patient specimens.
Immunofluorescence (IF)	Fluorescent-labeled antibodies bind to unlabeled (unknown) antigen, creating visible fluorescence in UV light if positive.	Detection of antigen in histologic sections or tissue specimens.

ABO Blood Typing

See Table below.

- All erythrocytes have alloantigens of the ABO type, which are important for blood typing and transfusions.
- Although there are only two genes (A and B) that encode for these antigens, there are four possible antigenic combinations: A, B, AB, or O.
- *Hemagglutination* occurs when blood types are mismatched.

ABO Blood Types

Blood Type	Erythrocyte Antigen	Plasma Antibody
A	A	Anti-B
B	B	Anti-A
AB (universal recipient)	Both A and B	Neither anti-A or anti-B
O (universal donor)	Neither A or B	Both anti-A and anti-B

> Type **O** blood is the universal d**o**nor because it contains n**o** A or B antigens.

Immunopathology

IMMUNODEFICIENCY DISEASES

See Table 21–10.

TABLE 21-10. Immunodeficiency Diseases

Disease	Cellular Pathology	Cause	Immunological Findings	Clinical Findings
Bruton's X-linked agammaglobulinemia	B-cells	Pre-B-cells do not differentiate into mature B-cells (*tyrosine kinase* mutation)	Poorly developed germinal lymph centers. Absence of B-cells, plasma cells, and Ig. T-cells are normal	Increased bacterial infections. Usually affects males. Presents after 6 months of age (maternal IgG initially protects). Also associated with lymphoma, leukemia, myeloma
Isolated IgA deficiency	B-cells	Mature B-cells do not differentiate into IgA-secreting plasma cells	Other Ig isotypes are normal	Most common inherited B-cell defect. Increased infection at mucosal surfaces
Common variable immunodeficiency	B-cells	Mature B-cells do not differentiate into plasma cells	Absence of various Ig isotypes	Associated with hemolytic anemias and lymphoid tumors

TABLE 21-10. Immunodeficiency Diseases (Continued)

Disease	Cellular Pathology	Cause	Immunological Findings	Clinical Findings
Ataxia-telangiectasia	B-cells	Defective DNA repair (especially to *ionizing radiation*)	Decreased IgA levels	**Ataxia:** Cerebellar problems (uncoordinated gait) **Telangiectasias:** Dilation of capillaries (sclera, ear, nose) Graying of hair Irregular skin pigmentation to sun-exposed areas Increased infections and malignancies
DiGeorge's syndrome	T-cells	Thymic hypoplasia (poorly developed thymus and parathyroids)	Absence of T-cells B-cells are normal Lip, ear, and aortic arch abnormalities	Defective development of 3rd and 4th pharyngeal arches Increased viral and fungal infections Decreased type IV hypersensitivity Associated with PTH deficiency (tetany from hypocalcemia)
Job's syndrome	T-cells	T$_H$-cells do not produce INF-γ	Elevated IgE levels. Poor PMN chemotaxis.	Increased bacterial infections (commonly *Staph aureus*)
Severe combined immunodeficiency disease (SCID)	B-cells and T-cells	Defective stem cell differentiation. ■ X-linked ■ Autosomal recessive (*adenosine deaminase* deficiency)	Absent or diminished lymphoid tissue Marked lymphopenia	Most severe inherited immunodeficiency Increased viral, bacterial, fungal infections Death generally occurs before age two
Wiskott–Aldrich syndrome	B-cells and T-cells	Defective IgM response to bacterial LPS	Decreased IgM levels Elevated IgA levels Normal IgE levels	X-linked (usually affects boys) Clinical triad: ■ Infections (from immunodeficiency) ■ Eczema ■ Thrombocytopenia

> **DiGeorge's syndrome:**
>
> **CATCH 22:**
>
> **C**ardiac defects, **A**bnormal facies, **T**hymic hypoplasia, **C**left palate, **H**ypocalcemia, microdeletion of chromosome **22**.

> **Thymus gland:**
>
> - Important for development of the immune system, beginning prenatally.
> - Involved in T-cell development and differentiation.
> - Located behind the sternum.
> - Functions in childhood then gradually atrophies with age.

AUTOIMMUNE DISEASES

- Caused by immune reactions verus self (host tissues).
- Usually involves auto-antibodies.
- HLA antigen association.
- Mechanisms:
  - Hypersensitivity reactions
  - Disordered immunoregulation
    - ↑ T_H-cell function
    - ↓ T_S-cell function
    - Nonspecific B-cell activation
- Examples:
  - Graves disease
  - Hashimoto's thyroiditis
  - Pernicious anemia
  - Sjögren's syndrome
  - Systemic lupus erythematosus
  - Scleroderma
  - Polyarteritis nodosa
  - Rheumatoid arthritis
  - Reiter's syndrome
  - Ankylosing spondylitis
  - Myasthenia gravis
  - Multiple sclerosis

CHAPTER 22

Systemic Pathology

Developmental Pathology	516
TERATOGENESIS	516
CHROMOSOMAL ABNORMALITIES	516
LYSOSOMAL STORAGE DISEASES	518
OTHER CHILDHOOD GENETIC DISORDERS	518
Dermatopathology	519
DISORDERS OF SKIN PIGMENTATION	519
SKIN INFECTIONS	520
IMMUNOLOGIC SKIN LESIONS	520
BENIGN (NONNEOPLASTIC) SKIN LESIONS	522
Cardiovascular Pathology	522
EDEMA	522
SHOCK	523
CONGESTION (HYPEREMIA)	524
THROMBOSIS	525
EMBOLUS	525
PHLEBITIS	526
ARTERIOSCLEROSIS	526
HYPERTENSION	527
AORTIC ANEURYSM	529
AORTIC DISSECTION	529
PATHOLOGY INVOLVING THE PERICARDIUM	530
RHEUMATIC FEVER	531
CORONARY ARTERY DISEASE (CAD)	532
HEART FAILURE	533
CV PULMONARY CROSS-CORRELATION	534
Respiratory Pathology	535
ASTHMA	535
CHRONIC OBSTRUCTIVE PULMONARY DISEASE	536
BRONCHIECTASIS	538
ATELECTASIS	538
PNEUMOCONIOSES	538

Sarcoidosis	539
Idiopathic Pulmonary Fibrosis	540
Pneumonia	540
Lung Abscess	541
Tuberculosis (TB)	542

Gastrointestinal Pathology — 542

Esophagus	542
Stomach	544
Small and Large Intestines	545
Pancreas	546
Liver Disease	548

Genitourinary Pathology — 550

Nephrolithiasis	550
Pyelonephritis	551
Diabetes Insipidus	552
Polycystic Kidney Disease (PCKD)	552
Medullary Cystic Disease	552
Medullary Sponge Kidney	552
Nephrosclerosis	552
Arteriosclerosis	553
Nephrotic Syndrome	553
Glomerulonephropathies	554

Blood–Lymphatic Pathology — 554

Anemia	554
Anemia from ↑ RBC Destruction	555
Anemia from ↓ RBC Production	557
↓↓ factors for RBC Production	557
Other Causes of ↓↓ RBC Production	559
Erythrocytes and Polycythemia (↑ RBCs)	559
Bleeding Problems	560
Disorders in Primary Hemostasis	561
Quantitative Platelet Deficiencies	561
Disorders in Secondary Hemostasis	563

Endocrine Pathology — 564

Antidiuretic Hormone (Vasopressin)	564
Insulin	564
Growth Hormone	565
Thyroid Hormone	566
Parathyroid Hormone	568
Cortisol	570

Muscoloskeletal Pathology — 571

Collagen Vascular Diseases	571
Osseous Pathology	573
Arthritis	579

Neuropathology 581
- NEUROLOGIC TRAUMA 581
- NEURODEGENERATIVE DISEASES 582
- DEMYELINATING DISEASES 583
- MYASTHENIA GRAVIS 583

DEVELOPMENTAL PATHOLOGY

Teratogenesis

- Induction of nonhereditary congenital malformations (birth defects) in a developing fetus by exogenous factors:
  - Physical
  - Chemical
  - Biologic agents
- Teratogens = Teratogenic agents
- **Physical agents**
  - Radiation
  - Hypoxia
  - CO_2
  - Mechanical trauma
- **Maternal infection**
  - TORCH complex (**T**oxoplasmosis, **O**ther agents, **R**ubella, **C**MV, and **H**SV)
- **Hormones**
  - Sex hormones
  - Corticosteroids
- **Vitamin deficiencies**
  - Riboflavin
  - Niacin
  - Folic acid
  - Vitamin E
- **Drugs**
  - Mitomycin
  - Dactinomycin
  - Puromycin

> - Effects of teratogens:
>   - Death
>   - Growth retardation
>   - Malformation
>   - Functional impairment
> - Mechanism of teratogens:
>   - Specific for each teratogen: inhibit, interfere, or block metabolic steps critical for normal morphogenesis.
>   - Most are site or tissue specific.
> - Susceptibility to teratogens is
>   - Variable.
>   - Specific for each developmental stage.
>   - Dose dependant.

Chromosomal Abnormalities

Autosomal Abnormalities

Down syndrome is the most frequent chromosomal disorder (1:700 births). People with Down syndrome can live into their 30s and 40s.

> Chromosomal abnormalities in decreasing order of incidence:
> - Down's = 1:700.
> - Edward's = 1:3000.
> - Patau's = 1:5000.

Syndrome	Chromosomal Abnormality	Findings
Down syndrome	Trisomy 21	Mental retardation Epicanthal folds Large protruding tongue Small head, low-set ears Broad flat face Simian crease **Complications** ↑ leukemia ↑ infection Alzheimer-like brain Δ

Autosomal Abnormalities (Continued)

Syndrome	Chromosomal Abnormality	Findings
Edward syndrome	Trisomy 18	Mental retardation Small head Micrognathia (small lower jaw) Pinched facial appearance Low-set, malformed ears Rocker bottom feet Heart defects Prognosis: months
Patau syndrome	Trisomy 13	Mental retardation Microcephaly Microphthalmia Brain abnormalities Cleft lip and palate Polydactyly Heart defects Prognosis: < 1 yr

Sex Chromosome Abnormalities

Syndrome	Chromosomal Abnormality	Findings
Klinefelter syndrome	XXY	1:500 men Manifests at puberty Hypogonadism, atrophic testes Tall stature Gynecomastia Female pubic hair distribution. Low IQ Associated with ↑ maternal and ↑ paternal age
Turner syndrome	XO	1:3000 live female births Diagnose at birth or puberty Female hypogonadism Primary amenorrhea Short stature Webbed neck Wide-spaced nipples Coarctation of aorta

Lysosomal Storage Diseases

LYSOSOMAL STORAGE DISEASES

- Tay–Sachs
- Gaucher
- Neimann–Pick
- Fabry
- See also Chapter 6, Biological Compounds.

Lysosomal storage diseases are most common in people of Eastern European ancestry.

Autosomal Recessive	X-linked
Tay–Sachs Gaucher Niemann–Pick	Fabry

Other Childhood Genetic Disorders

CYSTIC FIBROSIS

- Most common fatal genetic disease in white children.
- Occurs in both males and females (M = F).
- Life expectancy = 28 years.
- Generalized exocrine gland dysfunction. Problem with Cl- transporter
- Multiple organ systems.
    - Characterized by respiratory and digestive problems.
- **Pathogenesis:** Chromosome 7q.
    - Gene encodes CFTR (cystic fibrosis transmembrane regulator).
    - Regulates Cl^- and Na^+ transport across epithelial membranes.
- Affects Na^+ channels, especially mucous and sweat glands.
- **Test:** Sweat chloride test.
- **Findings**
    - Chronic pulmonary disease.
        - From thick mucous in airways:
            - Lung infections.
            - Bronchiectasis.
    - Pancreatic exocrine insufficiency.
    - Meconium ileus.
        - Intestinal obstruction in infants/newborns.

Cystic fibrosis
- Problem with Cl^- transporter
- Findings
    - Bronchiectasis
    - Meconium ileus

VON HIPPEL–LINDAU DISEASE

- Autosomal dominant
    - Chromosome 3
    - VHL gene
- **Findings**
- Hemangiomas
    - Retina
    - Cerebellum

- Cysts and adenomas
  - Liver
  - Kidney
  - Adrenal glands
  - Pancreas

MARFAN'S SYNDROME

- Uncommon hereditary connective-tissue disorder:
  - Fibrillin gene mutation.
- **Findings**
- Skeletal
  - Tall and thin patients
  - Abnormally long legs and arms
  - Spiderlike fingers
- Cardiovascular
  - Cystic medial necrosis of aorta
    - Risk aortic incompetence, dissecting aortic aneurysms.
  - Distensible mitral valve.
- Ocular: Lens dislocation.

▶ DERMATOPATHOLOGY

Disorders of Skin Pigmentation

HYPOPIGMENTATION

- **Albinism**
  - Failure in pigment production from otherwise intact melanocytes.
  - Usually tyrosinase problem; can't convert tyrosine to DOPA (in the pathway to form melanin).
- **Vitiligo**
  - Acquired loss of melanocytes.
  - Discrete areas of skin with depigmented white patches.
  - May be autoimmune.

HYPERPIGMENTATION

- **Freckle** (ephelis): Increased melanin pigment within basal keratinocytes.
- **Lentigo:** Pigmented macule caused by melanocytic hyperplasia in epidermis.
- **Pigmented nevi:** (See the section "Benign (Nonneoplastic) Skin Lesions" later in this chapter.)
- **Lentigo maligna:** (See the section "Benign (Nonneoplastic) Skin Lesions" later in this chapter.)
- **Café au lait spots:**
  - Increase in melanin content with giant melanosomes.
  - Conditions with café au lait spots include:
    - Neurofibromatosis type 1 (most frequent neurocutaneous syndrome).
    - McCune–Albright syndrome (See the section "Fibrous Dysplasia" later in this chapter).
    - Tuberous sclerosis.
    - Fanconi anemia.
- Diffuse hyperpigmentation with **Addison's disease.**
  - Secondary to ↑ melanocyte stimulating hormone.

Skin Infections

VIRAL SKIN ERUPTIONS

- Molluscum contagiosum (Poxvirus)
- Verruca vulgaris (common wart) (human papilloma virus [HPV])
- Herpes simplex
- Roseola
- Rubella
- Measles

BACTERIAL SKIN ERUPTIONS

IMPETIGO

- Common skin infection.
  - Common in preschool age children (2–5 years old).
  - Especially during warm weather.
- Etiology
  - Invasion of epidermis by *Staph. aureus* or *Strep. pyogenes*.
  - Similar to cellulitis, but more superficial.
  - Highly infectious.
- Signs/symptoms
  - Starts as itchy, red sore.
  - Blisters → breaks → oozes.
  - Ooze dries; lesion becomes covered with a tightly adherent crust.
  - Grows and spreads circumferentially (not deep); rarely impetigo forms deeper skin ulcers
  - Contagious; carried in the oozing fluid.
- Treatment
  - Topical antimicrobial (e.g., bactroban)
  - Oral antibiotic (e.g., erythromycin or dicloxacillin); rapid clearing of lesions.
- Course/prognosis
  - Impetigo sores heal slowly and seldom scar.
  - Cure rate is extremely high.
  - Recurrence is common in young children.

Note: Acute glomerulonephritis (renal disease) is an occasional complication (poststreptococcal glomerulonephritis [GMN]).

Immunologic Skin Lesions

HIVES

- Urticaria = wheals.
- Type I hypersensitivity.
- (See section on hypersensitivity in Immunology, Chapter 21.)

PEMPHIGUS VULGARIS

- Ages 30–60.
- Clinical
  - Oral mucosal lesions (often first sign).
  - Skin lesions follow.
  - Bullae rupture, leaving raw surface susceptible to infection.

- **Etiology**
  - Autoimmune: IgG antibodies against epidermal intercellular cement substance.
- **Histology**
  - Formation of intradermal bullae
    - Acantholysis: Tzanck cells.
    - Basal layer intact.
- Immunofluorescence shows encircling of epidermal cells.

BULLOUS PEMPHIGOID

- Resembles pemphigus vulgaris.
- Clinically less severe.
- **Etiology**
  - Autoimmune: IgG antibodies against epidermal basement membrane.
- **Histology**
  - Subepidermal bullae.
  - Characteristic inflammatory infiltrate of eosinophils in surrounding dermis.
  - Immunofluorescence shows linear band.

Pemphigus vulgaris = Intraepidermal bullae. Bullous pemphigoid = Subepidermal bullae.

ERYTHEMA MULTIFORME

- Peak incidence second and third decades.
- **Etiology**
  - Type III hypersensitivity
  - Response to:
    - Medications:
      - Sulfa drugs
      - Penicillins
      - Barbiturates
    - Infections
    - HSV
    - Mycoplasma
    - Other illnesses
- Damage to blood vessels of skin (because of immune complexes).
- **Clinical**
  - Classic "target," "bull's-eye," or "iris" skin lesion.
    - Central lesion surrounded by concentric rings of pallor and redness.
    - Dorsal hands.
    - Forearms.
  - No systemic symptoms.

STEVEN'S–JOHNSON SYNDROME

- Variant, more severe form of erythema multiforme.
- Severe systemic symptoms.
- Extensive skin target lesions
  - Involve multiple body areas, especially mucous membranes.

TOXIC EPIDERMAL NECROLYSIS

- Also called TEN syndrome and Lyell's syndrome.
- Multiple large blisters (bullae) that coalesce, sloughing of all or most of skin and mucous membranes.

Benign (Nonneoplastic) Skin Lesions

ACANTHOSIS NIGRICANS

- Cutaneous finding of velvety hyperkeratosis and pigmentation.
    - Flexural areas, most often
        - Axilla.
        - Nape of neck.
        - Other flexures.
        - Anogenital region.
- Often a marker of visceral malignancy.
    - > 50% have cancer.
        - Gastric carcinoma.
        - Breast, lung, uterine cancer
- Seen in diabetes.
- **Histology**
    - Acanthosis.
    - Hyperkeratosis.
    - Hyperpigmentation.

HEMANGIOMA

- Hamartoma (not true neoplasm).

XANTHOMA

- Associated with hypercholesterolemia.
- **Clinical**
    - Most common sites:
        - Eyelids (xanthelasma).
        - Nodules over tendons or joints.
- **Histology**
    - Yellowish papules or nodules composed of
        - Focal dermal collections of lipid-laden histiocytes.

▶ CARDIOVASCULAR PATHOLOGY

Edema

- Abnormal accumulation of fluid in interstitial spaces or body cavities.
- Fluid moves out of intravascular space.
- Results from some combination of:
- ↑ capillary permeability (as with histamine).
- ↑ capillary hydrostatic pressure.
- ↑ interstitial fluid colloid osmotic pressure.
- ↑ plasma colloid osmotic pressure.

(See also Chapter 20, Reactions to Tissue Injury.)

Types of Edema

Transudate	Exudate
More watery (serous) edema fluid	More protein-rich edema fluid
Usually noninflammatory	Usually inflammatory
From altered intravascular hydrostatic or osmotic pressure	From ↑ vascular permeability (with inflammation)

EXAMPLES OF TRANSUDATE

- **Anasarca:** Generalized edema.
- **Hydrothorax:** Excess serous fluid in pleural cavity.
- **Hydropericardium:** Excess watery fluid in pericardial cavity.
- **Ascites (hydroperitoneum):** Excess serous fluid in peritoneal cavity.

Remember: Right-side CHF results in peripheral edema; left-side CHF results in pulmonary edema.

CLINICAL EXAM OF EDEMA

- **Pitting:** Press finger for 5 s and quickly remove; an indentation is left that fills slowly.
- **Nonpitting:** No indentation left when finger is removed.

Edemas and Causes

Process	Cause
Congestive heart failure	↑ plasma/capillary hydrostatic pressure
Nephrotic syndrome	↓ plasma oncotic pressure
Cirrhosis	↑ capillary hydrostatic pressure ↓ plasma oncotic pressure
Elephantiasis	↑ plasma/capillary hydrostatic pressure Secondary to ↓ lymphatic return

Shock

- ↓ tissue perfusion.
- Hemodynamic changes result in:
  - ↓ blood flow, thereby
  - ↓ oxygen and metabolic supply to tissues.
- Can result in multiple organ damage or failure
- **Symptoms**
  - Fatigue
  - Confusion
- **Signs**
  - Cool pale skin (pallor)
  - Weak rapid pulse (tachycardia = ↑ HR)
  - ↓ BP (hypotension)
  - ↓ urine output
- Shock requires immediate medical treatment and can worsen rapidly.

↓ cardiac output is the major factor in all types of shock (because either ↓ HR, ↓ SV or both).

MAJOR CATEGORIES OF SHOCK

- Hypovolemic
- Cardiogenic
- Distributive
  - Septic
  - Neurogenic
  - Anaphylactic

Types of Shock

Type	Cause	Examples
Hypovolemic	↓ blood volume	Hemorrhage Dehydration Vomiting Diarrhea Fluid loss from burns
Cardiogenic	Pump failure Usually LV failure Sudden ↓ CO	Massive MI Arrhythmia
Septic	Infection (endotoxin release) Gram-negative bacteria Causes vasodilation	Severe infection
Neurogenic	CNS injury Causes vasodilation	CNS injury
Anaphylactic	Type I hypersensitivity Histamine release Vasodilation	Anaphylactic allergic reaction (e.g., insect sting)

Stages of Shock

Nonprogressive (Early)	Progressive	Irreversible
= compensated. ↑ sympathetic nervous system. ↑ CO ↑ TPR Try to maintain perfusion to vital organs	↓ cardiac perfusion. Cardiac depression. CO ↓ Metabolic acidosis. (Compensatory mechanisms are no longer adequate)	Organ damage. ↓ high energy phosphate reserves Death (even if restore blood flow)

Congestion (Hyperemia)

- ↑ volume of blood in local capillaries and small vessels.
- **Active congestion** (active hyperemia): ↑ arteriolar dilation (inflammation, blushing).
- **Passive congestion** (passive hyperemia): ↓ venous return (obstruction, increased back pressure),
    - Two forms:
        - Acute
            - Shock or right-sided heart failure.
        - Chronic
            - In lung (usually secondary to left-sided heart failure)
            - In liver (usually secondary to right-sided heart failure)

Thrombosis

- Blood clot attached to endothelial surface (blood vessel or heart (endocardium)
    - Usually a vein.
    - Virchow's triad.
- **Arterial thrombi**
    - Lines of Zahn (morphologically).
    - Alternating red and white laminations.
- **Venous thrombi**
    - Propagate: Enlarge while remaining attached to vessel wall.
    - Embolize.
    - Detach as large embolus.
    - Fragment off as many small emboli; shower emboli.

Thrombolysis = Breakdown of a clot.

Virchow's triad:
- Endothelial injury.
- Alteration in blood flow.
- Hypercoagulability of blood.

Types of Thrombus

Agonal	Intracardiac thrombi ▪ After prolonged heart failure
Mural	Thrombus from endocardial surface (or endothelium of large vessel) protrudes into lumen of heart or large vessel Forms after ▪ MI; damage to ventricular endocardium (LV most often) ▪ Atrial fibrillation ▪ Aortic atherosclerosis Can cause cerebral embolism
White	Thrombus composed mostly of blood platelets
Red	Thrombus composed of RBCs (rather than platelets) Occurs rapidly by coagulation with blood stagnation
Fibrin	Thrombus composed of fibrin deposits Does not completely occlude the vessel

Predisposing factors to thrombosis
- **Arterial thrombosis**
    - Atherosclerosis (major cause)
- Venous thrombosis:
    - Heart failure
    - Tissue damage
    - Bed rest (immobilization)
    - Pregnancy
    - Oral contraceptive pills
    - Age
    - Obesity
    - Smoking

Embolus

- Intravascular mass
    - Solid
    - Liquid
    - Gas
- Travels within a blood vessel.
    - Lodges at distant site.
    - Occludes blood flow to vital organs.
    - Possibly leads to infarction.
- **Thromboemboli** (most common): Blood clot.
    - Breaks off existing thrombus.
    - Forms and is released downstream in the circulation (e.g., from heart chambers in atrial fibrillation).
- **Fat embolism:** especially in long bone fractures.
- **Air embolism:** Air into circulation (e.g., Caisson disease).

- **Amniotic fluid embolism:** With delivery; can activate diffuse/disseminated intravascular coagulation (DIC).
- **Tumor embolism.**

Phlebitis

- Inflammation of the vein.
- Common sites
  - Legs.
  - Varicose veins.
- Common causes
  - Local irritation (e.g., IV).
  - Infection in or near vein.
  - Blood clots.

Thrombophlebitis

- Inflammation of the vein related to blood clot.
- Associated with
  - **Superficial thrombophlebitis:** Veins near skin surface.
  - **Deep venous thrombosis:** Deeper, larger veins.
  - **Pelvic vein thrombosis.**
- Clinical symptoms
  - Tenderness over vein.
  - Pain in body part affected.
  - Skin redness or inflammation.

Arteriosclerosis

- Hardening of the arteries
- General term for several diseases causing changes to artery wall:
  - Thicker
  - Less elastic

Atherosclerosis

- Degenerative changes in artery walls
- Most common cause of arteriosclerosis
- Atherosclerotic plaques: Fatty material accumulating under the arterial wall's inner lining
- Occurs in arteries (**not** veins)
- Risks
  - Men and postmenopausal women (estrogen may be protective)
  - Smoking
  - Hypertension
  - Heredity (familial hypercholesterolemia)
  - Nephrosclerosis
  - Diabetes
  - Hyperlipidemia
- Sites
  - Carotid
  - Coronary

> **Pulmonary embolism**
> - Embolism causing pulmonary artery obstruction.
> - Usually arises from
>   - Deep vein thrombosis (DVT); usually from lower extremities (above popliteal fossa).
> - **Course**
>   - Systemic vein.
>   - Right heart.
>   - Pulmonary artery.
> - **Causes**
>   - Right heart strain.
>   - Possibly infarction in the affected segment.
>   - Possibly pleurisy (pleuritic chest pain).
> - **Predisposing factors**
> - Virchow's triad
>   - Especially immobilization (leading to stagnation)
>   - Thrombophlebitis
>   - Hypercoagulable states

Saddle embolus: Large pulmonary embolus that obstructs the bifurcation of the pulmonary artery.

Paradoxical emboli
Begin in the venous system. End up in the systemic arterial system rather than the pulmonary artery. Most often allowed by an atrial septal defect. The only time a DVT can cause a stroke.

- Circle of Willis
- Renal and mesenteric arteries
- **Pathogenesis**
  - Fatty streak
    - Foam cells in intima (lipid laden macrophages)
  - Atheromas
    - Cholesterol
    - Fibrous tissue
    - Necrotic debris
    - Smooth muscle cells
- **Complications**
  - ↓ elasticity of vessel.
  - Ulceration of plaque; predisposing to thrombus formation.
  - Hemorrhage into the plaque; narrowing lumen, possibly occluding blood flow.
  - Thrombus formation.
  - Embolization; overlying thrombus or plaque material itself.
- **Symptoms**
  - Depend on site.
    - Visual changes, dizziness: Carotid or intracerebral arteries
    - Angina: Coronary arteries.
    - Leg pain (claudication): Lower extremity arteries.

Hypertension

- Primary (essential).
- Secondary (related to another disease).

Primary (Essential) Hypertension

- Accounts for 90–95% of hypertension.
- No identifiable cause; related to ↑ CO, ↑ TPR.
- **Risks**
  - Genetic
    - Family history
    - African Americans
  - Environmental
    - ↑ dietary salt intake
    - Stress
    - Obesity
    - Cigarette smoking
    - Physical inactivity
- **Pathologic findings**
  - Hypertrophy of arteries and arterioles **not** capillaries (because no smooth muscle).
  - ↑ Wall-to-lumen ratio.
    - ↑ smooth muscle cell growth (because of ↑ pressure, stretch).
  - ↓ arteriolar and capillary density.
  - ↓ total cross-sectional area of capillaries and arterioles.
- Three organs most often damaged.
  - Heart: 60% die of cardiac complications.
  - Kidneys: 25% die of renal failure.
  - Brain: 15% die of stroke or neurologic complications.

Atherosclerosis
- Most important contributor to arterial thrombosis.
- Most susceptible arteries—aorta and coronary arteries.

Atherosclerosis can lead to:
- Ischemic heart disease (CAD).
- Heart attack (myocardial infarction [MI]).
- Stroke or aneurysm formation.

Familial hypercholesterolemia
- Autosomal dominant disease.
- Anomalies of LDL (low-density lipoprotein) receptors.
- Atherosclerosis and its complications.
  - Xanthomas.
  - MI by age 20.

- Diet, exercise, and antihypertensive medications are used to treat hypertension.
- Untreated (or undertreated) hypertension can result in
  - "wear out" (cardiac failure).
  - "blow out" (CVA).
  - "run out" (renal failure).

Hypertension is the "silent killer"; usually has no symptoms.

Clinical Findings and Complications

Neurologic	Ophthalmologic	Cardiovascular	Renal
Headaches Nausea/vomiting Drowsiness Anxiety Mental impairment<ul><li>Intracerebral vessel damage</li></ul>	Retinal hemorrhage and exudates<ul><li>Damage to retinal arterioles</li></ul>	BP >140/90 **Arteriolar constriction** ↑ resistance. **Claudication** ↓ blood supply to legs. ↑ **cardiac workload** Angina ↓ coronary blood flow. Heart failure<ul><li>Dyspnea on exertion (LHF)</li><li>Peripheral edema (RHF)</li></ul>	Polyuria Nocturia ↓ urine concentration **Nephrosclerosis** Hardening of renal arterioles Proteinuria possible Hematuria possible

Renal disease is the most common cause of secondary hypertension.

Preeclampsia *occurs in pregnant patients:*
- *Hypertension: >140 systolic, or > 90 diastolic after 20 weeks gestation.*
- *Proteinuria.*
- *Edema.*

Eclampsia = *Preeclampsia + seizures.*

Predisposing conditions for preeclampsia and eclampsia:
- *Hypertension*
- *Diabetes*
- *Autoimmune diseases (e.g., SLE)*
- *Laboratory findings*
- *Hyperuricemia*
- *Thrombocytopenia*

SECONDARY HYPERTENSION

- Hypertension (HTN) from known causes.
    - 5–10% of HTN cases.
    - Identifiable, often correctable cause.
- **Renal disease**
    - Most common cause of secondary hypertension.
    - Renin–angiotensin–aldosterone system.
    - Two categories:
        - Renal parenchymal diseases.
        - Renal artery stenosis.
- **Endocrine disorders**
    - Hyperaldosteronism.
    - Cushing syndrome.
    - Hyperthyroidism.
    - Diabetes.
    - Pheochromocytoma.
- **Other causes**
    - Coarctation of the aorta.
    - Preeclamsia/eclampsia/toxemia of pregnancy.

MALIGNANT HYPERTENSION

- Severe form of high blood pressure.
    - Medical emergency.
    - Can lead to death in 3–6 months if untreated.
- Complication of either primary or secondary hypertension.
    - Most often with secondary hypertension from kidney disease.

- Occurs in
  - African American young adults
  - Women with toxemia of pregnancy (preeclampsia/eclampsia)
  - Patients with renal or collagen vascular disorders
- **Findings**
  - Sudden rapid ↑ BP, usually without a precipitating event
- Life-threatening consequences to multiple organ systems:
  - Cerebrovascular accident
  - Retinal hemorrhage and papilledema
  - Cardiac failure
  - Renal failure

Aortic Aneurysm

- Abnormal, localized dilation of the aorta
- True aneurysm = dilation of all three layers (intima, media, adventitia)
- **Causes**
  - Atherosclerosis
  - Cystic medial necrosis
    - Marfan's
    - Ehler's–Danlos
  - Infectious aortitis
    - Syphilitic aortitis
  - Vasculitis
- **Risk**
  - Rupture

Aortic Dissection

- Life-threatening
- Blood into medial layers of aorta
  - "Dissecting" the intima from the adventitia
- **Symptoms**
  - Ripping/tearing chest pain
  - Different BP measurement in each arm
- **Complications**
  - Rupture
    - Pericardial tamponade
    - Hemomediastinum or hemothorax
  - Occlusion of aortic branches
    - Carotid (stroke)
    - Coronary (MI)
    - Splanchnic (organ infarction)
    - Renal (acute renal failure)
  - Distortion of aortic valve
    - Aortic regurgitation

***Aortic dissection** most often ruptures into the pericardial sac (hemopericardium), causing fatal tamponade.*

Hemopericardium:
Can occur after MI.
- Ventricular rupture (necrotic myocardium).
- Blood into pericardial space.
- Can cause cardiac tamponade and death.

Pathology Involving the Pericardium

Infections of the heart

- Pericardium (pericarditis)
- Myocardium (myocarditis, often viral)
- Endocardium and heart valves (endocarditis, often bacterial or inflammatory)

Pericardial Effusion	Acute Pericarditis	Chronic (Constrictive) Pericarditis
Accumulation of fluid in the pericardial space ■ Hydropericardium = serous fluid ■ Hemopericardium = blood Can cause cardiac tamponade	Inflammation of the pericardium: ■ Serous ■ Fibrinous ■ Purulent ■ Hemorrhagic ■ Often painful ■ Can cause cardiac tamponade	Thickening and scarring of the pericardium Tb. ↓ elasticity Can cause tamponade-like picture

CARDIAC TAMPONADE

- Extrinsic compression of the heart
    - Fluid (accumulating quickly)
        - Pericardial effusion
        - Acute pericarditis
- Cardiac compression
    - ↓ venous return (↓ filling)
    - ↓ CO
    - Death
- Signs
    - Distended neck veins
    - Hypotension
    - ↓ heart sounds
    - Tachypnea
    - Weak/absent peripheral pulses

ENDOCARDITIS

Remember that the tricuspid valve is most often affected in IV drug users.

- Inflammation of endocardium and/or heart valves
- **Symptoms:** Develop quickly (acute) or slowly (subacute):
    - Fever (hallmark)
    - Nonspecific constitutional signs
    - Fatigue
    - Malaise
    - Headache
    - Night sweats
- **Findings**
    - Murmur (secondary to vegetations); may change with time.
    - Splenomegaly
    - Splinter hemorrhages (small dark lines) under fingernails

Types of Endocarditis

Infective	Rheumatic	Libmann–sacks
Usually bacterial Intrinsic bacteremia - Dental - Upper respiratory - Urologic - Lower GI tract - Introduced bacteremia - IV drug users	Complication of rheumatic fever Occurs in areas with greatest hemodynamic stress	Occurs in SLE
Valvular involvement Vegetations - Mitral - Tricuspid (in IVDU)	Mitral valve most often Calcification - Stenosis - Insufficiency - Both	Mitral valve most often Small vegetations on either or both surfaces of valve leaflets

> **Antibiotic prophylaxis before dental procedures**
> - Children with congenital heart disease
> - Adults with heart murmurs
> - To help prevent subacute bacterial endocarditis (SBE), *Streptococcus viridans,* from a dental/oral source.

Infective Endocarditis

Acute Endocarditis	Subacute (Bacterial) Endocarditis
Staphylococcus aureus (50%)	*Streptococcus viridans* (> 50%)
Usually secondary to infection elsewhere in body IVDUs	Patients with preexisting valve disease

> **Valvular vegetations can be dislodged and send septic emboli to organs:**
> - Brain
> - Lungs
> - Kidneys
> - Spleen

Rheumatic Fever

- Acute inflammatory disease.
- Develops after streptococcal infection, usually an URI with group A β-hemolytic strep.
- Most common in children 5–15 years old.
- **Onset**
    - Usually sudden, often after 1–5 weeks (asymptomatic) after recovery from sore throat or scarlet fever.
- **Course**
    - Mild cases = 3–4 weeks.
    - Severe cases = 2–3 months.
- **Etiology**
    - Due to cross-reactivity, not direct effect of the bacteria.
    - Type III hypersensitivity.
- **Sites**
    - Heart
    - Joints
    - Skin
    - Brain

> **Mnemonics for rheumatic fever**
>
> **PECCS**
>
> **P**olyarthritis
> **E**rythema marginatum
> **C**horea
> **C**arditis
> **S**ubcutaneous nodules
>
> **FEVERSS**
>
> **F**ever
> **E**rythema marginatum
> **V**alve damage
> **E**SR
> **R**ed-hot (polyarthritis)
> **S**ubcutaneous nodules
> **St**. Vitus dance (chorea)

*Though, rheumatic fever may follow a strep infection, it **is not** an infection. Rather, it is an inflammatory reaction to an infection.*

*Rheumatic carditis usually disappears within 5 months. However, permanent damage to the heart/heart valves usually occurs, leading to **rheumatic heart disease**. Valves involved are the mitral, aortic, and tricuspid. Pulmonic valve is rarely involved.*

- Pathology
  - Aschoff bodies
    - Focal interstitial myocardial inflammation: Fragmented collagen, and fibrinoid material
    - Anitschkow cells: Large unusual cells
    - Aschoff myocytes: Multinucleated giant cells
- Laboratory
  - ↑ ASO titers
  - ↑ ESR
- Findings/criteria for diagnosis = Jones criteria
  - Diagnose when two major or one major and one minor criteria are met. (See chart.)
- Treatment
  - Penicillin
  - Rest

Criteria for Diagnosis of Rheumatic Fever

Major Criteria	Minor Criteria
Carditis	Fever
Arthritis	Arthralgias
Chorea	History of rheumatic fever
Erythema marginatum	EKG changes
Subcutaneous nodules	

Coronary Artery Disease (CAD)

- CAD = Narrowing of coronary arteries
  - Atherosclerosis plaques
  - ↓ blood supply to myocardium
- Consequences
  - Ischemia
  - Infarction
- Symptoms
  - Classic symptom of CAD = angina
- Risks
  - Same as for atherosclerosis
  - Hypertension
  - Hyperlipidemia
  - Smoking
  - Obesity
  - Inactivity
  - Diabetes
  - Male gender

CAD causes

- ↓ blood flow to myocardium.
- ↓ O₂ and nutrients to myocardium.

In turn, this can lead to

- Ischemia (angina).
- Infarction (MI = heart attack with EKG changes and enzymes released from infarcted myocardial tissue).

Angina (stable angina) can be relieved by rest or nitrates.

ANGINA

- Squeezing (tight) substernal chest discomfort; may radiate to
  - Left arm
  - Neck
  - Jaw
  - Shoulder blade

- Caused by ↓ myocardial oxygenation
- Atherosclerotic narrowing
- Vasospasm

Stable Angina	Unstable Angina	Prinzmetal Angina
Most common type CAD/atherosclerotic narrowing Precipitated by exertion	Occurs even at rest More severe CAD Often imminent MI	Intermittent chest pain at rest Vasospasm

MYOCARDIAL INFARCTION (MI)

- Most important cause of morbidity from CAD.
- Prolonged interruption of coronary blood flow to myocardium; coagulative necrosis.
- **Cause:** Usually thrombus formation in the setting of a ruptured, unstable plaque.

Complete Occlusion	Partial Occlusion
Transmural infarction ST elevation MI	Subendocardial infarction Non-ST elevation MI

Most deaths from heart attack occur outside hospital; are due to arrhythmias causing ventricular fibrillation.

- **Symptoms**
  - Angina (that does not remit)
  - Sweating
  - Nausea, stomach upset
- **Signs**
  - EKG changes (ST elevation, ST depression, T waves, Q waves).
  - Enzyme leak.
- **Prognosis:** Good (if patient reaches hospital).
- **Complications**
  - Arrhythmia.
  - Myocardial (pump) failure.
  - Cardiac rupture.
  - Papillary muscle rupture.
  - Ventricular aneurysm

Cardiac enzymes elevated after an MI:
- *CK–MB (creatine kinase, MB fraction)*
- *TnT (troponin T)*
- *Myoglobin*

Creatine phosphokinase (CPK): Enzyme found in (↑ when damage to):
- *Heart*
- *Brain*
- *Skeletal muscle*
- *Not found in liver*

Heart Failure

- Heart's ability to pump does not meet needs of the body.
- Usually a chronic progressive condition.
- Can occur suddenly.
- **Causes:** Secondary to heart muscle damage
  - After MI
  - Cardiomyopathy
  - Valvular diseases

Pulmonary edema: *Life-threatening complication of left heart failure.*

> **Two earliest and most common signs of heart failure:**
> - Exertional dyspnea
> - Paroxysmal nocturnal dyspnea

> **Right heart failure**
> - Usually caused by left heart failure.
> - Isolated right heart failure (RHF) is uncommon.
> - When right heart failure does occur: **Corpulmonale.**
>   - Lung disease causes pulmonary hypertension, can lead to R heart failure.
>   - ↑ pulmonary vascular resistance causing ↑ R heart strain.
> - RHF leads to
>   - Systemic venous congestion.
>   - Peripheral edema (swollen ankles).

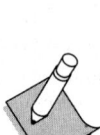

Cyanide poisoning poisons oxidative phosphorylation.

Pulmonary hypertension can lead to RV hypertrophy and R heart failure (corpulmonale).

- **Affects**
  - Left heart
  - Right heart
  - Both

Signs and Symptoms of Heart Failure

Left Heart Failure	Right Heart Failure
Exertional dyspnea Fatigue Orthopnea Cough Cardiac enlargement Rales Gallop rhythm (S3 or S4) Pulmonary venous congestion	Elevated venous pressure Hepatomegaly Dependent edema

Primary Pulmonary Hypertension	Secondary Pulmonary Hypertension
No known heart or lung disease Unknown etiology	Most common form<ul><li>COPD (most often)</li><li>Left to right shunt</li><li>↑ pulmonary resistance<ul><li>Embolism</li><li>Vasoconstriction from hypoxia</li></ul></li><li>Left heart failure</li></ul>

CV Pulmonary Cross-Correlation

Carbon Monoxide (CO) Poisoning

- Symptoms
  - Cherry-red discoloration of the skin, mucosa, and tissues
  - Mental status changes
  - Coma
  - Ultimately death

Pulmonary Edema

- Fluid in alveolar spaces of the lungs.
  - ↓ O_2 exchange.
- Cause
  - Usually left heart failure.
    - ↑ hydrostatic pressure.
      - Fluid extravasation into lung spaces.
- Mechanism
  - Backlog of blood in left heart (↑ volume).
  - ↑ left heart pressure.
  - ↑ pressure in pulmonary veins (transmitted backward from heart).
- Symptoms
  - Shortness of breath (SOB)/dyspnea
  - Orthopnea

- Cough
- Tachypnea
- Dependent crackles
- Tachycardia
- Neck vein distention
- **Treatment**
  - ↓ Vascular fluid
    - Diuretics
  - ↑ gas exchange and heart function
    - O_2
    - Antihypertensives
    - Positive inotropic agents
    - Antiarrhythmics

> *Mild CO poisoning can present with exhaustion and symptoms similar to a common cold or flu, delaying the diagnosis.*

> **CO** = *colorless, odorless gas.*
> **Sources:** *Automobile exhaust; home heating fumes.*
> **Mechanism:** *Competitive inhibition*
> - Much higher affinity for Hb than O_2.
> - Attaches to Hb and prevents O_2 carrying.

▶ RESPIRATORY PATHOLOGY

Asthma

- Chronic reactive airway disorder caused by episodic airway obstruction
- Any age
  - 3–5% of adults (usually < 30 years old)
  - 7–10% of children
  - 50% of asthma cases occur in children (<10 years old)
  - Boys > Girls (2:1)
- **Cause**
  - Bronchospasm (primary cause of airway obstruction)
  - Other contributors (↑ airflow resistance)
    - ↑ mucus secretion
    - Mucosal edema
- **Symptoms**
  - Dyspnea/SOB
  - Expiratory wheezes
  - Chest tightness
  - Cough
- **Pathology**
  - Bronchial smooth muscle hypertrophy
  - ↑ bronchial submucosal glands
  - Eosinophils
  - Charcot–Leyden crystals

> **Pulmonary edema from heart failure**
> - Transudate.
> - See heart failure cells (= heme-laden macrophages).

> **Pulmonary edema** *can be caused by*
> - ↑ intracapillary hydrostatic pressure
>   - Heart failure
> - ↑ capillary permeability
>   - Acute respiratory distress syndrome (ARDS)

Types of Asthma

Extrinsic (Allergic, Atopic, Immune)	Intrinsic (Nonimmune, Idiosyncratic)
Type I hypersensitivity Inhaled allergens (allergy triggers) - Pet dander - Dust mites - Cockroach allergens - Molds - Pollens	Exercise Cold air Tobacco smoke Respiratory infections Stress Other pollutants Drugs

> *Distinguish between*
> - Intraalveolar fluid: Pulmonary edema.
> - Intrapleural (between visceral and parietal pleura): Pleural effusion.

> **Status asthmaticus**
> - Severe asthma attack
>   - **Does not** respond to normal measures.
>   - Usually requires hospitalization.
> - Can lead to death from respiratory acidosis (obstruction).
> - Treat with epinephrine.

Mechanisms of Asthma Precipitation

Allergic (Immune)	Intrinsic (Nonimmune)		
Type I Hypersensitivity	Direct Bronchoconstrictor Release	↑ Vagal Stimulation	Cox Inhibitors (NSAIDs, ASA)
Atopic asthma ■ IgE vs. allergen ■ Fc binds mast cell ■ Reexposure to allergen ■ IgE cross-linked ■ Mast cells degranulate: 　■ Histamine 　■ Other substances Cause ■ Bronchospasm ■ More inflammatory cell recruitment	Caused by chemical inhalation or medications: ■ Chemicals ■ Resins ■ Plastics ■ Cotton fibers ■ Toluene ■ Formaldehyde ■ Penicillin	Respiratory threshold to vagal stimulation is lowered by ■ Viral infections. ■ URIs (cold or flu) Parasympathetic activity causes bronchoconstriction.	Cyclooxygenase pathway blocked ■ Arachidonic acid metabolism. Cause ■ ↑ Leukotrienes. ■ Bronchoconstrictors (as opposed to prostaglandins = bronchodilators).

> *Nitrous oxide is safe to administer to people with asthma, especially if their asthma is triggered by anxiety.*
>
> *Asthmatics taking chronic steroids may need corticosteroid augmentation.*
>
> *In children, asthma symptoms can decrease with time (children can outgrow it).*
>
> *COPD can overlap with asthma and bronchiectasis.*
>
> *Cigarette smoking is the greatest cause of COPD.*
>
> *Secondary pulmonary hypertension is most commonly caused by COPD.*

- Treatment
  - β_2 agonist inhalers.
    - Preferred treatment for acute asthma attack.
    - Terbutaline
    - Albuterol
  - Steroids
  - Mast cell stabilizers.
  - Epinephrine (sympathetic stimulation for status asthmaticus).

Chronic Obstructive Pulmonary Disease (COPD)

- Group of lung diseases characterized by ↑ airflow resistance.
  - Emphysema.
  - Chronic bronchitis.

Obstructive Lung Diseases	Restrictive Lung Diseases
↑ TLV	↓ TLV
Asthma COPD ■ Emphysema ■ Chronic bronchitis	Intrinsic lung diseases: ■ Pneumoconioses ■ Sarcoidosis ■ Idiopathic pulmonary fibrosis Extrinsic lung diseases: ■ Kyphosis ■ Obesity ■ Neuromuscular weakness

EMPHYSEMA
- "Pink Puffer"
- Adults, usually smokers.

Types of Emphysema

	Centrilobular	**Panlobular**
Cause	Cigarette smoking	Familial antiproteinase deficiency ↓ Alpha-1 antitrypsin
Region	Upper lobes of lungs	Upper and lower lobes

- **Pathophysiology**
  - Destruction of elastic fibers in alveolar walls (distal to respiratory bronchioles).
    - ↓ elastic recoil.
      - Distal airspaces enlarge (dilated alveoli) with inhalation.
      - Lungs overexpand (↑ total lung capacity [TLC]).
    - ↓ radial traction.
      - airways collapse with exhalation (leaving air behind, air trapping).
    - ↓ functioning parenchyma.
      - ↓ surface area for gas exchange.
- **Microscopic**
  - Enlarged air spaces.
  - Broken septae projecting into alveoli.
    - No fibrosis.
- **Clinical**
  - "Pink puffer."
  - Dyspnea.
  - Labored breathing.
  - No productive cough.
    - Scant clear mucoid sputum production.
    - ↑ infection susceptibility.
- **Findings**
  - PO_2 near normal.
    - No cyanosis (they are "pink").
    - Barrel chest on chest x-ray (CXR) (overexpansion).
    - Quiet chest to auscultation.
    - Adventitious sounds.
- **Pulmonary function tests (PFTs)**
  - ↑ TLC.
  - ↑ residual volume (RV).
  - ↓ FEV1/FVC (forced expiratory volume in 1 second/forced vital capacity).
- **Course**
  - Damage worsens with time.
    - ↑ as continue smoking.

Smoking related diseases:
- COPD
- Carcinoma
  - Oral cavity
  - Larynx
  - Lung
  - Esophagus
  - Pancreas
  - Kidney
  - Bladder
- Peptic ulcer disease (PUD)
- Low birth weight infants

Restrictive lung diseases:
- ↓ lung compliance.
- ↓ all lung volumes.
- ↑ FEV1/FVC.

Mechanisms of Airway Obstruction
- Airway hyperreactivity (bronchoconstriction): Asthma.
- ↓ elastic recoil (airways collapse): Emphysema.
- ↑ mucous: Chronic bronchitis.

Emphysema has two basic problems:

- Lungs are "fixed" in inspiration: Difficult to exhale (airways collapse, trapping air).
- ↓ gas exchange: ↓ respiratory surface area.

In emphysema, destruction of lymphatic structural support can lead to ↑ pigment deposition in the lungs.

Productive cough

- Cough contains sputum. Sputum can contain
  - Mucus
  - Cellular debris
  - Bacteria
  - Blood
  - Pus
- Common causes of productive cough:
  - Chronic lung abscess
  - Tb
  - Lobar PNA
  - Bronchogenic carcinoma
  - Pulmonary embolism

Atelectasis neonatorum: Alveolar collapse in newborn, usually due to ↓ surfactant (in premature infants).

CHRONIC BRONCHITIS

- "Blue bloaters"
- Adults with history of cigarette smoking
- **Definition:** Chronic productive cough for at least 3 months of the year for 2 years.
- **Microscopic**
  - Mucous hypersecretion.
    - Bronchi: Hypertrophy of mucous glands and smooth muscle.
    - Smaller airways: Goblet cell hyperplasia.
  - ↑ Reid index
    - ↑ ratio mucous gland thickness: bronchial wall thickness.
- **Clinical**
  - Productive cough.
    - ↑ sputum production.
  - Wheezing.
  - Auscultation.
    - Noisy chest.
    - Rhonchi.
- **Findings**
  - ↑ PO_2.
    - Cyanosis (look blue).
- **Complications**
  - Pulmonary hypertension.
    - RV overload; Cor pulmonale (R heart failure).
    - Peripheral edema (bloaters).
  - ↑ lung cancer risk (bronchogenic carcinoma).
    - Squamous metaplasia from chronic inflammation.

Bronchiectasis

- Permanent abnormal bronchial dilation.
- **Cause**
  - Bronchial obstruction.
    - Cystic fibrosis.
    - Lung tumor.
    - Kartagener syndrome.
    - Chronic sinusitis.
- **Clinical**
  - Chronic, productive cough.
    - Foul-smelling purulent sputum.
  - Hemoptysis.
  - Recurrent pulmonary infection.

Atelectasis

- Lung collapse (alveolar collapse)
- **Causes**
  - Failure of expansion
  - Bronchial obstruction
  - External compression

Pneumoconioses

- Caused by prolonged inhalation of foreign material.
- Named for the particle inhaled.

- **Symptoms**
  - Chronic dry cough
  - SOB
- Leads to pulmonary fibrosis.

ANTHRACOSIS

- Coal workers pneumoconiosis = black lung disease.
  - Inhalation of carbon dust.
- Two forms
  - Simple: Small lung opacities.
  - Complicated (= progressive massive fibrosis): Masses of fibrous tissue.
- **Findings**
  - Carbon-carrying macrophages.
  - Progressive nodular pulmonary disease (pulmonary fibrosis).

SILICOSIS

- Most common and most serious pneumoconiosis.
- Inhalation of silica (e.g., by miners, glass makers, stone cutters).
- **Findings**
  - Silica dust in alveolar macrophages.
  - Silicotic nodules (dense, made of collagen, can calcify).
    - Visualized silica within the nodules using polarized light.
  - Thick pleural scars.
  - ↑ susceptibility to Tb.
    - Silicotuberculosis.

ASBESTOSIS

- Inhalation of asbestos fibers.
- Can develop 15–20 years after cessation of regular asbestos exposure.
- **Results in:** Diffuse interstitial fibrosis.
- **Findings**
  - Asbestos in alveolar macrophages.
  - Ferruginous bodies (yellow-brown, rod-shaped).
    - Stain with Prussian blue.
  - Hyalinized fibrocalcific plaques on parietal pleura.
- **Course**
  - ↑ predisposition to
    - Bronchogenic carcinoma.
    - Malignant mesothelioma of pleura.

Sarcoidosis

- Unknown etiology
- Diagnosis/biopsy; noncaseating granulomas
- Black females
  - Manifests in teen or young adult years
- **Findings**
  - Interstitial lung disease

Mesothelioma
- Rare tumor.
- Involves parietal or visceral pleura.
- Associated with asbestos exposure; 25- to 45-year latency.
- Diffuse lesion; spreads over lung surface.

Byssinosis: Pneumoconiosis caused by inhalation of cotton particles.

Beryliosis
- Inhalation of berylium particle.
- **Causes**
  - Systemic granulomatous disorder.
    - Noncaseating granulomas.
    - Primary pulmonary involvement.
  - Mimics sarcoidosis.

- Enlarged hilar lymph nodes
- Uveitis
- Erythema nodosum
- Polyarthritis
- Hypercalcemia
- **Pathology**
  - Noncaseating granulomas.
    - Schaumann and asteroid bodies
- **Clinical**
  - Bilateral hilar lymphadenopathy on CXR
  - Interstitial lung disease (restrictive lung disease)
    - Cough
    - Dyspnea
  - Skin findings

Idiopathic Pulmonary Fibrosis

- Chronic inflammation and fibrosis of alveolar wall
- **Progression**
  - Alveolitis
  - Fibrosis
  - Fibrotic lung (honeycomb lung)
- Prognosis
  - Death within 5 years

Pneumonia

- Lung infection
  - Bacteria
  - Viruses
  - Fungi
- **Clinical**
  - Fever
  - Chills
  - Productive cough
  - Blood-tinged sputum
  - Dyspnea
  - Chest pain
- **Findings**
  - Hypoxia
  - Infiltrate on CXR
  - Crackles, other noises on auscultation

Interstitial fibrosis

- Usually the result of fibrosing alveolitis.
- Characterized by
  - Thickening/fibrosis of the alveolar interstitium.
    - Wall/space between the alveolus and the capillary.
  - Results in restrictive lung disease.
- **Causes**
  - Idiopathic.
  - Secondary to
    - Connective tissue disorders: SLE, PAN, RA.
    - Allergic extrinsic alveolitis.

Types of Pneumonia

	Lobar Pneumonia	**Bronchopneumonia**	**Interstitial Pneumonia**
Causes	*Pneumococcus*	*Staph. aureus* *H. flu* *Klebsiella* *Strep pyogenes*	Viruses; RSV, adenoviruses *Mycoplasma* *Legionella*
Findings	Exudate within alveolus Consolidation Lobe or entire lung	Bronchiole and alveolar infiltrates Patchy 1+ lobe	Diffuse patchy infiltrates (within interstitium) 1+ lobe
Age	Middle age	Infants Elderly	Young children

Viral Pneumonia	**Bacterial Pneumonia**
Most common cause of pneumonia in young children Peaks between age 2 and 3 yr	Most serious pneumonias (typically) Pneumococcus (*Strep pneumo*) is most common cause Most common fatal infection in the hospital

Lung Abscess

- Localized collection of pus in lung
- **Causes**
    - Aspiration
        - Altered mental status
    - Bronchial obstruction
        - Cancer
        - Pneumonia
        - Bronchiestasis
    - Septic emboli
- **Organisms**
    - Staphylococcus (most common)
        - Other organisms
            - Pseudomonas
            - Klebsiella (in alcoholics)
            - Proteus
            - Anaerobes
- **Clinical**
    - Productive cough; Large amounts of foul-smelling sputum
    - Fever
    - Dyspnea
    - Chest pain
    - Cyanosis
    - CXR with fluid-filled cavity

Lung abscess
- Most common predisposing factor = alcoholism.
    - In particular, aspiration.
- Aspiration predisposed by
    - Altered consciousness:
        - Alcoholic stupor.
        - Drug overdose.
        - Seizures.
        - Debilitated, comatose.
    - Neurologic dysfunction:
        - Impaired gag reflex.
        - Impaired swallowing.
    - Contents aspirated.
        - Bacteria (including anaerobes) from
            - Oral secretions.
            - Decayed teeth.
            - Vomitus.
            - Foreign material.

> **Hemoptysis** = Coughing up blood (or blood-streaked sputum).
> - Respiratory infections (minor URIs)
> - Bronchitis
> - Tb
> - Pneumonia
> - Bronchogenic carcinoma
> - Idiopathic pulmonary hemosiderosis (iron in lungs)

Remember: Ghon's complex = primary lesion + lymph node (LN) involvement.

> **Clinical presentation of TB**
> - Usually secondary TB; only 5% patients with primary TB have symptoms.
> - Secondary TB = reactivation of the primary Ghon's complex, which has remained quiescent (subclinical) and/or occurred years earlier.

Pott's disease = TB involving the vertebral body.

Tuberculosis (TB)

- Worldwide condition
- ↑ in conditions of
  - Poor sanitation
  - Poverty
  - Overcrowding
- Mycobacterium TB
  - Acid fast bacilli
  - Strict aerobe
- Transmitted by aerosolized "droplets"
- Pathology
  - Granulomas
    - Giant cells
    - Caseous necrosis
- **Clinical**
  - Hemoptysis
  - Weight loss
  - Night sweats
  - Malaise
  - Weakness

Types of Tuberculosis

	Primary TB	**Secondary TB**	**Miliary TB**
Site	Between upper and middle lobes Lower part of upper lobe or Upper part of lower lobe	Lung apices High O_2 tension	Widely disseminated
Characteristic	Ghon's complex: Parenchymal lesion Hilar LNs	Reactivation of Ghon's complex	Lesions like "millet seed" Multiple extrapulmonary sites

▶ **GASTROINTESTINAL PATHOLOGY**

Esophagus

Mallory–Weiss Syndrome

- Mild to major bleeding (usually painless) at the distal esophagus, proximal stomach.
  - Near or involving the LES (lower esophageal sphincter).
  - **Cause:** Longitudinal mucosal lacerations (tear in mucous membrane).
  - Occur because of severe retching or vomiting, especially following alcohol intake.
- Most common in:
  - Men > age 40.
  - Alcoholics.
  - Hiatal hernia.

- Clinical
  - Vomiting of blood (hematemsis).
- Treatment
  - Depends on amount/severity of bleeding.
  - Often stops spontaneously.
  - Tear usually heals in about 10 days without special treatment.
  - Local control.
    - Cautery.
    - Banding.

Achalsia

- ↓ propulsion of food down the esophagus (↓ peristalsis).
- Failure of lower esophageal sphincter (LES) to relax.
  - High pressure on manometry.
  - Difficulty opening.
  - Characteristic "bird's-beak appearance" on barium swallow.
- Cause
  - Nerve related.
- Clinical
  - Dysphagia to both solids and liquids.
  - Regurgitation of food.
- Treatment
  - Dilation.
  - Botox.

Gastroesophageal Reflux Disease (GERD)

- Acid reflux
- Backflow of acidic stomach contents up into esophagus
  - Lower esophageal sphincter leaky
- Risks
  - Hiatal hernia
  - Scleroderma
- Symptoms
  - Heartburn
  - Regurgitation of food
  - Hoarse voice
  - Wheeze
  - Cough
- Treatment
  - Proton pump inhibitors
  - Antacids
- Complications
  - Can lead to *Barrett's esophagus*
    - Premalignant condition

Hiatal Hernia

- Protrusion of part of the stomach through diaphragm into the thoracic cavity.
- Symptoms
  - Heartburn
  - Dysphagia
  - Belching

ESOPHAGEAL ULCERS

- Erosion on the esophageal lining mucosa.
- Usually caused by repeated regurgitation of stomach acid (HCL) to lower part of esophagus.
- Can also get esophageal infections causing erosion (e.g., candidal or viral).

BARRETT'S ESOPHAGUS

- Type of metaplasia.
- Change from normal columnar cells to intestinal epithelium.
- Precancerous condition.
- Complication of chronic heartburn.

Stomach

PEPTIC ULCER DISEASE (PUD)

Hemorrhage is the most common complication of PUD. It is most likely with duodenal ulcers.

- Erosion in the lining of the stomach or duodenum.
- Circumscribed lesions in the mucous membrane.
- Occur mostly in men age 20–50 years.
- ~80% are duodenal ulcers.
- Causes
    - Imbalance between acid and mucosal protection.
        - NSAIDs (↓ mucosal protection: ↓ prostaglandins).
        - Acid hypersecretion (e.g., Zollinger–Ellison).
    - Infection
        - Helicobacter pylori
- Risks
    - Aspirin, NSAIDs (as above)
    - Cigarette smoking
    - Older age
- Symptom
    - Pain
- Complications
    - Bleeding
        - When erode deep into blood vessels
        - Bleeding ulcer
    - Perforation
        - Ulcerate transmurally (through the entire wall).
        - Causes acute peritonitis; can lead to death.
        - Most often occurs with duodenal ulcers.
    - Malignant change is uncommon.
- Treatment
    - Antibiotics
    - Antacid medications
    - Proton pump inhibitors

Gastric Ulcer	Duodenal Ulcer
20% of PUD Peptic ulcer located in the stomach More common in middle-aged and elderly men	80% of PUD Peptic ulcer located in duodenum More associated with *H. pylori*

HEMATEMESIS

- Vomiting bright red blood
- Usually indicates upper GI bleeding
  - Esophageal varices
  - Peptic ulcers

Small and Large Intestines

MECKEL DIVERTICULUM

- Most common congenital anomaly of the small intestine.
- Remnant of the embryonic vitelline duct.
- Located in distal small bowel.
- May contain ectopic gastric, duodenal, colonic or pancreatic tissue.

INTESTINAL LYMPHANGIECTASIA

- In children, young adults in which lymph vessels supplying lining of small intestine become enlarged; fluid retention is massive

INFLAMMATORY BOWEL DISEASE

- Crohn's and ulcerative colitis (UC)
- Both can present with:
  - Abdominal pain
  - Obstruction
  - Bloody diarrhea (occult or gross)

Comparison of Crohn's Disease and Ulcerative Colitis

Crohn's Disease	Ulcerative Colitis
Can affect entire GI from mouth to anus Cobblestone appearance Transmural inflammation (giant cells)	Only the colon Inflammation limited to mucosa and submucosa ↑ risk of secondary malignancy

MALABSORPTION SYNDROMES

- Nutrients from food are not absorbed properly.
- Not absorbed across small intestine into the bloodstream.
- **Clinical**
  - Children
    - Growth retardation
    - Failure to thrive
  - Adults
    - Weight loss

Steatorrhea = *Soft, bulky, foul-smelling light colored stool.*

- Occurs when fat is not absorbed.
  - Pancreatic disease (↓ digestive enzymes).
  - Bile obstruction (↓ bile for emulsification).

Malabsorption Syndrome*	Cause	Comments
Celiac disease	Gluten sensitivity	Child or adult ↑ risk of GI lymphoma MALToma
Tropical sprue	Unknown Probably infection	Travelers to the tropics Steatorrhea Diarrhea Weight loss Sore tongue (↓ vitamin B)
Whipple's disease	*Tropheryma whippelii*	Middle-aged men Slow onset of symptoms: • Skin darkening • Inflamed painful joints • Diarrhea Can be fatal without treatment

*For vitamin and mineral deficiencies, see Chapter 16, "Nutrition."

Note: *In celiac disease, a longer duration of breastfeeding correlates to more atypical symptoms and later presentation of the disease.*

Pancreas

PANCREATITIS

- Inflammation or infection of the pancreas.
- Cause
  - Injury to pancreatic cells.
  - Obstruction of normal pancreatic outflow.
    - Autodigestion/autolysis by pancreatic enzymes.
    - Zymogens prematurely convert into their catalytically active forms.
    - These enzymes then attack the pancreatic tissue itself.
  - In chronic cases, inflammation and fibrosis cause destruction of functioning glandular tissue.
- Symptoms
  - Pain, destruction of pancreas.
- Laboratory
  - ↑ lipase (more important).
  - ↑ amylase.

	Acute Pancreatitis	**Chronic Pancreatitis**
Causes	Gallstones (#1) Other biliary disease Alcoholism Cystic fibrosis in children	Alcoholism (most often) Hyperlipidemia Hyperparathyroidism
Symptoms	Abdominal pain Knifelike Radiating to back Nausea and vomiting Jaundice (if gallstone) Pale or clay colored stools (if bile blockage too)	Abdominal pain Nausea and vomiting Fatty stools
Complications	Enzymatic hemorrhagic fat necrosis with calcium soap formation with resultant hypocalcemia	Pseudocyst* Pancreatic abscess Ascites

*Pancreatic abscesses occur in pancreatic pseudocysts that become infected.

CHOLELITHIASIS

- Stones in the gallbladder = gallstones.
- Almost all gallstones are formed in the gallbladder, where bile is stored after it is produced in liver.
- Bile is composed of
    - Water
    - Bile salts
    - Lecithin
    - Cholesterol
    - Small solutes
- Stone formation
    - Changes in relative concentration of bile components.
    - Precipitation from solution.
    - Nidus, or nest, around which gallstones are formed.
- Stone size
    - Ranges from small as a grain of sand to large as 1-inch diameter.
    - Depends on time elapsed since initial formation.
- Stone color
    - Depends on primary precipitated substance:
        - Yellow-white—cholesterol.
        - Red-brown—bilirubin.

Choledocholithiasis = Gallstones in the common bile duct (CBD).

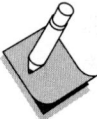

Gallstones that block the CBD result in obstructive jaundice, with yellow skin color caused by bile pigments being deposited in skin.

CHOLESTEROLOSIS

- Called strawberry gallbladder (GB).
- Small yellow cholesterol flecks against a red background in the lining of the gallbladder.
    - Polyps may form inside the GB.
    - May necessitate GB removal if outflow is blocked.

GALLBLADDER DIVERTICULOSIS

- Small fingerlike outpouchings of the GB lining may develop as a person ages; may cause inflammation and require GB removal.

Liver Disease

CIRRHOSIS (OF LIVER)

Cirrhosis is associated with increase in hepatocellular carcinoma.

- Most common chronic liver disease.
- Occurs twice as often in males as in females.
- Third most common cause of death among people age 45–65 (behind heart disease and cancer).
- **Characteristics**
  - Scarring/fibrosis
  - Loss of hepatic architecture
  - Formation of regenerative nodules
- **Causes**
  - Alcoholism (75%)
  - Viral hepatitis (hepatitis B, C)
  - Hemochromatosis
  - Wilson disease
  - Drugs/toxic injury
  - Biliary obstruction
  - Wilson's disease
  - Other inborn errors of metabolism:
    - Galactosemia
    - Glycogen storage diseases
    - Alpha-1 antitrypsin deficiency
- **Clinical findings/complications**
  - Ascites
  - Splenomegaly
  - Jaundice
  - Coagulopathy/bleeding disorders
  - Confusion/hepatic encephalopathy
  - Portal hypertension (and its complications)
  - Esophageal varices (with hematemesis)

Wilson's disease (hepatolenticular degeneration) is the hereditary accumulation of copper in liver, kidney, brain, and cornea. It is characterized by cirrhosis of the liver, degeneration of the basal ganglia in the brain, and deposition of green pigment in periphera of cornea.

PORTAL HYPERTENSION

- Abnormally high blood pressure in the portal vein/system
- Factors ↑ BP in portal vessels
  - ↓ volume of blood flowing through the portal system
  - ↑ resistance to blood flow through the liver
- **Causes**
  - Cirrhosis of liver—most common cause.
  - Splenic or portal vein thrombosis (prehepatic).
  - Schistosomiasis (intrahepatic).
  - Congestion distal hepatic venous circulation (Budd–Chiari syndrome) (posthepatic).
- **Results/complications**
  - Development of venous collaterals
    - Esophageal varices (common source of massive hematemesis in alcoholics).

Splenomegaly is the most important sign of portal hypertension.

- Hemorrhoids
- Enlarged veins on the anterior abdominal wall (caput Medusae)
- Spider angiomas
  - Ascites (fluid within abdominal cavity)
  - Splenomegaly (congestive)
- See Chapter 1 for the anatomy of the portal blood supply.

ASCITES

- Excess fluid in the space between the membranes lining the abdomen and abdominal organs.
  - Peritoneal cavity
    - Visceral peritoneum.
    - Parietal peritoneum.
- Ascites can be free serous fluid or protein-laden (like almost pure plasma).
- Disorders associated with ascites include:
  - Cirrhosis.
  - Hepatitis.
  - Portal vein thrombosis.
  - Constrictive pericarditis.
  - CHF.
  - Liver cancer.
  - Nephrotic syndrome.
  - Pancreatitis.

Hematemesis and bleeding from esophageal varices (dilated tortuous veins in submucosa of the lower esophagus) is often the first sign of cirrhosis and portal hypertension; it requires emergency treatment to control hemorrhage and prevent hypovolemic shock. This is an important cause of death in this group.

Liver disease is the most common cause of ascites.

JAUNDICE

- Yellow discoloration of skin, mucous membranes, eyes.
- **Mechanism**
  - ↑ bilirubin in blood.
  - Dissolves in subcutaneous tissues/fat.
- **Causes**
  - ↑ RBC destruction.
    - Release of bilirubin into blood (unconjugated).
  - Biliary obstruction.
    - Inability of bilirubin to be excreted into GI tract (conjugated).
  - Liver damage.
    - Bilirubin release into blood.
  - Any age, either sex.

Jaundice is a leading manifestation of liver disease.

BILIRUBIN

- Waste product from hemoglobin breakdown in RBCs.
- Excreted from body as chief component of bile.
- **Conjugated bilirubin**
  - Bilirubin conjugates with glucuronic acid in the liver.
- **Free bilirubin** (unconjugated) (converted to conjugated bilirubin in the liver).
  - Travels in blood bound to albumin.
  - Toxic

- **Kernicterus**
  - Newborn infants.
  - High levels of bilirubin accumulate in the brain.
  - Characteristic form of crippling.
    - Athetoid cerebral palsy.

HEPATITIS

- Inflammation of the liver.

TRANSAMINITIS

- Damage to liver cells → release enzymes into blood → ↑ serum levels of enzymes (transaminases = AST, ALT).
- ↑ transaminases used to diagnose liver disease.

VIRAL HEPATITIS

- Liver inflammation caused by a virus.
- See Chapter 16 for virology.

▶ GENITOURINARY PATHOLOGY

Nephrolithiasis

- Renal calculi (kidney stones).
  - Form within renal pelvis, calyces.
  - Pass into urinary system.
- Occurs more often in males than in females (M > F); rare in children.
- **Predisposing factors**
  - Dehydration
  - Infection
  - Changes in urine pH
  - Obstruction of urine flow
  - Immobilization with bone reabsorption
  - Metabolic factors (e.g., hyperparathyroidism with hypercalcemia)
  - Renal acidosis
  - ↑ uric acid
  - Defective oxalate metabolism
- **Stone composition**
  - Struvite
  - Calcium (most common)
  - Uric acid
  - Cystine
- **Clinical symptoms**
  - Usually asymptomatic (until stones pass into the ureter)
  - Renal colic (severe pain)
    - Once stone is in ureter, increased pressure and peristalsis from the ureter
- **Complications**
  - Obstruction of the ureter (with pressure and pain, renal colic)
  - Pyelonephritis (acute or chronic)
  - Hydronephrosis

STONE FORMATION

- Stones result from different processes or disease.
- But pathogenesis is the same: Supersaturation of the urine with a poorly soluble material.
- Renal stones grow on the surfaces of the papillae.
- Stones detach and flow downstream in the urine.
- Large stones will not fit through narrow conduits. Usually >1 cm to as large as staghorn stone.
- Obstruction → renal colic, hydronephrosis. Bilateral renal calculi are more apt to cause infection.

Calcium stones account for 80–90% of urinary stones. They are composed of calcium oxalate, calcium phosphate, or both.

HYDRONEPHROSIS

- Abnormal dilation of renal pelvis and calyces of one or both kidneys.
- Caused by urinary tract obstruction.
    - ↓ urine outflow.
    - Pressure ↑ behind the obstruction.
    - Renal pelvis and calyces dilates.
- Physical manifestation.
    - **Not** a disease process itself.
    - Disease = Stone, stricture, benign prostatic hyperplasia, etc.

Pyelonephritis

- Infection of the renal pelvis (kidney and ureters), usually *E. coli*.
- **Cause**
    - Most often from a urinary tract infection (UTI).
    - Retrograde/backflow bacteria-laden urine from bladder into ureters up to kidney pelvis.
        - *Vesicoureteral reflux*
- **Forms**
    - Acute
        - Active infection of the renal pelvis.
        - Abscess can develop; renal pelvis filled with pus (neutrophil rich).
    - Chronic
        - Scarring fibrosis; renal failure is possible.

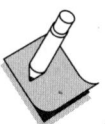

Kidney infections are usually caused by microorganisms ascending from the lower urinary tract.

Poststreptococcal GMN is the classic cause of blood in urine in children.

	Hematuria	Glucosuria	Ketonuria	Proteinuria
	Blood in urine **Women** Blood may come from vagina. **Men** Bloody ejaculation may be due to a prostate problem. **Children** Bleeding disorders. Recent strep infection may imply post-strep GMN.	Glucose in urine	Ketones in urine; acetonelike odor	Protein in urine
	Kidney or urinary tract disease	Diabetes mellitus	Starvation Uncontrolled DM Alcohol intoxication	Kidney disease

Bilirubinuria = Yellow-brown urine.

Frothy urine = Albumin or protein (> 2 gm/24 hr).

Diabetes Insipidus

See Chapter 17, "Endocrine Physiology."

Polycystic Kidney Disease (PCKD)

- **Adult form (APCKD)**
- Inherited disorder with multiple cysts on the kidneys.
- Exact mechanism is unknown.
- Course
  - Early stages
    - Kidney enlargement (as cysts form and grow)
    - Kidney function altered, resulting in:
      - Chronic high blood pressure; hypertension caused by polycystic kidneys is difficult to control.
      - Anemia
      - Erythrocytosis; if cysts cause ↑ erythropoietin (cause ↑ RBCs).
      - Kidney infections
      - Flank pain, if bleeding into a cyst occurs.
  - Later
    - Slowly progressive.
    - Ultimately results in **end-stage kidney failure.**
  - APCKD also associated with liver disease and infection of liver cysts.
- **Childhood form**
  - Autosomal recessive form of polycystic kidney disease.
  - More serious form.
  - Appears in infancy or childhood.
- Course
  - Progresses rapidly.
  - Resulting in ESRD.
    - Kidney failure leads to death in infancy or childhood.

Note: Kidney stones are less common in PCKD.

Medullary Cystic Disease

- Cysts in the kidney medulla (deep)
  - Results in kidney failure
- Uncommon
- Affects older children

Kidney disease is often associated with malignant hypertension.

Medullary Sponge Kidney

- Congenital disorder.
- Kidney tubules are dilated, causing the kidney to appear spongy.

Nephrosclerosis

- Renal impairment secondary to arteriosclerosis or hypertension.
- **Arterial nephrosclerosis**
  - Atrophy and scarring of the kidney.
  - Due to arteriosclerotic thickenings of the walls of large branches of renal arteries.

- **Arteriolar nephrosclerosis**
  - Arterioles thicken.
  - Areas they supply undergo ischemic atrophy and interstitial fibrosis.
  - Associated with HTN.
- **Malignant nephrosclerosis**
  - Inflammation of renal arterioles.
  - Results in rapid deterioration of renal function.
  - Accompanies malignant hypertension.

Arteriosclerosis

- Associated with chronic HTN.
- Reactive changes in the smaller arteries and arterioles throughout the body.

BENIGN NEPHROSCLEROSIS

- Arteriosclerosis affecting renal vessels.
- Result is a loss of renal parenchyma.
  - ↓ kidney function.

Nephrotic Syndrome

- **Not** a disease itself.
  - Glomerular defect underlies the process, indicating renal damage.
- **Demographics**
  - Any age
    - Children; usually age 18 mo–4 years; boys > girls.
    - Adults; males and females alike (M = F).
- **Characterized by**
  - **Proteinuria**; ↑↑ loss of protein in the urine (> 3.5 g per day).
  - **Hypoalbuminemia**
  - **Hyperlipidemia**
  - **Edema**; ↑ salt and water retention.
- **Cause**; ↑ glomerular capillary permeability.
  - Leads to ↓ blood protein (albumin).
  - Leads to ↑ protein in urine.
- **Associated diseases**
  - Amylodosis
  - Cancer
  - DM
  - HIV
  - Glomerulopathies
  - Leukemia
  - Lymphomas
  - Multiple myeloma
  - SLE
- **Clinical symptoms**
  - Loss of appetite
  - General sick feeling (malaise)
  - Puffy eyelids
  - Abdominal pain
  - Muscle wasting
  - Tissue swelling/edema
  - Frothy urine (protein-laden)

~75% of nephrotic syndrome are caused by primary glomerulonephropathies.

Hyperlipidemia in nephrotic syndrome is secondary to

- ↑ hepatic fat synthesis.
- ↓ fat catabolism.

Lipiduria: Cholesterol, triglycerides, lipoproteins leak into the urine.

Glomerulonephropathies

- Kidney disorders where inflammation affects mainly the glomeruli.
- Varied causes, but glomeruli respond to injury similarly.
- **Acute nephritic syndrome**
    - Example: Acute post streptococcal glomerulonephritis (acute glomerulonephritis).
        - Most common in boys 3–7; can occur at any age.
        - Starts suddenly and usually resolves quickly.
    - Acute glomerular inflammation.
    - Sudden hematuria.
        - Clumps of RBCs (casts).
        - Protein in urine.
- **Rapidly progressive nephritic syndrome**
    - Example: **Rapidly progressive glomerulonephritis (RPGN)**
        - Uncommon disorder; usually occurs at age 50–60.
        - Starts suddenly and worsens rapidly.
        - Most of the glomeruli are partly destroyed.
        - Results in kidney failure.
        - Idiopathic or associated with a proliferative glomerular disease (e.g., acute GN).
- **Nephrotic syndrome**
    - See earlier discussion.
    - Many disease processes can affect the kidney to cause **nephrotic syndrome**
        - **Findings**
        - Proteinuria (loss of large amounts of protein in the urine)
        - Hypoalbuminemia
        - Generalized edema
        - Hyperlipidemia
        - Hypercholesterolemia
- **Chronic nephritic syndrome**
    - Also called chronic glomerulonephritis
    - Examples of diseases causing:
        - SLE
        - Good pastures syndrome
        - Acute GN
        - Slowly progressive disease
        - Inflammation of the glomeruli
            - Sclerosis
            - Scarring
            - Eventual renal failure

▶ BLOOD–LYMPHATIC PATHOLOGY

Anemia

- ↓ RBCs and/or hemoglobin (absolute or qualitative).
- ↓ oxygen-carrying capacity
- ↓ energy
    - Fatigue
    - Weakness
    - Inability to exercise
    - Lightheadedness

Classification of Anemia

↑ RBC Destruction	↓ RBC Production
Blood loss Hemolytic (= RBC destruction) ■ Autoimmune hemolytic anemia ■ Erythroblastosis fetalis Hereditary spherocytosis ■ G6PD deficiency ■ Sickle cell anemia ■ Thalassemia	Hematopoietic cell damage ■ Aplastic anemia Deficiency of factors ■ B_{12} deficiency (pernicious anemia) ■ Folate deficiency ■ Fe deficiency Bone marrow replacement ■ Leukemia ■ Myelophthisis ■ Myelodyplasia

Anemia from ↑ RBC Destruction

BLOOD LOSS ANEMIA

- ↓RBCs because external loss.
- Hemorrhage.
- Symptoms are related to hypovolemia.

Note: Iron-deficiency anemia can be caused by both blood loss (↑ RBC destruction) and dietary deficiency (↓ RBC production).

HEMOLYTIC ANEMIA

- ↓ RBC lifespan (↑ RBC destruction).

AUTOIMMUNE HEMOLYTIC ANEMIA

- IgG antibodies combine with RBC surface antigens.
- Fc site of the bound antibody reacts with Fc receptor of phagocytic cells (and reticuloendothelial system).
- Antibody coated RBCs are sequestered in the spleen (where hemolysis occurs).
  - Splenomegaly.
- Diagnosis: Positive direct Coombs' test.
- Features (as with other hemolytic anemias):
  - Unconjugated hyperbilirubinemia.
  - Jaundice.

ERYTHROBLASTOSIS FETALIS

- Mother produces antibodies against fetal RBCs.
- Destruction of fetal RBCs.
- **Mechanism**
  - Occurs in cases where Mom = Rh⁻ and fetus = Rh⁺.
  - Rh+ is dominant trait (passed from father in this case).
  - Rh⁻ mom forms Abs against Rh⁺ fetal blood.
  - Antibodies cross placenta into fetus circulation where they attach and lead to destruction of fetal RBCs.
  - Anemia in the fetus.

Other causes of anemia:
- **Splenic sequestration**
  - Massive splenomegaly leads to ↑ repository of RBCs.
    - RBCs are sequestered in spleen so there are fewer in the bloodstream.
    - ITP and purpura occur with splenic sequestration too.
      - ↓ usable platelets (as they are sequestered in the spleen).
- **Renal failure**
  - ↓ synthesis of erythropoietin.
  - Normocytic, normochromic anemia.
  - Treat with Epo.

Coombs' test; positive implies hemolysis is mediated by antibodies attached to RBCs.

Hemolytic anemias
- Hyperbilirubinemia and hemoglobinuria.
- Broken down RBC:
  - Hb liberated.
  - Hb in urine.
  - Hb in blood.
    - Bilirubin (breakdown product of Hb).
    - ↑unconjugated bilirubin (water insoluble).
    - Jaundice (yellow under tongue = first sign; yellow sclera).
    - Conjugated bilirubin (water-soluble) forms when unconjugated bilirubin combines with albumin.

- Secreted with bile into the small intestine.
- Reduction of bilirubin in intestine to urobilinogen.
- ↑ urobilinogen.

Note: Erythroblastosis fetalis can also occur because of ABO incompatibility (e.g., Mom = O, fetus = type A or B). However, Rh incompatibility causes the most severe form.

HEREDITARY SPHREROCYTOSIS

- Sphere-shaped RBCs are selectively trapped in the spleen.
  - Sequestration splenomegaly.
  - Unconjugated hyperbilirubinemia.
- Autosomal dominant.
- Abnormality of RBC membrane protein (spectrin protein).
- ↑ erythrocyte fragility to hypotonic saline.

G6PD DEFICIENCY

*Toxic accumulation of unconjugated bilirubin in the brain and spinal cord is called **kernicterus**.*

- X-linked inheritance.
- ↓ activity of RBC G6PD.
- Failure of RBC hexose monophosphate shunt under oxidative stress.
- Leads to hemolysis (with hemoglobinemia, hemoglobinuria).

SICKLE-CELL ANEMIA

- Primarily in African Americans.
- Inherited autosomal recessive (inherited Hb-S from both parents).
- Abnormal type of hemoglobin Hb-S.
  - Globin portion: Valine substituted for glutamic acid in the sixth position.
- **Heterozygote (AS)** (less severe) = **Sickle-cell trait.**
  - One normal Hb (Hb-A).
  - One abnormal Hb (Hb-S).
- **Homozygote (SS)** (more severe) = **Sickle-cell disease.**
  - Two abnormal Hb (Hb-S).
  - Hb-S causes Hb instability when exposed to stress (e.g., ↓ O_2 (hypoxic conditions).
  - Lead to formation of fibrous precipitates.
  - Distort erythrocytes into sickle shape (crescent shape).
  - ↓ function.
- Sickle-cell pain crisis
  - Sickled cells form small blood clots.
  - Clots occlude blood vessels and give rise to painful episodes; usually affect bones of back, long bones, and chest.
  - Episodes can last hours to days.
- **Hemolytic crisis**
  - Life-threatening breakdown of damaged RBCs.
- **Splenic sequestration crisis**
  - The spleen enlarges because sickled RBCs are trapped.
- **Aplastic crisis**
  - Infection causes bone marrow to stop producing RBCs.

Patients with sickle-cell anemia can become functionally asplenic. As a result, they are prone to infections caused by encapsulated organisms (including Strep pneumonia and Hemophilus influenza). Salmonella bone infections/ osteomyelitis can occur.

Healing leg ulcers and recurrent bouts of abdominal and chest pain are characteristic of sickle-cell anemia.

Repeated sickle cell crises can damage kidneys, lungs, bones, eyes, and CNS.

THALASSEMIAS (MAJOR AND MINOR)

- Group of inherited Hb synthesis disorders (autosomal recessive).
- ↓ globin chain synthesis (one of the four amino acid chains that make up Hb).

- Abnormal Hb.
  - ↓ RBCs.
- Chronic anemia.

Anemia from ↓ RBC Production

HEMATOPOIETIC CELL DAMAGE

- Aplastic anemia
  - ↓ production of RBCs.
    - Inhibition or destruction of bone marrow.
  - Pancytopenia (↓ levels of all blood elements—cells and platelets).
  - BM biopsy.
    - Normal architecture, **but**
    - ↓ cellularity (< 25% normal).
  - Absolute neutrophil counts are extremely low.
- Causes
  - Hereditary
  - Acquired:
    - Radiation
    - Toxins:
      - Benzene
      - Insecticides
    - Viral infections
      - CMV
      - Parvovirus
      - Hepatitis
    - Medications:
      - Chloramphenicol
      - Anticonvulsants
      - Phenylbutazone

In drug-induced aplastic anemias, the RBCs appear normochromic (normal concentration of Hb) and normocytic (normal size).

↓ factors for RBC Production

B$_{12}$ DEFICIENCY

- **Pernicious anemia**
- Autoimmune disorder
  - Caused by **autoimmune gastritis** (failure production intrinsic factor).
    - Anti-intrinsic factor and antiparietal cell antibodies.
      - Lack of intrinsic factor (IF needed to absorb B$_{12}$).
    - Achlorhydria.
- Features
  - Megaloblastic (macrocytic) anemia.
  - Abnormal Schilling test.
    - Impaired absorption of B$_{12}$; corrected by adding intrinsic factor.
  - Hypersegmented neutrophils on peripheral blood smear.
  - Lemon-yellow skin.
  - Stomatitis and glossitis.
  - Subacute combined degeneration of the spinal cord.
- Symptoms
  - Fatigue, SOB, tingling sensations, difficulty walking, diarrhea.

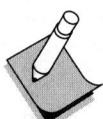

Intrinsic factor is a protein produced in gastric parietal cells. B$_{12}$ must be bound by IF to be absorbed in the GI. B$_{12}$ is necessary for RBC formation and is needed by nerves.

> *Major causes of B_{12} deficiency with the resultant megaloblastic anemia:*
> - *Pernicious anemia (↓ intrinsic factor because of autoimmune gastritis).*
> - *Dietary deficiency of B_{12} (strict vegetarian).*
> - *Gastric resection (remove cells that produce IF—parietal cells).*
> - *Ileal resection (remove intestinal cells that absorb B_{12}).*

- Other causes of vitamin B_{12} megaloblastic anemia:
  - Gastric resection (where IF is produced).
  - Strict vegetarian diet.
  - Distal ileum resection (where B_{12} is absorbed).

Note: Patients with atrophic gastritis are prone to gastric carcinomas.

FOLATE DEFICIENCY

- Megaloblastic (macrocytic) anemia.
  - Hypersegmented neutrophils.
  - Lack of folate results in delayed DNA replication.
- **Causes**
- Dietary deficiency
- Malabsorption syndromes (*sprue, Giardia lamblia*)
- Pregnancy
- Dilantin

Note: Folate deficiency has no neurologic abnormalities (in distinction to B_{12} deficiency)

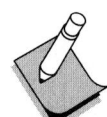

Plummer–Vinson syndrome: Fe deficiency anemia associated with upper esophageal web.

IRON DEFICIENCY

- Hypochromic microcytic anemia (pale small RBCs)
- **Causes**
  - Chronic blood loss (major cause of Fe deficiency anemia)
    - Excessive menstrual bleeding
    - GI bleeding
    - Results in:
      - ↓ or absent bone marrow Fe stores
      - ↓ serum ferritin
  - Dietary deficiency
    - Rare, except infants, elderly
    - ↓ Fe requirement
    - Pregnancy
    - Infants, fast-growing adolescents.
- **Findings**
  - Pallor
  - Fatigue
  - Shortness of breath
  - Glossitis, koilonychias

Microcytic versus Macrocytic Anemia

Microcytic	Macrocytic
Average size of RBC < normal Fe deficiency	Average size of RBC > normal B_{12} deficiency Folate deficiency

Other Causes of ↓ RBC Production

ANEMIA OF CHRONIC DISEASE

- Isolated ↓ RBC proliferation; may resemble Fe deficiency.

MYELODYSPLASTIC SYNDROMES

- Example: Myelodysplasia with myelofibrosis.
- Bone marrow is replaced by abnormal (dysplastic) stem cells or by fibrous tissue.
    - Ineffective hematopoiesis
    - ↑ immature RBCs and WBCs
    - Abnormally shaped RBCs (teardrop shaped)
    - Anemia
    - Splenomegaly
- Myeloproliferative disorders
    - Myeloid stem cells develop and reproduce abnormally in bone marrow
    - Peak incidence in middle age
    - ↓ blood basophils
    - ↑ serum uric acid
    - Splenomegaly

PURE RED CELL APLASIA

- Severe ↓ of RBC lineage only.

Erythrocytes and Polycythemia (↑ RBCs)

RELATIVE POLYCYTHEMIA

- ↓ Plasma volume.
- RBCs are more concentrated.
- Spurious polycythemia = Gaisbock syndrome.

TRUE POLYCYTHEMIA

- ↑ total blood volume
- ↑ RBC mass

TRUE POLYCYTHEMIA

- ↑ RBCs
- Opposite of anemia

PRIMARY POLYCYTHEMIA

- *Polycythemia vera* (a myeloproliferative disease).
- Genetic predisposition.
- ↓ sensitivity of myeloid precursors to erythropoietin.

- **Characteristics**
  - Erythrocytosis.
  - Leukocytosis.
  - Thrombocytosis.
  - Splenomegaly.
  - ↓ erythropoietin.

SECONDARY POLYCYTHEMIA

Remember: In polycythemia vera (primary polycythemia) erythropoietin levels are normal or low. In secondary polycythemia, erythropoietin levels are elevated.

Polycythemia is a myeloproliferative disorder, as is myelofibrosis (see above with anemia).

Remember: Erythropoietin is made by the kidney in the juxtaglomerular apparatus.

Aspirin inactivates cyclooxygenase (COX) by acetylation; causes ↓ production thromboxane A2 (a platelet aggregant). More prone to bleeding secondary to ↓ platelet aggregation.

- ↑ RBCs by conditions other than polycythemia vera.
- Secondary to ↑ erythropoietin.
- **Causes**
  - Renal disease
    - Polycystic kidney disease
    - Renal cell carcinoma
  - Chronic hypoxia
    - Pulmonary disease
    - Heavy smoking
    - High altitude (Osker's disease)
    - CHF
  - Tumors
    - Renal cell cancer (see above)
    - Hepatocellular carcinoma
    - Meningioma
    - Pheochromocytoma
    - Cerebellar hemangioma
    - Adrenal adenoma
  - Androgen therapy
  - Bartter syndrome
- **Features**
  - Plethora
    - Redness of skin and mucous membranes
  - ↓ blood viscosity
    - ↓ tissue perfusion
    - Propensity for thrombosis
  - No splenomegaly (this is a feature of polycythemia vera)

Bleeding Problems

- Bleeding occurs when there are abnormalities in:
  - Primary hemostasis (platelet plug); quantitative or qualitative platelet disorders.
  - Secondary hemostasis; disorder in the coagulation cascade.
  - Disorders affecting the structural integrity of blood vessels.

Bleeding Disorders

Primary Hemostasis (Platelet Plug)	Secondary Hemostasis (Coagulation)	Combined Primary and Secondary Defect	Vessel Damage
Quantitative ↓ *platelet (thrombocytopenia)* Marrow damage ■ Aplastic anemia Marrow replacement ■ Leukemia ■ Myelophthisis Splenic sequestration DIC ITP TTP *Qualitative ↓ platelet* Aspirin use Von Willebrand disease Bernard–Soulier syndrome Glanzman thrombasthenia	Hemophilias Vitamin K deficiency Anticoagulants ■ Heparin ■ Warfarin	Von Willebrand disease DIC Coagulopathy of liver disease	Scurvy Henoch–Schonlein purpura HHT Connective tissue disorders

Note: *DIC and von Willebrand's disease exhibit problems with both platelets and coagulation cascade.*

Disorders in Primary Hemostasis

Quantitative Platelet Deficiencies

THROMBOCYTOPENIA

- ↓ platelet count (quantitative ↓ platelets).
- ↑ bleeding time.
- **Features**
   - Mucosal oozing
   - Petechial cutaneous bleeding
   - Bruising
   - Hemorrhage into tissues
- **Causes**
   - Aplastic anemia (all blood cell elements, including platelets ↓).
   - Myelophthisis (marrow replaced by tumor cells).
   - Splenic sequestration.
   - Disseminated intravascular coagulation (DIC).
   - Idiopathic thrombocytopenic purpura (ITP).
   - Thrombotic thrombocytopenia purpura (TTP).

PURPURA

- Purplish spots produced by small bleeding vessels.
   - Skin (cutaneous).
   - Mucous membranes (mouth lining and in internal organs).

Platelets
- Primary hemostasis (platelet plug, prior to clotting).
- Help maintain the integrity of the capillary lining.

Thrombocytopenia is the most common cause of bleeding disorders.

- Sign of underlying causes of bleeding.
- **Nonthrombocytopenic purpura**
  - Normal platelet counts.
- **Thrombocytopenic purpura**
  - ↓ platelet counts.

Petechiae	Ecchymoses
Small purpura spots	Large purpura spots

DISSEMINATED INTRAVASCULAR COAGULATION (DIC)

- Life-threatening.
- Coagulation system widespread activation.
- Uncontrolled cycle of bleeding and clotting.
- Consumptive coagulopathy (platelets are depleted).
- Clotting: Extensive microclot formation.
- Bleeding: Accompanying fibrinolysis (see increased D-dimer and other fibrin split products).
- ↑ fibrinolysis = ↑ fibrin split products (e.g., D-dimer).
- Important indicators of DIC.
- **Laboratory**
  - ↓ platelet count.
  - ↑ PT.
  - ↑ PTT.
  - Hypofibrinogenemia (↓ fibrinogen).
  - ↓ levels of all clotting factors.
  - ↓ levels of fibrinolytic proteins.
- **Causes**
  - Amniotic fluid embolism.
  - Infection (gram-negative sepsis).
  - Malignancy.
  - Major trauma.

IDIOPATHIC THROMBOCYTOPENIC PURPURA

- ITP; immune TP.
- Antiplatelet antibodies coat and lead to destruction of platelets.
  - Platelets are opsonized in the spleen.
- Usually ensues after a viral URI.
- Acute form (usually in children).
  - Explosive but self-limited.
- Chronic form (in adults).
  - May respond to steroid therapy.

TTP = ↓ platelet count due to platelet consumption by thrombosis in the terminal arterioles and capillaries.

THROMBOTIC THROMBOCYTOPENIC PURPURA (TTP)

- Thrombocytopenia.
- Hyaline microthrombi in small vessels.
- Microangiothic hemolytic anemia.
  - Lesions in the microcirculation damage platelets and RBCs (become schistocytes) passing through.

Qualitative platelet disorders = von Willebrand's disease.

Von Willebrand's Disease

- Autosomal dominant.
- M = F.
- Platelet dysfunction secondary to ↓ von Willebrand factor (vWF).
- vWF
    - Large glycoprotein.
    - Allows adhesion of platelets to collagen.
        - Important in formation of platelet plug.
    - Binding sites for factor VIII.

Disorders in Secondary Hemostasis

- Bleeding caused by problems with the coagulation cascade

Hemophilia

- Hereditary bleeding disorder.
    - Takes a long time for blood to clot.
- ↓ plasma clotting factors.
- **Clinically**
    - Bleeding from larger vessels (unlike small vessel bleeding in platelet disorders).
- **Laboratory**
- ↑ PTT (PT and INR are normal).

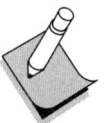

von Willebrand's disease and Bernard-Soulier disease are causes of qualitative platelet dysfunction.

von Willebrand disease = qualitative platelet defect resulting in impaired platelet adhesion. It can also affect coagulation by decreasing function of factor VIII.

Remember, clotting occurs when in the presence of thromboplastin and calcium ions, prothrombin is converted to thrombin, which in turn converts fibrinogen into fibrin. Fibrin threads then entrap blood cells, platelets, and plasma to form a blood clot.

Hemophilia is characterized by:
- *↑ PTT.*
- *Normal PT.*
- *Normal bleeding time.*

	Hemophilia A (Classic Hemophilia)	Hemophila B (Christmas Disease)	Hemophilia C (Rosenthal's Syndrome)
↓ factor	VIII (Antihemophilic factor)	IX (Plasma thromboplastin component)	XI (Plasma thromboplastin antecedent)
Features	X-linked (occurs in males) < 25 yr Excessive bleeding from minor cuts, epistaxis, hematomas, hemarthroses.	X-linked Clinically identical to hemophilia A 1/5 – 1/10 as common as hemophilia A	Not sex linked Less severe bleeding

All clotting factors are made in the liver. Factors II, VII, IX, X are vitamin K dependent.

Severe liver disease (e.g., cirrhosis), bleeding because:
- *↓ clotting factor production.*
- *↓ vitamin K (↓ production of factors II, VII, IX, X even more).*

Note: *↓ prothrombin (factor II) = hypoprothrombinemia. Prothrombin is formed and stored in parenchymal cells of liver; in cirrhosis there is profuse damage to these cells.*

Vitamin K Deficiency

- ↓ activity of vitamin K dependent factors (II, VII, IX, X)
- ↑ PT
- ↑ PTT
- Normal platelet count
- **Causes**
    - Fat malabsorption (pancreatic or GI disease)
    - Warfarin

ENDOCRINE PATHOLOGY

Antidiuretic Hormone (Vasopressin)

DIABETES INSIPIDUS

- See also Chapter 17, "Endocrine Physiology."
- Characterized by large volume of dilute urine.
- Central or nephrogenic.
- **Central DI**
  - Damage to hypothalamus; supraoptic nuclei or pituitary (post).
    - Lack or ↓ ADH secretion
      - Surgery
      - Infection
      - Inflammation
      - Tumor
      - Head injury
      - Rarely, idiopathic or genetic
  - Body fluid tonicity remains close to normal as long as patient drinks enough water to make up for ↑ water clearance in the urine.
- **Nephrogenic DI**
  - Kidney tubules are not sensitive to ADH.
  - ADH production and secretion is normal.
    - Resistance of ADH receptors.
  - Same result
  - Large volumes of dilute urine.
  - **Cause**
    - Genetic; sex-linked congenital DI
      - Affects men.
      - Women can pass it on to their children.
    - Lithium (or other medications).

Insulin

DIABETES MELLITUS (TYPE 1)

- Most common pancreatic endocrine disorder.
- Metabolic disease involving mostly carbohydrates (glucose) and lipids.
- **Causes**
  - Absolute deficiency of insulin (type 1) or
  - Resistance to insulin action (type 2)
- Classic symptom triad:
  - Polydipsia
  - Polyuria
  - Polyphagia

Warfarin (Coumadin) is an anticoagulant that interferes with vitamin K. It inhibits formation of prothrombin in liver. The effect of delayed blood clotting is useful to prevent and treat thromboembolic disease.

Review physiology: Hypothalamus makes ADH (vasopressin); it is then stored and secreted from the posterior pituitary. ADH is a hormone that causes kidneys to conserve water, creating concentrated urine. Absence of ADH results in urinary loss of water, lots of highly dilute urine.

Summary of Diabetes Type 1 vs. Type 2

	DM-1	DM-2
Symptoms	Polyuria Polydipsia Polyphagia Blurred vision Paresthesias Weakness/fatigue Weight loss	Polyuria Polydipsia Polyphagia Blurred vision Paresthesias Weakness/fatigue
Incidence	15%	85%
Age of onset	Childhood	Adulthood
Obese?	No	Usually
Insulin production	Minimal or none	May be normal or supranormal
Cause	Viral or immune destruction B cells	↑ insulin resistance (reduced sensitivity at target cells)
Genetic predisposition	Weak	Strong
Ketoacidosis	Common	Rare
Classic symptoms of polyuria, polydipsia, thirst, weight loss	Common	Sometimes
Rapidity of sexual development	Rapid	Slow
Treatment	Insulin injection Diet	Diet Weight loss Oral hypoglycemic drugs

Hyperglycemia = BGL > 126 mg/dL.

Glycosuria occurs when BGL > 160–180 mg/dL.

Blood insulin
- Absent in DM-1.
- Normal or ↑ in DM-2 (e.g., insulin resistance).

Ketoacidosis
- Accumulation of ketone bodies.
- Synthesized from free fatty acids
  - In cases of starvation or severe insulin deficiency.
- Usually in DM-1.
- (Rare in DM-2 unless advanced or improperly treated).

Blood ketones
- Acetoacetic acid
- Beta-hydroxybutyric acid

Growth Hormone

ACROMEGALY

- ↑ secretion of GH by anterior pituitary gland.
  - Usually secondary to a benign secreting pituitary tumor.
  - Ages 35–55.
  - After end plates/growth plates of bone have fused/closed.
  - After completion of skeletal growth.
    - Bones become deformed.
    - Long bones do not elongate.
- **Common findings**
  - Gradual marked enlargement of
    - Head/skull
    - Face

HbA1c (glycosylated Hb)

- Used to assess long-term diabetes control.
- Reflects glucose levels over past 2–3 months.
- Normal = 4–7%.

Nonenzymatic glycosylation
- Products formed
    - Schiff bases; reversible glycosylation products with proteins.
    - Amadori products; rearrangement of Schiff bases (more stable but still reversible).
    - Advanced glycosylated end products (AGE); irreversible (glycosylated HbA1c is an AGE).

Hashimoto's thyroiditis (autoimmune) is the most common cause of hypothyroidism.

Secondary hypothyroidism: Pituitary does not make enough TSH.

- Jaw
- Hands
- Feet
- Chest
- Excessive perspiration and an offensive body odor.
- Prognathism
- Enlarged tongue
- Deep voice

Causes	↑ GH	↑ GH	↓ GH
	Before end plates closed	After end plates closed	Before end plates close
Disease process	**Gigantism**	**Acromegaly**	**Dwarfism**
Findings	Abnormally large height, limbs, features	Enlargement of skin, soft tissue, viscera, bones of face	Arrested growth Small limbs and features

Thyroid Hormone

	Hypothyroidism	**Hyperthyroidism**
Causes	Myxedema Cretinism Hashimoto thyroiditis	Graves' disease Thyroid adenoma Pituitary adenoma (secondary hyperthyroidism)
Findings	Mental slowing, mental retardation Cold intolerance Weight gain Low-pitched voice Constipation Face, eyelid, hand edema Dry skin Hair loss, brittle hair	Restlessness, irritability Heat intolerance Weight loss, muscle wasting Tremor Diarrhea Sweaty, warm moist skin Fine hair

MYXEDEMIA

- Extreme hypothyroidism.
- Affects females more than males (M > F).
- **Risks**
    - Age > 50 yr
    - Female
    - Obesity
    - Past thyroid surgery or neck exposure to XRT
- **Causes**
    - Thyroid surgery, XRT.
    - Hashimoto's disease.

- Idiopathic
- Iodine deficiency.
- **Symptoms**
    - Slow basal metabolic rate.
        - Mental and physical sluggishness.
        - Fatigue
    - Puffiness of face and eyelids.
    - Swelling of tongue and larynx.
    - Dry, rough skin.
    - Sparse hair.
    - Poor muscle tone.
- **Treatment**
    - Exogenous thyroid hormone.

Myxedema = Extreme hypothyroidism in adults; *Cretinism* = extreme hypothyroidism in child. (during development)

CRETINISM

- Severe hypothyroidism in a child due to lack of thyroid hormone.
- **Findings**
    - Growth retardation.
    - Abnormal development of bones.
    - Mental retardation because of improper development of CNS.
- **Treatment**
- Thyroid hormone; recognized and treated early, cretinism can be markedly improved.

Note: See physiology section in Chapter 17 for discussion of TSH, TRH, T_3 (triiodothyronine), and T_4 (thyroxine).

Dental findings in child with hypothyroidism:
- Underdeveloped mandible.
- Delayed tooth eruption.
- Retained deciduous teeth.

HASHIMOTO'S DISEASE

- Autoimmune disease.
- Form of chronic thyroiditis.
    - Slow disease onset (months–years).
- Most common cause of hypothyroidism.
    - Affects 0.1–5% of adults in Western countries.
- Can occur at any age.
    - Often middle-aged women.
- **Risks**
    - Female
    - Family history of Hashimoto's disease
- **Clinical**
    - Typical symptoms of hypothyroidism:
        - Fatigue
        - Slowed speech
        - Cold intolerance
        - Dry skin
        - Coarse hair
        - Edema
        - Etcetera

HYPERTHYROIDISM

- Thyrotoxicosis.
- ↑ thyroid hormone production
- Role of thyroxine:

Dental findings (few, unless presents in childhood) are premature eruption of teeth and loss of deciduous dentition.

- ↑ cellular metabolism, growth, and differentiation of all tissues
- ↑ basal metabolism
  - Fatigue
  - Weight loss
  - Excitability
  - ↑ temperature
  - Generalized osteoporosis

GRAVES' DISEASE

- Most common form of hyperthyroidism; 85% of cases.
- Women age 20–40 most often affected.
- Autoimmune disease.
- Onset often after infection or physical or emotional stress.
- **Clinical**
  - Symptoms of hyperthyroidism +
  - **Exophthalmos**
    - Eyeballs protrude; retrobulbar tissue buildup
    - Irritation
    - Tearing

PLUMMER'S DISEASE

- Toxic nodular goiter.
- Usually arises from long-standing simple goiter.
- Most often in elderly.
- **Risks**
  - Female
  - Age > 60 yr
  - Never seen in children
- **Symptoms**
  - Typical symptoms of hyperthyroidism
  - No exophthalmos

Parathyroid Hormone

HYPERPARATHYROIDISM

- ↑ PTH

PRIMARY HYPERPARATHYROIDISM

- Common
- Usually caused by secreting adenoma
  - Benign productive tumor of parathyroid glandular epithelium
- **Clinical**
  - Cystic bone lesions
    - Osteitis fibrosa cystica (with giant cells)
    - von Recklinghausen's disease of bone
  - Nephrocalcinosis
    - Kidney stones (renal calculi)
  - Metastatic calcifications

- **Laboratory**
  - ↑ PTH.
    - ↓ Ca^{2+} (hypercalcemia)
    - ↑ phosphorus
    - ↓ alkaline phoshatase

SECONDARY HYPERPARATHYROIDISM

- Feedback for ↓ Ca^{2+} (hypocalcemia)
- Chronic renal disease
  - ↑ loss of calcium in urine
  - ↓ serum Ca^{2+}
  - ↑ parathyroid gland function (chief cells)
    - Hyperplasia
- **Clinical**
  - ↑ Same as primary hyperparathyroidism
  - Cystic bone lesions
  - Metastatic calcifications
- **Laboratory**
  - ↑↑ PTH
  - ↓ Ca^{2+}
  - ↑ phosphorus

HYPOTHYROIDISM

- ↓ PTH
- ↓ Ca^{2+} (hypocalcemia)
- **Causes**
  - Excision of parathyroid glands; usually accidental during thyroidectomy
  - DiGeorge's syndrome
- **Clinical**
  - Neuromuscular excitability
  - Tetany

TETANY

- Irritability of central and peripheral nervous system.
- Occurs when blood Ca^{2+} falls from 10 mg% (normal) to 6 mg% (4 mg% is lethal).
- **Causes**
  - ↓ Ca^{2+} = usual cause
    - Hypoparathyroidism
    - ↓ vitamin D
  - Alkalosis
- **Characterized by**
  - Muscle twitches
  - Cramps
  - Carpopedal spasm
  - Laryngospasm and seizures (if severe)
- **Tests for acute hypocalcemia and tetany**
  - Chvostek's sign
    - Tap facial nerve above mandibular angle (next to earlobe).
    - Upper lip twitches; facial nerve causes muscle spasm.
    - Confirms tetany.

Symptoms of hyperparathyroidism: bones, stones, moans, abdominal groans (mostly the result of PTH acting at the bone to liberate calcium (↑ Ca^{2+}), by activating osteoclasts: bone lesions, kidney stones, pain, peptic ulcers).

Hyperparathyroidism can be associated with MEN I and MEN III.

Remember: *The parathyroid glands are located on the sides and posterior surface of thyroid gland.*

Hypoparathyroidism is associated with congenital thymic hypoplasia (DiGeorge's syndrome).

- Trousseau's sign
  - BP cuff applied to arm and inflated.
  - Carpopedal spasm (thumb adduction and phalangeal extension).
  - Confirms tetany.

Cortisol

- Adrenal glands

Adrenal Cortex

↑ Cortisol	↓ Cortisol
Cushing's disease	Addison's disease
Cushing's syndrome	Waterhouse–Friderichsen syndrome

> Remember, the adrenal cortex also produces aldosterone and weak androgens (sex hormones).
>
> - ↑ Aldosterone = Conn's syndrome.
>   - HTN.
>   - ↑ Na⁺.
>   - ↑ H₂O.
>   - ↓ K⁺.
> - ↑ androgens = adrenal virilism (adrenogenital syndrome).

Note: See Chapter 17, "Endocrine Physiology," for discussion of Cushing's and further discussion of Addison's.

ADDISON'S DISEASE

- Primary adrenal hypofunction or adrenal insufficiency
  - Partial or complete failure of adrenocortical function
- ↓ Cortisol from adrenal cortex
  - Primary: Caused by damage to adrenal cortex (outer layer of the gland, zona fasiculata especially)
    - Autoimmune
    - Infection
    - Neoplasm
    - Hemorrhage within the gland
  - Secondary: Caused by ↓ ACTH from pituitary
- **Clinical findings**
- ↓ adrenocortical function by > 90% before obvious symptoms occur
  - Symptoms, insidious onset of
    - Weakness
    - Fatigue
    - Depression
    - Hypotension
    - Skin bronzing (with primary adrenocortical insufficiency)
    - Feedback to pituitary causing ↑ ACTH causes ↑ MSH to be released also
- **Laboratory**
  - ↓ cortisol
  - ↓ serum Na⁺
  - ↑ serum K⁺

> **Oral signs of Addison's disease (secondary Addison's):** Diffuse mucosal pigmentation:
> - Gingiva
> - Tongue
> - Hard palate
> - Buccal mucosa
>
> **Note:** Cutaneous pigmentation usually disappears following therapy, but the oral mucosal pigmentation tends to persist.

Waterhouse–Friderichsen syndrome: Hemorrhagic necrosis of the adrenal cortex; usually associated with meningococcal infection; catastrophic adrenal insufficiency and vascular collapse.

PRIMARY VS. SECONDARY ADDISON'S DISEASE

- Primary Addison's
  - ↓ ACTH : ↓ cortisol.

- Secondary Addison's
  - ↓ cortisol : ↑ ACTH.
- ACTH stimulation test (helps distinguish primary from secondary).
  - Administer exogenous ACTH.
  - Cortisol level ↑ (if adrenal cortex works).
    - Indicates primary Addison's.
  - Cortisol level does not change (adrenal cortex is damaged).
    - Indicates secondary Addison's.
- Treatment
  - Administer cortisol (as hydrocortisone).

▶ MUSCOLOSKELETAL PATHOLOGY

Collagen Vascular Diseases

- Autoimmune in origin
- ANA association (antinuclear antibodies)
- Collagen vascular diseases include:
  - Rheumatoid arthritis
  - Systemic lupus erythematosus (SLE)
  - Scleroderma
  - Dermatomyositis
  - Polyarteritis nodosa

> **Collagen vascular diseases** are characterized by
> - Inflammatory damage to connective tissues and blood vessels.
> - Deposition of fibrinoid material.

SYSTEMIC LUPUS ERYTHEMATOSUS (SLE)

- Prototypical autoimmune connective tissue disease.
- Women = > 90% SLE patients.
- Age of onset = late teens to 30s.
- **Cause**
  - Autoimmune
    - Mechanism poorly understood.
    - Hypersensitivity reactions (type III mostly).
- **Clinical**
  - Affects many organs (skin, tendons, joints, kidneys, heart, blood cells, and CNS).
  - Butterfly rash
    - Characteristic rash in 50% SLE patients.
    - Erythematous rash over cheeks and bridge of nose; worsened by sunlight
  - Diffuse skin rash
    - Other sun-exposed areas
  - Joint pain and arthritis
  - Raynaud's phenomenon (vasospasm in small vessels in finger)
    - Acrocyanosis
  - Pulmonary fibrosis
  - Immune complex vasculitis
  - Glomerulonephritis (from immune complexes)
    - Renal failure occurs and = usual cause of death
  - CNS involvement

See section on bone diseases and arthritis for discussion of rheumatoid arthritis (RA).

Drug-induced LE can be caused by certain drugs. It usually reverses when the medication is stopped.

Anti-DNA and anti-Sm antibodies are specific for SLE.

CREST syndrome
- Variant of scleroderma.
- Positive anti-Scl-70.

Characterized by
- **C**alcinosis.
- **R**aynaud phenomenon.
- **E**sophageal dysfunction.
- **S**clerodactyly.
- **T**elangiectasia.

- **Course**
  - Often begins with one organ system.
    - Later, other organs become involved.
  - Periods of remission and exacerbation.
  - Symptom severity ranges from mild and episodic to severe and fatal.
- **Laboratory**
  - Positive antinuclear antibody test (ANA).
    - Positive anti-double-stranded DNA; rim pattern on immunofluorescence.
    - Positive anti-Sm.
- **Treatment**
  - Immunosuppressive therapy.
  - Corticosteroids

SCLERODERMA

- Progressive systemic sclerosis
- Common in young women
- Widespread connective tissue fibrosis
- **Clinical**
  - Subcutaneous collagen hypertrophy
    - Fixed facial expression
  - Sclerodactyly
    - Clawed hands
  - Raynaud's phenomenon
  - Visceral fibrosis
    - Esophageal dysmotility
    - GERD; ↑ Barretts esophagus

POLYARTHRITIS NODOSA

Polyarteritis nodosa is the only autoimmune disease and only connective tissue disease to occur more often in men.

- Most common in men.
- Blood vessel disease.
  - Small and medium-sized arteries become inflamed and damaged.
    - Immune complex vasculitis mechanism.
    - ↓ blood supply to organs.
- Antigen implicated
  - Hepatitis B (30% of cases).
  - Drugs: Sulfa, PCN (penicillin).

POLYMYALGIA RHEUMATICA AND TEMPORAL ARTERITIS

- Other inflammatory diseases of unknown cause.
- Closely related and frequently occur together.

Polymyalgia Rheumatica	Temporal Arteritis
Pain and stiffness around large muscle groups. Involves muscles of the neck, shoulders, and hips.	Inflammation of large arteries (giant cells), Especially temporal artery. Causes headache, visual changes.

ANKYLOSING SPONDYLITIS

- Type of spondyloarthropathy.
- Inflammation of the spine and large joints.
    - Stiffness
    - Pain
- Associated with HLA-B27.
- More common in men.

REITER'S SYNDROME

- Associated with HLA-B27
- **Triad**
    - Arthritis: Inflammation of joints, tendon attachments
    - Eye inflammation: Conjunctivitis and uveitis
    - Urethritis

SJÖGREN'S SYNDROME

- Second most common autoimmune rheumatic disorder (RA is first.)
- 90% = women.
- Mean age = 50 yr.
- **Clinical triad**
    - Xerostomia (dry mouth)
    - Keratoconjunctivitis sicca (dry eyes)
    - Presence of other autoimmune disorder (e.g., SLE or RA)
- Glands ultimately become fibrotic and atrophy
    - Decrease salivation can cause rampant caries because shift to more acidogenic microflora

BEHÇET'S SYNDROME

- Most common in Turkey and Japan.
- Chronic, relapsing inflammatory disease.
- **Clinical**
    - Mouth sores
    - Skin blisters
    - Genital sores
    - Swollen joints
    - Hypopyon: Puslike fluid in the anterior chamber of the eye.
    - Pyodermas: Pus-producing disease of skin.
    - CNS involvement.

Osseous Pathology

OSTEOPOROSIS

- ↓ bone mass.
- Bone thinning (↓ bone density over time) from
    - ↑ bone resorption (osteoclastic)
    - ↓ bone formation (osteoblastic)
    - Both
- **Occurs in**
    - Females > males (F > M)
    - Age approximate 50 yr

Clinical triad with Reiter's = "Can't pee, can't see, can't climb a tree."

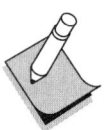

Uveitis = Inflammation of uveal tract of the eye (including iris, ciliary body, and choroids).

Sicca complex =
- Dry eyes (↓ lacrimal secretion).
- Dry mouth (↓ salivary secretion).
- Lymphocytic exocrine gland infiltration.
- Diagnose with two of these three symptoms.

Mikulicz's syndrome = Lymphocytic infiltration causing enlargement of the salivary and lacrimal glands; occurs in association with SLE, Sjögren's, leukemia; ↑ risk lymphoma.

- Clinical
  - Weak, brittle, fragile bones; subject to pathologic fractures (fxs), even in absence of trauma.
- Cause
  - ↓ estrogen in postmenopausal women.
  - ↓ testosterone in men.
- Risks
  - Postmenopausal.
  - Bed rest, immobilization.
  - Hypercoticism.
  - Hyperthyroidism.
  - ↓ calcium.

OSTEOMALACIA

Dental findings in children with Rickets:

- *Delayed eruption.*
- *Malocclusion.*
- *Dentin and enamel defects; ↑ caries.*

Bone softening from vitamin D deficiency =

- *Ricketts (children).*
- *Osteomalacia (adults, growth plates fused).*

- F > M.
- Bone softening secondary to ↓ vitamin D.
  - Osteoid matrix does not calcify without vitamin D.
- Causes of ↓ vitamin D:
  - ↓ dietary intake.
  - ↓ absorption (malabsorption).
  - ↓ sunlight exposure.
  - Hereditary or acquired disorders of vitamin D metabolism.
  - Kidney failure and acidosis.
  - Medication side effects.
  - ↓ phosphate intake.
- Radiologic findings
  - Diffuse radiolucency; mimics osteoporosis.
- Bone biopsy
  - Difficult to distinguish osteoporosis from osteomalacia.
- Clinical
  - Diffuse bone pain, especially hips.
  - Muscle weakness.
  - Fractures with minimal trauma.

RICKETS

- Osteomalacia in children (before growth plates fuse).
- More widespread effects.

Renal osteodystrophy = Osteomalacia secondary to renal disease.

	Ca^{2+}	Phosphorus	Alkaline Phosphate
Osteoporosis	–	–	–/↓
Brown tumor	↑	↓	↑
Rickets/osteomalacia	↓/–	↓/–/↑	↑/–
Paget's disease	–	–	↑↑

OSTEITIS FIBROSA CYSTICA

- Brown tumor = von Recklinghausen disease of bone.
- Bone lesion in hyperparathyroidism.
- Osteolytic lesions.
- Cystic spaces with multinucleated osteoclasts, fibrous stroma, brown discoloration from hemorrhage.
- **Laboratory**
  - ↑ PTH.
  - ↑ Ca^{2+}
  - ↓ Phosphorus.
  - ↑ Alkaline phosphatase.

Alkaline phosphatase is a marker of ↑ osteoblastic activity and bone formation.

PAGET'S DISEASE

- Osteitis deformans
- Metabolic bone disease
- Occurs mostly in the elderly
- Etiology unknown
  - Viral infection
    - possibly with mumps, measles, paramyxovirus
    - Intranuclear osteoclast inclusions
  - Genetic
- **Findings**
  - Cycle of bone destruction and regrowth of abnormal bone.
  - New bone is structurally enlarged, but weakened, filled with new vessels.
- **Sites**
  - Widespread.
  - Localize to one or two areas of skeleton.
    - Pelvis
    - Femur
    - Tibia
    - Vertebrae
    - Clavicle
    - Humerus
    - Skull
      - ↑ head size
      - Foraminal constriction (with CN compression, e.g., hearing loss).
      - Teeth displacement intraorally
- **Laboratory**
  - Anemia.
  - ↑↑ alkaline phosphatase.
  - ↑ urinary hydroxyproline.
- **Risks**
  - ↑ osteosarcomas.

Hydroxyproline is a marker of ↑ osteoclastic hyperactivity.

Note: *↑ serum acid phosphatase level with prostate cancer.*

FIBROUS DYSPLASIA

- Normal bone being replaced by fibrous tissue.
- Unknown etiology.
- **Clinical**
  - Bone enlargement (can be deforming)
  - Pain
  - Fractures

Café au lait spots are associated with

- Neurofibromatosis.
- McCune–Albright syndrome.
- Fanconi's anemia.
- Tuberous sclerosis.

- Three classifications (depending on involvement):
  - **Monostotic:** One bone.
  - **Polyostotic:** Multiple sites (> one bone).
  - **McCune–Albright:** Polyostotic fibrous dysplasia + endocrine abnormality.
    - Precocious puberty.
    - Café au lait spots.
    - Short stature.

OSTEOGENESIS IMPERFECTA

> **Prominent clinical findings of osteogenesis imperfecta:**
> - Blue sclera.
> - Multiple childhood fractures.

- "Brittle bones."
- Hereditary: Autosomal dominant is most common type.
- Defective collagen synthesis.
  - ↓ osteoid production.
  - General connective tissue abnormalities.
- Clinical
  - Skeletal fragility.
  - Thin skin.
  - Weak teeth: Malformation of dentin = dentinogenesis imperfecta.
  - Blue sclera.
  - Macular bleeding tendency.
  - Joint hypermobility.

OSTEOCHONDROSES

All osteochondroses occur M = F, except Freiberg's disease (F > M).

- Groups of diseases in children that cause areas of bone necrosis.
- **Cause**
  - Rapid bone growth/turnover during childhood.
    - ↓ Blood supply to bone (usually epiphyses, growing ends of bones).
      - Avascular necrosis of bone, usually near joints.
  - Necrotic areas self-repair over a period of weeks to months because bone is turning over rapidly (continually rebuilding).
- **Cycle of**
  - Necrosis.
  - Regeneration.
  - Reossification.
- Three common variants and locations:
  - **Articular**
    - Legg–Calvé-Perthes disease: At joints or articulations (e.g., hip).
    - Kohler's disease: Foot.
    - Freiberg's disease: Second toe.
    - Panner's disease: Elbow.
  - **Nonarticular**
    - Osgood–Schlatter disease: Tibia.
  - **Physeal**
    - Scheuermann's disease: Spine of intervertebral joints (physes) (especially chest/thoracic region)

Remember: Achondroplasia (dwarfism) is an autosomal dominant disorder manifesting with short limbs and normal-sized head and trunk.

OSTEOPETROSIS

- Albers–Schonberg disease.
- Autosomal dominant or recessive inheritance.

- **Types**
  - Adult type (mild).
  - Intermediate type.
  - Infantile (severe, often fatal).
- **Findings**
  - ↑ bone density.
    - Overgrowth and sclerosis of bone.
    - Thickening of the cortex.
    - Narrowing or even obliteration of the medullary cavity.
  - Brittle bones.
    - Trivial injuries may cause fractures due to abnormalities of the bone.
  - Skeletal abnormalities, sometimes.
- **Other symptoms**
  - Hepatosplenomegaly
  - Blindness
  - Progressive deafness
- **Cause**
  - Failure of osteoclastic activity

OSTEOMYELITIS

- Bone infection.
- Acute or chronic
- Usually caused by *Staph. aureus*.

ACUTE OSTEOMYELITIS

- Pyogenic bone infection
  - ↓ blood supply to bone
  - Abscess can develop
    - Pus
    - Pyogenic organisms (usually *Staph. aureus*)
  - Sequestrum (necrotic bone)
  - Involucrum (new bone formation surrounding sequestrum)

Etiology

Hematogenous	Direct Spread
Infection in other part of body spreads via blood to bone.	Direct inoculation after trauma, surgery, or nearby soft-tissue infection.

Sites Affected

Children	Adults
Long bones	Vertebra, pelvis

Salmonella osteomyelitis is seen commonly in sickle-cell patients.

Osteomyelitis of the vertebra with TB is called Pott's disease.

Condensing osteitis *(sclerosing osteitis) = Periapical bone reaction/inflammatory response from a low-grade pulpal infection.*

Fat embolism is a complication of bone fractures (usually long bones). Fat in the marrow is mechanically disrupted and enters bloodstream. Can be fatal.

Bisphosphonate medications have been associated with osteonecrosis of the jaws.

- **Symptoms**
  - Pain
  - Redness
  - Swelling of affected area
  - Fever
  - Malaise
- **Risks**
  - Trauma
  - Diabetes
  - Hemodialysis
  - Intravenous drug users (IVDU)
  - Splenectomy
  - Sickle-cell disease

CHRONIC OSTEOMYELITIS

- Longstanding osteomyelitis results in
  - Loss of blood supply.
  - Necrosis of bone tissue.
- Chronic infection can persist for years

FRACTURES

- Break in bone.
- Most common bone lesion.
- Force exerted overcomes bone strength.
  - Often with some surrounding tissue injury
- **Fracture classifications**
  - Complete: Bone broken into two pieces.
  - Greenstick: Bone cracks one side only (not all the way through).
  - Single: Bone broken in one place.
  - Comminuted: Bone is crushed into two or more pieces.
  - Bending: In children; bone bends but doesn't break.
  - Open: Bone pierces the skin.
- **Fracture healing**
  - Three phases:
    - Inflammatory phase: Formation of blood clot.
    - Reparative phase: Characterized by formation of cartilage callus; replaced by bony callus (compact bone).
    - Remodeling phase: Cortex is revitalized.
- Non-union: Fracture fails to heal.
  - Associated with
    - Ischemia: ↓ bone vascularity in some site subject to coagulation necrosis after a fracture.
      - Navicular bone of the wrist.
      - Femoral neck.
      - Lower third of tibia.
    - Excessive mobility: Pseudoarthrosis or pseudojoint may occur.
    - Interposition of soft tissue between the fractured ends.
    - Infection; more likely with compound fractures.
- Malunion
  - Bone heals/unites, but in abnormal position.

Arthritis

OSTEOARTHRITIS

- Degenerative joint disease.
- Most common form of arthritis.
- F > M.
- Age > 50 yr.
- Continual wear and tear (overuse).
  - Chronic inflammation
    - Articular cartilage gradually degenerates
- Overused joints affected:
  - Intervertebral joints
  - Phalangeal joints
  - Knees
  - Hips
- **Symptoms**
  - Those of inflammation:
  - Pain
  - Swelling
  - Stiffness
- **Findings**
  - Eburnation: Bone wearing on bone.
    - Polished, ivory like appearance
  - Osteophytes: Bone spurs.
    - Can break off and float into synovial fluid along with fragments of separated cartilage = *joint mice*.
    - Heberden's nodes: Nodules/bony swellings around DIP joints.
    - Produced by osteophytes at the base of the terminal phalanges.
    - Second or third fingers most oft affected.
  - Bouchard's nodes: Nodules affecting the PIP joints.

> **Remember:** Cardinal signs of inflammation:
> - Rubor (red)
> - Calor (hot)
> - Tumor (swelling)
> - Dolor (pain)

ACUTE GOUTY ARTHRITIS

- Uric acid deposits in the joints.
  - Causes painful arthritis.
    - Joints of feet, especially big toe.
    - Legs.
  - Overlying skin erythema.

GOUT

- M > F.
- ↑ uric acid.
- ↓ uric acid elimination by kidney.
- Inherited form: Disorder of purine metabolism.
  - Uric acid is product of purine metabolism (specifically xanthine metabolism).
- Other forms of gout associated with
  - DM
  - Obesity
  - Sickle-cell anemia
  - Kidney disease
  - Drugs that block uric acid excretion

- Four stages:
  - Asymptomatic
  - Acute
    - Symptoms develop suddenly.
    - Usually involve one or a few joints.
    - Pain begins at night and is throbbing, crushing, excruciating.
    - Joint appears with signs of inflammation (can be confused with infection).
      - Warmth
      - Tenderness
      - Redness (erythema)
      - Painful attack may subside in several days.
      - Recurs at irregular intervals.
      - Subsequent attacks have longer duration.
      - Some progress to gouty arthritis (others may have no further attacks).
  - Intercritical
  - Chronic
- Findings
  - Gouty arthritis.
  - Uric acid kidney stones (in ~25%).

PSEUDOGOUT

Gout = Uric acid deposits in joints.
Pseudogout =
Calciumpyrophosphate deposits in joints.

- Mimics acute gouty arthritis.
- Disorder of intermittent painful arthritis.
  - Deposition of calcium pyrophosphate crystals.
- M = F.
- Older people.

RHEUMATOID ARTHRITIS

Still's disease is type of RA that occurs in young people.

- Chronic inflammatory disease (autoimmune).
- Affects joints and surrounding tissues
  - Synovium
  - Muscles
  - Tendons
  - Ligaments
  - Blood vessels.
- *Proliferative inflammation of synovial membranes*
- Can affect organs systems
- **Demographics**
  - ~1–2% of population is affected
  - F 2.5 > M
  - Age = 25–55 yr (can occur any age)
    - More often in older people
- **Cause**
  - Likely autoimmune
    - Genetic predisposition (association with HLA-DR4)
- **Course**
  - Gradual onset
    - Fatigue
    - Morning stiffness (lasting >1 hr)
    - Diffuse muscle aches
    - Loss of appetite
    - Weakness

Note: *Osteophytes (bone spur) occur in OA **not** RA.*

Remember: *Collagen vascular diseases =*
- RA
- SLE
- Polyarteritis nodosa
- Dermatomyositis
- Scleroderma

- Progress to severe joint pain.
- Warmth
- Swelling
- Tenderness
- Stiffness after inactivity
- Ultimate condition
  - Permanent deformity
  - Ankylosis
  - Possible invalidism

NEUROPATHOLOGY

Neurologic Trauma

	Epidural Hematoma	**Subdural Hematoma**
Site	Overlying dura	Between dura and arachnoid
Vascular structure	Middle meningeal artery	Bridging veins
Time until symptoms develop	Immediate or hours (lucid interval)	Hours or days
CT	Lenticular, biconvex lucency	Crescent-shaped lucency

CONCUSSION

- Diffuse reversible brain injury.
  - Occurs secondary to trauma.
- Immediate and temporary disturbance of brain function.
- **Cause**
  - Shear strain from inertial force.
    - ↑ brain energy demand.
    - ↓ cerebral function (transient); involves reticular formation.
- **Characteristics**
  - Mental status change.
    - Loss of consciousness; resolution ranges from near immediate to several hours.
- **Signs**
  - Confusion
  - Amnesia
  - Headache
  - Visual disturbances
  - Nausea, Vomiting
  - Dizziness
  - Lack of awareness of surroundings
  - Cold perspiration

CEREBRAL INFARCTION

- Stroke = Infarction of cerebrum or other brain part.
- **Causes**

Symptoms with head trauma include:
- Headaches
- Disorientation
- Fluctuating levels of consciousness
- Coma

Epidural hematomas occur in ~1% of head traumas.

Subdural hematomas occur in ~15% head traumas.

Subarachnoid hemorrhage
- Blood in subarachnoid space.
- usually not traumatic (unlike epidural and subdural hematomas).
  - Most are caused by rupture of a saccular aneurysm.
- Prodromal/warning headache.

- **Postconcussion syndrome:** Can be a complication following concussion.
- Persistence of three of the following symptoms:
  - Headache
  - Dizziness
  - Fatigue
  - Irritability
  - Impaired memory and concentration
  - Insomnia
  - Lowered tolerance for noise and light

- Arterial occlusion.
  - Thrombus or embolism (brain or carotid).
  - Bleed; hemorrhagic stroke from rupture of vessel.
- **Symptoms**
  - Depend on area affected.
    - Often include sudden paralysis (hemiparesis) and numbness on side opposite the stroke.

SEIZURES

Epilepsy = Recurrent seizures.

- Temporary abnormal electrical activity of a group of brain cells.
- Usually manifesting as
  - Changed mental state.
  - Tonic or clonic movements.

Partial Seizures	Generalized (Diffuse) Seizures
Simple partial Complex partial	Absence Myoclonic Tonic–clonic (grand mal) Tonic Atonic

Neurodegenerative Diseases

Degenerative Diseases

Parkinson's is characterized clinically by

- Resting tremor.
- Cogwheel rigidity.
- Akinesia.
- Shuffling gait

Multiple sclerosis

- Autoimmune, demyelinating disease characterized by
  - Disparate lesions in time and space.
  - ↓ or blocked nerve transmission.
  - Affects 1:1000.
  - F > M.
  - Usually begins age 20–40.
  - ↑ IgG in CSF.
  - IV interferon ↓ the frequency of relapses.
- Triad
  - Scanning speech.
  - Intention tremor.
  - Nystagmus.

Disease	Signs and Symptoms
Alzheimer's	Dementia in elderly Plaques (amyloid) and neurofibrillary tangles
Pick's	Pick bodies
Huntington's	Autosomal dominant Chorea + dementia
Parkinson's	Lewy bodies Depigmentation of substantia nigra
ALS (amyotrophic lateral sclerosis or Lou Gehrig's disease)	Motor neuron disease
Werdnig–Hoffman	Floppy baby Tongue fasciculations
Poliomyelitis	Lower motor neuron
Shy–Drager syndrome (multiple system atrophy)	Symptoms similar to Parkinson's

Demyelinating Diseases

Disease	Signs and Symptoms
Multiple sclerosis	Damage to white matter Relapsing, remitting Symptoms may include visual changes, hemisensory findings, loss of bladder control
Progressive multifocal leukoencephalopathy (PML)	JC virus Seen in 2–4% of AIDs patients.
Guillain-Barré syndrome (acute idiopathic poylneuritis)	Peripheral nerve demyelination. Motor > sensory.

Myasthenia crisis = Life-threatening weakness in the respiratory muscles; ~10% MG patients.

Eaton–Lambert syndrome
- Similar to MG.
- Autoimmune disease.
- Causes weakness.
- Caused by ↓ release of Ach (**not** auto-antibodies versus Ach receptor, like MG).

Myasthenia Gravis

- MG = Neuromuscular disease.
- Affects 3:10000.
- Any age.
- Common in young women and older men.
- **Characterized by** variable weakness of voluntary muscles.
    - Improves with rest.
    - Worsens with activity.
- **Cause**: Autoimmune.
    - Auto-abs attack Ach receptors on postsynaptic (muscle side) of NMJ.
    - Decreases muscle fiber responsiveness.
- **Note**: Patients with MG have a higher risk of developing other autoimmune disorders.
    - Thyrotoxicosis
    - RA
    - SLE

Thymoma
- Tumor of thymus gland.
- Associated with myasthenia gravis.
- Clinical
    - Dyspnea (difficulty breathing).
        - Secondary to pressure on trachea.
    - Engorgement of deep and superficial neck veins.
        - Secondary to pressure on the SVC.

CHAPTER 23
Neoplasia

Dysplasia	587
Metaplasia	587
Neoplasms	587
INVASION AND METASTASIS	588
Malignant Tumors	589
CARCINOMA	589
SARCOMA	589
Benign Tumors	590
PAPILLOMA	590
ADENOMA	590
BENIGN TUMORS OF MESENCHYMAL ORIGIN	590
CHORISTOMA	590
HAMARTOMA	590
MYXOMA	590
APUDOMA	590
TERATOMA	591
Mutations and Carcinogenesis	591
RADIOSENSITIVITY	592
Neoplasia in Children	592
NEUROBLASTOMA	592
RHABDOMYOSARCOMA	592
Neoplasia in Women	592
LEIOMYOMA	592
BREAST CANCER	593
FIBROCYSTIC DISEASE (OF THE BREAST)	594
Neoplasia in Men	594
PROSTATE CANCER	594
BENIGN PROSTATIC HYPERPLASIA	594
Neoplasia of the Nervous System	595
Neoplasia of the Skin	595
BENIGN SKIN NEOPLASMS	595

Malignant Skin Neoplasms	597
SQUAMOUS CELL CARCINOMA (OF THE SKIN)	597
KERATOACANTHOMA	598
MALIGNANT MELANOMA	599
Lung Cancer	600
BRONCHOGENIC CARCINOMA	600
Gastrointestinal Cancer	601
ESOPHAGEAL CANCER	601
GASTRIC CANCER	601
COLORECTAL CANCER	602
MULTIPLE POLYPOSIS SYNDROMES	603
Neoplasia of the Genitourinary System	603
RENAL CELL CARCINOMA	603
BLADDER CANCER	604
Neoplasia of the Blood and Lymphatic Systems	604
LEUKEMIA	604
LYMPHOMAS	607
MULTIPLE MYELOMA	609
AMYLOIDOSIS	610
HISTIOCYTOSIS X	611
Neoplasia of the Adrenal Gland	611
ADRENAL MEDULLA	611
PHEOCHROMOCYTOMA	611
NEUROBLASTOMA	612
Neoplasia of Bone	612
OSTEOSARCOMA	612
CHONDROSARCOMA	613
MALIGNANT GIANT CELL TUMOR	613
Bone Tumors of Nonosseous Origin	613
EWING'S SARCOMA	613
FIBROSARCOMA	614
CHORDOMA	614

DYSPLASIA

- Nonmalignant cellular growth.
- Can be precursor to malignancy (e.g., cervical dysplasia).
- Reversible
- **Causes**
    - Chronic irritation.
    - Chemical agent.
    - Cigarette smoke.
    - Chronic inflammatory irritation.
    - Chronic cervicitis.
- **Characteristics**
    - Disorganized, structureless maturation and spatial arrangement of cells.
    - Atypical cells without invasion.
        - Pleomorphism (variability in size and shape).
        - ↑ mitoses.
    - Acanthosis in epithelium.
        - Abnormal thickening of prickle cell layer.

Neoplasia = Uncontrolled, disorderly proliferation of cells, resulting in a benign or malignant tumor or neoplasm.

METAPLASIA

- Replacement of one tissue cell type with another.
- Example: Squamous metaplasia.
    - Respiratory epithelium bronchi with long-term smoking.
        - Respiratory epithelium is replaced by squamous epithelium.
    - Barrett's esophagus.
- Associated with chronic irritation (helps host adapt to the stress/irritant).
- Can be associated with vitamin A deficiency.
- Often reversible.

NEOPLASMS

- Abnormal growth, independent of host control mechanisms.
- **Classification**
    - Malignant vs. benign
    - Well- or poorly differentiated
    - Based on appearance
    - Based on tissue of origin

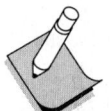

*Metastasis is most import characteristic distinguishing malignant from benign. Benign tumors do **not** invade or metastasize.*

Malignant vs. Benign Tumors

Benign	Malignant
Well-differentiated	Less well-differentiated (anaplastic)
Slow growth	Rapid growth
Encapsulated/well-circumscribed	Invasion
Localized	Metastasis
Movable	Immovable

Benign tumors cause harm by:

- Pressure
- Hormone overproduction
- Hemorrhage following ulcerations of an overlying mucosal surface

They usually do not recur after surgical excision.

Invasion and Metastasis

- Invasion
    - Aggressive infiltration of adjacent tissues by a malignant tumor.
        - Extension into lymphatics and blood vessels.
        - Can lead to metastasis.
    - However, tumor emboli within blood or lymph does **not** = metastasis.
        - Indicates only the penetration of basement membrane.
- Metastasis
    - Spread of tumor to secondary site distant and separate from primary site.
    - Implantation of tumor in distal site.
        - Liver
        - Lung
        - Brain
        - Bone marrow
        - Spleen
        - Soft tissue
- **Multiple steps**
    - Growth and vascularization.
    - Invasion (penetrate basement membrane to reach vessels, lymph).
    - Transport of tumor emboli in circulation (and survival).
    - Collection of tumor emboli in target tissue (again pierce basement membrane).
    - Avoid target tissue defense mechanism.
- **Routes of metastasis**
    - Bloodstream (usually venous at first) (hematogenous).
        - Sarcomas.
    - Lymph.
        - Carcinomas.

Malignant tumors spread by local invasion and metastasis. Metastasis is an absolute indicator of malignancy.

A malignancy will continue to grow even after removal of the irritating agent, as opposed to a benign lesion of inflammatory origin like an irritation fibroma (it may recede when the irritation is removed).

Immunologic response by the host to malignancy is reflected by lymphocytic infiltration at the tumor edge.

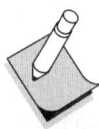

Cathepsin D is involved in invasion and metastasis.

HISTOLOGIC CHARACTERISTICS OF MALIGNANCY

- Anaplasia: Absence of differentiation.
    - Differentiation is a measure of a tumor's resemblance to normal. Tissue.
- Hyperchromatism.
- Pleomorphism.
- Abnormal mitosis.

PROGNOSIS OF MALIGNANT TUMORS

- Depends on:
    - **Degree of localization**
        - Most reliable indicator.
    - **Staging**
        - Helps determine treatment.
        - Helps determine chance for cure.
- Factors for staging:
    - Location of tumor
    - Size
    - Growth into nearby structures
    - Metastasis

Tumor Markers

Marker	Associated Cancer
AFP	Hepatoma / Yolk sac tumor
CEA	Adenocarcinoma
hCG	Choriocarcinoma
Desmin	Rhabdomyosarcoma
LSA	Lymphomas
Enolase	Neuroblastoma

Handwritten annotations: α fetoprotein; carcinoembrionic antigen; human chorionic gonadotropin; lymphocyte specific activity

▶ MALIGNANT TUMORS

Carcinoma

- Malignant tumor of epithelial cell origin.

SQUAMOUS CELL CARCINOMA

- Originates from stratified squamous epithelium.
- Examples: Skin, mouth, esophagus, vagina, bronchial epithelium (squamous metaplasia).
- Histologically marked by keratin production (keratin pearls).

TRANSITIONAL CELL CARCINOMA

- Arises from transitional cell epithelium of urinary tract.

ADENOCARCINOMA

- Carcinoma of glandular epithelium.
- Examples: GI tract glandular mucosa, endometrium, pancreas.
- **Desmoplasia**
  - Tumor-induced proliferation of nonneoplastic fibrous connective tissue.
  - Especially in breast, pancreatic, prostate adenocarcinomas.

Sarcoma

- Malignant tumor of mesenchymal origin.
- Prefix usually denotes tissue of origin.
- Examples:
  - Osteosarcoma (bone) (most common primary malignant tumor of bone).
  - Leiomyosarcoma (smooth muscle).
  - Rhabdomyosarcoma (skeletal muscle).
  - Liposarcoma (adipose).

Remember: Carcinomas usually spread by lymph. Sarcomas spread hematogenously.

▶ BENIGN TUMORS

Papilloma

- From surface epithelium (e.g., skin, larynx, tongue).
- Fingerlike epithelial processes overlying core of connective tissue stroma with blood vessels.
- May also form from transitional epithelium of urinary tract.

Adenoma

- Benign neoplasm of glandular epithelium; several variants.
- **Papillary cystadenoma**
  - Adenomatous papillary processes that extend into cystic spaces (e.g., cystadenoma of ovary).
- **Fibroadenoma**
  - Proliferation of connective tissue surrounding neoplastic glandular epithelium (e.g., fibroadenoma of the breast).

Benign Tumors of Mesenchymal Origin

- **Leiomyoma** (smooth muscle, e.g., uterine fibroid).
  - Most common neoplasm in women.
  - Rhabdomyoma
  - Lipoma
  - Fibroma
  - Chondroma

Choristoma

- Small benign nonneoplastic mass of normal tissue *misplaced* within another organ.
- Example: Pancreatic tissue in stomach wall.

Hamartoma

- Benign tumorlike overgrowth (nonneoplastic) of cell types regularly found in the affected organ
- Example: Hemangioma (accumulation of blood vessels).

Myxoma

- Benign tumor derived from connective tissue.

APUDoma

- Tumor characterized by amine precursor uptake and decarboxylation (APUD).
- Resultant production of hormonelike substances.

Teratoma

- *Can be malignant or benign.*
- Neoplasm comprised of all three embryonic germ cell layers.
    - Including tissues not normally found in the organ in which they arise.
    - May contain skin, bone, cartilage, teeth, hair, intestinal epithelium.
- Occurs:
    - Ovary (most frequently)
        - Mature teratoma = Dermoid cyst in ovary (benign).
    - Testes (can be malignant).

Tumors of Mesenchymal Origin

Benign	Malignant
Leiomyoma	Leiomyosarcoma
Rhabdomyoma	Rhabdomyosarcoma
Lipoma	Liposarcoma
Fibroma	Fibrosarcoma
Chondroma	Chondrosarcoma
Osteoma	Osteosarcoma

▶ MUTATIONS AND CARCINOGENESIS

See also Chapter 8, Molecular Biology.

- Results in alteration in the protein product coded for by the gene.
- Three types of mutation/molecular change:
- **Base substitutions**
    - One base inserted in place of another.
    - Results in either missense *mutation* or a *nonsense mutation*.
- **Frameshift mutations**
    - One or more base pairs are added or deleted.
- **Transposons**
    - Insertion sequences or deletions are integrated into the DNA.

Mutation = Stable, heritable change in the DNA nucleotide sequence.

Causes of Mutagenesis

Cause	Example	Mechanism
Chemicals	Nitrous oxide	Alters existing base
	Alkylating agents	Alters existing base
	Benzpyrene (found in tobacco smoke)	Binds to existing DNA bases and causes frameshift mutations
Ionizing radiation	Gamma and x-rays	Produce free radicals that can attack DNA bases
UV light		Cause cross-linking of adjacent pyrimidine bases to form
Dimers	Thymine dimers	Interfere with DNA replication.
Viruses	Bacterial virus Mu (mutator bacteriophage)	Frameshift mutations or deletions

Radiosensitivity

- Cells with high proliferation are more sensitive to radiation.
  - ↑ mutagenesis.
  - ↑ Response to therapy (with XRT).
- **High radiosensitive cells:** Cells with high turnover; more radiosensitive.
  - Lymphocytes.
  - Bone marrow blood-forming cells.
  - Reproductive cells (gonads).
  - Epithelial cells of GI tract.
- **Low radiosensitivty cells:** Cells with low turnover; more radioresistant.
  - Nerve cells.
  - Mature bone cells.
  - Muscle cells.

> **Sarcoma botryoides** = Embryonal type of rhabdomyosarcoma.
> - Resembles bunches of grades.
> - Protrudes into lumen.

All Neoplasms of muscle are rare; usually malignant when they occur.

▶ **NEOPLASIA IN CHILDREN**

Neuroblastoma

See also Chapter 17, "Endocrine Pathology."

- Most common malignancy in children.
- Usually affects adrenal medulla.

> **Rhabdomyoma**
> - Benign tumor of skeletal muscle.
> - Presents as mass in affected muscle.

Rhabdomyosarcoma

- Malignant tumor of muscle; striated muscle/skeletal.
- Infants/children
  - Throat
  - Bladder
  - Prostate
  - Vagina
- Elderly
  - Large muscle groups of the arm or leg.
  - Prognosis is poor.

Leukemia in children is usually acute lymphoblastic leukemia (ALL).

▶ **NEOPLASIA IN WOMEN**

Leiomyoma

- Uterine fibroid.
- Most common tumor in women
  - 25% of women older than 30 yr during reproductive years.
  - Most common pelvic tumor
  - 15–20% reproductive aged women and 30–40% of women > 30 years old.
  - Benign tumor
  - Derived from smooth muscle.
  - Can occur anywhere in body.
  - Most frequently in uterus (= uterine fibroid).
  - Less often in:
    - Stomach
    - Esophagus
    - Small intestine

*Remember leiomyoma is a **benign** process.*

- **Cause**
  - Unknown.
  - Growth depends on regular estrogen stimulation (reproductive age).
  - Menstruation.
    - Continues to grow as long as patient menstruates (though can grow quite slowly).
    - Fibroids are rare before age 20.
    - Shrink after menopause.
  - ↑ size with estrogen therapy.
    - OCPs (oral contraceptive pills).
    - Pregnancy.
- **Size**
  - Microscopic to macroscopic (e.g., weigh several pounds and fill uterine cavity).
  - Prognosis is good.

Malignant Neoplasia in Women

Cancer Incidence (Highest to Lowest)	Cancer Death (Highest to Lowest)
Breast	Lung
Lung	Breast
Colorectal	Colorectal
Uterine	Leukemia and lymphoma

Breast Cancer

- Most common cancer in women.
  - Rare before age 25.
  - ↑ age until menopause (incidence ↓ postmenopausal).
- **Cause/history**
  - Family history.
    - Strongest association.
    - Specifically in first-degree relatives (mother, sister, daughter).
  - BRCA-1, BRCA-2 genes.
- **Clinical**
  - Painless mass (in breast) (initially).
  - Breast skin or nipple retraction.
  - Peau d'orange (swollen, pitted surface).
  - Enlargement of the axillary lymph nodes (LNs).
  - Left breast > right.
  - Upper outer quadrant.
- **Spread/metastasis**
  - Chest wall.
  - Axillary LNs.
  - Distant metastasis (via lymphatic system and bloodstream) to:
    - Other breast.
    - Liver.
    - Bone.
    - Brain.
- **Histologic type**
  - Usually adenocarcinoma.
- **Prognosis**
  - LN involvement (most valuable prognostic predictor).

> **Breast cancer**
> *Can present as*
> - Axillary mass.
> - Paget's disease of the nipple: Eczematoid lesion.

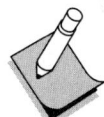

Distinguish breast cancer from fibrocystic disease. The latter is a benign process (but may increase breast cancer risk).

BRCA-1 is associated with both breast and ovarian cancer.

- 10-year survival rate (with adjuvant therapy):
  - Node-negative = 70–75% will survive 10 years or more.
  - Node positive = 20–25% will survive 10 years.

Fibrocystic Disease (of the Breast)

- **Not** malignant, but may ↑ risk of carcinoma.
- Most common cause of a clinically palpable breast mass in women 28–44 yr.
- **Signs/symptoms**
  - Lumpiness throughout both breasts.
  - Pain (especially prior to menstrual period).

▶ NEOPLASIA IN MEN

Lung cancer is the leading cause of cancer death in both men and women.

Distinguish prostate cancer from benign prostatic hyperplasia (BPH). The latter is a benign process, not thought to be premalignant.

Cancer Incidence (Highest to Lowest)	Cancer Death (Highest to Lowest)
Prostate	Lung
Lung	Prostate
Colorectal	Colorectal
Urinary tract	Leukemia and lymphoma

Prostate Cancer

- Common cause of death from cancer in men of all ages.
  - Most common cause of cancer death in men over age 75.
- Rare in men younger than 40.
- **Cause**
  - Unknown.
  - Possibly ↑ testosterone (hormonally dependent).
    - ↑ dietary fat leads to ↑ testosterone.
- **Laboratory**
  - ↑ PSA (prostate-specific antigen).
    - PSA testing helps detect prostate cancers prior to development of symptoms.
  - ↑ acid phosphatase.
- **Histology**
  - Adenocarcinoma
    - Usually arises in gland periphery.
    - May invade entire prostate.
- **Metastasis**
  - Common sites:
    - Bone
    - Lungs

Benign Prostatic Hyperplasia

- Nodular hyperplasia of the prostate.
- Benign enlargement of the prostate.
  - Hyperplastic nodules of stroma and glands (distorting the prostate).
  - This hyperplasia usually occurs in the center of the gland.

- Compresses the urethra.
- Causes urinary difficulty or obstruction.
- **Complications**
  - Pyelonephritis.
  - Hydronephrosis.
  - Painful or difficult urination (dysuria).
- **Not** considered premalignant.

NEOPLASIA OF THE NERVOUS SYSTEM

Brain Tumors

	Tumor	Signs and Symptoms
Adults	Glioblastoma multiforme	Most common primary brain tumor.
	Meningioma	2nd most common primary brain tumor Arises from arachnoid
	Pituitary adenoma	Usually secrete prolactin Can present as bitemporal hemianopia
Children	Craniopharyngioma	Benign Can cause bitemporal hemianopia Derived from Rathke's pouch
	Low-grade astrocytoma	Posterior fossa
	Medulloblastoma	Highly malignant cerebellar tumor Form of PNET (primitive neuroectodermal tumor)
	Ependymoma	Often in the 4th ventricle Can cause hydrocephalus

NEOPLASIA OF THE SKIN

Benign Skin Neoplasms

PIGMENTED NEVI

- **Nevocellular nevus** (common mole) = hamartoma (benign tumor); cluster of nevus cells (derived from melanocytes).
- **Junctional nevus:** Confined to epidermal–dermal junction.
- **Compound nevus:** Occurs at epidermal–dermal junction and in the dermis.
- **Intradermal nevi:** Within the dermis (often not pigmented).

BLUE NEVUS

- Present at birth.
- Nodular foci of dendritic, pigmented melanocytes in dermis.
- Blue appearance (because dermal location).

Spitz Nevus

- Children
- Benign
- Spindle-shaped cells

Dysplastic Nevus

- Atypical, irregularly pigmented lesion.
- Disordered proliferation of melanocytes.
- May transform into malignant melanoma, especially in dysplastic nevus syndrome (autosomal dominant).

Lentigo Naligna

- Precursor to lentigo maligna melanoma.
- Irregular macular pigmented lesion on sun-exposed skin.
- Atypical melanocytes in epidermal–dermal junction.

Basal Cell Carcinoma

Incidence of skin cancer is up, partly due to increased sun exposure (increased UV radiation).

Basal cell carcinoma is considered benign, even though "carcinoma" denotes malignancy.

- Most common skin cancer
  - 75% of all skin cancers
  - Most common form of cancer in U.S
- Derived from basal cells of epidermis
- **Clinical**
  - > 90% occur on sun-exposed areas of head and neck, including upper face.
  - Pearly papule
  - Overlying telangiectatic vessels (often)
  - Locally aggressive
  - Locally invasive and destructive
  - Ulcerate
  - Bleed
  - Nonhealing skin growth
- **Histology**
  - Clusters of darkly staining basaloid cells with a typical palisade arrangement of the nuclei at the periphery of the tumor cell clusters.
- **Prognosis/course**
  - Good when found and treated early.
    - Almost never metastasizes (benign).
    - Cured by surgical excision.
    - Radiosensitive if necessary.
  - When diagnosis or treatment is delayed:
    - Disability
    - Disfigurement
    - Destruction
    - Death (rarely)

Dermatofibroma

- Benign Neoplasms.
- **Clinical**

- Firm, red-brown nodules.
- Armpit or groin (usually).
- **Histology**
  - Acanthosis (sometimes).
  - Intertwining of collagen bundles and fibroblasts.

ACROCHORDON

- Skin tag = fibroepithelial polyp.
- Very common lesion.
- Most common sites:
  - Face (near eyelids).
  - Neck.
  - Armpit (axilla).
  - Groin.

ACTINIC KERATOSIS

- Seborrheic warts.
- Very common benign neoplasm.
- Premalignant epidermal lesion caused by chronic excessive sunlight.
- Older people.
- **Clinical**
  - Rough, scaling, poorly demarcated flesh-colored, brown, or black plaques.
    - "Stuck-on" appearance.
    - Anywhere on the skin, especially, face, neck, upper trunk, or extremities.

▶ MALIGNANT SKIN NEOPLASMS

Squamous Cell Carcinoma (of the Skin)

- Epithelial malignant tumor.
  - More aggressive than basal cell carcinoma.
  - Mean age = 50.
- **Causes**
  - Sun damage: Can arise within actinic keratosis.
  - Radiation
  - X-ray exposure.
  - Chemical carcinogens (e.g., arsenic).
- **Clinical:** Can occur in:
  - Normal skin
  - Damaged skin:
    - Burn
    - Scar
    - Site of chronic inflammation (as with skin disorders)
  - Sun-damaged skin areas (e.g., preexisting areas of actinic keratosis)
    - Face (lower face unlike basal cell carcinoma)
    - Dorsal hands
- **Lesion**
  - Scaling, indurated, ulcerative nodule.
  - Painless initially.
    - Pain may occur as if enlarges or ulcerates.

Skin cancer is the most common malignancy in the U.S.

Most to least common: Basal cell carcinoma > squamous cell carcinoma > malignant melanoma.

Malignant melanoma is the leading cause of death from skin cancer.

Squamous cell carcinoma (SCC) of the skin resembles cervical cancer in histologic appearance and biologic behavior.

- **Course**
- Usually is locally invasive.
  - May be relatively slow growing.
- Metastasis (unlike basal cell carcinoma).
  - < 5% metastasize (lymph).
  - Lymph nodes, internal organs.
- **Histology**
  - Sheets and islands of neoplastic epidermal cells (keratinocytes) in the middle portion of epidermis.
  - Keratin pearls.
- **Molecular properties**
  - Malignant epithelial cells have:
    - ↑ laminin receptors
    - Laminin (a glycoprotein) = Major component of basement membranes.
    - Biological activities:
      - Cell adhesion
      - Migration
      - Growth and differentiation.
- **Treatment**
- Excision usually curative.
- XRT may be used.

Keratoacanthoma

- Common low-grade malignancy.
- Originates in pilosebaceous glands and pathologically resembles SCC.
- Thought to be variant of invasive SCC.
- Was classified as benign, now as malignant.
- **Causes**
  - Sunlight
  - Chemical carcinogens.
  - Trauma
  - Human papilloma virus (HPV).
  - Genetic factors.
  - Immunocompromised status.
- **Clinical**
  - Sun-exposed areas:
    - Face
    - Neck
    - Dorsum of upper extremities.
- **Lesion**
  - Usually solitary.
  - Firm, roundish, skin-colored or reddish papules.
  - Rapidly progress to dome-shaped nodules.
    - Smooth shiny surface.
    - Central crateriform ulceration or keratin plug (that may project like a horn).
- **Course**
  - Rapid growth (over weeks to months), then
  - Spontaneous resolution over 4–6 months in most cases.
  - Can progress (rarely) to invasive or metastatic carcinoma.
- **Treatment**
  - Aggressive excision advocated due to possible progression to squamous cell carcinoma.

Malignant Melanoma
- Malignant tumor of melanocytes or nevus cells
- ↑ in incidence
- Median age 53
- Most common in:
  - Fair-skinned persons
  - Those with blue or green eyes
  - Those with red or blonde hair
- Causes
  - Sunlight exposure.
  - Particularly related to sunburns during childhood.
- Clinical
  - May appear on what was
    - Normal skin.
    - Mole (nevus). Some moles present at birth may develop into melanomas.
    - Other skin area that has changed appearance.
- Four major types:
- **Superficial Spreading**
  - Most common type.
  - Any age or site.
  - Most common in Caucasians.
  - Usually flat and irregular in shape and color; varying shades of black and brown.
- Nodular melanoma
  - Raised/nodular area
  - Blackish-blue or bluish-red (usually), although some lack color
  - Worst prognosis
- Lentigo maligna melanoma
  - Elderly (usually).
  - Develops from preexisting lentigo maligna (Hutchinson freckle).
  - Most common in sun-damaged skin (face, neck, arms).
  - Lesion: Large, flat, and tan with intermixed areas of brown.
- Acral lentiginous melanoma
  - Least common form.
  - Occurs on palms, soles, or under the nails (usually).
  - Most common in African Americans.
- Histology:
- Course
  - Can spread very rapidly.
  - Most deadly form of skin cancer.
  - **Growth phases**
  - **Radial (initial) phase:**
    - Growth in all directions but predominantly lateral (not invading deep).
    - Does not metastasize in this growth phase.
    - Radial growth is characteristic of spreading types.
  - **Vertical (later) phase:**
    - Growth into reticular dermis or beyond (deep).
    - Metastasis may occur.
    - Prognosis varies with depth of lesion.
    - Vertical growth is characteristic of nodular melanoma.

LUNG CANCER

Adenocarcinoma
- Less associated with smoking.
- Arises in periphery, usually in upper lobes.
- Develops in sites of prior pulmonary inflammation or injury:
  - Calcified TB granuloma.
  - Scars
  - Healed infarcts.

- **Metastatic**
  - Most common.
  - From primary tumors that occur elsewhere, then metastasize to the lung.
- **Primary**
  - Bronchogenic carcinoma (usually).

Bronchogenic Carcinoma

- Primary malignant neoplasm of the lung.
  - Develops in the wall or epithelium of the bronchial tree.
- M > F (4:1).
  - 50% of cases are inoperable at diagnosis.
  - Most common cause of cancer in men and women.
- **Causes**
  - Cigarette smoking.
    - Most common etiologic agent.
      - 90% of lung cancers are due to smoking.
      - Especially squamous cell and small cell carcinomas.
    - Benzpyrene is the carcinogen in cigarette smoke.
  - Carcinogenic exposure.
    - Industrial or air pollutants.
  - Familial susceptibility.
- **Clinical**
  - Persistent cough (smoker's cough).
  - Hemoptysis
  - Hoarseness
  - Wheezing
  - Dyspnea
  - Chest pain
  - Weight loss
  - Digital clubbing (fingers and toes)
    - Associated with chronic low oxygen tension
    - Proliferation of distal tissues; nail beds broaden and curve
  - Symptoms related to metastatic spread, especially to brain
- **Prognosis:** 14% survive 5 years + after diagnosis

Metastatic cancer to the lungs
- Via lymphatics
- Most often from:
  - Breast
  - Colon
  - Prostate
  - Kidney
  - Thyroid
  - Stomach
  - Cervix
  - Rectum
  - Testis
  - Bone
  - Skin
  - Brain

Types

Small Cell Carcinoma	Non-Small Cell Carcinoma (NSC)
Oat cell carcinoma (25%)	Squamous cell carcinoma (epidermoid) (35%) Adenocarcinoma (25%) Large cell carcinoma (anaplastic) (15%)

Sites

Peripheral	Central (Smoking-Associated)
Adenocarcinoma Large cell carcinoma	Small cell Carcinoma Squamous cell carcinoma

Pancoast tumor
- Tumor in apical segment of upper lung lobe.
- Hoarseness from compression of recurrent laryngeal nerve.
- Horner syndrome:
  - Ptosis
  - Miosis
  - Anhidrosis
  - From compression of cervical sympathetic plexus

Lung cancers associated with smoking; both arise centrally

Squamous Cell Carcinoma	Small (OAT) Cell Carcinoma
Appears as hilar mass. Often undergoes central cavitation. Paraneoplastic; PTH-like hormone with ↑Ca^{2+}	Most aggressive type bronchogenic carcinoma Highly malignant 80% are men 90% are smokers **Pathology** Oat cell: • Short, bluntly shaped, anaplastic cell • Large, hyperchromatic nucleus • Little or no cytoplasm • Paraneoplastic syndromes; production of ACTH, ADH

Causes of SVC Syndrome

Malignancy	Infection	Other
Bronchogenic carcinomas Lymphomas Leiomyosarcoma Plasmacytoma	Tuberculosis Syphilis Histoplasmosis	Goiter Thrombus Indwelling IV lines Pacemaker wires

▶ GASTROINTESTINAL CANCER

Esophageal Cancer

- **Type (in U.S.)**
- 50% squamous cell carcinoma.
- 50% adenocarcinoma (related to Barrett's esophagus).
- **Clinical findings**
  - Dysphagia
  - Weight loss
  - Anorexia
  - Pain
  - Hematemesis
- **Course**
  - Spreads by local extension.

Gastric Cancer

- Men > age 50.
- Japan
- **Risks**
  - *H. pylori*
  - Nitrosamines

Superior vena cava (SVC) syndrome

- ↓ Venous return from the head, neck, and upper extremities.
- Facial swelling.
- Cyanosis
- Dilation of head and neck veins.
- **Cause:** Compression of SVC
- \> 80% related to malignancy.
  - \> 80% = bronchogenic carcinomas.
    - Those that are located centrally:
      - Small cell carcinoma.
      - Squamous cell carcinoma.

Hypertrophic pulmonary osteoarthropathy

- Unknown etiology.
- Clinical syndrome of
  - Clubbing of the fingers and toes.
  - Enlargement of the extremities.
  - Painful swollen joints.
- X-ray shows new periosteal bone.
- Associated with
  - Bronchogenic carcinoma (not squamous cell).
  - Benign mesothelioma.
  - Diaphragmatic neurilemmoma.

- Salt intake.
- Achlorhydria
- Chronic gastritis.
- **Histology**
  - Adenocarcinoma (most often).
  - Signet-cell rings.
  - Intestinal type.
  - Infiltrating or diffuse carcinoma (linitus plastica).
- **Location**
  - Distal stomach.
    - Antrum, lesser curve, prepylorus.
- **Course**
  - Local spread.
  - LN metastases.
    - Virchow's node (supraclavicular node with metastatic gastric carcinoma).
  - Distant metastasis
    - Krukenberg tumor; metastatic gastric carcinoma to bilateral ovaries.

GASTRIC LYMPHOMA

Colon and rectum are most likely parts of GI to develop cancer.

- 4% malignant gastric tumors.
- Associated with *H. pylori*.
- MALToma
- Better prognosis than adenocarcinoma.

Colorectal Cancer

- Second most common cancer causing death in men.
- Third most common cancer causing death in women.
  - Lung cancer ranks first for both
- Rapidly increasing incidence after age 40.
- **Histology**
  - Adenocarcinoma
- **Cause**
  - No single cause for colon cancer.
  - Tumor progression: Most begin as benign polyps → develop into cancer over many years.
- **Risk factors**
  - Adenomatous polyps.
  - Inherited multiple polyposis syndromes.
  - Long-standing ulcerative colitis.
  - Family history.
  - Low-fiber, high-fat diet.
- **Clinical findings**
  - Rectal bleeding, possibly with diarrhea.
  - Abdominal pain.
  - Weight loss.
- **Site:**
  - Sigmoid colon is most common site.
- **Screening and diagnosis**
  - CEA (carcinoembryonic antigen).
  - Colonoscopy (treatable if caught early by colonoscopy).
  - Left (descending) colon cancers are diagnosed earlier (obstructing) than tumors of right colon (ascending) because they present as obstruction (constipation/obstipation).

Colon Polyps

- Benign polyps.
- Inflammatory polyps.
- Hamartomatous polyps.

Peutz–Jeghers Syndrome

- Hereditary
- Hamartomatous polyps.
  - Not true neoplasms.
  - Many lumps along GI.
    - Colon and small intestine (especially the jejunum).
- Melanin pigmentation of oral mucosa, especially lips and gingiva.
- **Course**
  - Presence of hamartomatous polyps.
  - Does **not** increase risk of GI cancer
    - However, increased risk cancer of pancreas, breast, lung, ovary, uterus.

Multiple Polyposis Syndromes

- Associated with ↑ risk malignant transformation

Familial Polyposis	Gardner's Syndrome	Turcot's Syndrome
Autosomal dominant Multiple adenomatous polyps Risk of malignant transformation is near 100%	True hereditary polyposis; autosomal dominant Numerous adenomatous polyps along intestine Osteomas Soft tissue tumors High risk of colon cancer	Adenomatous polyps + CNS tumors

▶ NEOPLASIA OF THE GENITOURINARY SYSTEM

Renal Cell Carcinoma

- Most common renal malignancy.
- Originates from renal tubules.
- Men 50–70
- Associated with
  - Cigarette smoking
  - Von Hippel–Lindau
- **Clinical**
  - Flank pain
  - Palpable mass
  - Hematuria
  - Erythrocytosis
  - Secondary polycythemia.
    - Tumor secretes erythropoietin.
      - Erythroid line stimulated in bone marrow.

Bladder Cancer

- Transitional cell carcinoma (usually).
- Hematuria

NEOPLASIA OF THE BLOOD AND LYMPHATIC SYSTEMS

Leukemia

- Leukemia = Group of malignancies that begin in the blood-forming cells of the bone marrow (lymphoid or hematopoietic cell origin).

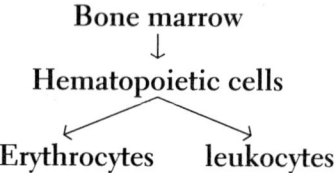

Leukemia can modify the inflammatory reaction.

Leukemia differs from other cancers by beginning in bone marrow and spreading to major organs (as opposed to beginning in major organs then spreading to bone marrow).

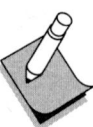

The principle organs involved in leukemia = bone marrow, then the spleen and liver.

LEUKOCYTES IN LEUKEMIA

- Normal leukocyte function
    - Immune cells
    - Fight against infection (viruses, and bacteria)
- Leukemic proliferation of leukocytes
    - ↑ immature leukemic cells.
    - Effects
        - ↓ function of leukocytes.
            - ↑ infection susceptibility.
        - Marrow replacement (↑ leukemic cells = ↓ space for other cell lines in marrow).
        - ↓ RBC (so ↓ O_2 carrying ability).
        - ↓ Platelets (↓ clotting = ↑ bleeding).
        - When ↑↑ leukemic proliferation, overwhelms bone marrow.
        - Leukemic cells into bloodstream.
        - Invade other parts of the body (LNs, spleen, liver, CNS).

LEUKEMIA ETIOLOGY

- Exact cause of leukemias remains unknown
- Evidence points to a combination of factors:
    - Familial tendency.
    - Congenital disorders/genetic predisposition.
        - Down's syndrome (↑ acute leukemias).
        - Philadelphia chromosome (in chronic myelogenous leukemia [CML]).
    - Viral infection
        - Herpes-like viral particles have been cultured.
        - High EBV antibody titers have been seen in leukemic patients.
        - HYLV-1 (adult T-cell leukemia).
    - Ionizing radiation (usually causes myelogenous).
    - Toxin exposures
        - Benzene
        - Alkylating agents.

LEUKEMIA CLASSIFICATION

- Dominant type cell:
  - Myeloid.
  - Lymphocytic.
- Duration from onset to death.
  - Acute
  - Chronic

Of all cases of leukemia, 50% are acute, 50% are chronic (evenly split). However, in children, ALL (acute lymphocytic leukemia) = two thirds of cases.

Leukemia Types

	ALL	AML	CLL	CML
Progression	Rapid	Rapid	Slow	Slow
WBC affected	Lymphocytes	Myelocytes	Lymphocytes	Myelocytes
Age	3–5 yr	Mostly adults	> 60	Any age
% diagnosed per yr	20	27	31	22
Features	Peak age = 4 yr. Form of acute leukemia most responsive to therapy	Responds poorly to treatment (vs. ALL)	2–3 × M > F Abnormal small lymphocytes Lymphoid tissue blood Bone marrow	Young and middle-aged adults. Rare in children. M > F (slightly) Philadelphia chromosome

ACUTE LEUKEMIAS

- Rapid onset (few months).
- Fatal unless treated quickly.
  - No treatment = Die within 6 months.
    - Death is usually due to hemorrhage (brain) or superimposed bacterial infection.
  - Intensive treatment can get remissions up to 5 years.
    - Chemotherapy
    - Radiation
    - Bone marrow transplants.
- Immature abnormal cells.
  - ↓ immune system functions.
  - ↓ bone marrow production of erythrocytes, platelets.
  - ↑ leukemic cells spill from bone marrow into peripheral blood and invade:
    - Liver
    - Spleen
    - Lymph nodes
    - Other parenchymal organs.
- **Clinical**
  - Anemia (usually severe).
    - Fatigue
    - Malaise

AML (acute myelogenous leukemia) and CLL (chronic lymphocytic leukemia) are the most common types of leukemia in adults.

In 75% of cases of ALL, the lymphocytes are neither B- nor T-cells and are called "null cells."

- ↑ infection.
  - No functioning granulocytes.
  - ↑ Bacterial infections are common.
  - ↑ bleeding (thrombocytopenia)
  - Petechiae and ecchymosis (in skin and mucous membranes).
  - Hemorrhage from various sites.
- Leukemic infiltration of organs.
  - Lymphadenopathy (enlarged LNs)
  - Splenomegaly (enlarged spleen)
  - Hepatomegaly (enlarged liver)
- Fever
- Bone and joint pain (common in children).
- **Laboratory**
  - Leukocytosis.
    - Leukocyte counts vary greatly in acute leukemias.
      - 30,000–1 million/mm^3.
      - Immature forms (myeloblasts and lymphoblasts) predominating.
    - ↑ ESR.

CHRONIC LEUKEMIAS

- Slower onset of progression.
- Longer, less devastating clinical course (versus acute leukemias).
  - CML median survival time is 4 years.
    - Death due to hemorrhage or infection.
  - CLL has a variable course.
    - Older patients may survive even without treatment
- Affected cells are more mature.
  - Perform some of their duties, but not well.
  - These abnormal cells proliferate at a slower rate.
    - Accounts for the slower disease progression.
- **Clinical**
  - Insidious onset (often diagnosed during examination for some other condition)
  - Weight loss
  - Anemia
    - Weakness/fatigue.
    - Malaise
    - **Note:** Lymphocytic anemia may be complicated by autoimmune hemolytic anemia.
  - ↑ infection
    - ↑ bacterial infections are common.
  - ↑ bleeding (thrombocytopenia)
    - Petechiae and ecchymosis (in skin and mucous membranes)
    - Hemorrhage from various sites (unexplained)
  - Leukemic infiltration of organs
    - Lymphadenopathy (enlarged LNs) (primary finding in CLL)
    - Massive Splenomegaly (enlarged spleen) (characteristic of CML)
    - Hepatomegaly (enlarged liver)
- **Laboratory**
  - Leukocytosis > 10,000/mm^3.
  - Mature forms on blood smear (granulocytes and lymphocytes predominating).

- CML
  - Philadelphia chromosome.
  - Low levels of leukocyte alkaline phosphatase.

Chronic Myelogenous Leukemia (CML)

- 90% of patients with CML have the Philadelphia chromosome.
- **Philadelphia chromosome** = Remnant of chromosome 22 + small segment of 9.
- Translocation:
  - Long arm of chromosome 22 (*bcr* [oncogene]).
  - Chromosome 9 (*c-abl* [proto-oncogene]).
- **Caused by:**
  - Radiation
  - Carcinogenic chemicals
- **Characterized by:**
  - ↑ granulocytic precursors (myeloblasts and promyelocytes).
    - Bone marrow.
    - Peripheral blood.
    - Body tissues.
  - Most common in young and middle-aged adults.
  - Men > women (slightly).
  - Rare in children.
- **Course**
  - Two distinct phases:
    - Insidious chronic phase: Anemia and bleeding disorders.
    - Blastic crisis or acute phase: Rapid proliferation of myeloblasts (the most primitive granulocyte precursors).
  - CML is invariably fatal.

Lymphomas

- Lymphoid neoplasms.
- **Hodgkin lymphoma** (Hodgkin disease)
- **Non-Hodgkin lymphoma**
  - B-cell neoplasms
  - T-cell neoplasms

Hodgkin Lymphoma

- Hodgkin's disease (HD).
- Cause unknown.
- **Theories**
  - Inflammatory or infectious process that becomes a neoplasm.
  - Immune disorder primarily.
  - M > F (2:1).
  - Usually between ages 15 and 35.
- **Signs/symptoms**
  - Painless lymph node enlargement (usually first sign).
    - Rubbery on exam.
    - Often without obvious/known cause.
  - Constitutional signs and symptoms may be present:
    - Fever
    - Diaphoresis

Hodgkin's lymphoma is characterized by painless, progressive enlargement of lymphoid tissue. Reed–Sternberg cells are the pathognomonic histological finding and are the actual malignant cells.

Hodgkin's lymphoma is classified as follows:
- Lymphocyte-rich (classical) Hodgkin's lymphoma.
- Mixed cellularity Hodgkin's lymphoma.
- Lymphocyte-depleted Hodgkin's lymphoma.
- Nodular sclerosis Hodgkin's lymphoma.

- Anorexia
- Weight loss
- Pruritis
- Low-grade fever
- Night sweats
- Anemia
- Leukocytosis
  - Can spread
    - Adjacent LNs
    - Extranodal organs
      - Lungs
      - Liver
      - Bones or bone marrow
  - Splenomegaly is common
- **Histology**
  - **Reed–Sternberg cells** (pathognomonic for HD).
    - Binucleated or multinucleated giant cells.
    - = the actual neoplastic cells.
- Prognosis is favorable with early diagnosis and limited involvement.
  - Lymphocyte predominance is linked with favorable prognosis.

Non-Hodgkin's Lymphoma (NHL)

NHLs can also be classified by morphology and clinical behavior as low-, intermediate-, or high-grade.

NHL is similar clinically to HD but Reed–Sternberg cells are not present (also the specific mechanism of LN destruction is different). So, biopsy differentiates NHL (malignant lymphoma) from HD.

- Malignant lymphoma.
- Heterogeneous group of malignant disease originating in lymph nodes or other lymphoid tissue
- Cause is unknown; some suggest a viral source.
- M > F (2–3:1).
- All ages
- **Signs/symptoms**
  - Lymph Node or other lymph tissue (e.g., tonsils or adenoids) (first indication).
  - Painless rubbery nodes in cervical or supraclavicular areas.
  - Symptoms specific to the area involved (as the lymphoma progresses).
- **Systemic signs/symptoms**
  - Fatigue
  - Malaise
  - Weight loss
  - Fever
  - Night sweats
  - Circumscribed solid tumor masses.
    - Composed of primitive cells or cells resembling lymphocytes, plasma cells, or histiocytes
- **Classification:** By cell type.
  - B-cell (85%).
    - Hairy cell leukemia
    - MALT lymphoma
    - Follicular lymphoma
    - Mantle cell lymphoma
    - Diffuse large cell lymphoma
    - Burkitt's lymphoma
  - T-cell (15%)
    - Adult T-cell leukemia (HTLV1+)
    - Mycosis fungoides (Sezary syndrome)

BURKITT'S LYMPHOMA

- High grade (aggressive) B-cell lymphoma (classified as a NHL).
  - Defective B-lymphocytes.
  - LNs tend to be spared.
  - **Etiology**
  - Closely linked to EBV infection (especially the African variety).
  - Closely related to B-ALL (acute lymphoblastic leukemia).
  - Cytogenic change = t(8; 14).
- **African type**
  - Middle African regions.
  - Large jaw mass.
  - Closely associated with EBV (95% of cases).
- **American type**
  - Abdominal mass.
  - Less closely associated with EBV.

There is a relationship between diffuse lymphocytic lymphoma and chronic lymphocytic lymphoma (CLL).

MYCOSIS FUNGOIDES

- Rare persistent slow-growing type of NHL that originates from a mature T-lymphocyte and affects the skin.
- **Clinical**
  - Skin lesions
    - Erythematous, eczematoid, or psoriasiform lesion.
    - Progress to raised plaques then to a tumor stage.
- **Histology**
  - Atypical CD4+ T cells with cerebriform nuclei.
  - *Pautrier microabscesses:* Small pockets of tumor cells within epidermis.
  - May progress to LNs and internal organs.

Multiple Myeloma

- ~1% of all cancers.
- Mostly in men > 40.
- Cancer of plasma cells.
  - Arises in the bone marrow.
- ↑ **Plasma cells**
  - Interferes with other bone marrow cell lineages.
    - ↓ RBC: Anemia.
    - ↓ platelets: Bleeding.
    - ↓ WBC: ↑ infection.
  - Abnormally functioning plasma cells: ↑ infection.
- **Osteolytic lesions**
  - As plasma cell proliferation ↑↑; expand in the bone marrow.
  - X-rays = "Punched-out" appearance.
    - Flat bones
    - Vertebrae
    - Skull
    - Mandible
    - Pelvis
    - Ribs
  - Severe, constant back and rib pain (early diagnostic sign).
    - ↑ with exercise.

Presence of Bence–Jones protein in the urine usually confirms the diagnosis of multiple myeloma. However, absence of Bence–Jones protein does not rule out multiple myeloma (sensitive but not specific).

Death in patients with multiple myeloma is most commonly related to the increased susceptibility to infection.

- ↑ at night.
- Pain is caused when malignant plasma cells create pressure on the nerves in the periosteum.
- Pathologic bone fractures can occur.
- **Renal failure**
  - Hypercalcemia (from bone destruction) leading to hypercalciuria.
  - Bence–Jones proteins (in the urine; is a diagnostic finding).
    - Caused by light chain dimers.
- **Amyloidosis**
  - May be seen in multiple myeloma.
  - Can also contribute to renal failure.

Amyloidosis

- Rare, chronic disease.
- Affects adults (middle-aged and older).
- Accumulation of abnormal fibrillar scleroprotein (amyloid).
  - Deposited in various organs and tissues of the body.
  - Organ function is eventually compromised (e.g., renal disease is a frequent manifestation.)
- Disease states associated with amyloidosis may be
  - Inflammatory
  - Hereditary
  - Neoplastic
- Deposition of amyloid may be
  - Local
  - Generalized
  - Systemic

Congo red stains amyloid.

Deposits of amyloid (amylin) in islet cells can cause DM-2.

	Primary Amyloidosis	**Secondary Amyloidosis**	**Hereditary Amyloidosis**
Cause	Unknown cause Associated w/plasma cell abnormalities Abnormal Ig production Multiple Myeloma	Secondary to another disease: - TB - RA - Familial Mediterranean fever - Alzheimer's disease - DM-2	Autosomal dominant Mutation of transtyretin protein Portugal, Sweden, and Japan
Sites of deposition	Heart Lung Skin Tongue Thyroid gland GI tract Liver Kidney Blood vessels	Spleen Liver Kidneys Adrenal glands Lymph nodes Heart rarely involved	Nerves GI tract

Histiocytosis X

- Langerhans cell histiocytosis, differentiated histiocytosis.
- Group of disorders characterized by abnormal ↑ histiocytes.
- **Treatment**
    - Radiation
    - Chemotherapy
- **Prognosis:** Poor

Histiocytes are immune cells include:

- Monocytes
- Macrophages
- Dendritic cells

Haberman's disease is **not** one of the histiocytosis X diseases. It a skin condition that manifests as sudden eruption polymorphous skin macules, papules, and occasionally vesicles with hemorrhage.

	Eosinophilic Granuloma	Letterer–Siwe Disease	Hand–Schuller–Christian Disease
Epidemiology	Most benign form Males ~20 yr	Fatal Infants < 2 yr	Early age (< 5 yr) Boys > girls
Clinical	Asymptomatic Local pain Mouth swelling Mandible most often affected Mobile teeth Periodontal inflammation	Skin rash Persistent fever, malaise Anemia Hemorrhage Splenomegaly Lymphadenopathy Localized tumefactions over bones Oral lesions uncommon	Triad of symptoms: Exophthalmos DI Bone destruction (skull and jaws affected) Oral signs: Halitosis (bad breath) Sore mouth Loose teeth

▶ NEOPLASIA OF THE ADRENAL GLAND

Adrenal Medulla

- **Tumors of the adrenal Medulla**
    - Pheochromocytoma
    - Neuroblastoma
- **Findings**
    - ↑ catecholamines

Pheochromocytoma

- Chronic chromaffin-cell tumor
    - Benign, usually
- Uncommon
- Affects men or women of any age
    - Most often ages 30–60
- Results in ↑catecholamines
    - ↑epinephrine and norepinephrine
- **Clinical**
    - Persistent or paroxysmal HTN (secondary HTN)
    - ↑ metabolism
    - Hyperglycemia

Pheochromocytoma may be associated with:

- MEN (multiple endocrine neoplasia) syndromes.
- Neurofibromatosis (von Reckinghausen's disease).
- Von Hippel–Lindau disease (multiple hemangiomas).

Catecholamine-secreting extra-adrenal chromaffin cell tumor = Paraganglioma.

Neuroblastoma

- Most common malignant tumor of childhood and infancy
- Adrenal medulla (most common site)
- **Etiology**
  - *N-myc* oncogene amplification.
- **Clinical presentation**
  - Abdominal mass.
    - Abdominal distention.
    - Sensation of fullness.
    - Abdominal pain.
  - 80% of neuroblastomas are productive of catecholamines.
    - ↑ epinephrine
    - ↑ HR
    - ↑ anxiety
- **Complications**
  - Invasion of abdominal viscera
  - Direct spread.
  - Metastasis to liver, lung, or bone.

▶ NEOPLASIA OF BONE

Osseous bone tumors arise from bony structure itself. Nonosseous tumors arise most often from hematopoietic, vascular, or neural tissues.

Bone Tumors

Primary Bone Tumors	Metastatic Bone Tumors
Rare (<1% all malignant tumors) M > F, young men ▪ Osteosarcoma	Majority of bone tumors Secondary; seeds from primary site ▪ Breast ▪ Lung ▪ Prostate ▪ Kidney ▪ Thyroid

Osseous	Nonosseous
Osteosarcoma Parosteal osteosarcoma Chondrosarcoma (actually from cartilage) Malignant giant cell tumor	Ewing's Chordoma Fibrosarcoma

Most common symptom of bone tumor = Bone pain.
- *Dull.*
- *Usually localized.*
- *↑ at night.*
- *↑ with movement.*

Most common type of bone tumors in children are
- *Osteosarcoma (osteogenic sarcoma).*
- *Ewing's sarcoma.*

Osteosarcoma

- Most common primary tumor of bone
- Malignant tumor
- Mesenchymal origin (bone)
  - Arise from osteoblast and osteoclasts
- Males 10–30
- **Common sites:**
  - Femur
  - Tibia
  - Humerus

- **Less frequent sites:**
  - Fibula
  - Ileum
  - Vertebra
  - Mandible

PAROSTEAL OSTEOSARCOMA

- Women aged 30–40.
- Most often affects the distal femur.
  - May occur in the humerus, tibia, ulna.
- Develops on bone surface.
  - Not endosseous (interior).
- Progresses slowly.

Chondrosarcoma

- Males aged 30–50.
- Arises from cartilage.
- **Common sites**
  - Pelvis
  - Proximal femur
  - Ribs
  - Shoulder girdle
- **Clinical**
  - Usually painless
- **Course**
- Grows slowly
- Locally recurrent and invasive

Malignant Giant Cell Tumor

- Females aged 18–50.
- Arises from benign giant cell tumor.
- **Most common site:** Long bones, especially knee area.

▶ BONE TUMORS OF NONOSSEOUS ORIGIN

Ewing's Sarcoma

- Nonosseous malignant bone tumor.
- Children
  - Usually males aged 10–20 yr.
  - Usually develops during puberty when bones are growing rapidly.
- Sites
  - Originates in bone marrow; invades long and flat bones.
  - Long bones upper and lower extremities
    - Femur
    - Tibia
    - Fibula
    - Humerus
  - Pelvis/innominate bones
  - Ribs

Ewing's is very radiosensitive.

- Vertebra
- Skull
- Facial bones
- **Histology**
  - Innominate; difficult to distinguish from neuroblastoma and reticulum cell sarcoma.
- **Symptoms**
  - Few symptoms
  - Pain: ↑ severity and persistence with time
  - Swelling at site
  - Fever
  - Pathologic fractures
- **Course**
  - Metastasis
  - One third of children have metastases at time of diagnosis.
  - To lungs and other bones.

Fibrosarcoma

- Males 30–40 yr
- **Sites**: Originates in fibrous tissue of bone
  - Invades long or flat bones:
    - Femur
    - Tibia
    - Mandible
  - Invades periosteum and overlying muscle.

Chordoma

- Males 50–60 years old.
- Derived from embryonic remnants of notochord.
- Slowly progressive.
- **Sites**
  - End of spinal column
  - Vertebra
  - Sacrococcygeal region
  - Spheno-occipital region
- **Symptoms** (depending on site)
  - Constipation
  - Visual disturbances

SECTION 4
Dental Anatomy and Occlusion

▶ Tooth Morphology
▶ Eruption
▶ Occlusion and Function
▶ Tooth Anomalies

CHAPTER 24
Tooth Morphology

Dental Anatomy	618
CLASSIFICATION OF DENTITIONS	618
DENTAL ANATOMIC TERMINOLOGY	618
INNERVATION	621
BLOOD SUPPLY	621
Permanent Tooth Form	621
GENERAL CONCEPTS	623
MAXILLARY PERMANENT TEETH	627
MANDIBULAR PERMANENT TEETH	633
Primary (Deciduous) Tooth Form	640
GENERAL CONCEPTS	640
MAXILLARY PRIMARY TEETH	642
MANDIBULAR PRIMARY TEETH	644

> **DENTAL ANATOMY**

Classification of Dentitions

BY MORPHOLOGY

- Homodont dentition: All teeth have the same morphology.
- Heterodont dentition: Teeth have different morphology (e.g., humans).

BY SETS OF TEETH

- Monophyodont dentition: One set of teeth.
- Diphyodont dentition: Two sets of teeth (e.g., humans).
- Polyphyodont dentition: Multiple sets of teeth.

Dental Anatomic Terminology

TOOTH LOCATION

- Anterior teeth: Incisors and canines. 12 total (6 per arch).
- Posterior teeth: Premolars and molars. 20 total (10 per arch).

CROWN TYPES

- Anatomic crown: The portion of the tooth that extends from the cementoenamel junction (CEJ) to the incisal edge or occlusal surface (enamel-covered portion of the tooth).
- Clinical crown: The portion of the tooth that extends incisally or occlusally from the gingival margin (clinically visible portion of the tooth).

CHEWING SURFACES

- Incisal edge: The chewing surface of anterior teeth.
- Occlusal surface: The chewing surface of posterior teeth consisting of cusps, ridges, and grooves.
- Occlusal table: The occlusal surface within the cusp and marginal ridges.

ENAMEL SURFACE ELEVATIONS

- Lobe: The primary center of enamel formation in a tooth. In fully formed teeth, lobes are represented by cusps, mamelons, and cingula, and are separated by developmental depressions (anterior teeth) or developmental grooves (posterior teeth).
- Mamelon: A round extension of enamel on the incisal edge of all incisors. (See Figure 24–1.) There are usually three mamelons per incisor (one for each facial lobe). They are often translucent because of a lack of underlying dentin. Mamelons are typically worn down by attrition and mastication; thus, their presence in adults is an indication of malocclusion.
- Cingulum: A bulbous convexity of enamel located on the cervical third of the lingual surface of all anterior teeth.

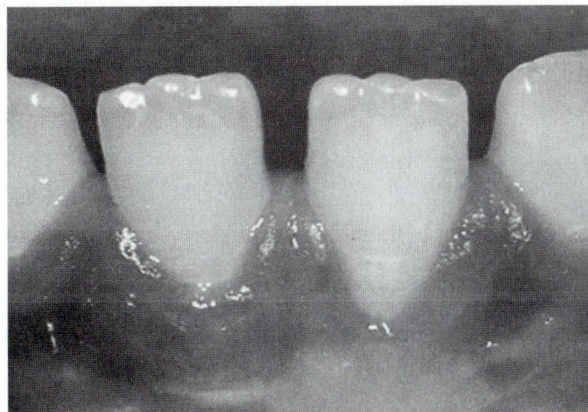

FIGURE 24-1. Mamelons.

- **Cusp:** A large elevation of enamel located on the occlusal surface of all posterior teeth and the incisal edge of canines.
- **Tubercle:** An extra formation of enamel on the crown of a tooth. Often manifests as a supernumerary cusp, such as the **cusp of Carabelli.**

RIDGES

See Figures 24–2 and 24–3.

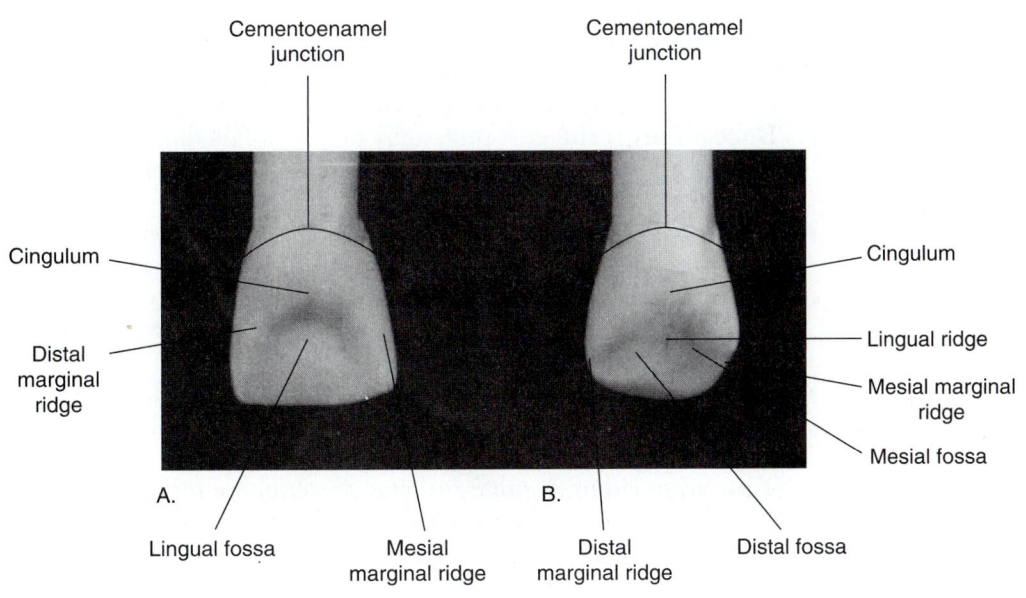

A. Maxillary right central incisor
B. Maxillarly right canine

FIGURE 24-2. Occlusal landmarks of two anterior teeth.

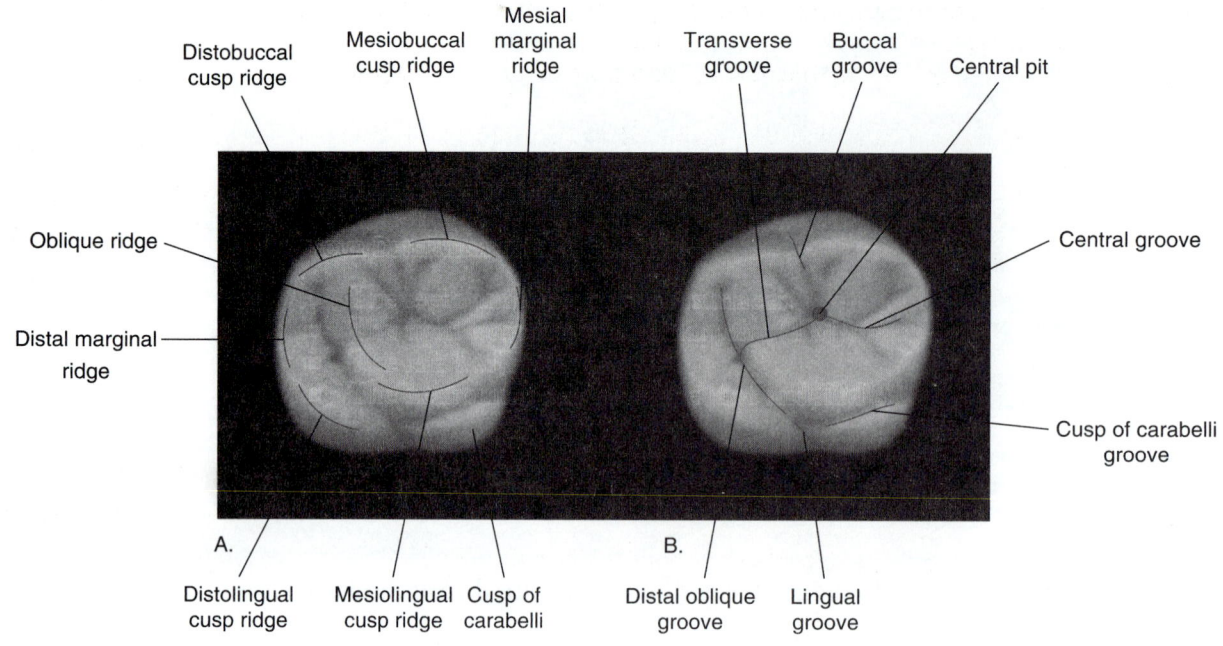

FIGURE 24-3. Occlusal landmarks of a posterior tooth.

A. Maxillary right 1st molar — ridges
B. Maxillary right 1st molar — grooves.

- **Ridge:** A linear elevation on the enamel surface.
- **Marginal ridge:** A ridge on *all teeth* that forms the mesial and distal margins of posterior occlusal surfaces and anterior lingual surfaces.
- **Labial ridge:** A ridge *only on canines* that runs incisocervically in the center of the facial crown surface. More prominent in maxillary canines.
- **Buccal (cusp) ridge:** A ridge *only on premolars* that runs occlusocervically in the center of the buccal crown surface. More prominent in first premolars.
- **Cervical ridge:** A ridge on *all primary teeth* and *permanent molars* that runs mesiodistally in the cervical third of the buccal surface of the crown.
- **Oblique ridge:** A ridge on *all maxillary molars* that extends from the mesiolingual (ML) to distobuccal (DB) cusps (it separates the mesiobuccal (MB) and distolingual (DL) cusps).
- **Triangular ridge:** A ridge on *all posterior teeth* that extends from the cusp tip to the central groove. The ML cusp of all maxillary molars has two triangular ridges.
- **Transverse ridge:** A ridge on *most posterior teeth* that runs buccolingually and connects opposing buccal and lingual triangular ridges. Most common on maxillary premolars and mandibular molars.

ENAMEL SURFACE DEPRESSIONS

- **Sulcus:** A V-shaped depression on the occlusal surface of posterior teeth between ridges and cusps.
- **Fossa:** An irregularly shaped depression in the enamel surface.

- **Developmental groove:** A well-defined, shallow, linear depression in enamel that separates the cusps, lobes, and marginal ridges of a tooth.
- **Fissure:** A narrow crevice at the deepest portion of the developmental groove in enamel.
- **Pit:** A small pinpoint concavity at the termination or junction of developmental grooves.
- **Supplemental groove:** An irregularly defined, short groove auxiliary to a developmental groove that does not separate major tooth parts.

ENAMEL SURFACE JUNCTIONS

- **Line angle:** An angle formed by the junction of *two* surfaces.
- **Point angle:** An angle formed by the junction of *three* surfaces.

INTERDENTAL SPACES

- **Contact area:** The location at which the proximal surfaces of adjacent teeth make contact.
- **Diastema:** A space between two adjacent teeth in an arch.
- **Embrasure:** A triangular space between the proximal surfaces of adjacent teeth that diverge in four directions from the contact area.
- **Interproximal space:** The cervical embrasure. In health, this space is completely filled with the gingival papilla.

INTRADENTAL SPACES

- **Furcation:** The area of a multirooted tooth where the roots diverge.

Innervation

Figure 24–4 illustrates the nerve supply to the teeth and gingiva.

- All dental and periodontal innervation arises from the **trigeminal nerve (CN V).**
- The maxillary nerve (V-2) supplies the maxillary teeth.
- The mandibular nerve (V-3) supplies the mandibular teeth.

Blood Supply

ARTERIAL SUPPLY

- All dental and periodontal arterial supply arises from the **maxillary artery.**
- The arterial supply generally parallels the corresponding nerves.

VENOUS RETURN

- All dental and periodontal venous return drains to the **pterygoid plexus of veins,** which eventually forms as the **maxillary vein.**

▶ PERMANENT TOOTH FORM

Table 24–1 compares the important characteristics of each permanent tooth.

Caries is most likely to occur in pits, fissures, and grooves. The teeth least likely to be lost to caries are mandibular incisors.

Anterior teeth have six line angles; posterior teeth have eight line angles. All teeth have four point angles.

There are four embrasures per contact area: buccal, lingual, occlusal, cervical. The cervical embrasure is also known as the interproximal space.

Maxillary molars are generally trifurcated; mandibular molars are generally bifurcated.

The DB root of the maxillary first molar is innervated by the posterosuperior alveolar nerve; the MB root receives its nerve supply from the middle superior alveolar nerve.

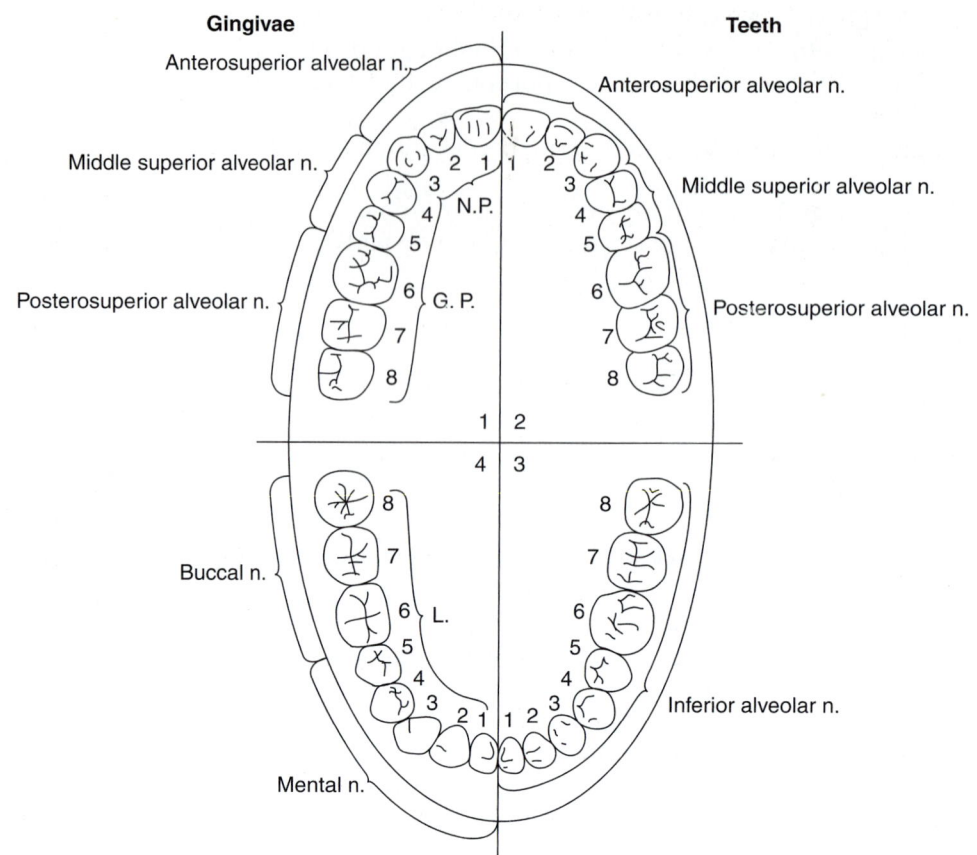

FIGURE 24-4. Nerve supply to maxillary and mandibular dental arches.

Reprinted, with permission, from Liebgott B. *The Anatomical Basis of Dentistry*. Toronto: BC Decker, 1986.

TABLE 24-1. Comparison of Permanent Tooth Forms

| | INCISO-CERVICAL DIRECTION | | | | ROOT LENGTH (MM) | CROWN LENGTH (MM) | # OF LOBES | # OF CUSPS | # OF ROOTS | # OF ROOT CANALS |
	MESIAL CONTACT	DISTAL CONTACT	FACIAL HOC	LINGUAL HOC						
				Maxilla						
Central incisor	Incisal 1/3	Junction	Cervical 1/3	Cervical 1/3 (cingulum)	13	10.5	4	1	1	1
Lateral incisor	Junction	Middle 1/3	Cervical 1/3	Cervical 1/3 (cingulum)	13	9	4	1	1	1
Canine	Junction	Middle 1/3	Cervical 1/3	Cervical 1/3 (cingulum)	17	10	4	1	1	1
First premolar	Middle 1/3	Middle 1/3	Cervical 1/3	Middle 1/3	14	8.5	4	2	2	2

TABLE 24-1. Comparison of Permanent Tooth Forms (Continued)

	INCISO-CERVICAL DIRECTION		FACIAL HOC	LINGUAL HOC	ROOT LENGTH (MM)	CROWN LENGTH (MM)	# OF LOBES	# OF CUSPS	# OF ROOTS	# OF ROOT CANALS
	MESIAL CONTACT	DISTAL CONTACT								
Second premolar	Middle 1/3	Middle 1/3	Cervical 1/3	Middle 1/3	14	8.5	4	2	1	1
First molar	Middle 1/3	Middle 1/3	Cervical 1/3	Middle 1/3	12–13	7	5	4 or 5	3	3 or 4
Second molar	Middle 1/3	Middle 1/3	Cervical 1/3	Middle 1/3	11–12	6.5	4	4	3	3 or 4
Third molar	Middle 1/3	N/A	Cervical 1/3	Middle 1/3	11	6	4 or 5	3	3	3
Mandible										
Central incisor	Incisal 1/3	Incisal 1/3	Cervical 1/3	Cervical 1/3 (cingulum)	12.5	9	4	1	1	1
Lateral incisor	Incisal 1/3	Incisal 1/3	Cervical 1/3	Cervical 1/3 (cingulum)	14	9.5	4	1	1	1 or 2
Canine	Incisal 1/3	Middle 1/3	Cervical 1/3	Cervical 1/3 (cingulum)	16	11	4	1	1 or 2	1
First premolar	Middle 1/3	Middle 1/3	Cervical 1/3	Middle 1/3	14	8.5	4	2	1	1
Second premolar	Middle 1/3	Middle 1/3	Cervical 1/3	Middle 1/3	14.5	8	5	2 or 3	1	1
First molar	Middle 1/3	Middle 1/3	Cervical 1/3	Middle 1/3	14	7.5	5	5	2	3 or 4
Second molar	Middle 1/3	Middle 1/3	Cervical 1/3	Middle 1/3	13	7	4	4	2	3 or 4
Third molar	Middle 1/3	N/A	Cervical 1/3	Middle 1/3	11	7	4 or 5	4 or 5	2	2 to 4

General Concepts

Tooth Numbering

See Figures 24–5 through 24–7.

- There are 32 permanent teeth (16 per arch).
- Teeth are numbered 1 through 32.

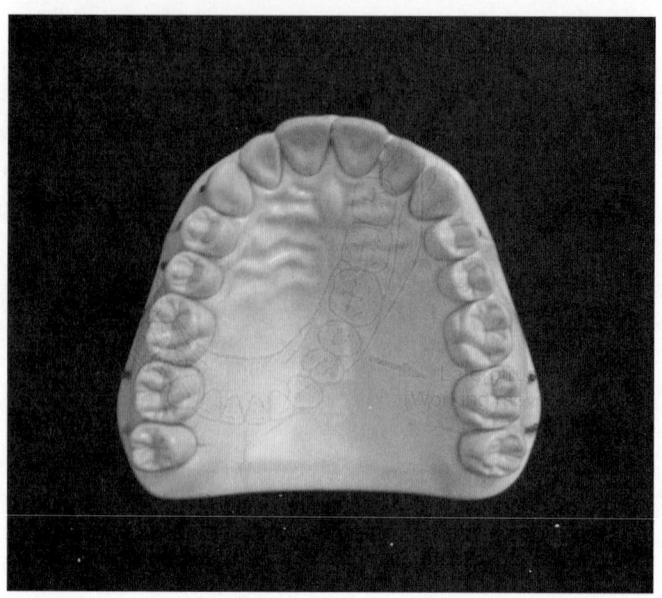

FIGURE 24-5. The maxillary arch.

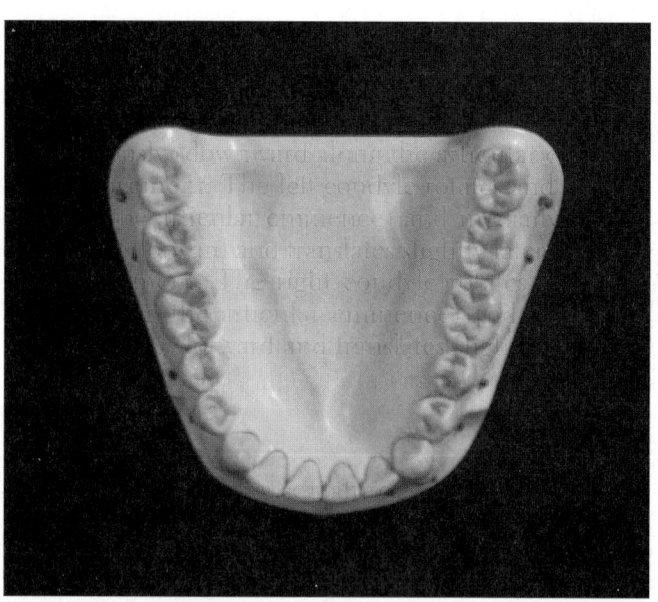

FIGURE 24-6. The mandibular arch.

```
                              Max
         1  2  3  4  5  6  7  8 | 9  10 11 12 13 14 15 16
Right  ─────────────────────────┼──────────────────────────── Left
        32 31 30 29 28 27 26 25 | 24 23 22 21 20 19 18 17
                              Mand
```

FIGURE 24-7. Tooth numbering of the permanent dentition.

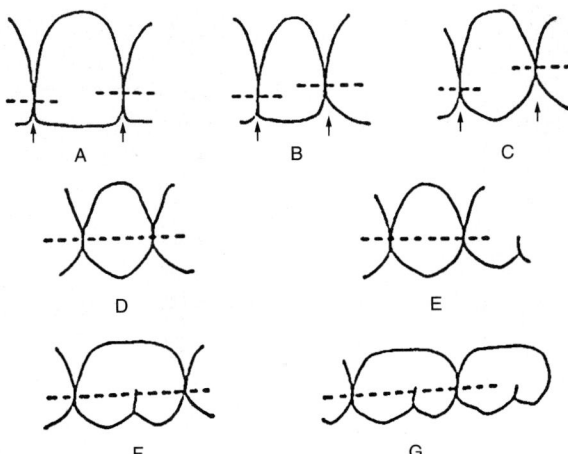

FIGURE 24-8. Proximal contacts of maxillary teeth.

Reprinted, with permission, from Ash MM. *Wheeler's Atlas of tooth form*, 5th ed. Elsevier, 1984:14.

PROXIMAL CONTACTS (VIEWED FROM THE FACIAL)

See Figures 24–8 and 24–9.

- Proximal contacts are generally located increasingly more incisally (occlusally) from the posterior to the anterior.
- The mesial contact is *always* located more incisally than the distal.
- Proximal contacts prevent rotation, mesial drift, and food impaction.
- As one ages, proximal wear creates a larger proximal contact area.

PROXIMAL CONTACTS (VIEWED FROM THE OCCLUSAL)

- The proximal contact is *always* located more buccally than lingually.

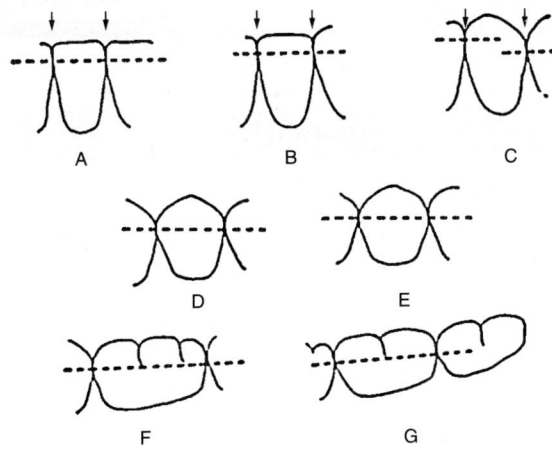

FIGURE 24-9. Proximal contact of mandibular teeth.

Reprinted, with permission, from Ash MM. *Wheeler's Atlas of tooth form*, 5th ed. Elsevier, 1984:14.

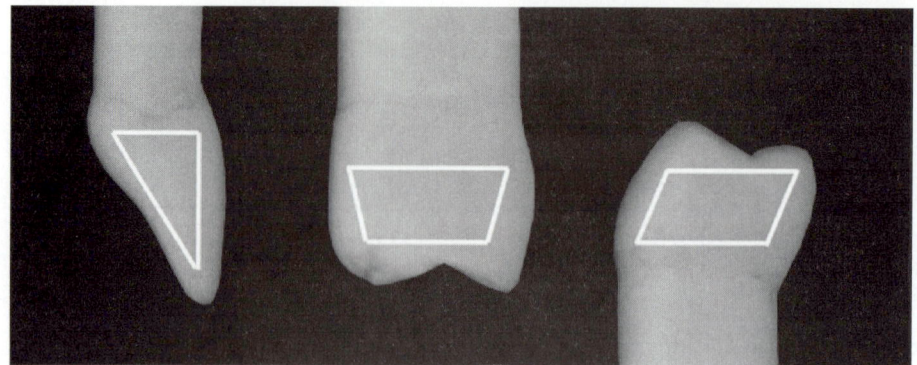

FIGURE 24-10. Proximal surface shapes.

PROXIMAL SURFACES

See Figure 24–10.

- Have specific shapes.
- Triangular: All anterior teeth.
- Trapezoidal: All maxillary posterior teeth.
- Rhomboidal: All mandibular posterior teeth.

HEIGHTS OF CONTOUR (HOC)

- The cingulum is the lingual height of contour for all anterior teeth and is *always* located at the cervical third of the crown.
- HOCs help form the mesial and distal contact areas.
- HOCs allow for adequate gingival health.

CEJ CONTOURS

See Figure 24–11.

- The maximum height of the proximal CEJ contour increases anteriorly.
- The mesial CEJ contour is *always* greater than the distal contour.
- The greatest CEJ contour is on the maxillary central incisor (mesial surface).

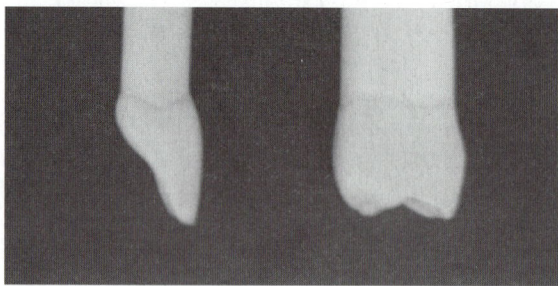

A.   B.

A. Maxillary right central incisor
B. Maxillary right 1st molar

FIGURE 24-11. Proximal CEJ contours.

- Facial and lingual CEJs curve apically.
- Mesial and distal CEJs curve coronally.

Lobes

- Incisors and canines: 4 lobes (3 labial [mamelons], 1 lingual [cingulum]).
- Premolars: 4 lobes (3 buccal, 1 lingual) **except** the mandibular second premolar, which has 5 lobes (3 buccal, 2 lingual).
- First molars: 5 lobes (one for each cusp).
- Second molars: 4 lobes (one for each cusp).
- Third molars: 4 or 5 lobes (one for each cusp, depending on variation).

Arch Lengths

- Maxillary: 128 mm (slightly longer).
- Mandibular: 126 mm.

Maxillary Permanent Teeth

Central Incisor

See Figure 24–12.

- Unique characteristics
    - Most prominent tooth.
    - Mesial CEJ contour is the greater than any other tooth.
    - Second longest crown length (next to mandibular canine).
    - Widest crown of all anterior teeth.
- Crown morphology
    - Mesiodistal dimension > faciolingual dimension.
    - Has narrowest incisal embrasures.
- Occlusal morphology
    - Has three mamelons and four developmental grooves.
    - Cingulum is located slightly distally.

Author's note: All references to pulp chamber shapes in this section are at the level of the CEJ.

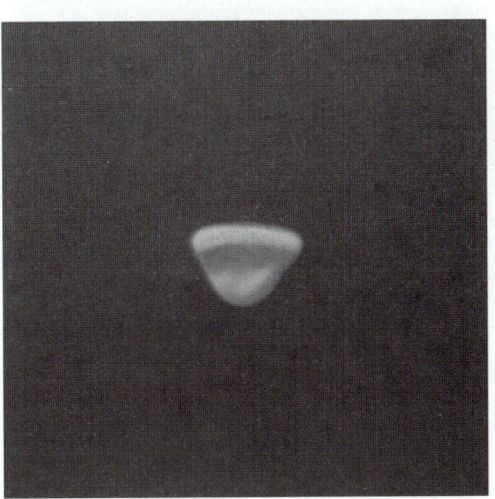

FIGURE 24–12. Maxillary central incisor.

- Pulp morphology
    - Pulp chamber is round.
    - Least likely to have a divided root canal.
- Root morphology
    - Roundest root form; can be rotated during extraction.
    - Has **greatest axial inclination.**
    - Sits almost vertically (mesiodistally) in alveolar bone.
- Occlusal contacts
    - Occludes with mandibular central and lateral incisors.

LATERAL INCISOR

See Figure 24–13.

- Unique characteristics
    - **Most common congenitally missing tooth.**
    - Second most variable tooth form (next to third molars).
        - Peg lateral (microdont)
        - Dens-in-dente
    - Most common tooth (2–5% prevalence) to have a **palatoradicular groove.**
- Crown morphology
    - Mesiodistal dimension > faciolingual dimension.
    - Lingual surface is the most concave of all incisors.
- Occlusal morphology
    - Cingulum is positioned centrally.
    - Pulp chamber is egg-shaped, with widest portion on the buccal.
- Root morphology
    - Root tip typically dilacerates to the distal.
- Occlusal contacts
    - Occludes with mandibular lateral incisor and canine.

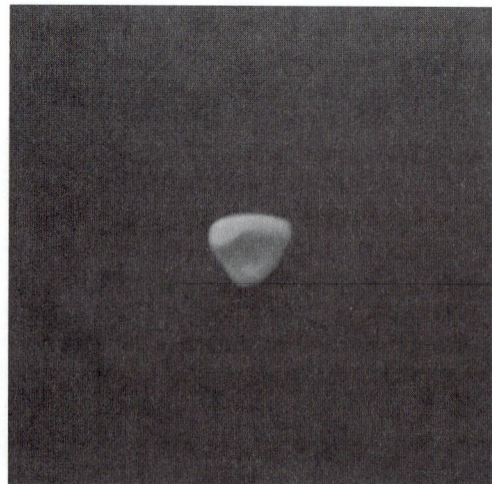

FIGURE 24–13. Maxillary lateral incisor.

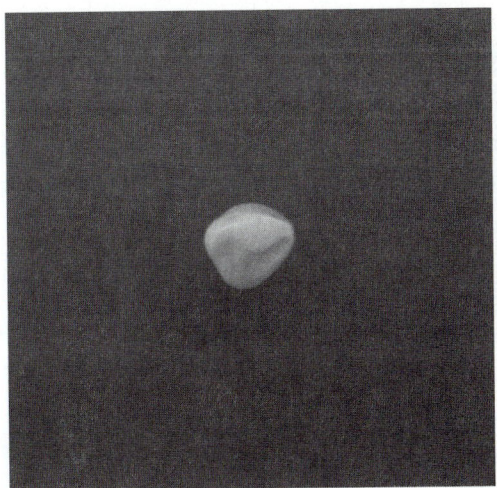

FIGURE 24-14. Maxillary canine.

Canine

See Figure 24-14.

- Unique characteristics
  - Longest tooth in the mouth.
  - Tooth least likely to be extracted (with mandibular canine).
- Crown morphology
  - Faciolingual dimension > mesiodistal dimension.
  - Mesial surface is straighter (less convex) than the distal.
  - Has a prominent **labial ridge**.
- Occlusal morphology
  - Occlusal surface has a prominent cingulum, lingual ridge, mesial and distal fossae, mesial and distal marginal ridges, and a **lingual-gingival groove**.
  - Cusp tip is located on the mesiofacial aspect of the crown.
  - Mesial cusp ridge is shorter than the distal.
  - Cingulum is positioned centrally.
- Pulp morphology
  - Pulp chamber is oval and flattened mesiodistally.
- Root morphology
  - Root is oval and flattened mesiodistally.
- Occlusal contacts
  - Occludes with mandibular canine and first premolar.

First Premolar

See Figure 24-15.

- Unique characteristics
  - Usually the largest premolar.
- Crown morphology
  - Occlusal shape is **rectangular**; proximal shape is **trapezoidal**.
  - Has a prominent **buccal ridge**.
  - Has a prominent **mesial root concavity**.
- Occlusal morphology
  - Occlusal table has a long central groove without pits.
  - Has a prominent **mesial marginal ridge groove**.
  - Mesial buccal cusp ridge is longer than the distal buccal cusp ridge.

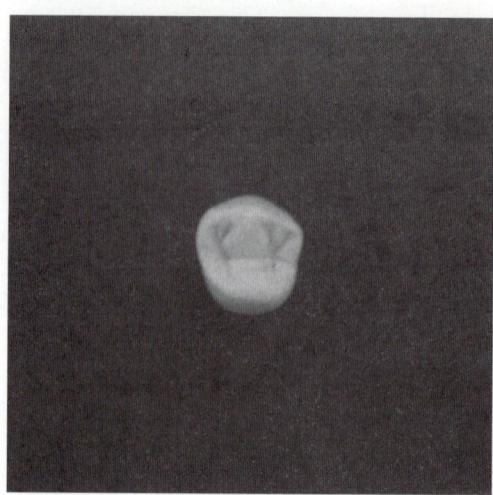

FIGURE 24-15. Maxillary first premolar.

- Has two cusps: Buccal (slightly distal), palatal (slightly mesial).
- Both cusps have steep inclines.
- Buccal cusp is longer than the lingual.
- Pulp morphology
  - Pulp chamber is oval and is usually pinched off mesiodistally creating two root canals, one for each root (B, P).
- Root morphology
  - Only premolar with **two roots.**
  - Sits almost vertically (buccolingually) in alveolar bone.
- Occlusal contacts
  - Occludes with mandibular first and second premolars.

Second Premolar

See Figure 24–16.

- Unique characteristics
- Crown morphology
  - Occlusal shape is **rectangular;** proximal shape is **trapezoidal.**
  - Has a **buccal ridge,** but not as prominent as first premolar.
- Occlusal morphology
  - Occlusal table is more ovoid and symmetrical than maxillary first premolar.
  - Occlusal table has a **short central groove with more supplemental grooves.**
  - Distal buccal cusp ridge is longer than the mesial buccal cusp ridge.
  - Has two cusps: Buccal, palatal (slightly mesial).
  - **Cusps have nearly similar heights.**
- Occlusal contacts
  - Occludes with mandibular second premolar and first molar.

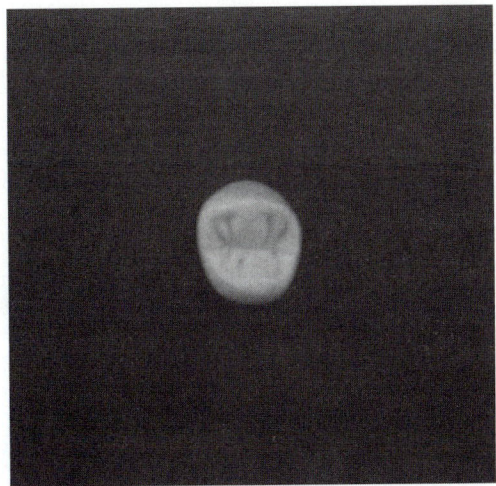

FIGURE 24-16. Maxillary second premolar.

First Molar

See Figure 24–17.

- Unique characteristics
    - Largest permanent tooth.
    - Only tooth that is **broader lingually than buccally**.
    - Only tooth with a **pronounced distal concavity** at the CEJ.
- Crown morphology
    - Occlusal shape is **rhomboidal**; proximal shape is **trapezoidal**.
- Occlusal morphology
    - Has a long buccal groove with a pit.
    - Has four cusps: MB, ML (largest), DB, DL (smallest).
    - The **primary cusp triangle** is formed by the ML, MB, and DB cusps (same for all maxillary molars).
    - Has a **distolingual groove** with a pit (on all maxillary molars).
    - Sometimes has fifth **cusp of Carabelli** lingual to ML cusp.
    - Has **most prominent oblique ridge** of all maxillary molars.
    - A **transverse groove** connects the central and distal pits (same for all maxillary molars).

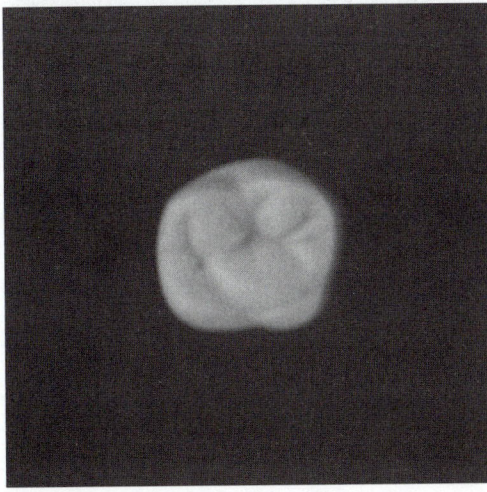

FIGURE 24-17. Maxillary first molar.

- Pulp morphology
  - Generally three root canals (MB, DB, P) but 30% have fourth canal in MB root.
- Root morphology
  - Has three roots: MB, DB (shortest), palatal (longest).
  - Distance from furcation entrance to CEJ: Mesial (3.6 mm) < buccal (4.2 mm) < distal (4.8 mm).
  - Roots are **closest to the maxillary sinus.**
  - MB and DB roots are often shaped like "plier handles."
  - MB root has more common (94%) and deeper (0.3 mm) concavities than other roots.
- Occlusal contacts
  - Occludes with mandibular first and second molars.

Second Molar

See Figure 24–18.

- Unique characteristics
  - Similar to maxillary first molar but smaller and more angular.
  - Second most common tooth to have **cervical enamel projections** (next to mandibular second molar).
  - Closest tooth to the opening of Stenson's (parotid) duct.
- Crown morphology
  - Occlusal table is usually **rhomboidal** but can be **heart-shaped** if the DL cusp is absent; proximal shape is **trapezoidal.**
- Occlusal morphology
  - Has smaller oblique ridge with a transverse groove.
  - Has a short buccal groove without a pit.
  - Has four cusps: MB, ML (largest), DB, DL (smallest).
- Root morphology
  - Roots are closer together than the maxillary first molar and typically turn distally.
  - Usually has a longer root trunk than the maxillary first molar.
- Occlusal contacts
  - Occludes with mandibular second and third molars.

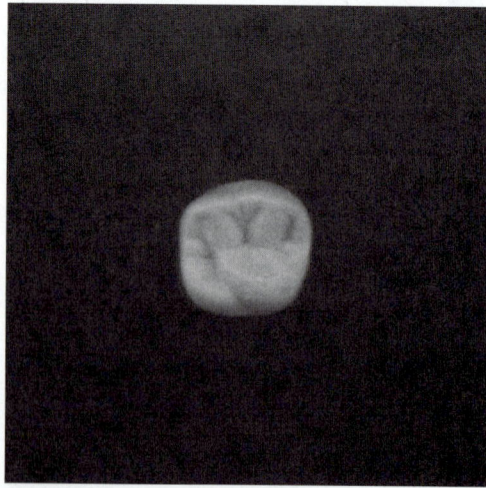

FIGURE 24-18. Maxillary second molar.

THIRD MOLAR

See Figure below.

- Unique characteristics
  - Has **most variable shape** of any other tooth (with mandibular third molar).
  - **Shortest** permanent tooth.
  - **Most common** tooth to have **enamel pearls** (with mandibular third molars).
  - Frequently congenitally missing or unerupted (similar to mandibular third molars).
- Crown morphology
  - Crown tapers lingually.
- Occlusal morphology
  - Has three cusps: MB, DB, Lingual.
  - DB cusp is smallest and often absent.
  - Oblique ridge is poorly developed and often absent.
- Root morphology
  - Roots are often fused.
- Occlusal contacts
  - Occludes only with mandibular third molar.

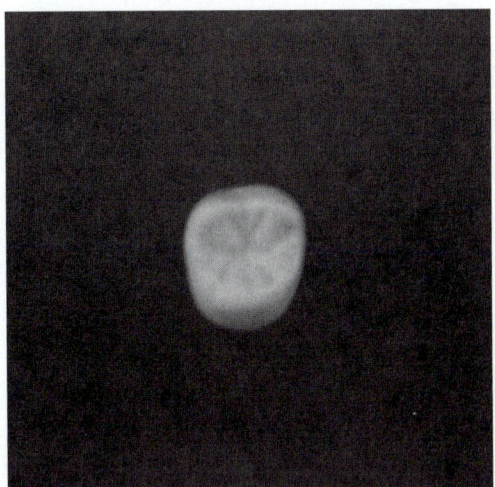

Maxillary third molar.

Mandibular Permanent Teeth

CENTRAL INCISOR

See Figure 24–19.

- Unique characteristics
  - Smallest permanent tooth.
- Crown morphology
  - **Most symmetrical** with its contralateral counterpart.
  - Disto-incisal angle is as sharp as the mesioincisal angle.
  - Faciolingual dimension > mesiodistal dimension.
  - Marginal ridges are the same length.

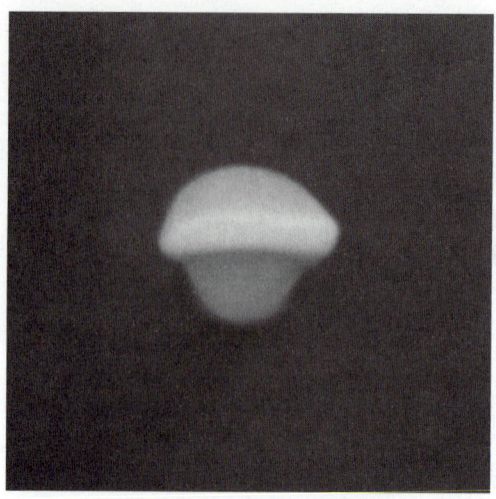

FIGURE 24–19. Mandibular central incisor.

- Occlusal morphology
  - Incisal edge is lingual to the long axis (same as mandibular lateral).
  - Cingulum (indistinct) is positioned centrally.
- Pulp morphology
  - Pulp chamber is oval and flattened mesiodistally.
- Occlusal contacts
  - Occludes with maxillary central incisor.
  - Only anterior tooth to occlude with one tooth.

LATERAL INCISOR

See Figure 24–20.

- Unique characteristics
  - Slightly larger in all dimensions than the mandibular central.
- Crown morphology
  - Not as symmetrical as the central; the crown is tilted distally on the root.
  - Faciolingual dimension > mesiodistal dimension.
  - Mesial marginal ridge is longer than the distal.
- Occlusal morphology
  - Incisal edge is **twisted distolingually.**
  - Incisal edge is lingual to the long axis (same as mandibular central).
  - Cingulum (indistinct) is positioned slightly distally.
- Pulp morphology
  - Pulp chamber is oval and flattened mesiodistally, sometimes pinched off creating two separate root canals (B, L).
- Root morphology
  - Root has mesial and distal concavities (hourglass-shaped).
- Occlusal contacts
  - Occludes with maxillary central and lateral incisors.

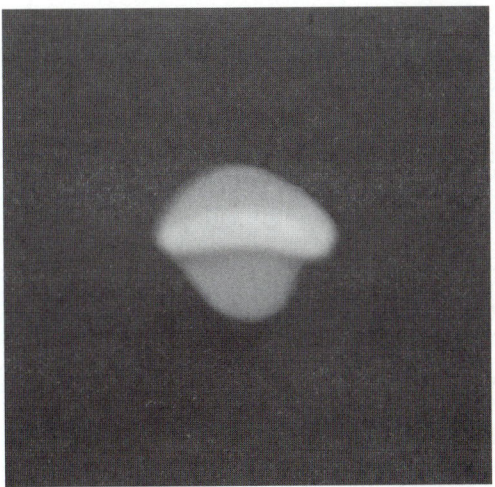

FIGURE 24-20. Mandibular lateral incisor.

CANINE

See Figure 24–21.

- Unique characteristics
    - **Longest crown** of any permanent tooth.
    - Longest tooth in mandible.
    - Tooth least likely to be extracted (with maxillary canine).
- Crown morphology
    - Faciolingual dimension > mesiodistal dimension.
    - Has a **labial ridge** but less prominent than the maxillary canine.
    - Mesial surface of the crown is nearly parallel with the long axis.
- Occlusal morphology
    - Cusp tip is on the lingual aspect of the crown.
    - Mesial cusp ridge is shorter than the distal.
    - Cingulum is positioned slightly distally (less prominent than maxillary canine); similar to the lingual cusp of mandibular first premolar.

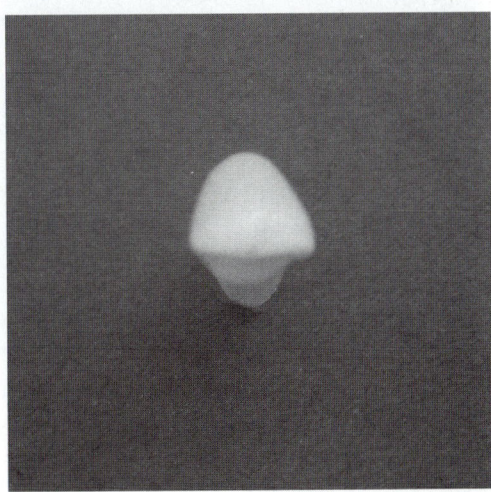

FIGURE 24-21. Mandibular canine.

- Pulp morphology
  - Pulp chamber is oval and flattened mesiodistally.
- Root morphology
  - Root is oval and flattened mesiodistally.
  - Root may have a mesial depression and may be bifurcated.
- Occlusal contacts
  - Occludes with maxillary lateral incisor and canine.

First Premolar

See Figure 24–22.

- Unique characteristics
  - Usually the smallest premolar.
- Crown morphology
  - Occlusal shape is **square**; proximal shape is **rhomboidal** (tilted lingually).
  - Has a prominent mesiolingual developmental groove.
- Occlusal morphology
  - Only posterior tooth with an **occlusal plane tilted lingually.**
  - Has a prominent **transverse ridge** without a central groove.
  - **Mesial marginal ridge is shorter** and less prominent than distal marginal ridge.
  - Has two cusps: Buccal (functional), lingual (nonfunctional).
  - Buccal cusp is larger (two thirds of occlusal surface) than the lingual.
- Pulp morphology
  - Pulp chamber is roundest of all premolars.
- Root morphology
  - Root is broader facially than lingually and may have proximal concavities.
- Occlusal contacts
  - Occludes with maxillary canine and first molar.

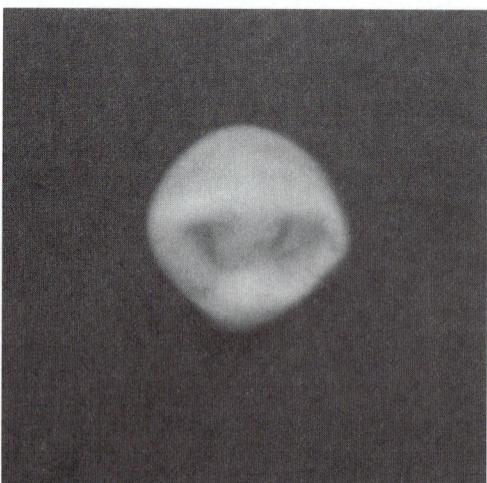

FIGURE 24-22. Mandibular first premolar.

Second Premolar

See Figure 24–23.

- Unique characteristics
    - The gingival papilla between the first and second premolar is the shortest.
- Crown morphology
    - Occlusal shape is **square**; proximal shape is **rhomboidal** (tilted lingually).
    - Lingual surface is wider than that of the mandibular first premolar.
    - From the buccal view, it is shorter and wider than the mandibular first premolar.
    - Only premolar with five lobes: three buccal and two lingual.
- Occlusal morphology
    - Occlusal surface can have three configurations:
        - Y (most common configuration): Three cusps—buccal (nonfunctional), ML, DL with a single central pit.
        - H: Two cusps—buccal and lingual with short central groove.
        - U: Two cusps—buccal and lingual with crescent-shaped central groove.
    - Buccal cusp is shorter and blunter than lingual cusps.
    - ML cusp is larger than the DL cusp.
    - Mesial marginal ridge has slight concavity.
- Root morphology
    - Root is longer than the first mandibular premolar.
    - Root is **closest to the mental foramen.**
- Occlusal contacts
    - Occludes with maxillary first and second premolars.

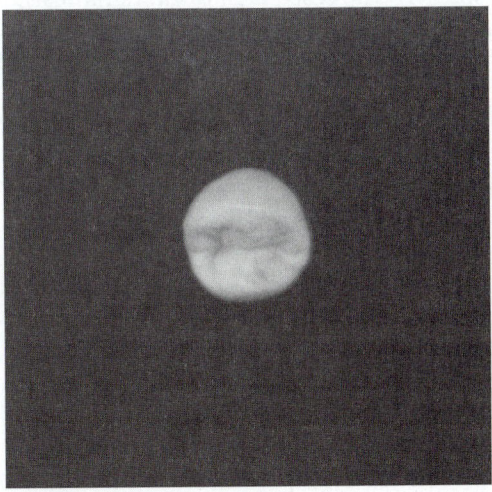

FIGURE 24-23. Mandibular second premolar.

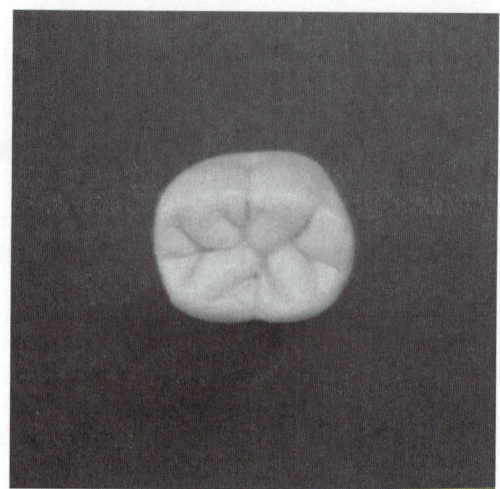

FIGURE 24-24. Mandibular first molar.

First Molar

See Figure 24–24.

- Unique characteristics
  - Largest mandibular tooth.
- Crown morphology
  - Occlusal shape is **trapezoidal;** Proximal shape is **rhomboidal** (tilted lingually 15–20°).
  - Largest mesiodistal dimension of any other tooth.
- Occlusal morphology
  - Has five cusps: MB (largest), DB, distal (smallest), ML, DL.
  - Buccal cusps are shorter and blunter then the lingual cusps.
  - Has two **transverse ridges,** three fossae with pits, **two buccal grooves** (MB and DB), and a short lingual groove.
  - Occlusal pattern resembles a +< with a twisted central groove.
- Pulp morphology
  - Pulp chamber is rectangular.
  - Generally three root canals (MB, ML, D) but 25% have a fourth canal in D root.
- Root morphology
  - Roots are usually widely separated.
  - The mesial root is broadest buccolingually.
  - Both roots will have root concavities (mesial slightly more prominent).
  - The root trunk is typically shorter than the mandibular second molar.
- Occlusal contacts
  - Occludes with the maxillary second premolar and first molar.

Second Molar

See Figure 24–25.

- Unique characteristics
  - Most symmetrical molar.
  - Most common tooth to have **cervical enamel projections.**
- Crown morphology
  - Occlusal shape is **rectangular;** proximal shape is **rhomboidal** (tilted lingually 15–20°).
  - The buccolingual dimension is greater at the mesial than distal.

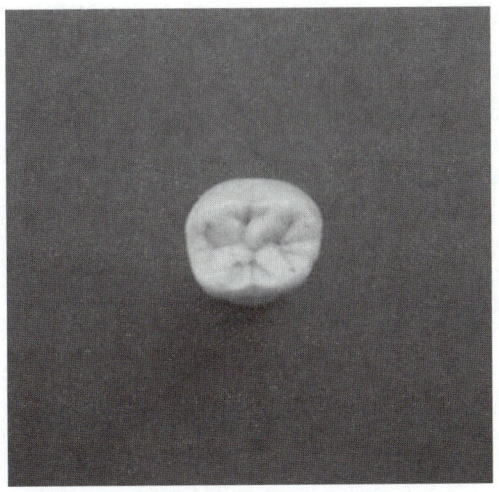

FIGURE 24-25. Mandibular second molar.

- Occlusal morphology
  - Has four cusps: MB, DB, ML, DL.
  - Occlusal pattern resembles a + with a straight central groove.
  - Has two **transverse ridges**, three fossae with pits, three secondary grooves, **one buccal groove** with a pit, and a short lingual groove.
- Pulp morphology
  - Pulp chamber is trapezoidal (tapers distally).
- Root morphology
  - Roots are closer together than the mandibular first molar and inclined distally.
  - The root trunk is typically longer than the mandibular first molar.
- Occlusal contacts
  - Occludes with the maxillary first and second molar.

THIRD MOLAR

See Figure 24–26.

- Unique characteristics
  - Has an extremely **variable morphology** (similar to maxillary third molar).
  - Most common tooth to have **enamel pearls** (with maxillary third molars).

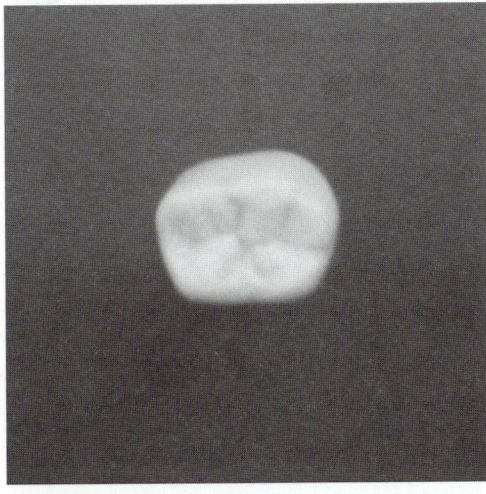

FIGURE 24-26. Mandibular third molar.

- Crown morphology
  - Has bulbous crown that tapers distally.
  - Occlusal shape can be similar to mandibular first or second molars; Proximal shape is **rhomboidal** (tilted lingually 15–20°).
- Occlusal morphology
  - Has an irregular groove pattern.
  - Has four or five cusps: MB, DB, distal (can be absent), ML, DL.
  - MB cusp is larger than DB cusp.
- Pulp morphology
  - Pulp chamber is trapezoidal (tapers distally).
- Root morphology
  - Roots are usually short, distally inclined, and often fused.
  - Typically has a **distally inclined root trunk.**
- Occlusal contacts
  - Occludes with maxillary second and third molar.

▶ PRIMARY (DECIDUOUS) TOOTH FORM

See Figure 24–27.

General Concepts

TOOTH LABELING

See Figure 24–28.

- There are 20 total primary teeth (10 per arch).
- There are no premolars.
- Teeth are labeled A through T.

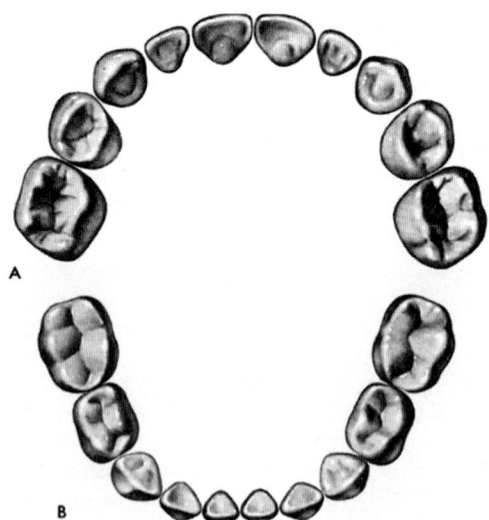

FIGURE 24–27. The primary dentition.

Reprinted, with permission, from ash MM. *Wheeler's Atlas of tooth form*, 5th ed. Elsevier, 1984:139.

```
                    Max
            A B C D E | F G H I J
Right      ----------+----------      Left
            T S R Q P | O N M L K
                    Mand
```

FIGURE 24-28. Tooth numbering of the primary (deciduous) dentition.

PRIMARY VS. PERMANENT TEETH

See Table 24–2.

- Typically lighter in color.
- Fewer grooves and pits (shallower and smoother).
- Crowns are more bulbous.
- Buccal and lingual surfaces are flatter above the height of contour.
- Enamel is thinner (only about 1 mm thick).
- Enamel stops abruptly at the CEJ.
- CEJs are more constricted.
- Anterior crowns are wider mesiodistally and shorter incisocervically.
- Posterior crowns are narrower mesiodistally and shorter occlusocervically.
- Pulp chambers are larger.
- Root trunks are shorter.
- Anterior roots are more tapered.
- Posterior roots are longer, more slender, broader buccolingually, and more divergent.

TABLE 24-2. Comparison of Primary (Deciduous) Tooth Forms

	Root Length (mm)	Crown Length (mm)	Number of Cusps	Number of Roots
Maxilla				
Central incisor	10	6	1	1
Lateral incisor	11.4	5.6	1	1
Canine	13.5	6.5	1	1
First molar	10	5.1	4	3
Second molar	11.7	5.7	4 or 5	3
Mandible				
Incisor	9	5	1	1
Lateral incisor	10	5.2	1	1
Canine	11.5	6	1	1
First molar	9.8	6	4	2
Second molar	11.3	5.5	5	2

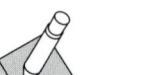

PRIMATE SPACE

- Allows for proper alignment of the permanent incisors.
- Occurs in about 50% of primary dentitions.
- Maxillary: Located between the lateral incisors and canines.
- Mandibular: Located between the canines and first molars.

The mesiodistal width of the primary molars is 2–5 mm greater than the width of the permanent premolars.

ARCH LENGTHS

- Maxillary: 68.2 mm (longer).
- Mandibular: 61.8 mm.

Maxillary Primary Teeth

See Figures 24–29 and 24–30.

CENTRAL INCISOR

- Straight incisal edge.
- No mamelons.
- Prominent facial and lingual cervical ridges.
- Occludes with mandibular central and lateral incisors.

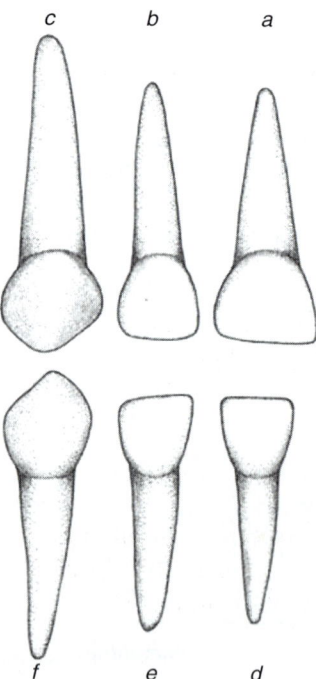

FIGURE 24–29. Primary anterior teeth.

Reprinted, with permission, from ash MM. *Wheeler's Atlas of tooth form*, 5th ed. Elsevier, 1984:139.

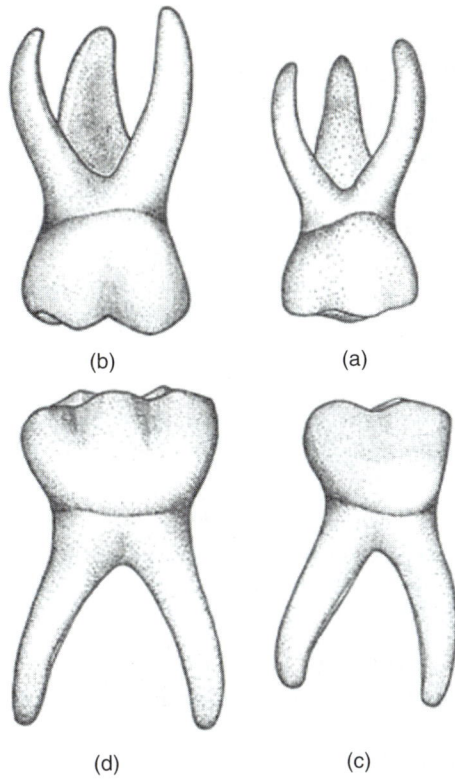

FIGURE 24-30. Primary posterior teeth.

Reprinted, with permission, from ash MM. *Wheeler's Atlas of tooth form*, 5th ed. Elsevier, 1984:146.

LATERAL INCISOR

- Straight incisal edge.
- No mamelons.
- Prominent facial and lingual cervical ridges.
- Occludes with mandibular lateral incisor and canine.

CANINE

- Facial shape is pentagonal.
- Longer and sharper cusp than permanent maxillary canine.
- Mesial cusp ridge is longer than the distal cusp ridge.
- Occludes with mandibular canine and first molar.

FIRST MOLAR

- Smallest primary molar.
- Generally **resembles a permanent maxillary premolar.**
- Occlusal shape is **rectangular.**
- Occlusal surface has **H-shaped** configuration.
- Has a prominent buccal cervical ridge.
- CEJ is more apical mesially than distally.
- Has four cusps: MB (largest), ML (sharpest), DB, DL (smallest).
- Occludes with mandibular first and second molars.

Second Molar

- Generally **resembles permanent maxillary first molar** but smaller.
- Occlusal shape is **rhomboidal.**
- Has a prominent buccal cervical ridge.
- Has an oblique ridge.
- Has four cusps: MB (largest), ML (almost as large as MB), DB, DL (smallest).
- May have a fifth cusp of Carabelli.
- Occludes with mandibular second molar.

Mandibular Primary Teeth

Central Incisor

- Straight incisal edge.
- No mamelons.
- Prominent facial and lingual cervical ridges.
- Occludes with maxillary central incisor.

Lateral Incisor

- Straight incisal edge.
- No mamelons.
- Prominent facial and lingual cervical ridges.
- Occludes with maxillary central and lateral incisors.

Canine

- Facial shape is pentagonal.
- Mesial cusp ridge is longer than the distal cusp ridge.
- Occludes with maxillary lateral incisor and canine.

First Molar

- **Most unique** primary or permanent tooth.
- Most difficult primary tooth to restore.
- Occlusal shape is **rhomboidal.**
- Has no central fossa (but has mesial and distal triangular fossae).
- Has a prominent buccal cervical ridge.
- Has a well-developed mesial marginal ridge.
- Has a prominent **transverse ridge** (connects MB and ML cusps).
- Has four cusps: MB (largest), ML (sharpest), DB, DL (smallest).
- Occludes with maxillary canine and first molar.

Second Molar

- Generally **resembles permanent mandibular first molar.**
- Occlusal shape is **rectangular.**
- Has a prominent buccal cervical ridge.
- Has five cusps: MB, ML, D (as large as MB and DB cusps), DB, DL.
- Occludes with maxillary first and second molars.

CHAPTER 25
Eruption

Definitions and General Concepts	646
DEFINITIONS	**646**
GENERAL CONCEPTS	**646**
Primary (Deciduous) Dentition	646
Mixed Dentition	647
Permanent Dentition	647

▶ DEFINITIONS AND GENERAL CONCEPTS

Definitions

- **Succedaneous teeth:** Permanent teeth that occupy positions held by primary teeth.
- **Exfoliation:** Shedding of the primary teeth. This is accomplished partly by the resorption of the deciduous roots by odontoclasts.
- **Mixed dentition:** A dentition having both primary and permanent teeth.
- **Active eruption:** Tooth movement from its germinative position until contact is made with opposing and/or adjacent teeth.
- **Passive eruption:** Tooth exposure secondary to the apical migration of the junctional epithelium.

Only the permanent incisors, canines, and premolars are succedaneous.

General Concepts

- Teeth erupt in pairs.
- Girls' teeth erupt before boys' teeth.
- Mandibular teeth generally erupt before maxillary teeth.
- Eruption starts once 50% of root formation is complete.

▶ PRIMARY (DECIDUOUS) DENTITION

NUMBER OF TEETH

- There are 20 total primary teeth (10 per arch).
- There are no premolars.

DENTAL FORMULA

- $I\,^2/_2 + C\,^1/_1 + M\,^2/_2$
  (*I*-incisors, *C*-canine, *M*-molar)

ERUPTION SEQUENCE AND TIMING

See Figure 25–1.

- Same sequence for both arches.

*Mandibular teeth generally erupt before maxillary teeth, **except** the lateral incisors.*

DEVELOPMENT

See Table 25–1.

- Begin to develop at 6 weeks in utero.
- Calcification starts at 4–6 months (18 weeks) in utero.
- Apices are complete 1–2 years after eruption (by age 3).

I1	I2	M1	C	M2
6	9	12	18	24

FIGURE 25–1. Eruption sequence and average timing (in months) of the deciduous dentition.

TABLE 25-1. Tooth Development of the Primary (Deciduous) Dentition

Tooth	Age at Enamel Completion	Age at Eruption Mandibular (mo)	Age at Eruption Maxillary (mo)	Age at Root Completion (yr)	Age at Exfoliation (yr)
Central incisor	6–10 wk	6	7	1.5	6–8
Lateral incisor	10–12 wk	7	9	1.5–2	7–9
First molar	6 mo	12	14	2–2.5	10–12
Canine	9 mo	16	18	3–3.5	9–12
Second molar	10–12 mo	20	24	3	10–12

▶ MIXED DENTITION

- Occurs from ages 6 through 12 years.
- Usually starts with the eruption of the permanent first molar.
- Usually ends with the exfoliation of the primary maxillary canine.
- Permanent incisors often erupt *lingual* to their primary counterparts.

▶ PERMANENT DENTITION

Number of teeth:

- There are 32 total permanent teeth (16 per arch).

Dental formula:

- $I\,^2/_2 + C\,^1/_1 + PM\,^2/_2 + M\,^3/_3$

Eruption sequence and timing:

See Figures 25–2 and 25–3.

- Different sequence for each arch.

*Mandibular teeth generally erupt before maxillary teeth, **except** the premolars.*

DEVELOPMENT

See Table 25–2.

- Begin to develop at 4 months in utero.
- Calcification starts at birth (of mandibular first molar).
- Apices are complete 2–3 years after eruption.

M1	I1	I2	C	PM1	PM2	M2	M3
6	6	7	10	10	11	12	20

FIGURE 25-2. Eruption sequence and average timing (in years) of the mandibular permanent dentition.

M1	I1	I2	PM1	PM2	C	M2	M3
6	6	7	10	10	11	12	20

FIGURE 25-3. Eruption sequence and average timing (in years) of the maxillary permanent dentition.

TABLE 25-2. Tooth Development of the Permanent Dentition

Tooth	Age at Enamel Completion (yr)	Age at Eruption (yr) Mandibular	Age at Eruption (yr) Maxillary	Age at Root Completion (yr)
First molar	2.5–3	6–7	6–7	9–10
Central incisor	3.5	6–7 yr.	7–8	9–10.5
Lateral incisor	4–5	7–8	8–9	10–11
Canine	4–7	9–10	11–12	12–14
First premolar	5–6	10–12	10–12	12–13.5
Second premolar	5.5–7	10–12	10–12	12.5–14
Second molar	6–8	11–13	12–13	14–15
Third molar	13–16	17–21	17–21	18–25

CHAPTER 26
Occlusion and Function

Occlusion	650
Occlusal Terminology	650
Occlusal Relationships	652
Mandibular Movements	654
Concepts to Remember	654
Mandibular Positions	654
Posselt's Envelope of Motion	654
Mandibular Movement and Guidance	654
Occlusal Interferences	655
Condylar Movements	656
Occlusal Musculature	656

OCCLUSION

Occlusal Terminology

GENERAL TERMS

- **Occlusion:** The contact relationships of the teeth. The contacts are generally edges or points touching other edges, points, or areas.
- **Functional occlusion:** Occlusion during mandibular movement (mastication, swallowing, etc.).
- **Plane of occlusion:** An imaginary plane anatomically related to the cranium that theoretically touches the incisal edges of incisors and the cusp tips of posterior teeth.
- **Occlusal adjustment (equilibration):** Reshaping the occlusal surfaces of teeth to create harmonious contacts between the maxillary and mandibular teeth.

OCCLUSAL DIMENSIONS

- **Vertical dimension:** A vertical measurement of the face between any two arbitrary points (usually in the midline), one above and one below the mouth.
- **Vertical dimension of occlusion (VDO):** The vertical dimension of the face when the teeth are in centric occlusion.
- **Vertical dimension of rest (VDR):** The vertical dimension of the face when the mandible is in the rest position.

OCCLUSAL CURVATURES

- **Curve of Spee:** The anteroposterior curvature of the occlusal surfaces. (See Figure 26–1.)
- **Curve of Wilson:** The mediolateral curvature of the occlusal surfaces. (See Figure 26–2.)
- **Compensating curve:** The anteroposterior curvature (in the median plane) and the mediolateral curvature (in the frontal plane) in the alignment of the occluding surfaces and incisal edges of *artificial teeth* that are used to develop *balanced occlusion*.

OCCLUSAL CONTACTS

- **Functional contacts:** Contacts made during functional occlusion.
- **Parafunctional contacts:** Abnormal contacts; typically result from habits such as bruxism and include *area-to-area contacts*.

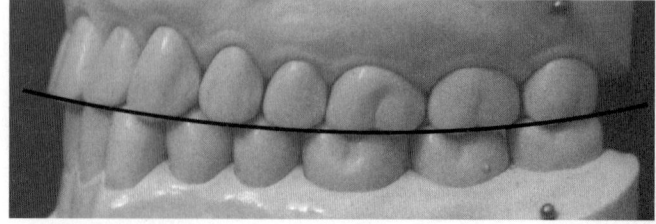

FIGURE 26–1. Curve of Spee.

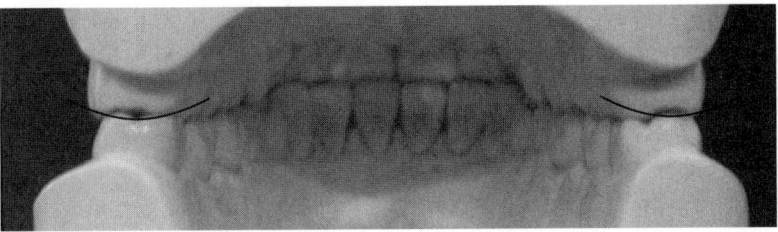

FIGURE 26-2. **Curve of Wilson.**

- **Protrusive contacts:** Contacts made when the mandible has moved anteriorly from centric occlusion (protrusive movement). These are usually *edge-to-edge contacts* for anterior teeth.
- **Working side contacts (laterotrusive contacts):** Contacts on the side toward which the mandible has moved from centric occlusion (working side movement).
- **Nonworking side contacts (mediotrusive contacts):** Contacts on the side away from which the mandible has moved from centric occlusion (nonworking side movement).

Occlusal Relationships

- **Overbite:** The *vertical* overlapping of the mandibular incisors by the maxillary incisors when the jaws are in centric occlusion. (See Figure 26–3.)
- **Overjet:** The *horizontal* overlapping of the mandibular incisors by the maxillary incisors when the jaws are in centric occlusion.
- **Open bite:** A condition in which opposing teeth do not occlude.
- **Cross-bite:** An abnormal relation of one or more teeth in one arch to its antagonist in the other arch due to a deviation of tooth or jaw position.

In cross-bite occlusions, the working and nonworking cusps are reversed for the affected teeth.

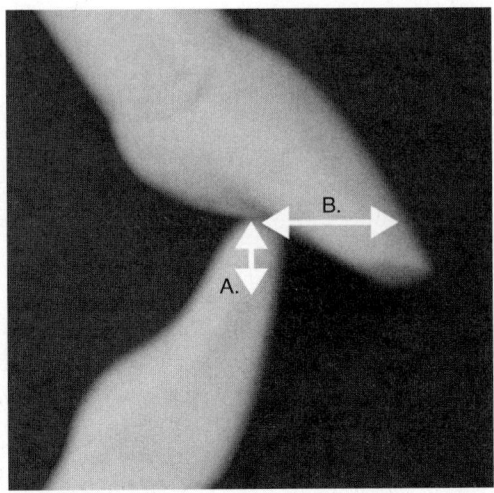

A. Overbite
B. Overjet

FIGURE 26-3. **Overbite and overjet.**

- **Anterior cross-bite:** One or more maxillary incisors are positioned lingually to the mandibular incisors when in centric occlusion.
- **Posterior cross-bite:** One or more maxillary posterior teeth are positioned palatally to the mandibular posterior teeth when in centric occlusion.

Occlusal Relationships

FOUR DETERMINANTS OF OCCLUSION

- The teeth and their occlusal surfaces.
- The right temporomandibular joint (TMJ).
- The left TMJ.
- The neuromusculature of the jaws and TMJs.

ANGLE'S CLASSIFICATION

Angle's classification is based on molar and canine relationships.

Chronic thumb sucking can cause an anterior open bite, flaring/rotation of the maxillary incisors, crowding of the mandibular incisors, constriction of the maxillary arch, a high palatal vault, and class II, division I malocclusions.

- **Class I:** 70% of population.
  - Molar: MB cusp of the maxillary first molar occludes with the MB groove of the mandibular first molar.
  - Canine: Maxillary canine occludes between the mandibular canine and first remolar.
  - See Figure 26–4 for class I occlusion.
- **Class II:** 25% of population.
  - Molar: MB cusp of the maxillary first molar occludes mesially to the MB groove of the mandibular first molar.
  - Canine: Maxillary canine occludes mesially to the distal surface of the mandibular canine.
    - **Division I:** All maxillary anterior teeth are proclined (flared). (See Figure 26–5.)
    - **Division II:** The maxillary laterals are proclined, and the central incisors are typically retroclined. (See Figure 26–6.)
- **Class III:** 5% of population. (See Figure 26–7.)
  - Molar: MB cusp of the maxillary first molar occludes distally to the MB groove of the mandibular first molar.
  - Canine: Maxillary canine occludes distally to the distal surface of the mandibular canine.

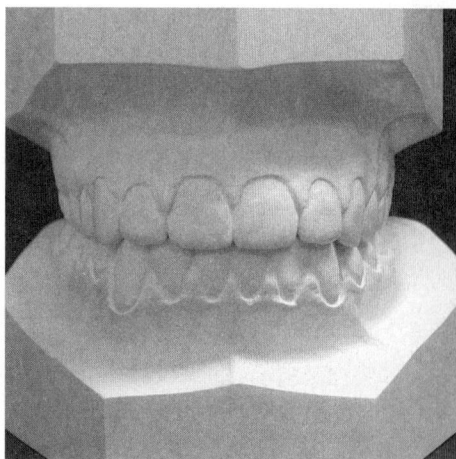 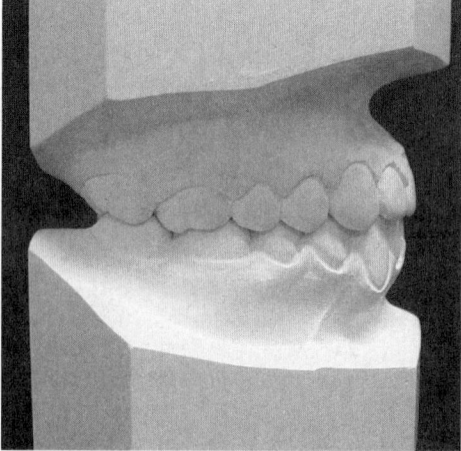

FIGURE 26–4. Class I occlusion.

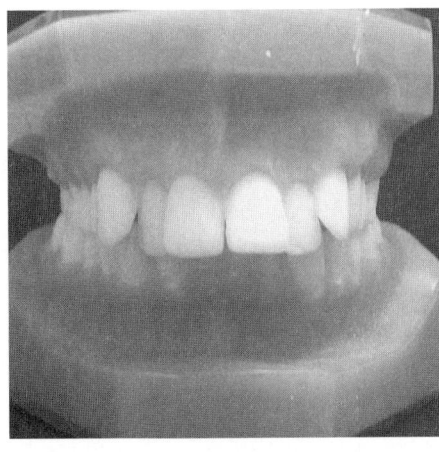 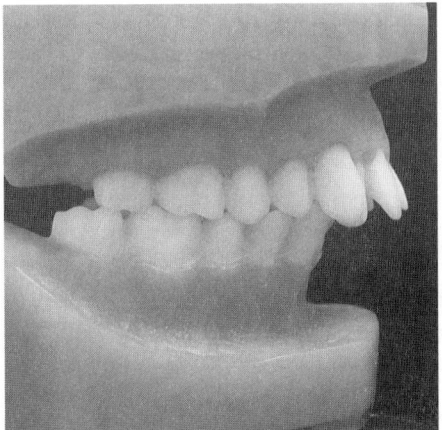

FIGURE 26-5. Class II, division I occlusion.

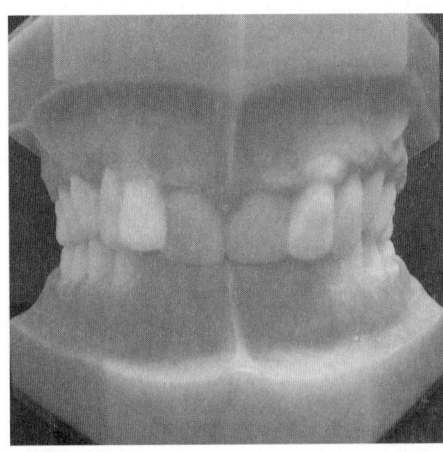 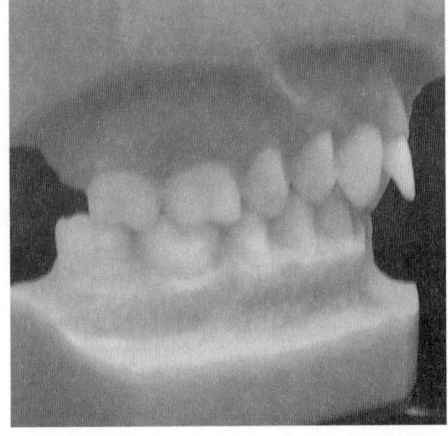

FIGURE 26-6. Class II, division II occlusion.

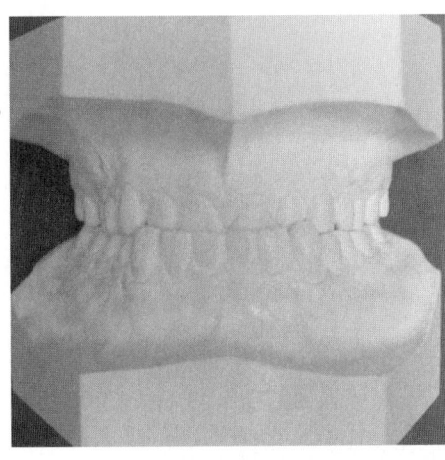 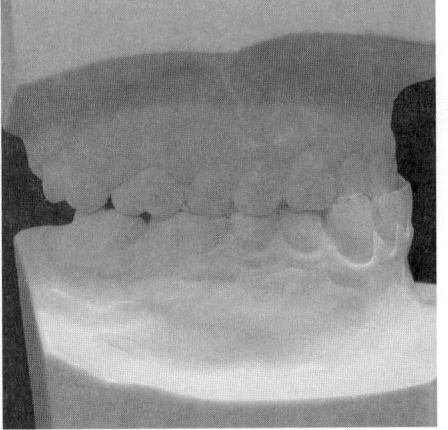

FIGURE 26-7. Class III occlusion.

IDEAL OCCLUSION AND INTERCUSPAL RELATIONSHIP

*An **ideal occlusion** is a class I occlusion with a smooth plane of occlusion.*

- **Working (supporting, holding) cusps:** *Maxillary lingual* and *mandibular buccal cusps.* Occlude with opposing fossae or marginal ridges. They are generally broader and rounder and support the vertical dimension of the face.
- **Nonworking (balancing, guiding) cusps:** *Maxillary buccal* and *mandibular lingual cusps.* Do **not** contact opposing teeth, but oppose grooves and embrasure spaces. They are generally sharper.

▶ MANDIBULAR MOVEMENTS

Concepts to Remember

- The mandible acts as a class III lever.
- Movement occurs in three planes (frontal, horizontal, sagittal).
- There are two mandibular motions (rotation and translation).

Mandibular Positions

- **Centric occlusion (CO):** The maximum intercuspation of the opposing arches. It is a purely *tooth-guided* position. This creates the **vertical dimension of occlusion (VDO).**
- **Centric relation (CR):** The most anterior and superior position of the mandibular condyles within the glenoid fossae (**terminal hinge position**). By maintaining this position, only rotational movements around a horizontal (hinge) axis can occur. It is a purely *ligament-guided* position.
- **Rest (postural) position (RP):** The position of the mandible when it is in a physiologic rest position. There are no tooth contacts in this position; it is a purely *muscle-guided* position. This creates the **vertical dimension of rest (VDR).** The resulting space between the teeth in this position (about 1–3 mm) is called the **freeway space (FS).**
- **Maximum opening (MO):** The maximum separation of the opposing arches. Creates the greatest amount of space between the teeth (about 40–50 mm).

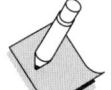

VDR = VDO + FS.

During the act of swallowing, the mandible meets the maxilla in centric occlusion and the tongue touches the palate.

Posselt's Envelope of Motion

See Figure 26–8.

- Sagittal plane
- Horizontal plane
- Frontal plane

Posselt's envelope of motion illustrates the range of motion of the mandible in three planes.

Mandibular Movement and Guidance

- **Protrusive movement:** The anterior movement of the mandible. As the mandible moves anteriorly, the posterior teeth disarticulate. This is known as **anterior guidance.** The maximum posterior disarticulation occurs when the anterior teeth are edge-to-edge. Anterior guidance depends largely on the horizontal and vertical relationship of the maxillary and mandibular incisors and canines. Cusp length varies on the extent of this relationship.

Effects of Anterior Tooth Relationship on Cusp Height

	↑ Overjet	↓ Overjet
↑ Overbite	Variable	Longest cusps
↓ Overbite	Shortest cusps	Variable

- **Lateral movement:** The lateral movement of the mandible. The side toward which the mandible moves is the **working side;** the side away from which the mandible moves is the **nonworking side.** Lateral movements occur via two types of guidance:
  - **Canine guidance:** The contact between the opposing canines on the working side disarticulates all posterior teeth. Any premature contacts on the working or nonworking sides are working and nonworking interferences, respectively.
  - **Group function:** The contact between the opposing canines and posterior teeth on the working side disarticulates the posterior teeth on the nonworking side. Any contacts on the nonworking side are nonworking interferences.

Occlusal Interferences

- **Occlusal interference:** Any contact that inhibits the remaining occlusal surfaces from achieving harmonious contacts.
- **Protrusive interference:** Premature contact between the mesial aspects of mandibular posterior teeth and the distal aspects of maxillary posterior teeth.
- **Working interference:** Premature contact on the working side during lateral mandibular movement.
- **Nonworking interference:** Premature contact on the nonworking side during lateral mandibular movement.

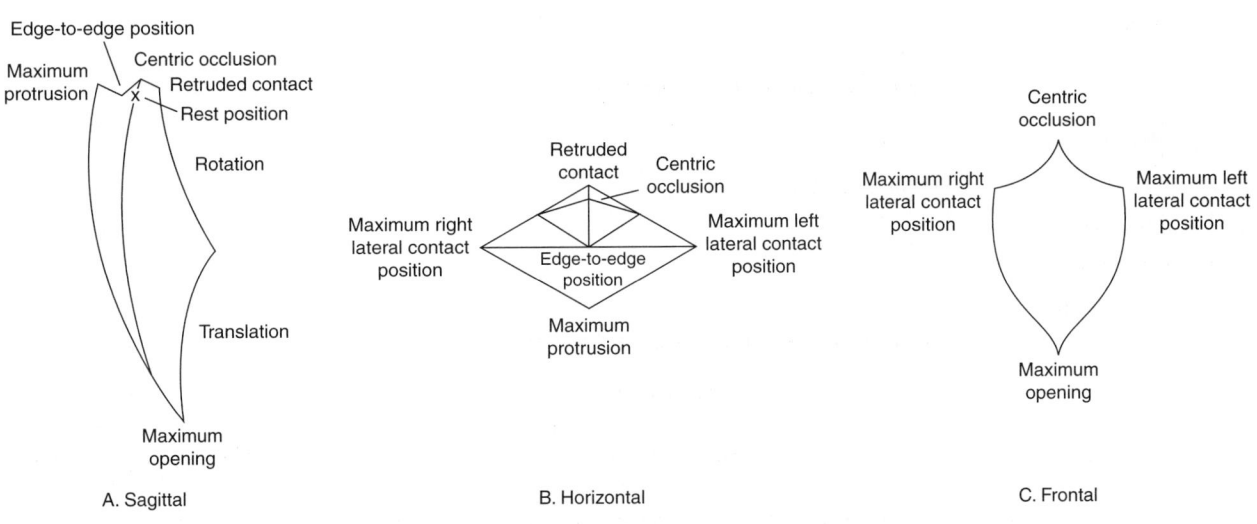

FIGURE 26-8. Three planes of Posselt's envelope of motion.

A **Bennett movement** occurs during lateral excursive movements in which the working side condyle bodily shifts laterally (toward the working side). It has been reported to occur in about 86% of lateral movements, and its average length ranges from 0.5 to 3 mm. (See Figure 26–10.)

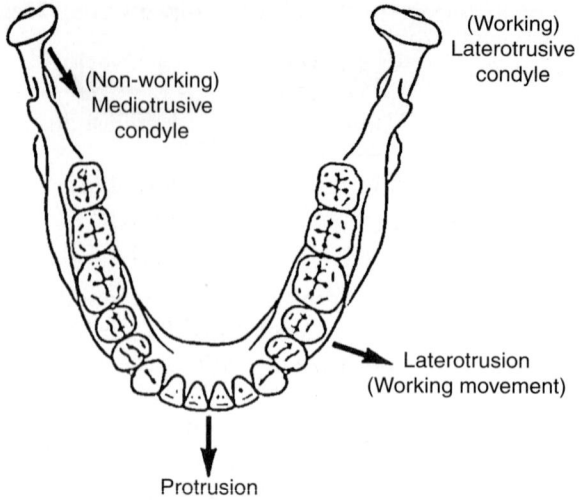

FIGURE 26–9. Condylar movements.

Reprinted, with permission, from Carranza FA. *Clinical Periodontology*, 8th ed. Elsevier, 1996:175.

The **buccinator** is considered the accessory muscle of mastication.

Protrusive movements are caused by contraction of both lateral pterygoids. Lateral excursive movements to the working side are caused by the contraction of the lateral pterygoid on the contralateral (nonworking) side.

If a muscle of mastication becomes paralyzed or injured, the mandible will always deviate to the same side as the muscle injury.

The suprahyoid muscles generally act to elevate the hyoid, especially during swallowing.

Condylar Movements

See Figure 26–9.

- **Protrusive movement:** Both right and left condyles rotate and translate anteriorly simultaneously (downward along the articular eminence).
- **Right working movement:** The left condyle rotates and translates anteriorly (downward along the articular eminence) and medially (to the right). The right condyle rotates forward and translates slightly laterally (to the right).
- **Left working movement:** The right condyle rotates and translates anteriorly (downward along the articular eminence) and medially (to the left). The left condyle rotates forward and translates slightly laterally (to the left).

Occlusal Musculature

See Chapter 1 for details of oral musculature.

Muscles of Mastication

- Temporalis
- Masseter
- Medial pterygoid
- Lateral pterygoid

Suprahyoid Muscles

- Mylohyoid
- Geniohyoid
- Digastric
- Stylohyoid

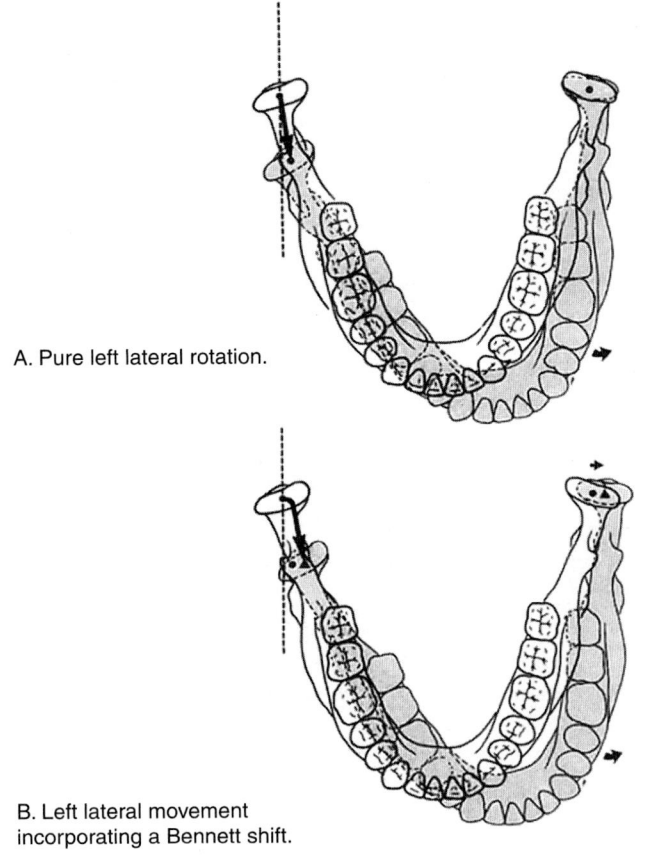

A. Pure left lateral rotation.

B. Left lateral movement incorporating a Bennett shift.

FIGURE 26-10. **Lateral condylar movements.**

Reprinted, with permission, from Carranza FA. *Clinical Periodontology*, 8th ed. Elsevier, 1996:175.

INFRAHYOID MUSCLES

- Omohyoid
- Sternohyoid
- Thyrohyoid
- Sternothyroid

EXTRINSIC MUSCLES OF THE TONGUE

- Genioglossus
- Hyoglossus
- Styloglossus
- Palatoglossus

INTRINSIC MUSCLES OF THE TONGUE

- Longitudinal
- Vertical
- Transverse

The infrahyoid muscles generally depress the hyoid and larynx, especially after swallowing.

Extrinsic tongue muscles bodily move the tongue.

If the hypoglossal nerve becomes paralyzed or injured, the tongue will always deviate to the same side as the muscle injury.

Intrinsic tongue muscles change the shape of the tongue.

CHAPTER 27
Tooth Anomalies

Developmental Anomalies	660
SIZE	660
NUMBER	660
MORPHOLOGY	660
Acquired Anomalies	661
DENTAL INJURIES	661

DEVELOPMENTAL ANOMALIES

Size

- **Microdontia:** Having one or more teeth that are smaller than normal.
- **Macrodontia:** Having one or more teeth that are larger than normal.

The most common congenitally missing teeth are third molars, maxillary lateral incisors, and second premolars.

Number

- **Complete anodontia:** Congenital absence of teeth; generally due to developmental abnormalities such as ectodermal dysplasia.
- **Partial anodontia:** Congenital absence of one or more teeth.
  - **Hypodontia:** Congenital absence of a few teeth.
  - **Oligodontia:** Congenital absence of a large number of teeth.
- **Supernumerary teeth:** Teeth in excess of the normal number. Most common in maxilla.
- **Mesiodens:** A supernumerary tooth located between the maxillary central incisors.

Morphology

- **Ankylosis:** Fusion of the tooth and alveolar bone.
- **Dilaceration:** A bend in the root of a tooth.
- **Taurodontism:** A molar with an elongated root trunk. Generally occurs in patients with amelogenesis imperfecta, Klinefelter syndrome, or Down's syndrome.
- **Dens invaginatus (dens in dente):** Developmental abnormality of *maxillary lateral incisors* in which the focal crown is invaginated for various distances.
- **Dens evaginatus:** Developmental abnormality in which a focal portion of the crown projects outward, creating an extra cusp. A prominent dens evaginatus often seen on *maxillary lateral incisors* is called a **talon cusp**. (See Figure 27–1.)
- **Hypercementosis:** Excessive deposition of cementum.

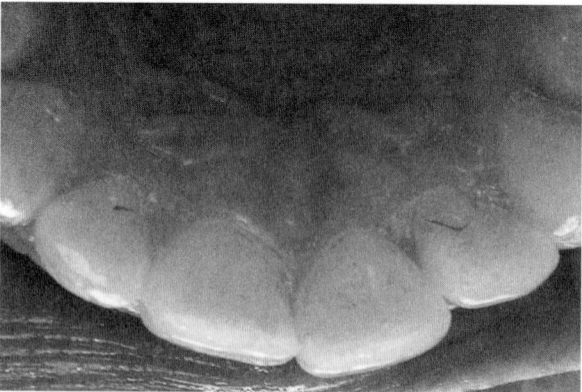

FIGURE 27–1. Talon cusp.

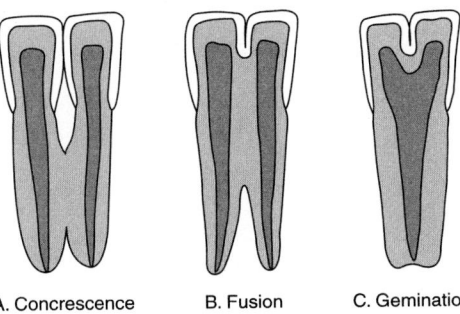

FIGURE 27-2. Concrescence, fusion, and gemination.

- **Cervical enamel projection:** An apical extension of enamel usually located at furcation entrances on molar teeth.
- **Enamel pearl:** A small, focal mass of enamel formed apical to the CEJ.
- **Concrescence:** Fusion of two completely formed teeth at their roots; must have *confluent cementum*.
- **Fusion:** Fusion of two unique tooth buds; must have *confluent dentin*. Its severity depends on the stage of tooth development at which the fusion occurs.
- **Gemination:** Development of two crowns from one tooth bud; *share a single root and root canal*. (See Figure 27–2.)

▶ **ACQUIRED ANOMALIES**

Dental Injuries

Acquired Dental Injuries

Acquired Injury	Definition	Common Cause
Attrition	Loss of tooth structure due to physiologic *tooth-to-tooth contact*, creating **wear facets**	Parafunction (bruxism)
Abrasion	Loss of tooth structure due to abnormal *mechanical* means	Overzealous use of oral hygiene aids Detrimental oral habits (fingernail biting)
Erosion	Loss of tooth structure due to abnormal *chemical means*	Consumption of acidic foods and drinks (facial/buccal surfaces) Bulimia, GERD (lingual/palatal surfaces)
Abfraction	Loss of tooth structure due to abnormal *mechanical stresses*	Occlusal trauma Parafunction (bruxism)

INDEX

A

A band, skeletal muscle and, 331, 331*b*
A fibers, 172
abdomen, 83–88
    regions of, 85
abdominal aorta, 96
abdominal muscles, 85–86
abdominal viscera, 88–113
    pelvic splanchnic nerves and, 147
abducens nerve, 125, 126*f*
    pituitary tumor and, 25
abfraction, 661
ABO blood typing, 510
abrasion, 661
abscess, 436
    acute inflammation and, 491
absolute refractory period, 313
    heart and, 350, 351*f*
absorption, and digestion, 393
acanthosis nigricans, 522
accessory canals, 204
accessory hemiazygos vein (superior hemiazygos vein), 97
accessory nerve (CN XI), schematic illustration, 147*f*
accommodation, pupillary light reflex and, 128
acetone, ketone bodies and, 278
acetylcholine metabolism, 319
acetyl-CoA fate, metabolic fates of, 278
ACh metabolism, enzymes in, 319*b*
achalasia, 543
achlorhydria, pernicious anemia and, 557
achondroplasia (dwarfism), 576
acid-base balance
    control of, 380–381
    respiratory changes and, 372
acquired dental injuries, 661
acquired immunity, 498
    classification of, 498–499
acral lentiginous melanoma, 599
acrochordon, 597
acromegaly, 413, 565
    GH and, 566
acrosome, egg fertilization and, 216
ACTH, negative feedback loop and, 419
actin, 161, 330
    skeletal muscle contraction and, 332, 332*f*
actinic keratosis, 597
Actinomyces species
    plaque induced gingivitis and, 480
    root caries and, 480*b*
Actinomyces viscosus, plaque induced gingivitis and, 480
action potential, 313
    of cardiac muscle, 334

activation energy, 268
    reaction rate, 268, 269*t*
active eruption, 646
active immunity, 454, 498
    viruses and, 469
acute gouty arthritis, 579
acute hypocalcemia, Chvostek's sign and, 569
acute inflammation
    chronic inflammation v., 492
    signs of, 491*b*
    stages of, 491, 491*t*
acute leukemias, 605–606
acute lymphoblastic leukemia (ALL), 592
acute myelogenous leukemia (AML), 605
acute nephritic syndrome, 554
acute osteomyelitis, etiology of, 577
acute pancreatitis, 547
acute pericarditis, 530
Addison's disease, 421–422, 430
    cortisol and, 570
    hyperpigmentation, 519
adenine, 284*b*
adenocarcinoma, 589, 600, 601
    prostate cancer and, 594
    smoking and, 600*b*
adenohypophysis, 179
adenoma, 590
adenomatous polyps, colorectal cancer, 602
adenovirus, 465, 465*t*
ADH. *See* antidiuretic hormone
adipocytes, triglyceride lipolysis and, 276, 277*f*
adipose tissue, lipids and, 264
adjuvants
    immunity and, 499
    vaccines and, 469
adrenal cortex, 111, 423*f*, 570–571
    aldosterone and, 430
    atrophy of, ACTH and, 420
    histologic layers, 419*b*
    precocious puberty, 416
    zones of, 180*b*
adrenal glands, 110, 180, 570–571
    neoplasia of, 611–612
adrenal hormones, 407
adrenal insufficiency, 420
adrenal medulla, 111, 422, 423*f*
    tumors of, 611
adrenal-ACTH axis, exogenous cortisol and, 420
adrenergic agonists, 424
adrenergic neurons, 303
adrenergic receptors, 305
ADUDoma, 590
adult periodontitis, 480
adult polycystic kidney disease (APCKD), 552
adults, brain tumors, 595

afferent nerves, 331
aflatoxins, 471
afterload, 346, 347
ageusia, 326
aggressive periodontitis
    characteristics of, 481
    microbial flora in, 481
aging
    cementum and, 206
    dentin and, 202
    enamel matrix and, 204
    PDL and, 210
    presbycusis and, 142
    pulp and, 205
agranular leukocytes, 501
agranulocytes, 174
air embolism, 525
airway, CN XII paralysis and, 147
airway obstruction, mechanisms of, 537*b*
Albers-Schonberg disease, 576–577
albinism, 519
albumin, function of, 257
albuterol, asthma and, 536
alcoholism, lung abscess and, 541, 541*b*
aldoses, 248*f*
aldosterone (mineralocorticoid), 430
    kidney function and, 386
alkaline phosphatase
    bone formation and, 575
    bone mineralization and, 169
ALL. *See* acute lymphoblastic leukemia
allantois, formation, 219
allergic response, fungi and, 471
allografts, 506
allosteric inhibitor, 268
allosteric regulation, 270*f*, 271
alpha globulins, function of, 257
alpha toxin, host tissue destruction and, 443
alpha-adrenergic receptors, 305
alpha-ketoacids, oxidative deamination and, 278
ALS. *See* amyotrophic lateral sclerosis
alveolar bone
    clinical implications and, 207
    components of, 207
    proper, 207
alveolar epithelial cells, 181
alveolar pressure, 363
alveolar septum, 181
alveolar surface area, gas exchange and, 365
alveolar ventilation, 364
alveolar wall, epithelial cells of, 364
alveoli, 181
alveologingival fibers, 199
Alzheimer's disease, 582
amelogenesis imperfecta, 204
amelogenin, enamel matrix protein and, 203
amine hormones, 407

663

amino acids, 253, 253t–254t
  carbon skeletons of, metabolic intermediates formed, 278, 279f
  derivatives, 254, 254f
    amine hormones, 407
  by dietary necessity, classification of, 253t
  metabolic end product, classification of, 253t
  metabolism, disorders of, 255
  mnemonic, 254
  by R-Group, classification of, 253t
  structure, 254f
  transamination, 278
amino sugar, 250
aminoglycosides
aminotransferases, transamination, 278
AML. See acute myelogenous leukemia
ammonia
  kidney function and, 381
  oxidative deamination and, 278
amniotic fluid embolism, 526
  DIC and, 562
amoxicillin
amphiarthrosis, 170
amphipathic lipid bilayer, membranes and, 294
ampicillin, 455
ampulla of Vater, 185
amygdala, limbic system and, 301
amylases
  starch catabolism and, 249
  starch hydrolysis and, 249
amyloidosis
  multiple myeloma and, 609
  types of, 610
amyotrophic lateral sclerosis (ALS), 582
ANA. See antinuclear antibody test
anal canal, blood supply and description, 109
anaphase, 162
anaphylactic shock, 524
anastomosing vessels of gingiva, PDL and, 209
anatomic crown, 618
anemia(s), 357, 554–559
  of chronic disease, 559
  classification of, 555
  compensations with, 357
  consequences, 357
  erythropoietin and, 358
  from red blood cell destruction, 555–557
  from red blood cell production, 557–559
  types of, 357
aneurysm, atherosclerosis and, 527b
angina, CAD and, 532–533
angioedema, 507
Angle's classification, occlusal relationships, class I-III, 652, 652f–653f
angular artery, 67
ankylosing spondylitis, 573
ankylosis, teeth and, 660
anosmia, 327
ANS. See autonomic nervous system
ansa cervicalis, 65
antacid mediations, peptic ulcer disease, 544
anterior cranial fossa
  contents of, 8
anterior cross-bite, 652
anterior facial vein. See also facial vein
  connections, 25
anterior guidance, mandible and, 654
anterior hard palate, nasopalatine artery and, 68

anterior pituitary
  hormones, 413
  hypothalamic control of, 409
anterior teeth, 618, 621
anterior triangle, of neck, subsets of, 60–62, 61f
anterior/ventral horn, 149
anthracosis, 539
anthrax toxin, host tissue destruction and, 443
antibiotic drugs, 454–459, 455t
  classification of, 454
  comparison of, dentistry and, 455t
  oral, impetigo and, 520
  peptic ulcer disease, 544
  topical, 458
antibiotic prophylaxis, 458, 458t–459t
antibody-mediated immune response, 499
  acquired immunity and, 498
anticonvulsants, aplastic anemia and, 557
antidiuretic hormone (ADH; vasopressin), 407, 564–565
  diabetes insipidus and, 412
  kidney function and, 386
  pituitary gland and, 179
antifungal drugs, for candidiasis, 473t
antigenic shifts, viruses and, 461
antigen-presenting cells (APCs), 499, 502
  immune system and, 502
antigens, immunity and, 499
antinuclear antibody test (ANA), systemic lupus erythematosus, 571
antiseptics, 438, 439t
antitoxin vaccine, 454
aortic aneurysm, 529
aortic arch derivatives, embryology and, 228, 228f
aortic body, respiratory chemoreceptors and, 371, 372f
aortic dissection, pericardial sac and, 529
aortic valve, 91
APCKD. See adult polycystic kidney disease
APCs. See antigen-presenting cells
apical foramen, pulp and, 204
apical vessels, PDL and, 209
aplastic anemia, 557
aplastic crisis, sickle-cell anemia and, 556
apnea, 374
aponeurosis, 166
apoprotein, 262
apoptosis, 490
appositional growth, cartilage and, 168
aqueous humor, 193
arachnoid barrier, 27
arboviruses, 462
arch lengths
  mandibular teeth, 642
  maxillary teeth, 642
arginine, 254
  histones and, 287
Argyll Robertson pupil, 128
arm movement, at shoulder, 81–82
arterial constriction system, mean systemic filling pressure and, 343
arterial nephrosclerosis, 552–553
arterial supply
  dental, 621
  liver and, 106
arterial thrombi, 525
arterial thrombosis, predisposing factors for, 525b
arteries, 342
  of brainstem, Circle of Willis and, 28f

arteriolar nephrosclerosis, 553
arterioles, 176
  oxygen exchange and, 342
arteriosclerosis, 526, 553
arthritis, 579–581
articular capsule (bursa), 51, 170
articular disk of TMJ. See meniscus
articular eminence, 50
articular osteochondroses, 576
artificial teeth, compensating curve and, 650
asbestosis, 539
ascending pharyngeal artery, 67, 67f
ascites, 549
  disorders associated with, 549
  liver disease and, 549
asexual reproduction, spores, 471
aspiration, right lung and, 89
aspirin
  bleeding problems and, 560
  cyclooxygenase and, 262
  irreversible inhibition, 268
  Reye's syndrome and, 466
assembly, viral replication and, 460
asthma, 235–236
  mechanisms of precipitation, 236
  treatment, 536
  types of, 235
astigmatism, 323
atelectasis, 538
atelectasis neonatorum, 538
atherosclerosis, 347, 526–527, 527b
atlanto-axial joint, 54
atlanto-occipital joint, 54
atopic allergies, 507
ATP
  molecule, skeletal muscle contraction and, 332, 332f, 333, 333b
  production, metabolic pathway and, 272
atria, 91
atrial septal defect, embryology and, 228b
atrioventricular valves, 91
atrophic candidiasis, 482
attached gingiva, 197
attachment, viral replication and, 460
attrition, 661
Auerbach's plexus. See myenteric plexus
auricular branch of vagus, distribution, 135, 136f
auriculotemporal nerve, 51
  distribution, 130, 135, 136f
autoclaving, hepatitis viruses and, 468
autograft, 506
autoimmune diseases, 512
  polyarthritis nodosa, 572
  RA as, 580
  systemic lupus erythematosus, 571–572
autoimmune gastritis, pernicious anemia and, 557
autoimmune hemolytic anemia, 555
autolysis, enzymatic cellular degradation and, 488
automaticity, heart and, electrical conduction of, 350, 351f
autonomic ganglia, ANS and, 303
autonomic nervous system (ANS), 299–301, 303
  autonomic ganglia, 303
  basic pathway, 303
  pathway, 154
  smooth muscle and, 335, 335f
  summary of, 305
autoregulation of blood flow, exercise and, 356

664

autosomal abnormalities, 516–517
AV node, nodal/pacemaker conduction system and, 352
avascular connective tissue, 168
axilla, boundaries of, 77–78
axillary artery, 78
axillary nerve, 80
axillary vein, 78
axon, 171
axoneme, 161
axonotmesis, 316
azithromycin, 456
AZT, reverse transcriptase function and, 291
azygous system, 96–97, 97f

B

bacilli, plaque induced gingivitis and, 480
Bacillus, 445
bacitracin, 458
bacteria, 441
    classification of, 444–445, 444f
    gram positive v. gram negative, 445, 445t
    medically relevant, 446–453
bacterial adhesion/attachment, mediators of, 442
bacterial colonization, 478
bacterial endocarditis, antibiotic prophylaxis and, 458, 458t–459t
bacterial genetic exchange, 441–442
bacterial growth curve, 441, 441f
bacterial infection, neutrophilia and, 492
bacterial pneumonia, 541
bacterial polysaccharides, 251
bacterial structures, specialized, 444
bacterial virulence factors, 442–445
bacteriology, 441–459
bacteriophages, 469
    replication, 470f
bactroban, impetigo and, 520
Bainbridge reflex, 354
balance, hair cells and, 308
baroreceptor reflex, 354
    sudden standing and, 355
baroreceptors, 143, 354
Barr body, 161
Barrett's esophagus, 544
    GERD and, 543
    scleroderma, 572
basal cell carcinoma, 596
basal ganglia, motor behavior and, 301
basal nuclei, 115
base pairing
    DNA and, 284–287
    organization of, 284
base substitutions, mutation and, 591
basement membrane, 191
    components, 165
    functions of, 165
basilar artery, 27
basilic vein, 78
basophils, 502
BBB. *See* blood-brain barrier
B-cell, 500, 500t
    maturation, bone marrow and, 177
    NHL and, 608
B-complex vitamins, nonprotein enzyme components, 266
Behcet's syndrome, 573
Bell's palsy, 139
Bence-Jones protein, multiple myeloma, 609
benign nephrosclerosis, 553

benign prostatic hyperplasia, 594–595
benign tumors
    harm of, 587b
    malignant tumors v., 587
    of mesenchymal origin, 590
    types of, 590–591
Bennet movement, 656, 657f
Bernard-Soulier disease, 563
berylliosis, causes, 539b
beta$_2$ agonist inhalers, asthma and, 536
beta-adrenergic receptors, 305
beta-globulins, function of, 257
beta-oxidation, lipid metabolism and, 276, 277f
Bezold-Jarisch reflex, 373
BGL. *See* blood glucose level
bifid tongue, 241
bilaminar disc, 217
bile, 107, 184–185
    composition, 186, 547
    duodenum and, 110
    pHs of, 395
    pigment, 174
    salts, 263
    secretion pHs, 395
biliary flow, 186, 186f
biliary tree, 185, 186f
bilirubin, 398, 549–550
    jaundice and, 397
    levels, 185
bilirubinuria, 552
binary fission, bacteria and, 441
biofilm, 478
biologic width, 198
bisphosphonate drugs, osteonecrosis of jaws and, 578
black lung disease, 539
bladder. *See* urinary bladder
bladder cancer, 604
bleeding
    disorders, 561
    problems, 560
blood
    components of, 173f
    formation, primitive embryology, 221
    formed elements of, 173
    functions of, 172
    neoplasia of, 604–611
    oxygen in, 366
    oxygen-carrying capacity in, 366, 366b
    PO$_2$ and, oxygen transfer in, 367b
    type O, 510b
    in urine, children and, 551
blood flow, 339
    autoregulation, exercise and, 356
    cardiodynamics and, 339–342
    properties of, 340, 340f
    velocity of, 340, 340f
    changes in, 341f
blood glucose level (BGL), normal, 419
blood ketones, 565b
blood pressure, 344
    arterioles, 342
    changes in, 341f
    pulmonary circulation, systemic circulation v., 343
blood supply
    buccinator, 140
    dental arterial, 621
    to face, 66
    meninges and, 22
    to nasal cavity, 17

    stomach, 105, 106f
    tongue, 66
blood typing. *See* ABO blood typing
blood vessel(s)
    bleeding problems and, 560
    damage, intrinsic/extrinsic pathways and, 358, 359f
    oxytalan fibers and, 209
    types
        and characteristics, 342
        histologic differences, 176
    walls, layers of, 175f
blood volume, systemic venous circulation and, 342
blood-brain barrier (BBB), 27
blood-CSF barrier, 27
blood-loss anemia, 555
blood-lymphatic pathology, 554–564
bloodstream, endocrine glands and, 166
blue bloaters, chronic bronchitis and, 538
blue nevus, 595
body cavities, posterior and anterior, 88
body fluid, distribution, 376
Bohr effect, 366
    anemia and, 357
bone
    formation, alkaline phosphatase and, 575
    fracture, fat embolism and, 578
    functions of, 169
    remodeling, 170
    resorption, 428
    surfaces, 169
    types of, 169
bone marrow, 170, 177, 500, 500t
    leukemia and, 604
    multiple myeloma, 609
bone spurs, osteoarthritis and, 579
bone tumors, of nonosseous origin, 613–614
botox, achalasia and, 543
botulinum toxin, host tissue destruction and, 442
Bouchar's nodes, osteoarthritis and, 579
Bowman's capsule, filtration and, 382, 383
brachial arches
    derivatives of structures for, 235f
    embryology, 231
brachial artery, 78
brachial plexus, 153
    actions, by roots, 81
    branches of, 79, 79f
    nerves, 81
    terminal nerves of, 80
    and upper extremities, 77–83
brachial vein, 78
brachiocephalic artery, 95
brachiocephalic veins, 95
brain, 113–115, 114f
    drainage of, IJV and, 24
    embryology of, 227
    hypoxia and, 486b
    injury, 581
    neurocranium and, 6
    tumors, 595
        adults, 595
brainstem, 116–117, 117f, 227
    components, 302
branched amylopectin, starch, 249
branchiomeric nerves, 231
BRCA-1 gene, breast cancer and, 593
breast, 86–87
breast cancer, 593–594, 593b
    fibrocystic disease v., 593b

665

breastfeeding, celiac disease and, 546
bronchial arteries, 89
bronchiectasis, 538
bronchoconstrictor release, asthma and, 536
bronchodilation
    epinephrine and, 254
    norepinephrine and, 254
bronchogenic carcinoma, 600
bronchopneumonia, 541
bronchus, pulmonary artery v., 89
brown tumor, blood chemistry values, 574
brownish-gray banding, tetracycline and, 204
buccal ridge, 620
    first premolar, 629, 630f
buccinator nerve, 656
    blood supply to, 140
    of V-3, 129
budding, viruses and, 459
buffer, 380
buffer systems, 380
bullate papillae, 326
    pemphigoid, 521
Burkitt's lymphoma, 609
bursa. *See* articular capsule
butterfly rash, systemic lupus erythematosus, 571
byssinosis, 539

C

C fibers, 172
CA^{2+}-Na^+ exchange system, cardiac muscle and, 334
CAD. *See* coronary artery disease
Café au lait spots, 519
    disease association with, 575b
    tuberous sclerosis, 575b
calcification, 169
calcinosis, 489b
calcitonin, 170
    calcium regulation and, 428
    parafollicular cells and, 72
calcium
    deficiency, 403
    hyperparathyroidism and, 429
    hypoparathyroidism and, 429
    metabolism, 427–429
    regulation, 170
    skeletal muscle contraction and, 333
    stones, 551
calcium channel blockers, gingival overgrowth and, 487b
calculus, formation, 479
calicivirus, 461
calmodulin, smooth muscle contraction and, 335
caloric test, vestibuloocular reflex, 143b
calorimetry, 246
cAMP protein kinases
    cardiac muscle and, 334
    hormones and, 408
    mechanism, 408, 409f
Campylobacter rectus, plaque induced gingivitis and, 480
canaliculi, 185, 206
cancellous bone, 169, 207
cancer. *See specific type cancer i.e. prostate cancer*
Candida albicans, candidiasis, 482

candidiasis
    antifungal drugs and, 472, 473t
    characteristics and classification, 482
canine guidance, mandible and, 655
canines, 629, 629f
    lobes of, 627
    mandibular permanent teeth, 635–636, 635f
    mandibular primary teeth, 644
    maxillary permanent teeth, 629, 629f
    maxillary primary teeth, 643
capacitance, 342
capillaries, 176
    oxygen exchange and, 342
capillary permeability, edema and, 378
capsid, viruses and, 459
capsular polysaccharide vaccine, 454
capsulated joint receptors, nonencapsulated joint receptors v., 307
carbohydrate(s), 248–256
    cell membranes and, 295
    classification, 248
    complexes, calculus and, 479
    digestion and absorption, 393
    metabolism, 272–276
    structure, 248
carbon dioxide (CO_2), blood and, 368, 368f
carbon monoxide poisoning, 357, 534
carbonic anhydrase
    reaction, 246, 246f
    serum and, 368
carcinogenic bacteria, dietary sucrose and, 251
carcinomas, 589
cardiac compensation, anemia and, 357
cardiac conduction, 176
    tissues, 350
cardiac cycle, 348, 349f
cardiac demand, compensatory hypertrophy and, 334
cardiac enzymes, after MI, 533b
cardiac esophageal sphincter, 105
cardiac function, determinants of, 345–350
cardiac glands, gastric secretion and, 392
cardiac muscle. *See also* heart
    action potential, 334
    contraction, 334
    histology, 334
    innervation, 334
    skeletal muscle v., refractory period and, 350b
cardiac myocytes, cardiac conductive tissues and, 350
cardiac output (CO), 345
    high HR and, 347
    shock and, 523
cardiac system, embryology of, 227–228, 230f
cardiac tamponade, 530
cardiac veins, 93
cardiodynamics, blood flow and, 339–342
cardiogenic shock, 524
cardiovascular pathology, 522–535
cardiovascular pulmonary cross-correlation, 534–535
cardiovascular tissue, 175–176
caries, 621
    characteristics of, 479
    classification, 479
    Stephan curve and, 479, 480f
carnitine-mediated enzyme system, fatty acids, 278
carotid body, respiratory chemoreceptors and, 371, 372f

carotid body O_2, pH levels and, 308
carotid sheath, 57, 57f
carotid sinus, 355
carotid sinus syndrome, 355
carrier infection, 436
cartilage, 168
    ECM of, 168
    growth of, 168
    surface of, 168
    types of, 168
cartilaginous joints, 170
catabolism, glycogen synthesis and, 276, 277f
catalase, 503
catecholamines, 407
    tyrosine metabolism and, 424
cathepsin D, malignant tumors and, 588
cauda equina, 149
cavernous sinus, 24, 24f, 25f
    infection and, 71
CD3-associated T-cell receptor (TCR), T-cells and, 499, 500t
CD8 lymphocytes, 500b
CDC. *See* Centers for Disease Control and Prevention
cecum, blood supply and description, 109
cefadroxil, 456
cefazolin, 456
cefepime, 456
cefixime, 456
cefoxitin, 456
cefpodoxime, 456
cefprozil, 456
CEJ contours, 626
    proximal, 626–627, 626f
celiac disease, 546
cell(s)
    cardiac muscle and, 334
    of small intestine, 183t
    turnover, tissue types and, 162
    types, comparison, 435, 435t
cell cycle, 162, 162f
cell death
    necrosis, types of, 490, 490t
    nuclear changes with, 490
cell injury
    chemical, 486
    chemical-induced, 486
    free-radical, 486–487
    modes of, 486
    reactions to, 487t
    types of, 487
cell membranes, triglycerides in, 260
cell morphology, 164
cell surface appendages, 161
cell-mediated immune response, 499
    acquired immunity and, 498
    fungal infection, 471
cell-to-cell contacts, 163t
cellulitis, 436
cellulose, 251
cementicles, 209f
cementoblasts, 206
cementogenesis, 206
cementum, 205–206
    aging effects on, 206
    classifications of, 206
    functions of, 206
    morphology, 207f
Centers for Disease Control and Prevention (CDC), 439
central diabetes insipidus, 412, 564
central hearing connections, deafness and, 143

central incisor, 627–628, 627f
  mandibular permanent teeth, 633–634, 634f
  maxillary permanent teeth, 627, 627f
  maxillary primary teeth, 642
central nervous system (CNS), 299
  embryology of, 225, 225f
  hypercarbia, 369
  nervous tissue, 171
centric occlusion (CO), mandible and, 654
centric relation (CR), mandible and, 654
centroacinar cells, 187
centrocytes, 206
cephalexin, 456
cephalic vein, 78
cephalosporins, 456
cerebellum
  function and components, 116
  motor control, 302
cerebral arteries, major, 28f
cerebral circulation, CO_2 effect on, 370
cerebral cortex, 114, 114f, 299
  functions of, 114, 114f
  hemispheres, lobes of, 299
cerebral infarction, 581–582
cerebral medulla, 114, 114f
cerebrospinal fluid (CSF)
  ependymal cells and, 26
  spinal cord and, 149
cerebrospinal fluid (CSF) circulation pathway, 26
cerebrum, 114
cervical cancer, squamous cell carcinoma v., histologic appearance, 598
cervical enamel projection, 661
cervical loop, root formation and, 213, 214f
cervical plexus, 65f, 153
cervical ridge, 620
cervical vertebrae, 54
cGMP, hormones and, 408
chemical neurotransmitters, 318
chemical plaque control, 483, 483t
chemical synapse, 317
chemokines, 502
chemoreception, 143
chemoreceptor, 308, 354, 355
  pathway, 356
chewing surfaces, of teeth, 618
CHF. See congestive heart failure
children
  acute osteomyelitis, 577
  bone tumors, 613–614
  brain tumors in, 595
  cretinism and, 567
  dental findings
    hypothyroidism and, 567b
    rickets, 574
  genetic disorders of, 518–519
  histiocytosis X and, 611
  intestinal lymphangiectasia, 545
  leukemia and, 592
  osteomalacia and, 574
  PCKD and, 552
  Reye's syndrome and, 466
  skin eruptions, impetigo, 520
chitin, 251
  fungi cells and, 470
chloramphenicol, 458
  aplastic anemia and, 557
chlorhexidine gluconate, 478
chloride shift, 368
cholecystokinin, stimulus and control, 390
cholelithiasis, 547

cholesterol
  membranes and, 294
  as steroid, 261
  synthesis, liver and, 396
cholesterolosis, 547
cholinergic neurons, 303
chondroblasts, 168
chondrocytes, 168
chondroma, 590
chondrosarcoma, 613
chorda tympani nerve
  components of, 31
  course of, 31
  lingual nerve and, 132
chordae tendinea, valves and, 92
chordoma, 614
choristoma, 590
choroid, 193
choroid plexus, intracranial pressure and, 25
Christmas disease, 563
chromatin, 161
  DNA, 287, 288f
chromosomal disorders, 516–517, 516b
chronic bronchitis, 538
chronic hyperplastic candidiasis, 482
chronic infection, 436
chronic inflammation
  acute inflammation and, 491
  acute inflammation v., 492
  stages of, 492
chronic leukemias, 606
chronic lymphocytic lymphoma (CLL), diffuse lymphocytic lymphoma and, 609
chronic myelogenous leukemia (CML), 607
chronic nephrotic syndrome, 554
chronic obstructive pulmonary disease (COPD), 537–538
  hypoxemia in, 368
chronic osteomyelitis, 578
chronic pancreatitis, 547
chronic pericarditis, 530
chronic periodontitis
  characteristics, 480
  predominant microbial flora in, 481
Chvostek's sign, tetany, 569
chylomicrons, 394
chyme, 392
  segmentation, 392, 393
cigarette smoking
  adenocarcinoma, 600b
  emphysema and, 537
  lung cancers and, 601
  related diseases, 537b
cilia, 161
ciliary body, 193
  of eyeball, 320
ciliary zone, 194f
cingulum, 618
ciprofloxacin, 457
Circle of Willis, 27, 28f
  arteries of brainstem and, 28f
  of brainstem, 28f
  middle cerebral artery v., 29
circuit, pulmonary circulation, systemic circulation v., 343
circulation, blood vessels in, arrangement of, 175f
circumferential fibers
circumpulpal dentin, 201
  formation, 201
circumvallate papillae, 32

cirrhosis, 548
  edema and, 523
  proteins and, 358
cisterna chyli, 100
citrate-malate shuttle, fatty acid synthesis, 276, 277f
citric acid cycle, 274, 275f
clarithromycin, 456
class I MHC surface proteins, nucleated cells and, 499
class II MHC proteins, immune system and, 502
classic hemophilia, 563
clavicle, 83
cleavage stages, morula and blastula, embryology and, 219f
cleft lip, formation and variations, 237, 238f, 239
cleft palate, formation and variations, 237
clindamycin, 457
clinical crown, 618
CLL. See chronic lymphocytic lymphoma
clonal selection, 500
Clostridium, 445
clotting factors, liver and, 563
cloxacillin, 455
CML. See chronic myelogenous leukemia
CN II. See facial nerve
CN III injury, lesions and, 128
CN III. See levator palpebrae superioris
CN IX. See glossopharyngeal nerve
CN V. See trigeminal nerve
CN VII. See orbicularis oculi
CN VIII. See vestibulococholear nerve
CN X. See vagus nerve
CN XI. See accessory nerve
CN XII. See hypoglossus nerve
CNs. See cranial nerves
CNS. See central nervous system
CO. See centric occlusion;
  See cardiac output
CO_2. See carbon dioxide
coagulase, 442
coagulation, intrinsic and extrinsic pathways, 358, 359f
coagulative necrosis, 490
coal workers pneumoconiosis, 539
coenzyme Q, ubiquinone as, 275
coenzymes, 400
cold caloric test, 143, 143b
collagen, 169
  structure, 256f
  synthesis, 256, 257f
  type I, dentogingival connective tissue and, 199
  type II, 168
  type IV, oral mucosa and, 196
collagen remodeling, wound repair and, 496
collagen vascular diseases, 571–573, 571b
  types, 580b
collagenases (metalloproteinases), host tissue destruction and, 442
collapsing forces, lung and, 363
colloid osmotic pressure. See oncotic pressure
colon
  blood supply and description, 109
  GI cancer and, 602
colon polyps, 603
colonoscopy, colorectal cancer and, 602
colony stimulating factors (CSFs), 493, 493t–494t

667

colorectal cancer, screening and diagnosis, 602
commensalism, 436
common bile duct, 107
   choledocholithiasis and, 547
common carotid, 95
common central vein, 106
common facial vein, 71
common iliac artery
   pelvic kidney and, 98
   ureter and, 111
communicating-obstruction, in subarachnoid space, 26b
compensating curve, 650
compensatory hypertrophy, cardiac demand and, 334
competitive inhibition, 268, 270f
complement protein system, 505f
complement proteins, 504
   activation, pathways of, 505t
   function of, 257, 505t
complete anodontia, 660
complete bilateral cleft, 239
complex carbohydrates, 251–252
compliance
   pulmonary circulation, systemic circulation v., 343
   venus return and, 347
concrescence, 661, 661f
concussion, 581
condensing osteitis, 578
conductance, 339
conducting zone, lung and, 364
conduction velocity, 316b
conductive loss, 143
condylar movements, 656, 656f
condyle, 20
   of mandible, 50
cones, 193, 321
confluent cementum, concrescence and, 661, 661f
congenital syphilis, enamel and, 204
congestion (hyperemia), 524
congestive heart failure (CHF), edema and, 523
congo red, amyloid stain and, 610
conidia, 471
conjugated bilirubin, 549
conjugation, bacterial cell and, 441
connective tissue (CT)
   attachments, 166
   cells of, 166
   classification of, 165
   skeletal muscle and, 332
contact area, 621
continuous conduction, 316
contour lines of Owen, 202
contractility, HR and, 346
contraction (twitch), of skeletal muscle, 332, 332f
contraction (twitch) speed
   pneumonic for, 333b
   skeletal muscle, comparison by, 333
contralateral tracts, 306b
conus medullaris, 149
convergence, pupillary light reflex and, 128
COPD. See chronic obstructive pulmonary disease
copper, transferrin and, 404
cor pulmonale, right heart failure and, 534b
Cori cycle, lactic acid and, 273, 274f
cornea, 192
corneal reflex, 136, 136b

corneoscleral coat, 192
coronary arteries, 92–93, 92f
coronary artery disease (CAD), 532–533
   causes of, 532b
coronary ligaments, 106
coronary sinus, 93
coronavirus, 462
coronoid process, 20
corpora cavernosa, 189
corpus callosum, 114, 114f, 299
corpus luteum, 418
corpus spongiosum, 189
cortex, medullary rays and, 187
cortical bone, 169, 207
cortical sinuses, lymph and, 177
corticospinal tract (pyramidal system), 311, 312f
corticosteroids, 419
   phospholipase A2 and, 262
cortisol, 420, 570–571
cough reflexes, 89
Coumadin. See Warfarin
countercurrent exchange, 384
countercurrent multiplier, 384
coupled, transport proteins and, 295
covalent bonds, 246
covalent modification, enzyme regulation and, 269
COX (cyclooxygenase)
   aspirin and, 262
   inhibitors, asthma and, 536
coxsackieviruses, 462
CPE. See cytopathic effect
CR. See centric relation
cranial base, of internal skull, 11, 11f
cranial foramina, 20–21
   important, 8–9
cranial fossae, 8. See also internal skull
cranial nerve (CN), 118–119, 124–155
   brainstem and, 117, 117f
   chart, 120t–124t
   components, 118
   motor nuclei, unilateral corticonuclear connections and, 117
   sensory nuclei, hearing and, 117
   taste sensation, tongue and, 30
craniopharyngioma, 595
cranium, 6
   bones of, 6
creatine phosphate, skeletal muscle contraction and, 333
creatine phosphokinase (CPK), 533b
cremaster muscle, 86
CREST syndrome, 572b
cretinism, 179b, 426, 566, 567
Creutzfeldt-Jakob disease, 470
CRH-ACTH-Cortisol axis, 419
cricothyroid membrane, 74
Crohn's disease, 545
   Ulcerative colitis v., comparison of, 545
   vitamin B_{12}, 402
cross-bite, 651
cross-striations, skeletal muscle and, 331
crown, 618
CSF. See cerebrospinal fluid
CSFs. See colony stimulating factors
CT. See connective tissue
curve of Spee, 650, 650f
curve of Wilson, 650, 651f
Cushing's disease
   cortisol and, 570
   Cushing's syndrome v., 421

Cushing's syndrome, 420, 420f
   cortisol and, 570
   Cushing's disease v., 421
cusp, 619
   height, anterior tooth relationship and, 655f
cusp of Carabelli, 619
cutaneous innervation, face/scalp/auricle, 135f
cyanide poisoning, oxidative phosphorylation and, 535
cyanosis, 357
Cyclooxygenase. See COX
cyclosporin, gingival overgrowth and, 487b
cyst, 436
cystic fibrosis, 518, 518b
cysticercosis, 476
cytochrome oxidase, 275
cytochromes, 274
   complexes, 274
cytokeratin, 161
cytokines, 493, 493t–494t
cytopathic effect (CPE), 460
cytoplasm, 160
   viral replication and, 460
cytosine, guanine and, 284b
cytoskeleton, 171
cytosol, fatty acid synthesis, 276, 277f
cytotoxic hypersensitivity, 508f

D

DAG, hormones and, 408
daily imbrication line of von Ebner, 202
dead space, 364
dead tracts, 201
deafness, central hearing connections and, 143
death phase, bacteria and, 441
decidual reaction, week 2, 219
deciduous tooth form. See primary tooth form
deep cervical fascia, investing layer of, 55
deep facial vein, connections, 25
deep venous thrombosis, 526
defecation, 113
degenerative diseases, 582
DEJ. See dentino-enamel junction
delayed hypersensitivity, 509f
delayed passive eruption, 214
deltavirus, 462
dendrites, 171
dendritic cells, 501
dens evaginatus, 660
dens invaginatus (dens in dente), teeth and, 660
dense connective tissue
   irregular, 166
   regular, 166
dental anatomy, 618–621
dental findings
   child and, hypothyroidism and, 567–568
   rickets, 574
dental follicle, 213
dental formula
   permanent dentition, 647
   primary dentition, 646
dental injuries, 661
dental papilla, 213
   differentiated ectomesenchymal cells, 200
dental treatment, antibiotic prophylaxis and, 458, 458t–459t
denticles, 205

dentifrice, gingivitis and, 483, 483t
dentin, 200
    aging and, 202
    classifications of, 201–202
    deformities, 202
    formation, chronological order of, 213b
dentin dysplasia, 202
dentinal hypersensitivity, 202
dentino-enamel junction (DEJ), 203–204
dentinogenesis imperfecta, 202
dentist, universal precautions and, 440
dentitions. *See also* permanent dentition; primary dentition
    classification of, 618
dentogingival connective tissue, type I collagen and, 199
dentogingival epithelium, 198
dentogingival fibers
dentogingival junction, 198
    tooth eruption, 214, 214f
dentoperiosteal fibers, 199
dermatofibroma, 596–597
dermatomes, 87, 87f
    derivatives, 223f
dermatomyositis, calcinosis and, 489b
dermis, 191
descending colon, 108
descending motor tracts (descending pathways), 310–311
descending pathways. *See* descending motor tracts
desmin, 161
desmoplasia, 589
desmosome (macula adherens), 162
    cardiac muscle and, 334
developmental groove, 621
developmental pathology, 516–519
dextran, 251
ΔG. *See* Gibbs free energy change
diabetes insipidus, 419, 564
    causes of, 412
    diabetes mellitus v., 412
diabetes mellitus
    pancreas and, 419
    type 1, diabetes type 2 v., 565
diabetic coma, 278
diapedesis, 502.502t
diaphragm muscles, 84, 101
diaphragma sella, 22
diarrhea, clindamycin and, 457
diarthrosis, 170
diastema, 621
diastole
    cardiac cycle and, 348
    fibrous pericardium and, 345b
diastolic pressure, 344
dicloxacillin, 455
    impetigo and, 520
diencephalon, 299
diffuse lymphocytic lymphoma, chronic lymphocytic lymphoma and, 609
DiGeorge's syndrome, 512b
    hypoparathyroidism and, 569
digestion, absorption and, components, 393
dilaceration, teeth and, 660
Dilantin. *See* phenytoin
dilation, 543
dimorphism, molds and, 471
diphtheria toxin, host tissue destruction and, 443
diphyodont dentition, 618
diploic veins, 24
dipolar ions. *See* Zwitterions

direct calorimetry, 246
disaccharide absorption, 394
disaccharides, 248
disease. *See specific type disease i.e. degenerative diseases*
disinfectants, 438, 438t
disinfection, 438
disseminated intravascular coagulation (DIC)
    causes, 562
    laboratory indications, 562
distolingual groove, first molar, 631, 631f
disulfide bonds, immunoglobulins and, 503
DNA
    backbone structure of, 286, 286f
    base pairing and, 284–287, 285f
    ligases, 291
        DNA synthesis and, 289, 289f
    metronidazole and, 457
    organization, 287–288, 288f
    polymerase, 291
        DNA synthesis and, 289, 289f
    synthesis, 289, 289f
    transduction and, 442
    transfer, bacteria and, 441
    transformation and, 442
    viruses, 459
        viral replication and, 460
domains, protein structures and, 255
dorsal column system, pathway, 309
dorsal root ganglion, afferent/sensory nerves and, 150
dorsal scapular artery, 79f
Down syndrome, 516
    chromosomal disorders and, 516b
doxycycline, 457
drug-induced lupus erythematosus, 571
drugs
    antiviral, 469
    teratogenesis and, 516
duct of Wirsung, 110
ductus deferens, 113
duodenal ulcer, 544
duodenum, 96, 184
    blood supply and description of, 108
dura mater, dural folds of, 22, 23f
dural folds, of dura mater, 22, 23f
dural sinuses
    list of, 23, 23f
    tributaries of, 24
dust cells, 181, 501
dwarfism, 413, 576
dysarthria, hypoglossus nerve and, 147
dysgeusia, 326
dysosmia, 327
dysplasia, 587
dysplastic nevus, 596
dyspnea, 374
dystrophic calcifications, 205

E

ear, anatomy, 141, 142f, 323
Eaton-Lambert syndrome, 583b
eburnation, osteoarthritis and, 579
ecchymoses, petechiae v., 562
ecchymosis, leukemias and, 606
eclampsia, secondary HTN and, 528, 528b
ECM. *See* extracellular matrix
ectomesenchyme, tooth type and, 212
edemas
    cause of, 378, 523
    clinical exam of, 523

nephrotic syndrome and, 553
types of, 522–523
Edward syndrome, 517
EFC. *See* extracellular fluids
effective renal plasma flow (ERPF), 385
efferent nerves, 331
efferent pathways. *See* descending motor tracts
egg, stages of meiosis in, 215
eggshell calcification, 489b
eicosanoids, pathways, 262
ejaculatory duct, 113
ejection fraction, 345
elastic arteries, 176
elastic cartilage, 168
elastin, hydroxylsine and, 256
electrical synapse, 317, 318
electrocardiogram (EKG), 352–353
    leads, 352
    waves, 353, 353f
electron transport chain, 274
elephantiasis, edema and, 523
embolus, 525
embrasures, 621
    contact area and, 621
embryo development
    pituitary gland, 410, 410f
    week 1, 218f
    week 4, 225b
embryology, 215–242
    brain, 227
    forebrain, 227
    gametogenesis, 215, 215f–217f
    heart, 231f
    kidney, stages of, 232f
    pancreas, 233f
    patent foramen ovale, 228b
    tongue and, 30
embryonic body axis, 221, 221f
emissary veins, 24
emphysema
    problems with, 538b
    types of, 537
enamel
    aging effects on, 204
    amelogenesis of, 203
    cross striations and incremental lines, 203
    deformities of, 204
    formation, chronological order of, 213b
enamel hypoplasia, 204
enamel knot, 213
enamel matrix formation, defect, 204
enamel maturation defect, 204
enamel organ, 212
enamel pearl, 661
enamel surface depression, 620–621
enamel surface elevations, 618–620
enamel surface junctions, 621
encapsulated joint receptors, types of, 307b
endemic infection, 436
endocarditis, 530
    types of, 531
endochondral ossification, 169
endocrine disorders, secondary HTN and, 528
endocrine glands, 178–180, 187
    function and excretions of, 166
endocrine pancreas, 187
endocrine pathology, 564–571
endogenous pigments, 488
    comparison of, 488t
endomysium, CT and, 332
endopeptidases, 256

endosomes, 161
endosteum, 169
endothelium, 165
endotoxin
    host tissue destruction and, 443
    mode of action, 443f
    structure, 443f
end-stage kidney disease, APCKD, 552
enolase, fluoride and, 273
enteric nervous system, 390
entero gastrone, 390
enterohepatic circulation, lipoproteins and, 262
enterotoxins, host tissue destruction and, 442
enteroviruses, 462
enthalpy, 246
entropy, 246
envelope, viruses and, 459
enzymatic cellular degradation, 488
enzyme(s)
    in ACh metabolism, 319b
    biomechanics, induced-fit model, 266, 266f
    classification of, 266
    digestion and absorption, 393
    host tissue destruction and, 442
    inhibition, 268
    in intestinal villi, 108b
    kinetics, 267–268
        ΔG and, 267, 267f
        reaction equilibrium, 268, 269f
        reaction rate, 268
    regulation of, 186
        covalent modification and, 269
    triglycerides and, digestion and, 394
eosinophilia, parasitic infections and, 492
eosinophilic granuloma, clinical symptoms, 611
eosinophils, 502
ependymal cells
    cerebrospinal fluid and, 26
    ventricular system and, 25
ependymoma, 595
epidemic infection, 436
epidermal cells, specialized, 191
epidermal layers, of skin, mnemonic for, 191b
epidermis, 191
epididymis, 189
    sperm and, 216
epidural hematoma, 22b, 581
epiglottis, 75
epilepsy, 582
epimysium, CT and, 332
epinephrine, 305, 424
    adrenal medulla and, 254
    asthma and, 536
    smooth muscle and, 335
    status asthmaticus and, 536b
epiploic foramen of Winslow, 102
epistaxis (nosebleed), 68
    Kiesselbach's plexus and, 18
epithalamus, 115
epithelial cells
    of alveolar wall, 364
    specialized, 196
epithelial intercellular junctions, 163f
epithelial migration, wound repair and, 495
epithelial rests of Malassez, 209f
    root formation and, 213, 214f
epithelial rests of Serres, 213
epithelial types, 164t
epithelium, 164

epitope, immunity and, 499
ergosterol
    fungal cell membranes and, 473
    fungi cells and, 470
erosion, 661
ERPF. See effective renal plasma flow
ERV. See expiratory reserve volume
erythema multiforme, 521
erythroblastosis fetalis, 555–556
erythrocytes, 173, 174
    and polycythemia, 559–560
    red pulp and, 178
erythrogenic toxin, host tissue destruction and, 443
erythromycin, 456
    impetigo and, 520
erythropoietin, 358, 429–430
    kidney and, 560
    polycythemia, 560
Escherichia coli, sepsis and, 436
esophageal cancer, 601
esophageal plexus, vagus nerves and, 145
esophageal ulcers, 544
esophageal varices, hematemesis and, 549
esophagus, 104, 182
    disorders of, 542–544
estradiol, hCG and, 417
estrogens, 414, 415
ETC. See inner mitochondrial membrane
ethmoid bones, 6
    components and functions of, 12
ethmoid sinuses, 18
    location of drainage, 19
euchromatin, 161
eukaryotic cells, 70s ribosomes and, 290
eustachian tube, 142
EV. See residual volume
Ewing's sarcoma, 613–614
excitable cells, 314b
excitatory neurotransmitters, 315
excretion rate, 386
exercise, physiologic response to, 356
exfoliation, 646
    host tissue destruction and, 442
exocrine glands
    classification of, 167, 167f
    function and excretions of, 166
exocrine pancreas, 187, 394–395
exogenous cortisol, adrenal-ACTH axis and, 420
exonuclease, 291
    DNA synthesis and, 289
exotoxin A, host tissue destruction and, 443
exotoxin B, host tissue destruction and, 442
expanding forces, lung and, 363
expiration, lung mechanics and, 363
expiratory reserve volume (ERV), lung volumes, 362, 362f
external basal lamina, 199
external carotid artery, 66–69, 67f
    branches of, mnemonic for, 66
    course of, 66
    supply, 66
external ear, 141, 142f
    anatomy, 323
    innervation of, 65, 136f
    sensation of, nerves for, 135
external jugular vein, 70
external nose, 20, 20f
    anatomy, 20f
external oblique fibers, 86
external thorax, 83–88
exteroreceptors, CNS and, 307

extracellular fluids (EFC), 376
    expansion, edema and, 378–379
extracellular matrix (ECM), cartilage, 168
extracellular spaces, paracrine glands, 166
extrafusal fibers, 333
extraocular movements, muscles and nerves in, 125
extrapyramidal system, 311
extra-testicular duct system, 189
extrinsic asthma, 535
extrinsic muscles of tongue, 657
exudate, 491
exudate edema, 522–523
eye, 192–194
    layers, 192
    ophthalmic artery and, 13
    structures, 192f
eye chambers, 193
eye elevators, eye muscle action and, 126, 127f
eye muscle action, eye elevators and, 126, 127f
eyeball, 319–323
    components, 320–321
    segments, 319–320

F

Fabry's disease, 264, 518
face
    blood supply, 66
    development of, 238f–239f
    formation, 236–242
    lymph nodes in, 71, 71f, 72f
    orbital bones of, 12–13, 13f
    venous drainage from, 69–71, 69f, 70f
    viscerocranium and, 6
facial artery, 67, 67f
    ECA and, 42
    facial expression and, 67
    portions of, 68
    supply, mnemonic for, 66
facial expression, facial musculature and, 138, 138f, 139
facial musculature, facial expression, 138, 138f
    CN VII and, 139
facial nerve (CN VII)
    chorda tympani nerve and, 31
    components of, 138
    course of, 137, 137f
    facial expression, muscles of, 139
    lesions, 139
    nuclei, 138
facial paralysis, total and partial, 140f
facial reflexes, CN V and, 136
facial sensation, CN V distribution, 134f
facial vein (anterior facial vein), 70
factor I. See fibrinogen
facultative anaerobic, bacteria, 445
falciform ligament, 102, 106
fallopian tubes. See oviducts
falx cerebelli, 22
familial hypercholesterolemia, 262, 527b
familial polyposis, 603
Fanconi's anemia, Café au lait spots and, 575b
fascia, 86
fascial spaces, 46–47, 46f
fasting, glucose and, 397
fat(s)
    digestion and absorption, 393
    excess vitamins in, 400
fat catabolism, hyperlipidemia, 553b

fat embolism, 525
  bone fracture and, 578
fatal tamponade, 529b
fatty acids
  classification, 260
  structure, 260
  synthesis, lipid metabolism and, 276, 277f
  types, 260
fauces, 37
F_c site, immunoglobulins and, 504
feedback regulation, 270f, 271
females, urinary infections and, 111
femoral triangle, 88, 88f
fertilization, 215
fetal circulation, 220f, 221
fetus
  erythroblastosis fetalis and, 555–556
  stages of, 224f
Feulgen reaction, DNA v. RNA, 285
fever, 492
FFAs. See free fatty acids
fibrin, coagulation, 358, 359f
fibrin clot, wound repair and, 495
fibrinogen (factor 1)
  coagulation, 358, 359f
  function of, 257
fibrinolysis, wound repair and, 495
fibroadenoma, 590
fibroblasts, PDL and, 208
fibrocartilage, 168
fibrocystic disease, 594
  breast cancer v., 593b
fibroma, 590
fibrosarcoma, 614
fibrous dysplasia, 575–576
fibrous joints, 170
fibrous pericardium, diastole, 345b
filaments, 161
filiform papillae, 32
filovirus, 462
filtration, 383, 384f
  glomerulus and, 382
  kidney function and, 381
filum terminale, 149
fimbriae. See pili
first arch, embryology and, 231b
first molar
  mandibular permanent teeth, 638, 638f
  mandibular primary teeth, 644
  maxillary permanent teeth, 631–632, 631f
  maxillary primary teeth, 643
first premolar
  mandibular permanent teeth, 636, 636f
  maxillary permanent teeth, 629–630, 630f
fissure, 621
flagella, 161, 444
flavivirus, 462
fluid capillary exchange, 377, 377f
fluid mosaic model, plasma membrane and, 294, 294f
fluid movement, 377–378
fluoride, enolase and, 273
fluoroquinolones, 457
fluorosis, 204
folate deficiency, 558
foliate papillae, 32
folic acid, neural tube formation, 402
follical-stimulating hormone (FSH), 407
  corpus luteum and, 418
follicular cells. See thyroid cells
food
  mastication and, 47
  pharynx and, 41

foramen cecum, 8
foramen lacerum, 9
foramen magnum, 9
foramen ovale, 9
foramen rotundum, 9, 144f
forebrain, embryology of, 227
foregut, 103
formen ovale, 144f
fossa, 620
fovea, 194f
fractures, 578
  healing phases, 578
frameshift mutation, 291, 591
Frank-Starling mechanism, 345, 345f
FRC. See functional residual capacity
freckle, 519
free bilirubin, 549
free fatty acids (FFAs)
  ketoacidosis and, 565b
  triglycerides and, digestion and, 394
free gingiva, 197
free gingival groove, 197
free nerve endings, 307
freeway space (FS), mandible and, 654
Freiberg's disease, 576
Freund's adjuvant, 499
frontal bone, 6
frontal lobe, 114, 114f, 299
frontal nasal processes, formation, 236
frontal sinuses, 18
  location of drainage, 19
frontonasal process, nasal placodes and, 237
fructose, insulin, 249
FS. See freeway space
FSH. See follical-stimulating hormone
functional contacts, 650
functional occlusion, 650
functional residual capacity (FRC), lung mechanics and, 363
functional syncytium, smooth muscle and, 335
fundus, gastric secretion and, 392
fungal cell membranes, ergosterol and, 473
fungal infection
  opportunistic, 473t
  pathogenesis of, 471
  systemic and cutaneous, 472t
fungi, 470–473
  classification, 471, 471t
  medically relevant, 472, 472t, 473t
  reproduction, 471
fungiform papillae, 32, 325
furcation, 621
fusion, 661, 661f
Fusobacterium nucleatum, plaque induced gingivitis and, 480

G

G6PD. See glucose-6-phosphate dehydrogenase
gag reflex, 143
gallbladder, 107, 186
  lipoproteins and, 262
gallbladder diverticulosis, 548
gallstones, 547
GALT. See gut-associated lymphatic tissue
gametogenesis, 215, 215f–217f
gamma globulins, function of, 257
ganglia, 152–153
gap junction, 162
Gardner's syndrome, 603
gas poisoning, colorless/odorless, 535, 535b

gas solubility, 365
gastric acid secretion
  H_2 receptors and, 255
  pHs of, 395
gastric cancer, 601–602
gastric emptying, 392
gastric gland secretion
  by region, 391
  stages of, 392
gastric lymphoma, 602
gastric pits, 182
gastric resection, B_{12} megaloblastic anemia, 558, 558b
gastric ulcer, 544
gastrin
  as gastric secretion, 392
  stimulus and control, 390
gastrocolic ligament, 102
gastroduodenal ligament, 102
gastroesophageal reflux disease (GERD), 543
  scleroderma and, 572
gastrohepatic ligament, 102
gastrointestinal cancer, 601–603
gastrointestinal contractions, 392–393
gastrointestinal pathology, 542–550
gastrointestinal system
  ectodermal derivatives to, 229b
  embryology of, 229–230
  hormonal control, 390
  nervous control, 390
gastrointestinal tract, 102–103, 102f
gastrosplenic ligament, 102
Gaucher's disease, 264, 518
GCF. See gingival crevicular fluid
gemination, 661, 661f
gene transcription, thyroid hormones and, 425
general visceral efferent motor system (GVE), 153
generalized seizures, 582
genetic disorders, childhood, 518–519
genitourinary pathology, 550–554
genitourinary system, neoplasia of, 603–604
Gentamycin, 457
GERD. See gastroesophageal reflux disease
germ layer derivatives, 222t
GFR. See glomerular filtration rate
GH. See growth hormone
Ghon's complex, 542
Gibbs free energy change (ΔG), 267, 268f
  enzyme kinetics and, 267, 267f
gigantism, 413
gingiva, 196–198
  anatomy, 197f, 198f
  calculus, 479
  nerve supply to, 621, 622f
  zones of, 197
gingival col, 198
gingival crevicular fluid (GCF), 199
gingival fiber groups, 199, 199f
gingival overgrowth, 487b
gingivitis
  plaque-induced, characteristics, 480
  sex steroids and, 480
GIP, stimulus and control, 390
glands
  of stomach, 183t
  types of, 166
glandular tissue, 166–167
glenoid/mandibular fossa, 50
glioblastoma multiforme, 595
glomerular filtrate, 381

671

glomerular filtration rate (GFR), 385
  kidney function and, 386
glomerulonephritis, systemic lupus erythematosus, 571
glomerulonephropathies, 554
glomerulus, filtration and, 382, 383
glossopharyngeal nerve (CN IX)
  components of, 143, 144f
  parotid gland and, innervation of, 44f
glottis, 74
glucagon, pancreas and, 418
gluconeogenesis, 397
  stoichiometry of, 276, 277f
glucose, 248
  carbohydrate metabolism, 272
  concentration, filtration and, 383
  liver and, 396–397
  metabolism, liver and, 396
  molecule, ATP production, 272
  polymers, absorption and, 394
glucose-6-phosphate dehydrogenase (G6PD), 276
  deficiency, 556
glucosuria, 383, 551
glutamate, oxidative deamination of, 278, 279f, 280
glutamate dehydrogenase, oxidative deamination and, 280
glycine, 254
glycine-x-y, proelastin polypeptide chain and, 256
glycocholic acid, lipoproteins and, 262
glycogen, 249
  metabolism, enzymatic regulation of, 276, 277f
glycogen storage diseases, 249
glycogen synthesis, catabolism and, 276, 277f
glycogenesis, 397
glycolipids, 251
glycolysis, 272
  major reactions of, 273, 273f
  stoichiometry of, 273, 273f
glycoprotein hormone, erythropoietin and, 358
glycoproteins, 251
  viral replication and, 469
glycosaminoglycans (GAGs), 250, 251t
glycosphingolipids, membranes and, 294
glycosuria, 565
glycosylated Hb (HbA1c), 566b
goblet cells, conducting zone airways and, 364
Golgi tendon organs, 334
gomphosis, 170
gout, 579–580
  stages, 580
graft
  rejection, 506
  types of, 506
graft-versus-host reaction, 506
gram stain, 445, 445t
gram-negative bacilli, comparison of, 448, 448t–449t, 450, 450t–451t
gram-negative cocci, major, comparison of, 449t
gram-positive cocci, 446, 447t
  plaque induced gingivitis and, 480
granulocytes, 174
granuloma, 436
granulomatous inflammation, 492

Grave's disease, 179b, 426, 427, 568
gray rami, spinal nerve and, 154
great auricular nerve, 66
great cardiac vein, 93
great extensor nerve, 81
greater auricular nerve, distribution, 135, 136f
greater omentum, 101
greater palantine artery, 18, 36
greater petrosal nerve, 42, 141
  pterygopalatine ganglion and, 141
greater palatine foramen, 8
gross anatomy, 3–155
group function, mandible and, 655
growth hormone (GH), 407, 565–566
  actions of, 413
  pituitary gland and, 179
guanine, 284b
  cytosine and, 284b
Guillain-Barré syndrome, 583
gut-associated lymphatic tissue (GALT), 184
GVE. See general visceral efferent motor system

H

H band, skeletal muscle and, 331, 331b
H1 receptors, type I hypersensitivity and, 255
H2 receptors, pepsin secretion, 255
hair, 191
hair cells, 308
hair follicle receptors, 307
haldane effect, 366
hamartoma, 590
Hand-Schuller-Christian disease, clinical symptoms, 611
handwashing, infection control and, 440
hantavirus, 462
hapten, immunity and, 499
hard palate, 16
  composition of, 37
  lateral, 17
Hashimoto's thyroiditis, 179b, 426, 566, 567
Haversian canal, 169
Haversian systems, 169
HBV. See hepatitis B virus
hCG. See human choriogonadotropin
HCL, as gastric secretion, 392
HCV. See hepatitis C virus
HD. See Hodgkin disease
head, cranial anatomy and osteology of, 6–54
head and neck
  arteries of, 67f
  vagus nerve branches in, 120t–124t, 145, 146f
  veins of, 69f
head injury
  diabetes insipidus and, 564
  symptoms, 581b
hearing, 323–325
  cranial nerve sensory nuclei and, 117
  hair cells and, 308
hearing loss, 142–143
hearing pathway, 324–325
heart
  autonomic control of, 354
  electrical conduction of, 350, 351f
  great vessels and, 90, 90f
  hypoxia and, 486b
  Laplace's law in, 341

layers of, 176
  receptors, 354
heart attack, atherosclerosis and, 527b
heart embryology, 231f
heart failure. See also left heart failure; right heart failure
  pulmonary edema from, 535b
  signs and symptoms of, 534, 534b
heart murmurs, with valvular disease, 350
heart rate (HR)
  CO and, 345
  and contractility, 346
heart valves, 91
heat loss, ANS and, 300
heat regulation, ANS and, 300
heat transfer, ANS and, 301
heavy polypeptide chains, 503
Heberden's nodes, osteoarthritis and, 579
Hehring-Breur reflex, 373
heights of contour (HOC), teeth and, 626
helical amylose, starch, 249
helicase, DNA synthesis and, 289
helminths. See metazoa
hemagglutination, ABO blood typing and, 510
hemagglutinin, influenza virus and, 461
hemangioma, 522
hematemesis, 544
  esophageal varices and, 549
hematocrit (HCT), 173, 339, 356
hematopoiesis, 175, 175f
hematopoietic cell damage, 557
hematuria, 551
heme, structure, 259, 259f
hemiacidrin concentration, 356–357
hemiazygos vein (inferior hemiazygos vein), 97
hemidesmosome, 162
hemochromatosis, 489
hemoglobin, 365–370
  concentration, normal values for, 366
  myoglobin v., 258, 258t
  oxygen-binding curves of, 259
  types of, 258, 258t
hemolytic anemias, 555, 555b–556b
hemolytic crisis, sickle-cell anemia and, 556
hemopericardium, 529b
hemophilia, 563
  characterization, 563b
hemoptysis, 542b
hemorrhage
  baroreceptor reflex and, 355
  chronic leukemias and, 606
  PUD and, 544
hemosiderin, accumulation, 489
hemosiderosis, 489
hemostasis, 358–359
Henderson-Hasselbach equation, 380
hepadnavirus, 466, 466t–467t
hepatic fat synthesis, hyperlipidemia, 553b
hepatic sinusoids, 106
hepatic veins, IVC and, 106
hepatitis, 550
  infections, serological profiles of, 468t
  viral, 550
  viruses, 467–469
    comparison of, 467t
hepatitis A virus, 462
hepatitis B virus (HBV)
  serological findings, 468f
  vaccine, 468
    preexposure protocol and, 440
hepatitis C virus (HCV), liver transplantation and, 468

hepatocellular carcinoma, cirrhosis, 548
hepatocytes, 185
hepatoduodenal ligament, 102
hereditary amyloidosis, cause and sites of, 610
hereditary spherocytosis, 556
heredity, aplastic anemia and, 557
Hering-Breuer reflexes, 89
herpesvirus, 466, 466t–467t
Hertwig's epithelial root sheath (HERS), root formation and, 213, 214f
heterochromatin, 161
heterodont dentition, 618
heterolysis, enzymatic cellular degradation and, 488
heterophile test, Burkitt's lymphoma and, 466t
heteropolymer chains, 250
heterozygote, sickle-cell anemia and, 556
Hfr. See high-frequency recombination cells
hiatal hernia, 543
high altitude, respiration and, 374
high radiosensitive cells, 592
high-frequency recombination cells (Hfr), 441
hindbrain, embryology of, 227
hindgut, 103, 108
hippocampus, limbic system and, 301
His-Purkinje system, nodal/pacemaker conduction system and, 352
histamine, 255
histidine, 254
histiocytes, 501, 611b
histiocytosis X, 611
histones, 287
HIV
    environmental surfaces and, 438
    RNA strands and, 464, 464f
    universal precautions and, 440
hives, 520
HLA-B27
    ankylosing spondylitis, 573
    Reiter's syndrome and, 573
Hodgkin disease (HD), 607
Hodgkin's lymphoma, 607–608, 608b
homodont dentition, 618
horizontal fold, 22
hormone(s). See also parathyroid hormone
    calcium regulation and, 428
    endocrine glands and, 166
    kidney and, 381, 386, 429–430
    mechanisms, 408
    pancreas and, 418
    regulation, triacylglycerol lipase and, triglyceride lipolysis and, 276, 277f
    second messengers and, 408
    smooth muscle and, 335
    teratogenesis and, 516
    types and classification, 407–408
Horner's syndrome, 128
host defenses, evasion of, mediators of, 442
host tissue destruction, mediators of, 442
HR. See heart rate
HTN. See hypertension
human choriogonadotropin (hCG), 417
Hunter's syndrome, 251
Hunter-Schreger bands, 203
Huntington's disease, 582
Hurler's syndrome, 251
Hutchinson incisors, enamel and, 204
hyaline, 168
    external nose and, 20

hyaline cartilage, 169
hyaluronidase, host tissue destruction and, 442
hydrocephalus, CSF and, 26b
hydrocortisone, 420
    primary Addison's disease and, secondary Addison's disease v., 571
hydrogen bonds, 246, 284b
hydrolasestransferases, 266
hydronephrosis, 551
hydrostatic pressure, fluids and, 377
hydroxyapatite, 169, 479
hydroxylysine, elastin and, 256
hydroxyproline, osteoblastic hyperactivity and, 575
hyoglossus muscle, relationships to, 35
hyoid bone, 62
    attachments, 63
hyperapnea, 374
hypercalcemia, 427
hypercapnea, 374
hypercarbia, 369
hypercementosis, 206, 660
hyperemia. See congestion
hyperglycemia
    diabetes mellitus, 419
    values for, 565
hyperlipidemia, 553b
    nephrotic syndrome and, 553
hyperopia, 323
hyperparathyroidism, 568
    signs of, 569b
    symptoms of, 429
hyperpigmentation, 519
hyperplasia, cell injury and, 487
hyperpolarization, 314
hypersensitivity, 506–509
    reactions, types I-IV, 508f–509f
hypertension (HTN), 344, 527–529
    treatment, 527b
hyperthyroidism, 179b, 569
    causes and findings, 566
    hypothyroidism and, diseases and symptoms, 426
hypertrophic pulmonary osteoarthropathy, 601b
hypertrophy, cell injury, 487
hyperventilation, 374
    symptoms of, 370
hypoalbuminemia, nephrotic syndrome and, 553
hypocalcemia, 427
hypocapnea, 374
hypochromic microcytic anemia, 558
hypodermis, 191
hypodontia, 660
hypoglossal nerve
    relationships to, 35
    tongue, 657
hypoglossus nerve (CN XII)
    course of, 147, 148f
    lesions, 148
    paralysis, 148
hypoparathyroidism, symptoms of, 429
hypopigmentation, 519
hyposmia, 327
hypothalamic neurosecretory cells, hormones by, 410
hypothalamic-pituitary-endocrine organ axis, 410, 411f
hypothalamic-pituitary-thyroid axis (TRH-TSH-thyroid hormone axis), 424
hypothalamus, 115, 300
    BBB and, 27

    pituitary gland and, 409–416
    posterior pituitary hormones and, 412
hypothenar region, ulnar nerve and, 81
hypothyroidism, 179b, 567–568
    causes and findings, 566
    hyperthyroidism and, diseases and symptoms, 426
hypoventilation, 374
hypovolemia
    baroreceptor reflex and, 355
    veins/venules in, 343
hypovolemic shock, 524
hypoxemia, 368–369
hypoxia, 486b
hypoxic vasoconstriction, 369

I

I band, skeletal muscle and, 331, 331b
IC. See inspiratory capacity
ICA. See internal carotid artery
ICF. See intracellular fluids
ideal occlusion, intercuspal relationship and, 654
idiopathic pulmonary fibrosis, 540
idiopathic thrombocytopenic purpura (ITP), 562
idiotype, immunoglobulins and, 504
IEE. See inner enamel epithelium
IgA protease, 442
IgG antibodies, NK cell and, 501
IJV. See internal jugular vein
IL. See interleukins
ileum, 184
    blood supply and description of, 108
immediate anaphylactic hypersensitivity, 508f
immune globulin vaccine, viruses and, 469
immune response, hypersensitivity and, 506, 507t
immune system, 498
    cellular components of, 499–502
    lines of defense in, 498
immune-complex hypersensitivity, 508f
immunity
    live attenuated vaccine, 469
    zinc and, 94
immunodeficiency diseases, 510t–511t
immunoglobulin, 503–504, 503f, 504f
immunologic response, malignant tumors and, 588
immunology, 498–512
immunosuppression, necrotizing periodontal diseases, 481
impetigo, 520
implantation, 216, 218f
incisal edge, 618
incisive canal, 8
incisors, lobes, 627
indirect calorimetry, 246
INF. See interferons
infarction, 490
infection. See also inflammation; viralinfections
    antibiotic prophylaxis and, 458, 458t–459t
    DIC and, 562
    enamel and, 204
    epidemiology and, 436
    of heart, 530b
    interactive associations of, 436
    latent, 436
    maternal, teratogenesis and, 516

infection (Cont.):
  metazoa and, 476t
  opportunistic, 472
  opportunistic fungal, 473t
  protozoa and, 475t
  retrograde flow and, 71
  rheumatic fever v., 532
  skin, 520
  states of, 436
  subclinical, 436
infection control
  regulations v. recommendations, 439
  universal precautions, 440
infectious diseases, microorganisms in, 435, 435t
infectious swellings, 436
infective endocarditis, acute v. subacute, 531
inferior alveolar nerve, distribution, 130
inferior alveolar nerve block, needle course, 131, 131f
inferior hemiazygos vein. See hemiazygos vein
inferior meatus, 41, 42f
inferior mediastinum, 93
inferior mesenteric vein, 99
inferior nasal conchae, 12
inferior oblique muscle, 126
inferior orbital fissure, 9
inferior vena cava (IVC), 93
  paired branches of, 98
inflammation
  cardinal signs, 579b
  repair and, 486–496
  systemic effects of, 492
  tissue injury and, responses to, 490
inflammatory bowel disease, 545
inflammatory cytokines, 493, 493t–494t
inflammatory infiltrate, 199
inflammatory mediators, 493–495, 494t–495t
inflammatory reaction, leukemia and, 604
influenza virus, 461
infrahyoid muscles, 63–64, 63f, 657
infraorbital foramen, 8
infraspinatus, 83
infratemporal fossae, 14f
  boundaries of, 15t
inguinal canal, males v. female, 113
inhibitory neurotransmitters, 315
injury, to left lateral pterygoid muscle, 47
innate immunity, 498
inner ear, 142, 142f
  anatomy, 323, 324f
inner enamel epithelium (IEE), 213
inner medulla (of ovary), 190
inner mitochondrial membrane (ETC), ATP production and, 272
innervation, dental, 621
inspiration, lung mechanics and, 363
inspiratory capacity (IC), lung volumes, 362, 362f
inspiratory reserve volume (IRV), lung volumes, 362, 362f
insulin, 249, 418
  DM and, 565
insulin clearance, 386
integral proteins, 295
integument, 190–192
interalveolar septum, 207
intercalated disc, cardiac muscle and, 334
intercostal artery, 83
intercostal muscles

orientation of, 84
respiration and, 83
intercostal nerves, 83
  intercostal muscles and, 85
intercostal space, 83
intercostal vein, 83
intercuspal relationship, ideal occlusion and, 654
interdental papilla, 198
interdental spaces, 621
interferons (INF), 469, 493, 493t–494t
interglobular dentin, 201
interleukins (IL), 493, 493t–494t
intermediate filaments, 161
intermediate junction (zonula adherens), 162
intermediolateral horn, gray matter, 149
internal acoustic meatus, 9
internal basal lamina, 199
internal carotid artery (ICA), 27
internal cranial skull base, 10, 10f
internal jugular vein (IJV), 71
  brain, 24
internal oblique fibers, 86
internal skull, 10, 10f
  cranial base of, 11, 11f
internal thoracic artery, 96
internodal pathways, nodal/pacemaker conduction system and, 352
internuclear ophthalmoplegia, 128
interoreceptors, CNS and, 307
interphase, cell cycle and, 162
interproximal space, 621
interradicular septum, 207
interstitial fibrosis, 540b
interstitial growth, cartilage and, 168
interstitial lamellae, 169
interstitial lung disease, sarcoidosis and, 539
interstitial pneumonia, 541
interstitial space, edema and, 378–381
intertubular dentin, 201
intestinal glands, 184
intestinal lymphangiectasia, 545
intestinal secretions, pHs of, 395
intestinal villi, enzymes in, 108
intraalveolar fluid, intrapleural fluid v., 536b
intracellular fluids (ICF), 376
intracranial circulation, 27
intracranial pressure, choroid plexus and, 25
intradental spaces, 621
intradermal nevi, 595
intrafusal fibers, 333
intramembranous growth, 6
intramembranous ossification, 169
intraperitoneal colon, 110b
intrapleural fluid, intraalveolar fluid v., 536b
intrapleural pressure, 363
intra-testicular duct system, 189
intrathoracic lymph nodes, eggshell calcification and, 489b
intrathoracic pressure, compliance, 347
intrinsic asthma, 535
intrinsic factor
  as gastric secretion, 392
  pernicious anemia and, 402, 557
intrinsic muscles of tongue, 657
invasion, metastasis and, 588
inverse myotatic reflex. See tendon reflex
iodopsin, 193
ionic bonds, 246
IP3, hormones and, 408
ipsilateral motor loss, 312
ipsilateral tracts, 306b
iris, 193, 320

iron
  deficiency, 558
  transferrin and, 404
iron atom, heme, 259, 259f
irreversible cell injury, 487
irreversible inhibition, 268, 270f
IRV. See inspiratory reserve volume
ischemic injury, middle cerebral artery and, 29
Islets of Langerhans, 187
isoelectric point, 380
isograft, 506
isomaltase, 249
isotonic solutions, membrane and, 379
isovolumetric contraction, cardiac cycle and, 348
isovolumetric relaxation, cardiac cycle and, 348
isozymes, 266
Ito cells, 185
ITP. See idiopathic thrombocytopenic purpura
IV drug users, tricuspid valve and, 530
IVC. See inferior vena cava

J

jaundice, 549
  bilirubin levels and, 185
  causes, 397
  liver disease and, 549
jaw jerk reflex, 136
jejunum, 184
  blood supply and description of, 108
JG cells. See juxtaglomerular cells
JGA. See juxtaglomerular apparatus
joint receptors, types of, 307b
joints. See also rheumatoid arthritis
  classification of, 170
jugular foramen, 9
jugular lymph trunk, 71
  venous emptying of, 72
junctional complex, 162b, 163f
junctional epithelium, 198–199
junctional nevus, 595
juxtaglomerular apparatus (JGA), 188
juxtaglomerular cells (JG cells), 188

K

K^+ leak, 313
K^+ permeability, repolarization and, 313
karyolysis, cell death and, 490
karyorrhexis, cell death and, 490
keratinocytes, 196
keratoacanthoma, 598
keratohyalin granules, 196
keratoses, 248f
kernicterus, 550, 556
ketoacidosis, 278, 565b
ketone bodies
  fatty acids and, 278
  ketoacidosis and, 565b
ketonuria, 551
ketosis, 278
kidney(s), 98, 111
  components of, 188
  diseases, nephrotic syndrome and, 554
  embryology, stages of, 232f
  erythropoietin and, 560
  function, 381–383
  functions of, 188

hormones and, 386, 429–430
infections, lower urinary tract and, 551
structure of, 112f
Kiesselbach's plexus, arteries and, 18
killed vaccine, 454
viruses and, 469
Klinefelter syndrome, 517
Kohler's disease, 576
Kupffer cells, 106, 185, 501

L

labial ridge, 620
laboratory tests, antigen-antibody, 509, 509t
lacrimae, 169
lacrimal canals, 41, 42f
lacrimal gland, 41, 42, 42f
lacrimal nerve, 42
lacrimal puncta, 41, 42f
lacrimal sacs, 41, 42f
lactate, glycolysis, 273
lactic acid
    caries and, 479
    Cori cycle and, 273
    gluconeogenesis and, 276, 277f
lactic acid cycle, 274, 274f
Lactobacillus species, root caries and, 480b
lactogenesis, 413
lacunae, 168, 206
lamina densa, 165
lamina lucida, 165
laminar flow, 341f
laminin, oral mucosa and, 196–198
Langerhans cells, 196, 501
LaPlace's law, 341, 346
large cell carcinoma, 600, 601
large intestine, 108–109, 184
    disorders, 545–546
laryngeal muscles, extrinsic v. intrinsic, 75
laryngeal nerves, 76
laryngeal skeleton, cartilages of, 74
larynx, voice production and, 74
latent infection, 436
lateral cleft lip, 237
lateral incisor, 628, 628f
    mandibular primary teeth, 644
    maxillary permanent teeth, 628, 628f
    maxillary primary teeth, 643
lateral movement, mandible and, 655
lateral nasal branches of facial artery, 18
lateral pterygoid muscle, 48, 49f
    damage, 50
laterotrusive contacts. *See* working side contacts
lecithinase, host tissue destruction and, 442
left atrium, 91
left gastric artery, 105
left gonadal vein, 98
left heart failure, signs and symptoms of, 534
left lateral pterygoid muscle, mandible and, 47
left vagus nerve, 145
    AV node innervation and, 354
left ventricle, 92
left working movement, condylar movements as, 656, 656f
Legg-Calvé-Perthes disease, 576
leiomyoma, 590, 592–593
lens, 320
lentigo maligna, 519, 596
lentigo maligna melanoma, 599
lesions
    CN VI, 128
    CN VI, 139
    lower motor neuron, 148
    optic nerve, 128
    squamous cell carcinoma, 597–598
lesser occipital nerve, 66
    distribution, 135, 136f
lesser palatine artery, soft palate and, 68
lesser palatine foramen, 8
Letterer-Siwe disease, clinical symptoms, 611
leukemia
    childhood and, 592
    classification, 605
    etiology, 604
    types, 605
leukocidins, 442
leukocytes, 173, 174
    comparison of, 174t
    in leukemia, 604
leukocytosis, 492
levan, 251
levator palpebrae superioris (CN III), eyelids and, 136b
levator veli palatini, tensor veli palatini v., 38
LH. *See* luteinizing hormone
Libmann-sacks endocarditis, 531
ligament, 166
ligases, 266
light polypeptide chains, 503
limb muscles. *See* muscle(s)
limbic system, ANS and, 301
limbus, 192
line angle, 621
linea alba, 86
lines of defense, immune system and, 498
lingual artery, 67, 67f, 68
    branches of, 36f
    ECA and, 42
    lingual nerve v., 131
    relationships to, 35
lingual frenulum, 31
lingual nerve
    course of, 132
    cutting of, 131
    damage, third molar extraction and, 132
    distribution, 130
    lingual artery v., 131
    relationships to, 35
lingual tongue, branches of
lingual tonsils, 37
lingula, 21
lip formation, 236
lipid(s)
    membranes and, 174, 294, 295f
    metabolism, 276, 277f, 278
        β-oxidation and, 276, 277f
        fatty acid synthesis and, 276, 277f
        triglyceride lipolysis and, 276, 277f
    structure, 259–261
    transport, 262
    types, 260
lipid storage diseases, 264
lipiduria, urine and, 553
lipoma, 590
lipopolysaccharide (LPS), host tissue destruction and, 443
lipoproteins, 262
    major, 263
    structure, 262f
    viruses and, 459
lithium, nephrogenic diabetes insipidus, 564
live attenuated vaccine, 454
    viruses and, 469
liver, 106, 184
    cholesterol synthesis in, 396
    clotting factors and, 563
    complement proteins, 504
    functions, 395–396
        tests, 468
    glucose metabolism and, 396
    glycogen, 249
    leukemia and, 604
    lipoproteins and, 262
    lobules, 185
    plasma proteins, 257
    synthesis, 397
    transplantation, hepatitis C virus and, 468
    urea cycle in, 381, 396
liver disease, 548–550
    jaundice and, 549
lobar pneumonia, 541
lobes, 618
    canines, 627
    incisors, 627
    molars, 627
    premolars, 627
local anesthetics, neurophysiology of, spinal tract and, 314
log phase
    antibacterial activity during, 454
    bacteria and, 441
loose connective tissue, 165
low radiosensitive cells, 592
lower digestive system, 184–189
lower jaw, components of, 20
lower motor neuron lesion, 148
lower urinary tract, kidney infections and, 551
low-grade astrocytoma, 595
LPS. *See* lipopolysaccharide
Ludwig's angina, 436
lumbar plexus, 153
lung(s)
    abscess, 541, 541b
    gas exchange in, 365
    hilum, 89
    hyperinflation, 373
    hypoxia and, 486b
    mechanics, 363–364
    metastatic cancer to, 600b
    right and left, 89, 89f
    volumes, 362–363, 362f
    zones, 364
lung cancer, 600–601
    chronic bronchitis and, 538
    types of, 600
luteinizing hormone (LH), 407
    corpus luteum and, 418
    follicle and, 417
luxated TMJ, 51
lyases, 266
Lyell's syndrome, 521
lymph, 176
    drainage, 177
    gallbladder and, 107
lymph nodes, 177
    facial, 71, 71f, 72f
    thymus and, 94
lymphatic drainage, 42
lymphatic system, 100, 176–178
    components of, 177
    functions of, 177
    neoplasia of, 604–611
lymphatic vessels, 176
lymphocytes
    lymph and, 177
    white pulp, 178

675

lymphocytosis, viral infections, 492
lymphomas, 607–609
lysine
   collagen synthesis and, 256
   histones and, 287
lysosomal storage diseases, 518
lysosomes, 161
   contents, 503

M

M protein, 442
macrocytic anemia, microcytic anemia v., 558
macrodontia, 660
macrolides, 456
macrophages, 174t, 501
   lymph and, 177
macula adherens. *See* desmosome
macula densa, 188
macula lutea, 194
mad cow disease, 470
magnetic resonance imaging (MRI), TMJ and, 51
malabsorption syndrome, 546
malignancy. *See also* multiple polyposis syndromes
   DIC and, 562
   histologic characteristics of, 588
   malignant tumors and, 588
malignant epithelial cells, 598
malignant giant cell tumor, 613
malignant hypertension (HTN), 528–529
   kidney disease and, 552
malignant melanoma, histology of, 599
malignant neoplasia, in women, cancer incidence and death, 593
malignant nephrosclerosis, 553
malignant skin neoplasms, 597–599
malignant tumors
   benign tumors v., 587
   prognosis, 588
   spread of, 588
   types of, 589
Mallory-Weiss syndrome, 542–543
malunion, fractures, 578
mamelons, 618, 619f
mammary glands, 190
mandible, 20. *See also* Lower jaw
   formation, 236
   guidance, 654–655
   left lateral pterygoid muscle and, 47
   movements, 654–656
   positions, 654
   Posselt's envelope of motion, 654, 655f
   TMJ ligaments and, 51–52
mandibular arch, permanent dentition, 647
mandibular artery, 69
mandibular canal, 20
mandibular capsule, 54f
mandibular condyle
   meniscus and, 53f
   palpation of, 50
mandibular foramen, 9, 20
mandibular nerve (V3), 129f, 130
   branches of, 129f, 130
mandibular permanent teeth
   canine, 635–636, 635f
   central incisor, 633–634, 634f
   first molar, 638, 638f
   first premolar, 636, 636f
   lateral incisor, 634, 635f
   second molar, 638–639, 639f
   second premolar, 637, 637f

mandibular primary teeth, 644
   central incisor, 644
mandibular teeth
   primate space and, 642
   proximal contacts of, 625, 625f
mantle dentin, 201
   formation, 201
Marcus-Gunn pupil, 128
Marfan's syndrome, 519
marginal ridge, 619f, 620, 620f
masseter muscle, 48, 48f, 49
mast cells, 502
mastication
   mandibular functions for, 50
   muscles of, 48f–49f
   TMJ and, 47–54
masticator space, boundaries and contents, 46f, 47
materia alba, 479
maternal infection, teratogenesis and, 516
matrix vesicles, 201
maturation, plaque formation and, 478
mature bone, 169
maxilla, 14
   formation, 236
   processes of, 14
maxillary arch, permanent dentition, 647, 648f
maxillary artery, 67, 67f, 621
   parts of, 68–69
maxillary central incisor, 627f
maxillary nerve (V2), 129f, 130
maxillary permanent teeth
   canine, 629, 629f
   central incisor, 627, 627f
   first molar, 631–632, 631f
   first premolar, 629–630, 630f
   lateral incisor, 628, 628f
   second molar, 632, 632f
   second premolar, 630, 631f
maxillary primary teeth, 642–644, 642f, 643f
   canine, 643
   central incisor, 642
   first molar, 643
   lateral incisor, 643
   second molar, 644
maxillary sinus, 18
   Sniderian membrane and, 18
maxillary teeth
   primate space and, 642
   proximal contacts of, 625f
maxillary vein, 70, 621
maximum opening (MO), mandible and, 654
McCune-Albright syndrome, Café au lait spots and, 575b
mean arterial pressure (MAP), TPR and, 343, 343b, 344
mean systemic filling pressure, arterial constriction system and, 343
mechanoreceptor, 308
Meckel diverticulum, 545
medial lemniscus system, pathway, 309
medial pterygoid muscle, 48, 49f
   mandible and, 50
median nerve, 80
mediastinum, 93–94
mediotrusive contacts. *See* nonworking side contacts
medulla
   PCO_2 and, 371
   pyramids and, 188
medulla oblongata, 116, 302

medullary cystic disease, 552
medullary rays, cortex and, 187
medullary sponge kidney, 552
medulloblastoma, 595
megaloblastic anemia, 402
meiosis II, fertilization and, 216
Meissner's corpuscles, 307
Meissner's plexus. *See* submucous plexus
melanocytes, 196
membrane(s)
   capacitance, 315
   carbohydrates and, 295
   components, 294–295
   isotonic solutions and, 379
   phospholipids, 295f
   transport, 295, 296f
membrane-bound organelles, 161
membranous urethra, 189
meningeal veins, 24
meninges, 149
   space and description of, 22
meningioma, 595
meningitis, 22
meniscus
   articular disk of TMJ, 50–51
   damage, 50
   mandibular condyle and, 53f
menstruation, 416, 417f
mental foramen, 9, 21
mental nerve, 21
   distribution, 130
Merkel cells, 196
Merkel's disc, 307
mesencephalic nucleus, 132
mesencephalon. *See* midbrain
mesenchyme, thymus and, 94
mesentery, adult v. embryonic, 101
mesial root concavity, first premolar, 629, 630f
mesiodens, 660
mesoderm, cardiovascular system from, 228
mesothelioma, 539b
mesothelium, 165
messenger RNA (mRNA), 286
metabolic acidosis, respiratory compensation for, 372
metabolic alkalosis, respiratory compensation for, 372
metabolic intermediates, 272, 272f
metabolic pathways, 271–280, 271f
metalloproteinases. *See* collagenases
metals, nonprotein enzyme components, 266
metaphase, 162
metaplasia, 587
metastasis, 587
   breast cancer and, 593
   gastric cancer and, 602
   and invasion, 588
   routes of, 588
   squamous cell carcinoma and, 598
metastatic cancer, to lungs, 600b
metazoa (helminths), 474
   human infection and, 476t
methemoglobinemia, 259
methicillin, 454
metronidazole, 457
MG. *See* myasthenia gravis
MI. *See* myocardial infarction
micelles, 161, 394
Michaelis-Menten equation, enzyme kinetics and, 267, 267f
microbial flora, plaque induced gingivitis and, 480

microbodies. *See* peroxisomes
microcytic anemia, macrocytic anemia v., 558
microdontia, 660
microorganisms, infectious diseases and, 435, 435t
microtubules, 161
microvilli, 161, 182
midbrain (mesencephalon), 116, 302
    embryology of, 227
middle cerebral artery, 29
middle cranial fossa
    contents of, 8
    middle meningeal artery and, 7
middle ear, 141, 142f
    anatomy, 323
    muscles in, 142
middle meatus, sinus openings and, 19
middle meningeal artery, 68
    middle cranial fossa and, 7
midgut, 103
Mikulicz's syndrome, 573
miliary tuberculosis, 542
milk, pasteurization of, 438
mineralocorticoid. *See* aldosterone
minerals
    major, 403, 402t
    minor, 404, 403t
minocycline, 457
minor salivary glands, 44
minute ventilation, 364
miosis, eyeball and, 320
missense mutation, 290
mitochondria, 161
mitosis, 162
mitral valve, 91
mixed dentition, 646, 647
MO. *See* maximum opening
molar(s)
    extraction, lingual nerve damage and, 132
    lobes, 627
molds, yeasts v., 471, 471t
molecular bonds, 246
monoamine oxidase (MAO), monamines and, 305
monocytes, 501
monoglycerides, triglycerides and, digestion and, 394
monophyodont dentition, 618
monosaccharides, 248, 248f
motor branches, distribution, 130
motor control, and coordination, 301–302
motor innervation, skeletal muscle and, 332
motor nerve, 129
motor nucleus, 132
motor pathway, 302
motor units, 331b
mouth, formation, 236, 237, 238f–239f, 241f
mouth breathing, chronic, 197
mouthrinses, plaque control, 483, 483t
movement disorders, motor pathway, 302
MRI. *See* magnetic resonance imaging
mucopolysaccharide storage diseases, 251
mucous, 252
    as gastric gland secretion, 392
mucous cells, conducting zone airways and, 364
mucous membranes, antiseptics and, 438, 439t
mulberry molars, enamel and, 204
multiple myeloma, 609–610

multiple polyposis syndromes, 603
multiple sclerosis, 582b, 583
muscle(s), 330–331
    cellular components, 330
    controlling tongue, 33, 34f, 35
    exercise, 356
    innervation, 331
    of limbs
        arm movement, at elbow, 82
        functions by joint, 81–83
        hand movement, at elbow, 82
    of mastication, 48f–49f, 656
    middle ear, 142
    receptors, 334
    spindles, 334
    tone, stretch reflex and, 334
    Trichinella spiralis and, 476t
    types of, comparison of, 330
muscle fiber, 333
muscular arteries, 176
musculocutaneous nerve, 80
musculoskeletal pathology, 571–581
mutagenesis, 591
mutagenic chemicals, mutations by, 290–291
mutations, 290–291, 591
    and carcinogenesis, 591–592
    change, 591
mutualism, 436
myasthenia gravis (MG), 331, 583
mycobacteria, 452
    cell walls, mycolic acid and, 445
Mycobacteria species, comparison of, 452t
mycolic acid, mycobacteria cell walls and, 445
mycosis fungoides, 609
mycotoxicosis, fungi and, 471
mydriasis, eyeball and, 320
myelin, 315
myelin sheath, 172
myelination, 172, 172t
myelodysplastic syndromes, 559
myeloproliferative disorders, 559
myenteric plexus (Auerbach's plexus), 184, 390
Myobacterium tuberculosis, 438
    disinfectant and, 438
myocardial infarction (MI), complete v. partial occlusion in, 533
myocardial oxygen demand, cardiac function and, 346
myocardial oxygen supply, cardiac function and, 346
myofibril, skeletal muscle and, 331
myofilaments, 330
myoglobin, 259
    hemoglobin v., 258, 258t
    oxygen-binding curves of, 259
myopia, 323
myosin, 161, 330
myosin light-chain kinase, smooth muscle contraction and, 335
myotome, derivatives, 223f
myxedema, 179b, 426, 566, 567
myxoma, 590

N

Na^+ permeability, repolarization and, 313
nafcillin, 454
Na^+/K^+ pump, 313

nasal cavity
    blood supply of, 17
    boundary and contributing structures to, 16
    formation, 240f
    lateral, 17f
    sensory innervation of, 17
nasal conchae, function, 17
nasal meatuses, function, 17
nasal placodes
    formation, 236
    frontonasal process and, 237
nasal septum, cartilaginous and bone components of, 18, 18f
nasolacrimal apparatus, 41, 42f
    location of drainage, 19
nasolacrimal duct, 41, 42f
natural killer (NK) cells, 501
NE. *See* norepinephrine
neck
    anatomy, 54–77
    ICA, 28
    layers and facia of, 55
    triangles of, 59–64
necrotizing periodontal diseases
    characteristics of, 481
    classification of, 482
    microbial flora in, 482
necrotizing ulcerative gingivitis (NUG), 482
necrotizing ulcerative periodontitis (NUP), 482
negative feedback, erythropoietin and, 358
negative feedback loop
    adrenal gland and, 419
    hypothalamic-pituitary-thyroid axis, 424, 425f
neomycin, 458
neonatal line, 202
neoplasia
    adrenal gland, 611–612
    blood, 604–611
    genitourinary system, 603–604
    lymphatic systems, 604–611
    in men, 594–595
        cancer incidence and death and, 594
    nervous system, 595
    skin, 595–597
    in women, 592–594
neoplasms, 587–588
nephrogenic diabetes insipidus, 412, 564
nephrolithiasis, 550–551
nephron
    functions and components, 188
    kidney function and, 381–382
    types, 188
nephron segments, 383
nephrosclerosis, 552–553
nephrotic syndrome
    associated diseases, 553
    edema and, 523
    kidney diseases and, 554
    symptoms, 553
nerve(s)
    dermatomes and, 87, 87f
    to masseter, 51
nerve conduction, 315–317
    problems with, 316–317
nerve fiber, 152
nerve impulse, 315, 317
nervous system, 113
    myelin-producing cells of, 172t
nervous tissue, 171
    supporting cells of, 172t
net reabsorption, 386
net secretion, 386

neural crest
　　adrenal medulla, 422, 423f
　　neuroectoderm forms, 226f
neural plate, embryonic life and, 225
neural retina, 193
neural tube
　　folic acid and, 402
　　neuroectoderm forms, 226f
neuraminidase, influenza virus and, 461
neurapraxia, 316
neurilemma, 172
neuroanatomy, 113–155
neurocranium
　　brain and, 6
　　formation, 231, 233f
neurodegenerative diseases, 582–583
neuroectoderm, 225
　　neural crest and, 226f
　　neural tube and, 226f
neurofibromatosis, Café au lait spots and, 575b
neurogenic shock, 524
neurohypophysis, 179
neurologic trauma, 581–583
neuromuscular junction (NMJ), sequence, 318–319
neuromuscular spindles, 307b
neuronal excitability, 317
neurons, 171
neuropathology, 581–583
neurotmesis, 317
neutrophilia, bacterial infection and, 492
nevocellular nevus, 595
NHL. See non-Hodgkin's lymphoma
Niemann-Pick disease, 264, 518
nitrates, angina and, 533
nitrogenous base, nucleotides, 284
NK cells. See natural killer cells
nodal/pacemaker
　　conduction system, 352
　　tissue, 350
nodes of Ranvier, 172, 316
nodular melanoma, 599
nonarticular osteochondroses, 576
noncommunicating obstruction,
　　in ventricular system, 26b
noncompetitive inhibition, 268, 270f
noncovalent bonds, 246
nonencapsulated joint receptors
　　capsulated joint receptors v., 307
　　types of, 307b
non-Hodgkin's lymphoma (NHL), 608
non-membrane-bound organelles, 161
nonprotein nitrogen, urea and, 396
nonsense mutation, 290
non-small cell carcinoma (NSC), 600
nonsteroidal antiinflammatory drugs
　　(NSAIDs), cyclooxygenase and, 262
non-union, fractures, 578
nonworking cusps, 654
nonworking interference, 655
nonworking side contacts (mediotrusive contacts), 651
　　mandible and, 655
norepinephrine (NE), 424
　　adrenal medulla and, 254
　　alpha-adrenergic receptors, 305
　　release, 422b
normal values
　　hemoglobin concentration, 366
　　oxygen content, 366
nose. See external nose
nosebleed. See epistaxis

NSAIDs. See nonsteroidal antiinflammatory drugs
NSC. See non-small cell carcinoma
nuclear bag fibers, 333
nuclear chain fibers, 333
nuclear membrane, 161
nucleic acids, DNA v. RNA, 285–286
nucleoplasm, 161
nucleosomes, DNA and, 287, 288f
nucleotides, 284
　　biosynthesis of, 284, 285f
nucleus, 161
nucleus ambiguous, swallowing and, 41
NUG. See necrotizing ulcerative gingivitis
null cells, 605–606
NUP. See necrotizing ulcerative periodontitis
nutritional deficiency, enamel and, 204
nystagmus, 143

O

oat cell carcinoma, 600, 601
obligate aerobic, bacteria, 445
obligate anaerobic, bacteria, 445
obligate intracellular bacteria, 453t
oblique ridge, 620
obstructive jaundice, gallstones and, 547
obstructive lung diseases, 536
occipital artery, 67, 67f
occipital bone, 6
occipital lobe, 114, 114f, 299
occlusal adjustment, 650
occlusal contacts, 650–651
occlusal dimensions, 650
occlusal interferences, 655
occlusal musculature, 656–657
occlusal relationships, 651–652
　　Angle's classification, 652, 652f–653f
　　determinants of, 652
occlusal shape, first premolar, 629, 630f
occlusal surface, 618
occlusal table, 618
occlusion, 650–654
Occupational Safety and Health
　　Administration (OSHA), 439
ocular muscles, 126f
oculomotor nerve, 125, 126f
odontogenesis
　　Appositional stage, 213
　　bell stage, 212f, 213
　　bud stage, 212, 212f
　　cap stage, 212, 212f
　　initiation, 212, 212f
　　mineralization stage, 214
OEE. See outer enamel epithelium
ofloxacin, 457
Okazaki fragments, DNA synthesis and, 289, 289f
olfactory nerve (CN I), primary
　　olfactory cortex and, 17
oligodontia, 660
oligosaccharides, 248
olivospinal tract, 311
oncotic pressure (colloid osmotic pressure), fluids and, 377
oocyte, maturation of, 217
oogonia, 417–418
open bite, 651, 651f
ophthalmic artery
　　ICA and, 28
　　orbit and, 13
ophthalmic nerve (V1), 129f, 130
ophthalmic veins, retrograde flow and, 24b

ophthalmoplegia, 128
opsonins, 502
opsonization, 502
optic canal, 8
optic disc, 193
optic nerve (CN II), 124, 125f
oral cavity, 29–41, 29f
　　antifungal drugs and, 472
　　origin, 237, 238f–239f
oral cavity proper, 29
oral microbiology, 478–479
oral mucosa
　　layers, 196
　　types of, 196, 197t
oral pathology, 479–482
oral vestibule, 29
orbicularis oculi (CN VII), eyelids and, 136b
orbit, 13, 13f
organelles, 160, 160f
organogenesis, 225
orthomyxovirus, 462
OSHA. See Occupational Safety and Health Administration
osmoreceptors, pH levels and, 308
osmosis, 378, 378f
osseous pathology, 573–581
osteitis fibrosa cystica, 575
osteoarthritis, 579
osteoblasts, 169
　　alkaline phosphatase and, 575
osteochondroses, 576
osteogenesis imperfecta, clinical findings, 576, 576b
osteoid bone matrix, 169
osteolytic lesions, multiple myeloma, 609
osteomalacia, 574
　　blood chemistry values, 574
osteomyelitis, 577. See also acute
　　osteomyelitis; chronic osteomyelitis
　　sickle-cell anemia and, 556
osteonecrosis of jaws, bisphosphonate drugs and, 578
osteopetrosis, 576–577
osteophytes, RA and, 580
osteoporosis, 573–574
　　blood chemistry values, 574
otitis externa, 142
otitis media, 142
outer cortex, of ovary, 190
outer enamel epithelium (OEE), 212
ovale foramina, of splenoid bone, 12
ovarian cancer, BRCA-1 and, 593
ovarian follicle, maturation of, 217
ovary, 190
overbite, 651
overjet, 651, 651f
oviducts (fallopian tubes), 190
ovulation, 416b
oxacillin, 455
oxidative deamination, glutamate and, 278, 279f
oxidative phosphorylation
　　ATP and, 272
　　cyanide poisoning and, 535
oxidoreductases, 266
oxygen
　　in blood, 366
　　Laplace's law, 341
oxygen content, 366
　　normal values for, 366
oxygen exchange, 342
oxygen narcosis, hypercarbia, 369
oxygen saturation, 366

oxygen-hemoglobin dissociation curve, 365–366, 365f
oxytalan fibers, blood vessels and, 209
oxytocin, 407
  breast-feeding and, 413
  smooth muscle and, 335

P

Pacinian corpuscles, 307
Paget's disease, 575
  blood chemistry, 574
pain
  CN V sensory distribution for, 133
  spinal lesions and, 312
palatal aponeurosis, tongue muscles and, 37
palatal foramen, 16
palatal salivary glands, location, 36
palate, 36–37. *See also* hard palate; soft palate
  blood supply, 36
  formation, 237, 241f
  formation defects, 241f
  innervation, 36
palate close, swallowing and, 41
palatine tonsils, 37
palmar digital nerves, 81
pampiniform veins, 113
Pancoast tumor, 600b
pancreas, 110, 418
  amylases and, 249
  disorders, 546–547
  embryology, 233f
pancreatic acinar cells, triglycerides and, digestion and, 394
pancreatic acini, 187
pancreatic digestive enzymes, 186
  duodenum and, 110
  trypsin, 186
pancreatic ducts, 110
pancreatic hormones, 407
pancreatic islets, cells of, 187t
pancreatic secretion, pHs of, 395
pancreatitis, 546–547
Panner's disease, 576
papillary cystadenoma, 590
papillary layer, of dermis, 191
papillary muscles, valve closure and, 92
papilloma, 590
papovavirus, 465, 465t
paracrine glands, function and excretions of, 166
paradoxical emboli, 526
parafollicular cells, calcitonin and, 72
parafunctional contacts, 650
parallel resistance, 339
paramyxovirus, 462
paranasal sinuses, 18, 19f
parapharyngeal space, 47
parasites
  classification of, 474
  common metazoa, 476t
  common protozoa, 475t
  medially relevant, 475t
  phylogeny of, 474t
parasitic infections, eosinophilia and, 492
parasitology, 474–476
parasympathetic cranial nerves, 119
parasympathetic ganglia, 119
parasympathetic nervous system, composition of, 304
parasympathetic preganglionics, 140

parathyroid cells, major, 179t
parathyroid glands, 74, 179, 179t, 569
parathyroid hormone (PTH), 407
  bone resorption, 170
  calcium and phosphorus, normal values, 427
  calcium regulation and, 428
  disorders, 568–570
  effects of, 179b
parietal lobe, 114, 114f, 299
parietal pericardium, 92
parietal peritoneum, 101
parietal pleura, 89
Parkinson's disease, 582b
parosteal osteosarcoma, 613
parotid gland, 42, 44f
  amylases and, 249
  innervation schematic of, 44f
  salivary fluid and, 44
  serous only saliva and, 44
parotid space, boundaries and contents, 46, 46f
partial anodontia, 660
partial pressure gradient, 365
partial seizures, 582
parvovirus, 465, 465t
passive eruption, 646
passive immunity, 454, 498–499
pasteurization, 438
Patau syndrome, 517
patent foramen ovale, embryology and, 228b
pathologic calcifications, 489, 489t
Pautrier microabscesses, 609
PCKD. *See* polycystic kidney disease
PDL. *See* periodontal ligament
pectoral girdle, muscles of, 85
pellagra, 402
pellicle formation, 478
pelvic cavity, female v. male, 112
pelvic kidney, common iliac artery and, 98
pelvic splanchnic nerves, 108
  abdominal viscera and, 147
pelvic vein thrombosis, 526
pemphigus vulgaris, 520–521
penetration, viral replication and, 460
penicillin(s), 454–455, 499
  combinations, 455
  polyarthritis nodosa, 572
  rheumatic fever, 532
penicillin G, 454
penicillin V, 454
penile urethra, 189
penis, 189
pentose phosphate pathway, 276
pentose sugar, nucleotides, 284
pepsin secretion, H2 receptors and, 255
pepsinogen, as gastric secretion, 392
peptic ulcer disease (PUD), 544
peptide bonds
  by dietary necessity, 253t, 254
  metabolic end product, 254, 254t
  by R-group, 253t, 254
peptide hormones, 407–408
peptidoglycan cell wall, bacteria and, 441
Peptostreptococcus micros, plaque induced gingivitis and, 480
perfusion pressure, 339
perianal pruritis, metazoa and, 476
pericardial effusion, 530
pericardial sac, aortic dissection and, 529
pericardioperitoneal canal, 101
pericardium, 92
  diastole and, 345b
  pathology involving, 530

Perikaryon cell body, 171
perimysium, CT and, 332
periodontal health, 478
periodontal ligament (PDL), 208, 208f
  collagen fibers, 209, 209f
  contents of, 208
  functions of, 208
  nerve fibers, 210
periodontium, 208b
periorbital edema, *Trichinella spiralis* and, 476t
periosteal vessels, PDL and, 209
periosteum, 169
peripheral edema, right-side CHF and, 523
peripheral nerve, 151
peripheral nervous system (PNS), 151, 299
  nervous tissue, 171
  subdivisions of, 303
peripheral proteins, 295
perisinusoidal space, 185
peristalsis, 182, 392
peritoneal fluid, 101
peritoneal ligaments, 101
peritoneum, 101
peritubular dentin, 201
permanent dentition
  dental formula, 647
  eruption sequence and timing, 647
  mandibular arch, 647
  maxillary arch, 647, 648f
  number of teeth, 647
  primary teeth v., 641, 641t
  tooth development in, 647, 648t
  tooth numbering, 623, 624f
permanent tooth forms, 621, 622t–623t
pernicious anemia, 557
  schilling test, 557
  vitamin B_{12} and, 402
peroxisomes (microbodies), 161, 185, 503
petechiae
  ecchymoses v., 562
  leukemias and, 606
petrosal nerve, course and components of, 140–141
petrotympanic fissure, 9
petrous temporal bone, 7
Peutz-Jeghers syndrome, 603
Peyer's patches, 109
PFK. *See* phosphofructokinase
PFTs. *See* pulmonary function tests
pH levels, 308
phagocytes, 501
phagocytosis, 106
  stages of, 502, 502t
phagosome formation, 502, 502t
pharyngeal arches, tongue and, 241, 242f
pharyngeal derivatives, 236f
pharyngeal muscles, 39
pharyngeal plexus, 41
pharyngeal pouches, 234, 436f
pharyngeal region, derivatives, 231, 234f
pharyngeal tonsils, 37
pharynx, 29–41, 29f, 39, 40f, 41t
  external view, 40f
  food, 41
  parasagittal view, 38f
  posterior view, 40f
phenylalanine, 254, 254f
phenylbutazone, aplastic anemia and, 557
phenytoin (Dilantin), gingival overgrowth and, 487b
pheochromocytoma, 611–612, 611b
phlebitis, 526

phosphate
  hyperparathyroidism and, 429
  hypoparathyroidism and, 429
phosphate groups, nucleotides, 284
phosphatidic acid, structure, 261
phosphodiester bonds, 285
phosphodiesterase, second messenger and, 408
phosphofructokinase (PFK), glycolysis and, 273, 273f
phospholipase A2, corticosteroids and, 262
phospholipids
  membrane lipids and, 294, 295f
  types and structure, 261
phosphorus metabolism, 427–429
photophosphorylation, 274
photopigments, of eyeball, 321
photoreceptor, 308
phrenic nerve, 65, 66
physeal osteochondroses, 576
Pick's disease, 582
picornavirus, 461
pigment epithelium, 193
pigmented nevi, 595
pili (fimbriae), 444
pineal gland, BBB and, 27
pitch, 621
  sound wave and, 324
pituitary adenoma, 595
pituitary gland, 115, 178–179, 178b, 410, 410f
  functional components of, 178t
  hormones, 179
  hypothalamus and, 409–416
  insulin and, 418
  secondary hypothyroidism and, 566
  surgical approach to, sphenoid sinus and, 19
  tumor, abducens nerve and, 25
placenta, immunoglobulins and, 503
placentation, 219
plane of occlusion, 650
plaque, 478, 478t, 480. See also chemical plaque control
  formation, 478
plasma, body fluid and, 376
plasma cell membrane, 160, 294
  bacteria and, 441
  fluid mosaic model of, 294, 294f
  protein types, 295
plasma cells, multiple myeloma, 609
plasma proteins
  functions of, 257
  liver and, 257
  protein types, 295
platelets, 173
platysma muscle, 55, 56f
pleura, 101
plexuses, major, 153
plica fimbriata, 31
plicae circulares, 182
Plummer's disease, 426, 427, 568
PML. See progressive multifocal leukoencephalopathy
pneumoconioses, 538–539
pneumolysin, host tissue destruction and, 442
pneumonia, 541
PNS. See peripheral nervous system
point angle, 621
point mutations, 290–291
Poiseuille's law, resistance and, 339
poliovirus, 462
polyarthritis nodosa, 572

polycystic kidney disease (PCKD), 552
polycythemia, 559–560
  erythropoietin and, 358
  as myeloproliferative disorder, 560
polycythemia vera, 559–560
polydipsia, 412
polymorphonuclear neutrophils, 501, 501t
polymyalgia, temporal arteritis v., 572
polymyxin B, 458
polyphyodont dentition, 618
polysaccharide capsule, cell wall and, 441
polysaccharides, 248
  storage of, 249
polyuria, 412
  diabetes mellitus and, 419
pons, 116
portal blood, 99
portal hypertension, 548–549
  splenomegaly and, 548
portal system, capillary beds of, 179
portal systemic anastomoses, 100f
portal triad, 99, 106, 185
portal vein, and branches, 98–99, 99f
portal venous blood, liver, 106
portocaval shunt, 99
Posselt's envelope of motion
  mandible and, 654, 655f
  planes of, 655f
postconcussion syndrome, 581b
posterior abdominal muscles, innervation of, 110
posterior auricular artery, 67, 67f
posterior belly of digastric, CN VII and, 140
posterior belly of stylohyoid, CN VII and, 140
posterior cord, nerves and, 81
posterior cranial fossa, contents of, 8
posterior cross-bite, 652
posterior deep temporal nerve, 51
posterior pituitary
  hormones, 407, 412
  hypothalamic control of, 410
posterior rectus sheath, 86
posterior teeth, 618
posterior triangle of neck, 60
posterior/dorsal horn, 149
postexposure protocol, 440
postganglionic autonomic fibers, 154
postganglionic autonomic systems, cholinergic effects, 304
postganglionic nerves, lacrimal gland and, 42
postganglionic neurons, 304
  sympathetic nervous system, 305
postsynaptic neurons, 317
Pott's disease, 542, 578
poxvirus, 466, 466t–467t
precocious puberty, 416
predontoblasts, 213
preeclampsia, secondary HTN and, 528, 528b
preexposure protocol, 440
preganglionic autonomic systems, cholinergic effects, 304
preganglionic neuron, 304
  sympathetic nervous system, 304–305
preganglionic parasympathetic nerve, 31
preganglionic parasympathetics, cranial nerves and, 118
preganglionic receptors, nicotinic and muscarinic, 304
preganglionics, brainstem and, 119
pregnancy, preeclampsia and, 528b
preload, 346
premolars, lobes, 627

premyeloblasts, 213
presbycusis, 142
presbyopia, 323
pressure, CN V sensory distribution for, 133
pressure-volume loop, cardiac cycle and, 348, 349f
presynaptic neurons, 317
pretracheal layer, of deep cervical facia, 56, 56f
prevertebral layer
  of deep cervical facia, 56, 56f, 58
Prevotella intermedia, plaque induced gingivitis and, 480
primary Addison's disease, 422
  secondary Addison's disease v., 570–571
primary amyloidosis, 610
primary cusp triangle, first molar, 631, 631f
primary dentition
  dental formula, 646
  development, 646, 647t
  eruption sequence and timing, 646, 646f
  number of teeth, 646
  primate space and, 642
  tooth labeling, 640, 641f
primary glomerulonephropathies, nephrotic syndrome and, 553
primary hemostasis
  bleeding problems and, 560
  disorders in, 561–563
primary hyperparathyroidism, 568–569
primary hypertension, clinical findings and complications, 528
primary olfactory cortex, olfactory nerve and, 17
primary palate, formation, 237
primary polycythemia, 559
primary pulmonary hypertension, heart failure and, 534
primary response, immunoglobulins and, 503
primary structure, protein structures and, 255
primary teeth, permanent teeth v., 641, 641t
primary (deciduous) tooth form, 640–644, 640f
primary tuberculosis, 542
primate space, primary dentitions and, 642
Prinzmetal angina, 533
prions, 470
productive cough, 538b
proelastin polypeptide chain, glycine-x-y and, 256
progesterone
  hCG and, 417
  ovaries and, 414
progressive multifocal leukoencephalopathy (PML), 583
prokaryotic cells, 70s ribosomes and, 290
prolactin, breast-feeding and, 413
proline, collagen synthesis and, 256
prophase, 162
proprioception, CN V sensory distribution for, 133
proprioceptors, CNS and, 307
prostate cancer, 594
  serum acid phosphatase level and, 575
prostate gland, 189
prostatic urethra, 189
prosthetic implants, antibiotic prophylaxis and, 458, 458t–459t
protease, 269, 270f
proteins, 252, 266
  absorption, 394
  cirrhosis and, 358
  digestion and absorption, 393

immunity and, 499
kinases, 408
metabolism, 278–280, 397
peripheral, 295
physiologically relevant, 256–264
plasma membranes and, 295
structure, 255
viral, 459
proteinuria, 551
nephrotic syndrome, 553
proteoglycans, 250
prothrombin, coagulation and, 358, 359f
proton pump inhibitors, peptic ulcer disease, 544
protozoa, 474
human infection and, 475t
protrusive contacts, 651
protrusive interference, 655
protrusive movement
condylar movements as, 656
mandible and, 654
proximal contacts
of mandibular teeth, 625, 625f
of maxillary teeth, 625f
proximal convoluted tubule, glomerular filtrate and, 381
proximal surfaces, shapes, 626, 626f
PSA testing, prostate cancer, 594
pseudogout, 580
pseudomembranous candidiasis (thrush), 482
pseudomembranous colitis, clindamycin and, 457
pterygoid plexus of veins, 25, 69, 621
connections, 25
pterygopalatine artery, 69
pterygopalatine fossae
boundaries of, 15t
lateral scheme of, 14f
major communications, 15
pterygopalatine ganglion, greater petrosal nerve and, 141
PTH. *See* parathyroid hormone
ptosis, lesions and, 128
puberty. *See also* precocious puberty
hormones and, 414–416
in male, 414, 415f
PUD. *See* peptic ulcer disease
pulmonary artery, bronchus v., 89
pulmonary capillaries, ACE, 373
pulmonary chemoreflex, 373
pulmonary circulation, systemic circulation v., 343
pulmonary edema, 534–535
causes, 535b
heart failure and, 535b
left-side CHF and, 523
pulmonary embolism, 526b
pulmonary fibrosis, coal workers pneumoconiosis, 539
pulmonary function tests (PFTs), emphysema, 537
pulmonary hypertension, 534
pulmonic valve, 91
pulp, 204–205
aging and, 205
classifications of, 205
functions of, 205
pulp calcifications, 205
pulp chamber, 204
pulp zones, 205
pulse pressure, narrow v. wide, 344
pupil, 320

pupillary light reflex, 126, 127f, 128
pure Ag (silver), 284b
pure red cell aplasia, 559
purines, pyrimidines v., 284
purpura, 561–562
pus, 436
pyelonephritis, 551
pyknosis, cell death and, 490
pyloric sphincter, 105
pylorus, gastric secretion and, 392
pyramidal system. *See* corticospinal tract
pyramids, medulla and, 188
pyriform recesses, food and, 41
pyrimidines
mnemonic, 284b
purines v., 284
pyruvate
to alanine, transamination of, 278, 279f
metabolic fates, 273

Q

quantitative platelet deficiencies, 561–563

R

RA. *See* rheumatoid arthritis
radial nerve, 80, 81
deficit, 81
radiation
aplastic anemia and, 557
mutations by, 290–291
radiosensitivity, 592
RADIUS, vascular resistance and, 339
rami, 20
rapidly progressive glomerulonephritis (RPGN), 554
rapidly progressive nephritic syndrome, 554
Rathke's pouch, diencephalon and, 115
Raynaud's phenomenon, scleroderma and, 572
reabsorption, 383
reaction equilibrium, 269f
enzyme kinetics and, 268, 269f
reaction rate
enzyme kinetics and, 268
factors influencing, 268, 269t
receptors
CNS, 307
of heart, 354
by stimulus type, 308
recombinant DNA technology, clinical considerations and, 291
recombination, bacterial cell and, 441
rectum
blood supply and description, 109
GI cancer and, 602
rectus sheath, 86
recurrent caries, 479
recurrent laryngeal nerve, 76, 76f
recurrent periodontitis, 481
red marrow, 170
red pulp, of spleen, 178
reduced enamel epithelium (REE), appositional stage, 213
Reed-Sternberg cells, HD and, 608
reflex arc, pathway, 127, 127f
reflexes, 87
refractory period, 313. *See also* relative refractory period
heart and, electrical conduction of, 350, 351f

skeletal muscle and, cardiac muscle v., 350b
refractory periodontitis, 481
regeneration
acute inflammation and, 491
wound healing and, 496
Reiter's syndrome, 573
clinical triad with, 573
relative afferent pupil, 128
relative polycythemia, 559
relative refractory period, 313
heart and, 350, 351f
renal blood
flow, 385
supply, 382, 382f
renal cell carcinoma, 603
renal clearance, 386
renal disease, secondary HTN and, 528
renal failure
anemia and, 555b
multiple myeloma and, 609
renal osteodystrophy, 574
renal sodium, edema and, 378
renin
JG cells and, 188
kidney function and, 386
repair, acute inflammation and, 491
reparative dentin, formation, 201
repeat mutation, 291
repolarization, 313, 314f
reproductive system, 189–190, 416–418
female, 416, 417b, 417f
male, components of, 189
rER. *See* rough endoplasmic reticulum
residual volume (EV), lung volumes, 362, 362f
resistance to blood flow, 339
heart and, 92
pulmonary circulation, systemic circulation v., 343
respiration
accessory muscles of, 85
intercostal muscles and, 83
muscles of, 84–85
respiratory acidosis, status asthmaticus and, 536b
respiratory arrest, 374
respiratory chemoreceptors, 371
respiratory compensation, anemia and, 357
respiratory conditions, 374
respiratory drive pathway, 370–371
respiratory rate, 364
respiratory regulation, 370–374
function of, 371
respiratory system, 180–181
components, 76
divisions, 180
functions, 180
pathology, 535–540
segments, 180, 181t
respiratory zone, 364
rest position (RP), mandible and, 654
resting membrane potential, neurophysiology and, 312–313
restriction endonucleases, 291
restrictive lung diseases, 536, 537b
reticular lamina, 165
reticular layer, of dermis, 191
reticuloendothelial system, components of, 501
reticulospinal tract, 311
retina, 193, 320–321
layers of, 193
vitamin A and, 193

681

retrograde flow
    infection and, 71
    ophthalmic veins and, 24b
retromandibular vein, 70
retroperitoneal structures, 109, 110b, 110f
retropharyngeal space, 58, 58f
retroviruses, 461, 462
    reverse transcriptase and, 460
reverse transcriptase
    AZT and, 291
    clinical considerations and, 291
    retroviruses, 460
reversible cell injury, 487
Reye's syndrome, aspirin and, 466
rhabdomyoma, 590, 592b
rhabdovirus, 462
rheumatic carditis, rheumatic heart disease and, 532b
rheumatic endocarditis, 531
rheumatic fever, 531–532
    diagnosis criteria for, 532
    mnemonics for, 531b
rheumatic heart disease, rheumatic carditis and, 532b
rheumatoid arthritis (RA), 580–581
rhodopsin, 193
ribosomes, 161
ribs, 83
    spleen injury and, 83
rickets, 574
    blood chemistry values, 574
ridges, 619–620, 619f, 620f
right atrium, 91
right gastric artery, 105
right gastroepiploic, 105
right heart failure, signs and symptoms of, 534, 534b
right lymphatic duct, 101
right vagus nerve, 145
    SA node and, 354
right ventricle, 92
right working movement, condylar movements as, 656, 656f
right-side CHF, peripheral edema and, 523
Rivian ducts, 31
RNA, 285
    backbone structure of, 287f
    protein translation, 290, 290f
    transcription, 289, 290f
    types of, 286
    viruses and, 459, 461–463
RNA viruses, viral replication and, 460
roboviruses, 462
rods, 193, 321
Rokitansky-Aschoff sinuses, 186
root formation, 213, 214f
rootless teeth, 202
Rosenthal's syndrome, 563
rotator cuff, 83
    muscles of, mnemonic for, 83
rotundum foramina, of splenoid bone, 12
rough endoplasmic reticulum (rER), 161
RP. *See* rest position
RPGN. *See* rapidly progressive glomerulonephritis
rubrospinal tract, 311
Ruffini's corpuscles, 307
rugae, 182

S

SA node. *See* sinuatrial node
sacral plexus, 153
saddle embolus, 526
saliva
    components of, 252
    secretions, 252
salivary control, 252
salivary fluid
    parotid gland and, 44
    submandibular gland and, 44
salivary glands, 42–43
    primary secretions of, 252
salmonella bone infections, sickle-cell anemia and, 556
saltatory conduction, 315–316, 316
sanitization, 439
Santorini's duct, 110
sarcoidosis, 539–540
sarcolemma, 330
sarcoma, 589
sarcoma botryoides, 592b
sarcomere, skeletal muscle and, 331
sarcoplasm, 330
sarcoplasmic reticulum (SR), 330
scalene muscles, 78
scalp
    components of, mnemonic for, 21, 21f
    venous drainage and, 70
scar, wound repair and, 496
Scheuermann's disease, 576
sclera, 192
scleroderma, 572
    calcinosis and, 489b
sclerotic dentin, 201
sclerotome, derivatives, 223f
sebaceous glands, 192
sebum, 192
second messenger, 408
second molar
    mandibular permanent teeth, 638–639, 639f
    mandibular primary teeth, 644
    maxillary permanent teeth, 632, 632f
    maxillary primary teeth, 644
second premolar
    mandibular permanent teeth, 637, 637f
    maxillary permanent teeth, 630, 631f
secondary Addison's disease, 422
    primary Addison's disease v., 570–571
secondary amyloidosis, cause and sites of, 610
secondary hemostasis, 561
    bleeding problems and, 560
    disorders in, 563
secondary hyperparathyroidism, 569
secondary hypertension (HTN), 528
secondary hypothyroidism, 566
secondary palate, 237
secondary polycythemia, 560
secondary pulmonary hypertension, heart failure and, 534
secondary response, immunoglobulins and, 503
secondary sex characteristics, male v. female, 415, 415f
secondary structure, protein structures and, 255
secondary tuberculosis, 542
secretin, stimulus and control, 390
segmentation, 392

seizures, 582
semilunar valves, 91
seminiferous tubules, 189
senses, 319–328
sensorineural loss, 143
sensory distribution, CN V and, 133–134, 134f, 135f
sensory nerve, 129
    branches, 66
    fibers, taste buds and, 325
sensory nucleus, 132
sensory spinal tract pathway, 306
sensory tracts, ascending, 308–310
sepsis, signs and symptoms, 436
septic shock, 524
sER. *See* smooth endoplasmic reticulum
series resistance, 339
serous, 252
serum, 173
    carbonic anhydrase, 368
serum sodium (Na^+), edema and, 378
severe liver disease, 563b
sex chromosome abnormalities, 517
sex hormones, 407, 414
sex pilus, 441
sex steroids, gingivitis and, 480
sexual cycle, female, 417b
sexual reproduction, spores, 471
Sharpey's fiber, 166, 209
Sherman classification, bacteria and, 446
shivering, ANS and, 300
shock
    categories of, 523
    stages of, 524
    types of, 524
Shy-Drager syndrome, 582
SIADH. *See* syndrome of inappropriate ADH secretion
sicca complex, 573b
sickle-cell anemia, 556
sickle-cell crisis, organ damage and, 556–557
sickle-cell pain crisis, sickle-cell anemia and, 556
silica dust, silicosis and, 539
silicosis, 539
    eggshell calcification and, 489b
silver. *See* pure Ag
sinuatrial (SA) node, 176
    heart and, 334
    nodal/pacemaker conduction system and, 352
sinusoids, 185
Sjögren's syndrome, 573
skeletal muscle, 331–334
    cardiac muscle v., refractory period and, 350b
    contraction, venus return and, 347
    contraction of, 332, 332f
    fiber types, 333
    histology, 331, 331f
    motor innervation of, 332
    twitch speed, comparison by, 333
skin
    antiseptics and, 438, 439t
    epidermal layers of, mnemonic for, 191b
    epidermis, intracellular fluids, 376
    eruptions
        bacterial, 520
        viral, 520
    functions of, 190
    infections, 520
    layers of, 191

lesions
    benign, 522
    immunologic, 520–521
  neoplasia of, 595–597
  neuronal endings of, 191
  pigmentation, disorders of, 519
skin cancer, sun exposure, 596–597
skull
  anterior aspect of, 6, 6f
  lateral aspect of, 7, 7f
  posterior aspect of, 7, 7f
sliding filament model, skeletal muscle contraction and, 332
small cell carcinoma, 600
small intestine, 108, 182–184
  cells of, 183t
  disaccharides, 248
  disorders, 545–546
  hormones and, 391
  pancreatic digestive enzymes and, 186
smell, 326–328
  disturbances of, 327
  pathway, 326–327, 328f
smoking. *See* cigarette smoking
smooth endoplasmic reticulum (sER), 161
smooth muscle
  contraction, 335, 335f
  histology, 335
  innervation, 335
Sniderian membrane, maxillary sinus and, 18
sodium reabsorption, countercurrent multiplier and, 384
soft oral tissues, 196–199
soft palate
  composition of, 37
  lesser palatine artery and, 68
  parasagittal view, 38f
solitary toxic adenoma, 426
somatic nervous system, 303
somatosensory cortex, 310, 310f
somatosensory pathways, 308–312, 308f
somatostatin, 414
sound wave, characteristics, 324
spatial summation, 315
specialized epithelial cells, 196
sperm, 189
  development, 216f
  mature, 216f
  stages of meiosis in, 215
spermatic cord, layers and contents of, 113
spermatogenesis, 189
sphenoid bones, 6
  components and functions of, 12
  spinosum foramina, 12
sphenoid sinuses, 18
  location of drainage, 19
sphenomandibular ligament, 54f
sphenopalatine artery, 18
sphenopalatine vessels, 36
sphincter of Boyden, 185
sphincter of Oddi, 185
  gallbladder and, 107
spinal accessory nerve, damage to, trapezius and, 62
spinal cord, 149–155
  anatomy, 306b
  cross section, 149, 149f, 150f
  lesions, 312
  tracts, 150
spinal nerves, 151
spinal reflexes, stretch, 334
spinal tracts, 306–308

spinal trigeminal nucleus, 132
spinosum foramina, of sphenoid bone, 12
spinothalamic tract (anterolateral system), pathway, 309
spirochete bacteria, comparison, 453t
spirochetes, plaque induced gingivitis and, 480
spitz nevus, 596
splanchnic nerves, 97, 153
spleen, 178
  embryology of, 107
  histology of, 107
  leukemia and, 604
spleen injury, ribs and, 83
splenic artery, 105
splenic sequestration, anemia and, 555b
splenic sequestration crisis, sickle-cell anemia and, 556
splenic vein, 99
splenomegaly, portal hypertension and, 548
splenorenal ligament, 102
spongiform encephalopathies, prions and, 470
spore, 445
  sterilization and, 445
  tests, 438
squamous cell carcinoma, 589, 600, 601
  of skin, 597–598
SR. *See* sarcoplasmic reticulum
stab wound, intercostal space and, 83
stable angina, 533
staging, malignant tumors and, 588
standing, sudden, 355
stapedius, 141
Staphylococci, 446, 447t
  comparison of, 447t
Staphylococci aureus
  osteomyelitis and, 577
  sepsis and, 436
staphylokinase, host tissue destruction and, 442
starch, 249
starch hydrolysis, amylases in, 249
Starling mechanism, 344
Starling's curve, 345b
status asthmaticus, 536b
steatorrhea, 545b
stellate reticulum, 213
Stephan curve, caries and, 479, 480f
stereocilia, 161
sterilization
  disinfection and, 437–439
  spores and, 445
  techniques, 437t
sternum, 83
steroids, 261, 407
  asthma and, 536
Steven's-Johnson syndrome, 521
Still's disease, 580–581
stomach, 104–105, 104f, 182
  blood supply to, 105, 106f
  disorders of, 544–545
  gastric secretion and, 392
  glands of, 183t
  sphincters of, 105
stomodeum, 237
stone formation
  gallstones and, 547
  nephrolithiasis and, 551
stratified squamous epithelium, 196
stratum basale, 191
stratum corneum, 191
stratum granulosum, 191
stratum intermedium, 213

stratum lucidum, 191
stratum spinosum, 191
strawberry gallbladder, 547
Streptococci, 446, 447t
  classification of, by hemolysis, 446, 446t
  comparison of, 447t
Streptococcus mitis, plaque induced gingivitis and, 480
Streptococcus sanguis, plaque induced gingivitis and, 480
Streptococcus species, root caries and, 480b
streptodornase, host tissue destruction and, 442
streptokinase, host tissue destruction and, 442
streptolysin O, host tissue destruction and, 442
streptolysin S, host tissue destruction and, 442
streptomycin
stress, TSH secretion and, 424
stretch reflexes, spine and, 334
striae of Retzius, 203
stroke, 29
  atherosclerosis and, 527b
  leticulostriate arteries and, 29
stroke volume (SV), 345, 345b
structural polysaccharides, 250–251
stylopharyngeus muscle, 41
subarachnoid hemorrhage, 22b, 581b
subarachnoid space, communicating-obstruction in, 26b
subclavian arteries, 96
  branches of, 96
  upper extremities and, 77
  vertebral arteries and, 28
subclinical infection, 436
subcondylar fracture, 47
subdural hematoma, 22b, 581
subepithelial connective tissue, oral mucosa and, 196
subgingival plaque, supragingival plaque v., 478, 478t
sublingual gland, 43, 45f
sublingual space, boundaries and contents, 46, 46f
submandibular duct, 131
  relationships to, 35
submandibular gland, 61f
  innervation of, 43, 45f
  salivary fluid and, 44
submandibular space, boundaries and contents, 46, 46f
submandibular triangle, 60, 61f, 62
submucosa
  gallbladder and, 107
  oral mucosa and, 196
submucosal glands of Brunner, 184
submucous plexus (Meissner's plexus), 390
suboccipital triangle, vertebral arteries and, 62
subscapularis, 83
substrate concentration, effect of, enzyme kinetics and, 267, 267f
subunit vaccine, viruses and, 469
subunits, protein structures and, 255
succedaneous dental lamina, 213
succedaneous teeth, 646
sucrose, cariogenic bacteria, 251
sulcular epithelium, 198
sulcus, 620
sulfa drugs, polyarthritis nodosa, 572
sulfadiazine, 458

683

sulfamethoxazole, 458
sulfonamides, 458
sun exposure, skin cancer and, 596–597
superficial temporal artery, 67, 67f
superficial temporal vein, 70
superficial thrombophlebitis, 526
superior epigastric artery, 96
superior hemiazygos vein. *See* accessory hemiazygos vein
superior labial artery, 18
superior laryngeal nerve, 76
superior mesenteric vein, 99
superior orbital fissure, 9
superior petrosal sinus, connections, 24
superior rectus, 126, 127f
superior salivatory nucleus, 42
superior thyroid artery, 67, 67f
superior vena cava, 98
superior vena cava (SVC), 93
   causes of, 601, 601b
supernumerary teeth, 660
supplemental groove, 621
supporting alveolar bone, 207
supporting cells, 171
   of nervous tissue, 172t
supraclavicular nerves, 65
supragingival plaque, v. subgingival plaque, 478, 478t
suprahyoid muscles, 63–64, 63f, 656
supraspinatus, 83
suture, 170
SV. *See* stroke volume
SVC. *See* superior vena cava
swallowing, infrahyoid muscles, 657
swallowing center, sensory information and, 41
sweat chloride test, cystic fibrosis and, 518
sweat glands, 192
swinging flashlight test, 128
symbiosis, 436
sympathetic ganglia of head and neck, 119
sympathetic nervous system, 304–305
   compliance, 347
   exercise, 356
symphysis, 170
synapses, 171, 317–318
synaptic cleft, 317
synaptic transmission, 318
synarthrosis, 170
synchondrosis, 170
syndesmosis, 170
syndrome of inappropriate ADH secretion (SIADH), 413
synovial cavity, 170
synovial fluid, 170
synovial joints, 170
synovial membrane, 170
synovium, 51
systemic circulation, pulmonary circulation v., 343
systemic lupus erythematosus, 571–572
systemic venous circulation, blood volume in, 342
systole, cardiac cycle and, 348
systolic pressure, 344

T

talon cusp, dens evaginatus, 660, 660f
target cells, 408
taste pathways, 326
   chorda tympani nerve and, 31, 32f
   diagram, 32f
taste sensation(s), 325–326
   basic, 326b
   disturbances, 326, 327f
   nerves for, 141
   tongue and, CNs and, 30
tastebuds
   receptors, 325–326
   type and description of, 32
taurocholic acid, lipoproteins and, 262
taurodontism, teeth and, 660
Tay-Sachs disease, 264, 518
TB. *See* tuberculosis
TBW. *See* total body water
TCA cycle, 272
   stoichiometry of, 275f
T-cell-mediated immune response, graft rejection and, 506
T-cells
   immune system and, 499, 500t
   NHL and, 608
TCR. *See* CD3-associated T-cell receptor
tectospinal tract, 311
teeth
   formation, 240f
   nerve supply to, 621, 622f
   staining, tetracyclines, 457
telophase, 162
temperature, CN V sensory distribution for, 133
temperature loss, spinal lesions and, 312
temporal arteritis, polymyalgia v., 572
temporal lobe, 114, 114f, 299
temporal summation, 315
temporalis muscle, 48, 49f
temporomandibular joint (TMJ), 170
   bony components of, 50–51
   disc placement, 52
   dislocation, 52
   imaging, 51
   ligaments of, 51–52
   mastication and, 47–54
   movements, 53, 53f–54f
   nerves of, 51
   noises, 52
temporomandibular ligament, 54f
TEN syndrome, 521
tendon, 166
tendon (inverse myotatic) reflex, 334
tensor veli palatini, levator veli palatini v., 38
teratogens, 516b
teratoma, 591
terbutaline, asthma and, 536
teres minor, 83
tertiary structure, protein structures and, 255
testis, 189–190
testosterone, 189, 415
tetanus toxin, host tissue destruction and, 443
tetany, 569–570
tetracyclines, 457
   brownish-gray banding and, 204
thalamus, 115, 300
thalassemias, 556–557
thermodynamics, laws of, 246
thermoreceptor, 308
thick filaments, skeletal muscle and, 331
thin filaments, skeletal muscle and, 331
third arch, embryology and, 231b
third molar
   mandibular permanent teeth, 639, 639f
   maxillary permanent teeth, 633, 633f
third ventricle, BBB and, 27
thoracic aorta, and branches, 95, 95f
thoracic duct, 100
thoracic outlet syndrome, 78
thoracic viscera, 88–113
thorax, muscles of, 85
3 ATP, urea cycle, 280
thrombocytopenia, 561
thromboemboli, 525
thrombolysis, 525
thrombophlebitis, 526
thrombosis, 525
   predisposing factors to, 525b
thrombotic thrombocytopenic purpura (TTP), 562
thrombus, 525
thrush. *See* pseudomembranous candidiasis
thymic hormones, 94
thymine/uracil, hydrogen bonds, 284b
thymoma, 583b
thymus gland, 177
   anatomy, 94
   function, 94
   immune system and, 512b
   location of, 93
   lymph nodes and, 94
   T-cells and, 499, 500t
thyroglobulin, 425
thyroglossal duct, 72
thyroid cells (follicular cells), 72, 425
thyroid follicles, cellular components of, 179t
thyroid gland, 72–74, 73f, 179, 424, 425f
   blood supply and drainage, 73–74
thyroid hormone, 407, 566–570
   production, 425
   secretion, 425–426
thyroid-stimulating hormone (TSH), 407
   stress and, 424
thyroxine, hypothyroidism and, 567–568
tidal volumes (TV), 364
   lung volumes, 362, 362f
tight junction (zonula occludens), 162
tissue factor, extrinsic pathway and, 358, 359f
tissue types, cell turnover rate, 162
TLV. *See* total lung volume
TMJ. *See* temporomandibular joint
TNF. *See* tumor necrosis factors
togavirus, 462
tongue
   blood supply, 66
   development, 241, 242f
   dorsal view, 33f
   extrinsic muscles of tongue, 657
   function and innervation of, 30
   hard palate v., 37
   inferior surface of, 31
   jaundice and, 397
   lymphatic drainage of, 33, 34f
   muscles controlling
      boney attachments of, 33, 34f
      extrinsic v. intrinsic, 35
   sensory innervation of, 30, 31f
   shape, intrinsic muscles of tongue, 657
   soft palate v., 37
   speaking sounds and, 35
   surface components of, 33
   taste pathway of, 30, 31f
tonic contractions, GI system and, 393
tonsillar space, boundaries and contents, 46f, 47
tonsils
   lesser palatine artery and, 68
   location and description, 37

tooth
  acquired anomalies, 661
  developmental anomalies, 660–661
  eruption, 214, 214f, 646
  location, 618
  and periodontium, 208f
  tissues, comparison of, 200
tooth germ, 213b
tooth labeling, primary dentition, 640, 641f
tooth numbering, 623, 624f
  of permanent dentition, 623, 624f
topical antimicrobial, impetigo and, 520
topoisomerase, DNA synthesis and, 289
TORCH complex, 516
torticollis, 62
total body water (TBW), 376
total lung volume (TLV), 363
total peripheral resistance (TPR), 339, 343–344
touch, CN V sensory distribution for, 133
toxic epidermal necrolysis, 521
toxic shock syndrome toxin (TSST), host tissue destruction and, 443
toxins
  aplastic anemia and, 557
  host tissue destruction and, 442
toxoid vaccine, 454
TPR. See total peripheral resistance
trabecular sinuses, lymph and, 177
trachea, branching pattern of, 77
transalveolar vessels, PDL and, 209
transaminases, medically relevant, 278, 279t
transamination, protein metabolism and, 278
transcription, viral replication and, 460
transduction, DNA and, 442
transfer RNA (tRNA), 286
transferrin, blood plasma and, 404
transformation, DNA and, 442
transfusions, ABO blood typing and, 510
transition mutation, 291
transitional cell carcinoma, 589
translation, viral replication and, 460
transplantation, 506
transport proteins, 295
transposons, 591
  bacterial cell and, 441
transudate, 491
transudate edema, 523
transverse cervical nerve, 65, 66
transverse groove, first molar, 631, 631f
transverse mutation, 290
transverse ridge, 620
trapezius muscles, 62
trapezoidal proximal shape, maxillary first premolar, 629, 630f
trauma. See also neurologic trauma
  DIC and, 562
trench mouth, 481
TRH-TSH-thyroid hormone axis. See hypothalamicpituitary-thyroid axis
triacylglycerol lipase, hormone regulation and, triglyceride lipolysis and, 276, 277f
triacylglycerols (triglycerides)
  digestion and absorption, 394
  structure, 260
triangle of face, danger area, 71
triangular ridge, 620
tricuspid valve, 91
  IV drug users and, 530
trigeminal nerve (CN V), 129–136, 621
  branches of, 129f
  divisions of, 129–130

facial reflexes and, 136
facial sensation from, 133–134, 134f, 135f
lesions, type and findings, 135
trigeminal nuclei, 132
triglyceride lipolysis, 276, 277f
triglycerides. See triacylglycerols
trimethoprim, 458
trochlear nerve, 125, 126f
tropical sprue, 546
tropomyosin, 330
  skeletal muscle contraction and, 333
troponin, 330
  smooth muscle and, 335
Trousseau's sign, tetany and, 569
true polycythemia, 559
trypsin, pancreatic digestive enzymes and, 186
tryptophan, 254, 407
TSH. See thyroid-stimulating hormone
TSH-secreting pituitary tumor, 426
TSST. See toxic shock syndrome toxin
TTP. See thrombotic thrombocytopenic purpura
t-tubules
  skeletal muscle contraction and, 332, 332f
  smooth muscle, 335, 335f
tubercle, 619
tuberculosis (TB), 542
  types of, 542
tuberculum impar, tongue and, 241, 242f
tuberous sclerosis, Café au lait spots and, 575b
tubuloalveolar glands, 190
tumor cells, NK cells and, 501
tumor markers, 589
tumor necrosis factors (TNF), 493, 493t–494t
tumors, 588. See also lesions; metastasis; neoplasia
  of adrenal medulla, 611
  of mesenchymal origin, benign v. malignant, 591
tunica albuginea, 189
turbulent flow, 341f
Turcot's syndrome, 603
Turner syndrome, 517
TV. See tidal volumes
twinning, 220f
twitch speed. See contraction speed
tympanum plexus, 144f
type 1 sensitivity, asthma and, 536
tyrosine, 407
tyrosine metabolism, pathway, 424

U

ubiquinone, coenzyme Q as, 275
ulcerative colitis (UC), 545
  Crohn's disease v., comparison of, 545
ulnar nerve, 80
  hypothenar region and, 81
uncoating, viral replication and, 460
uniport, transport proteins and, 295
universal precautions, 440
unstable angina, 533
upper digestive system, 181–184
  esophagus, 182
  functions, 181
  layers, 182
  stomach, 182
upper extremities, subclavian arteries and, 77
upper motor neurons, 311
  lesion of, 148

urea
  formation of, reactions and intermediates in, 280f
  nonprotein nitrogen and, 396
urea cycle, 280
  liver and, 396
  stoichiometry of, 280f
ureter, 111
urethra, 111, 189
uric acid synthesis, 284, 285f
urinary bladder, 111
urinary infections, females and, 111
urinary system, 111, 187–189, 381–383
urinary tract infection (UTI), pyelonephritis, 551
urine
  characteristics and contents, 381
  lipiduria and, 553
uronic acid, 250
uterine tube, fertilization and, 215
uterus, 190
UTI. See urinary tract infection
UV light, mutations by, 290–291
uvea, 193
uveitis, 573b
uvula, 37

V

V1. See ophthalmic nerve
V2. See maxillary nerve
vaccination, hepatitis B virus and, 468
vaccines. See also specific type vaccine i.e. killed vaccine
  bacterial, 454
  preexposure protocol and, 440
  viral, 469
vagal stimulation, asthma and, 536
vagina, 190
vagotomy, salivary production and, 252
vagus nerve (CN X), 90
  cardiac branches of, 147
  course of, 145
  lesions, 147
vallecula recesses, food and, 41
valves, head and neck, 71
valvular disease, heart murmurs with, 350
van der Waals bonds, 246
vancomycin, 456
vascular compliance, 344
vascular resistance, 339
vascular-endothelial barrier, 27
vasoconstriction, epinephrine and, 254
vasopressin. See antidiuretic hormone
VC. See vital capacity
VDO. See vertical dimension of occlusion
VDR. See vertical dimension of rest
veins, 176, 343
veins of heart. See cardiac veins
velopharyngeal incompetence, prevention of, 41
vena cava, aorta v., velocity of blood flow and, 340
venous anastomoses, 100, 100f
venous drainage, from face, 69–71, 69f
venous return, 347, 347f
  CO and, 345
  dental, 621
  exercise, 356
venous sinuses, 23, 23f
venous thrombi, 525

venous thrombosis, predisposing factors for, 525b
ventricles, 92
  nearby anatomical structure, 25
ventricular fibrillation, 533
ventricular system, 26f
  parts of, 25
venules, 176, 342
vertebral arteries, 27
  subclavian artery and, 28
  suboccipital triangle and, 62
vertebral canal, spinal cord and, 149
vertical dimension, 650
vertical dimension of occlusion (VDO), 650
vertical dimension of rest (VDR), 650
  mandible and, 654
vertical fold, 22
vessels, Laplace's law in, 341
vestibular folds, 75
vestibular lamina, embryo and, 237
vestibulocochlear nerve (CN VIII), 141–143, 141f
  course of, 141, 141f
  lesions, 142–143
vestibulo-ocular reflex, caloric test and, 143b
vestibulospinal tract, 311
villi, 182
vimentin, 161
Vincent's disease, 481
viral cells, NK cells and, 501
viral hepatitis, 550
  signs and symptoms of, 467
viral infections
  aplastic anemia and, 557
  lymphocytosis and, 492
viral pneumonia, 541
viral proteins, 459
Virchow's triad, 358, 525b
virology, 459–469
viruses, 459
  antigenic changes, 461
  DNA non-enveloped, 465, 465t
  DNA-enveloped, 466, 466t–467t
  enveloped v. non-enveloped, 459f
  growth curve, 460, 460f
  mutations by, 290–291
  pathogenesis of, 460, 460f
  replication and, 460, 461f
    glycoproteins, 469
  RNA non-enveloped, 461, 462t
  RNA-enveloped, 462, 463t–464t

skin eruptions and, 520
visceral pericardium, 92
visceral peritoneum, 101
visceral pleura, 89
viscerocranial region of head, 233f
viscerocranium
  bones of
    face and, 6
    formation, 231, 233f
    orbital bones of, 12–13, 13f
vision, 319–323
  disturbances, 323
vision pathway, 321–322, 322f
  lesions along, 322
vital capacity (VC), 363
vitamin(s), 400
  deficiencies, teratogenesis and, 516
  fat-soluble, 400
  water soluble, 401–402, 401t
vitamin A, retinal and, 193
vitamin B_6, transamination, 278
vitamin B_{12}
  Crohn's disease and, 402
  deficiency, 557–558
  megaloblastic anemia, causes, 558, 558b
  pernicious anemia and, 402
vitamin C, collagen synthesis and, 256
vitamin D, 574
  biologically active, synthesis of, 400f
  calcium and phosphorus, normal values, 427
vitamin K
  deficiency, 563
  warfarin and, 564
vitiligo, 519
vitreous humor, 193
vocal cords, 74
vocal folds, 74
voice production, larynx and, 74
Volkmann's canals, 169
volume changes, hormonal response to, 386–387, 387f
von Ebner glands, serous only saliva and, 44
von Willebrand's disease, platelet disorders and, 562, 563
Von-Hippel-Lindau disease, 518–519

W

Waldeyer's ring, 38
Wallerian degeneration, 316

wall-less bacteria, comparison of, 453t
Warfarin (Coumadin), vitamin K and, 564
water, 246
water retention, edema and, 378
Waterhouse-Friderichsen syndrome, cortisol and, 570
Wharton's ducts, 31
Whipple's disease, 546
white pulp, of spleen, 178
Wilson's disease, 548
Wolffian duct, 229
working cusps, 654
working interference, 655
working side contacts (Laterotrusive contacts), 651
  mandible and, 655
wound healing, methods, primary v. secondary, 496
wound repair, stages of, 495–496
woven bone, 169

X

xanthoma, 522
xenograft, 506
x-ray, eggshell calcification and, 489b
x-ray diffraction analysis, protein structures and, 255

Y

yeasts, molds v., 471, 471t
yellow marrow, 170

Z

Z line, skeletal muscle and, 331, 331b
zinc, immunity and, 94
zonula adherens. *See* intermediate junction
zonula occludens. *See* tight junction
Zwitterions (dipolar ions), 380
zygoma bone, 13
zygomatic arch, 13
zymogens, 269
  protease function and, 269